HISTORY OF
THE SECOND WORLD WAR

UNITED KINGDOM MEDICAL SERIES

Editor-in-Chief

Sir Arthur S. MacNalty, k.c.b., m.a., m.d., f.r.c.p., f.r.c.s.

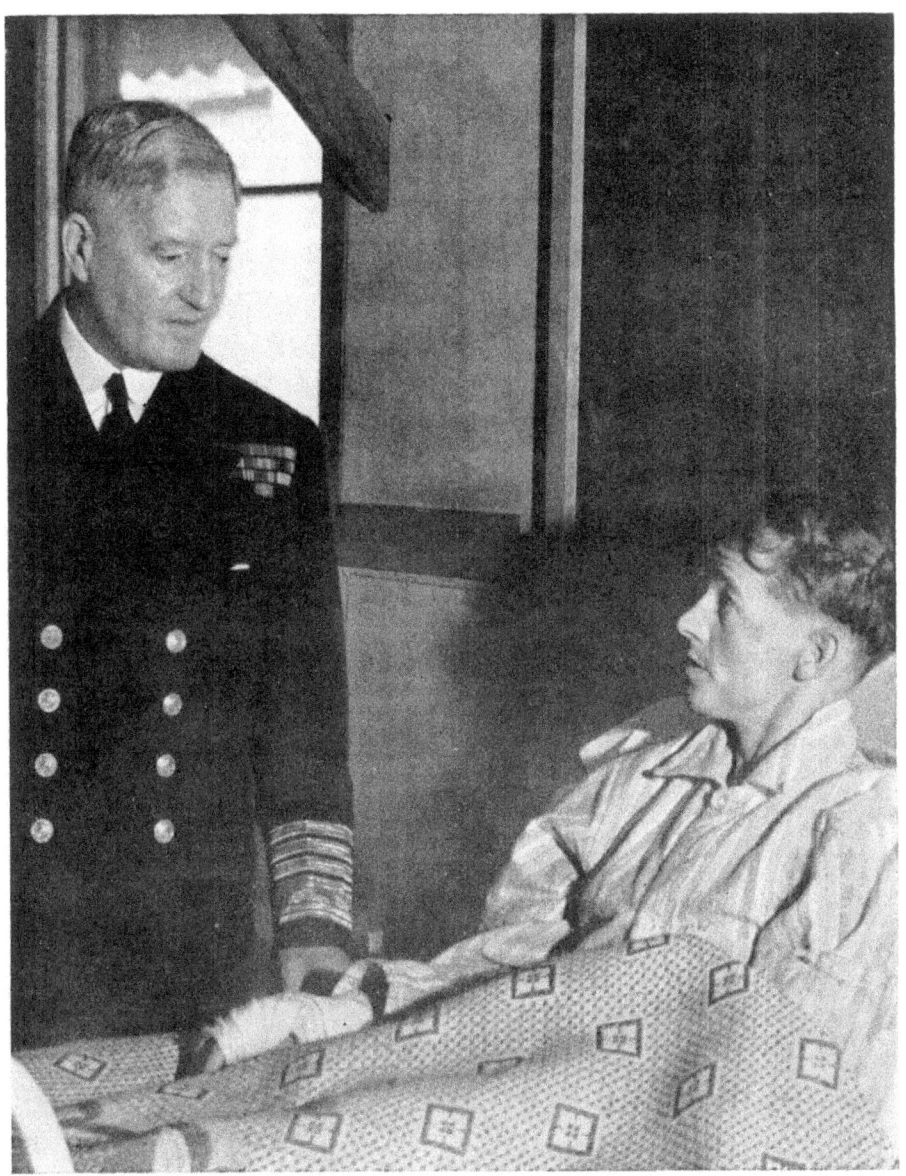

PLATE I. Admiral Sir Bruce Fraser, Commander-in-Chief, British Pacific Fleet, during his inspection of the Royal Naval Hospital at Herne Bay, Sydney, Australia.

THE ROYAL NAVAL MEDICAL SERVICE

BY
Surgeon Captain J. L. S. COULTER, D.S.C., R.N.
Barrister-at-Law

VOLUME II

Operations

The Naval & Military Press Ltd

Published by

The Naval & Military Press Ltd
Unit 5 Riverside, Brambleside
Bellbrook Industrial Estate
Uckfield, East Sussex
TN22 1QQ England

Tel: +44 (0)1825 749494

www.naval-military-press.com
www.nmarchive.com

In reprinting in facsimile from the original, any imperfections are inevitably reproduced and the quality may fall short of modern type and cartographic standards.

PREFATORY NOTE
by the Editor-in-Chief

THE ROYAL NAVAL MEDICAL SERVICE
VOLUME II
Operations

THIS is the second volume devoted to the Royal Naval Medical Service in the Official Medical History of the War. It deals with the medical aspects of the chief naval events of the war afloat and ashore and gives a complete and even at times a dramatic account of the injuries and diseases that assailed British sailors throughout the Seven Seas, and of the way in which medical officers of the Navy, sometimes single-handed, prevented, fought and overcame them.

This book is not only a narrative of stirring events. The Editor, whenever possible, has not omitted to introduce constructive criticism, which should be found helpful in planning for the future.

The extreme importance of the development and maintenance of the morale of individual officers and ratings in action at sea is dealt with by the Editor in a searching analysis of the many factors which tend to lower and even destroy the efficiency of the sailor unless this danger is foreseen and adequate steps taken to combat it. It constitutes a valuable study of the application of the principles of psychology.

A review of the contents of the book will be found in the Medical Director-General of the Navy's Foreword.

To Surgeon Vice Admiral Sir Alexander Ingleby MacKenzie and to the Editor thanks are due for their co-operation in our task here of seeing the work through the Press.

The volume has been prepared under the direction of an Editorial Board appointed by H.M. Government, but the Editor alone is responsible for the presentation of the facts and the opinions expressed.

ARTHUR S. MACNALTY

February 1955

EDITORIAL BOARD

Sir Cyril Flower, C.B., F.S.A., (*Chairman*)

Sir Weldon Dalrymple-Champneys, Bart., D.M., B.Ch., F.R.C.P.
Sir Francis R. Fraser, M.D., F.R.C.P.
} *Ministry of Health*

Sir Andrew Davidson, M.D., F.R.C.P. Ed., F.R.C.S. Ed.
A. K. Bowman, M.B., Ch.B., F.R.F.P.S.
} *Department of Health for Scotland*

J. Boyd, C.B.E., M.D., F.R.C.P.I.
} *Government of Northern Ireland*

Sir Harold Himsworth, K.C.B., M.D., F.R.C.P., F.R.S., Q.H.P.
Janet Vaughan, O.B.E., D.M., F.R.C.P.
} *Medical Research Council*

Surgeon Vice Admiral Sir Alexander Ingleby MacKenzie, K.B.E., C.B., B.M., B.Ch., Q.H.P.
} *Admiralty*

Lt. General Sir Frederick Harris, K.B.E., C.B., M.C., M.B., LL.D. Q.H.S.
Major General A. Sachs, C.B., C.B.E., M.Sc., M.D., M.R.C.P., Q.H.P.
} *War Office*

Air Marshal Sir James M. Kilpatrick, K.B.E., C.B., M.B., B.Ch., Q.H.P.
} *Air Ministry*

Brigadier H. B. Latham
A. B. Acheson, Esq., C.M.G.
} *Cabinet Office*

Editor-in-Chief: Sir Arthur S. MacNalty, K.C.B., M.D., F.R.C.P., F.R.C.S.

Secretary: W. Franklin Mellor

The following persons served on the Editorial Board for varying periods: The Rt. Hon. R. A. Butler, P.C., M.A., F.R.G.S., M.P. (*Chairman*); Brigadier General Sir James E. Edmonds, C.B., C.M.G., D.Litt. (*Committee of Imperial Defence*); Surgeon Vice Admiral Sir Sheldon F. Dudley, K.C.B., O.B.E., M.D., F.R.C.P., F.R.C.S. Ed., F.R.S.; Surgeon Vice Admiral Sir Henry St. Clair Colson, K.C.B., C.B.E., F.R.C.P.; Surgeon Vice Admiral Sir Edward Greeson, K.B.E., C.B., M.D., Ch.B. (*Admiralty*); Lt. General Sir William P. MacArthur, K.C.B., D.S.O., O.B.E., M.D., B.Ch., D.Sc., F.R.C.P.; Lt. General Sir Alexander Hood, G.B.E., K.C.B., M.D., F.R.C.P., LL.D.; Lt. General Sir Neil Cantlie, K.C.B., K.B.E., M.C., M.B., F.R.C.S.; Major General H. M. J. Perry, C.B., O.B.E., F.R.C.P.; Major General L. T. Poole, C.B., D.S.O., M.C., M.B., Ch.B.; Brigadier J. S. K. Boyd, O.B.E., M.D., F.R.S.; Brigadier H. T. Findlay, M.B., Ch.B. (*War Office*); Air Marshal Sir Harold E. Whittingham, K.C.B., K.B.E., M.B., Ch.B., F.R.C.P., F.R.C.S., LL.D.; Air Marshal Sir Andrew Grant, K.B.E., C.B., M.B., Ch.B.; Air Marshal Sir Philip C. Livingston, K.B.E., C.B., A.F.C., F.R.C.S. (*Air Ministry*); Sir Edward Mellanby, G.B.E., K.C.B., M.D., F.R.C.P., F.R.S. (*Medical Research Council*); Professor J. M. Mackintosh, M.A., M.D., F.R.C.P. (*Department of Health for Scotland*); Lt. Colonel J. S. Yule, O.B.E., Philip Allen, Esq., G. Godfrey Phillips, Esq., M. T. Flett, Esq., A. M. R. Topham, Esq., D. F. Hubback, Esq. (*Cabinet Office*).

EDITORIAL COMMITTEE

Sir ARTHUR S. MACNALTY, K.C.B., M.D., F.R.C.P., F.R.C.S.
(*Chairman*)

Surgeon Captain J. L. S. COULTER, D.S.C., M.R.C.S., L.R.C.P. (Barrister-at-Law) } *Admiralty*

Professor F. A. E. CREW, D.Sc., M.D., F.R.C.P. Ed., F.R.S. } *War Office*

Squadron Leader S. C. REXFORD-WELCH, M.A., M.R.C.S., L.R.C.P. } *Air Ministry*

A. K. BOWMAN, M.B., Ch.B., F.R.F.P.S. { *Department of Health for Scotland*

J. BOYD, C.B.E., M.D., F.R.C.P.I. { *Government of Northern Ireland*

F. H. K. GREEN, C.B.E., M.D., F.R.C.P. — *Medical Research Council*

J. ALISON GLOVER, C.B.E., M.D., F.R.C.P. — *Ministry of Education*

A. SANDISON, O.B.E., M.D. — *Ministry of Pensions*

Lt. Colonel C. L. DUNN, C.I.E., I.M.S. (ret.)
Sir ZACHARY COPE, B.A., M.D., M.S., F.R.C.S. } *Ministry of Health*

Secretary: W. FRANKLIN MELLOR

The following persons served on the Editorial Committee for varying periods:

Surgeon Commander J. J. Keevil, D.S.O., M.D.; Surgeon Lieutenant L. D. de Launay, M.B., B.S.; Surgeon Lieutenant Commander N. M. McArthur, M.D.; Surgeon Commander A. D. Sinclair, M.B., Ch.B. (*Admiralty*); Colonel S. Lyle Cummins, C.B., C.M.G., LL.D., M.D. (*War Office*); Wing Commander R. Oddie, M.B., B.Ch.; Wing Commander E. B. Davies, M.B., B.Ch.; Squadron Leader R. Mortimer, M.B., B.S.; Squadron Leader H. N. H. Genese, M.R.C.S., L.R.C.P. (*Air Ministry*); Charles E. Newman, M.D., F.R.C.P.; N. G. HORNER, M.D., F.R.C.P., F.R.C.S. (*Ministry of Health*).

CONTENTS

PREFATORY NOTE BY THE EDITOR-IN-CHIEF

                                                                                       Page

FOREWORD by *Surgeon Vice Admiral Sir Alexander Ingleby MacKenzie, K.B.E., C.B., B.M., B.Ch., Q.H.P.*   xv

CHAPTER 1: THE NAVAL MEDICAL OFFICER AFLOAT IN TIME OF WAR

(i)

THE MEDICAL ORGANISATION OF H.M. SHIPS . .   1

(ii)

THE DAILY JOURNAL OF A MEDICAL OFFICER AFLOAT   31

A record of the day to day problems of the naval medical officer at sea on active service.

(iii)

THE LESSONS TO BE LEARNED FROM THE JOURNAL .   77

CHAPTER 2: THE NAVAL MEDICAL OFFICER ON ACTIVE SERVICE ASHORE

(i)

SOME MEDICAL OPERATIONS ASHORE . . .   120

A selection from the records of the more important shore units:

The Mobile Naval Base Defence Organisation . .   120
M.N.B.D.O. (1)   123
The First Royal Naval Tented Hospital . . .   124
The Second Royal Naval Tented Hospital . . .   135
M.N.B.D.O. (2)   144
Mobile Landing Craft Advanced Bases (MOLCAB)   150
H.M.S. *Landswell* (MOLCAB 1) . . .   151
H.M.S. *Landlock* (MOLCAB 2) . . .   164
Activities with the Special Operations Executive .   168

CONTENTS

Page

(ii)

SOME MEDICAL EVENTS OF SPECIAL INTEREST	176

Selected narratives of certain Naval Medical Personnel captured by the enemy.

The loss of H.M.S. *Gloucester* and subsequent events	177
The loss of H.M.S. *Exeter* and subsequent events	202
The escape from Singapore	223
The fall of Hong Kong	256

CHAPTER 3: MEDICAL ASPECT OF THE CHIEF NAVAL EVENTS 1939–41

THE YEAR 1939	283
The Battle of the River Plate	285
THE YEAR 1940	290
Norwegian Operations	290
Evacuation of the B.E.F. from the Continent	308
Medical Organisation for the Evacuation	319
Action off Calabria	331
Action off Crete	331
Operations off Dakar	332
Actions involving Armed Merchant Cruisers	333
Effects of Particular Weapons	335
Rescues at Sea	343
Clinical Practice in Convoy	344
THE YEAR 1941	347
Operation 'Excess'—Convoys Gibraltar to Greece	347
The Sinking of the *Bismarck*	359
Greek and Cretan Operations	364
Operations in the Red Sea, East Africa and the Persian Gulf	375
North African Coastal Operations	376
The Loss of H.M.Ss. *Prince of Wales* and *Repulse*	383
Air Raids affecting Naval Establishments ashore and ships in Harbour	387
Effects of Particular Weapons	392

CHAPTER 4: MEDICAL ASPECT OF THE CHIEF NAVAL EVENTS 1942–3

SOME MINOR NAVAL OPERATIONS 1942	400
Naval Operations off Ceylon	400
The Loss of H.M.Ss. *Dorsetshire* and *Cornwall*	401
The Loss of H.M.Ss. *Hermes*, *Vampire* and *Hollyhock* and the R.F.A. *Athelstone*	408

CONTENTS

	Page
Naval Operations at the Capture of Diego Suarez, May 1942	410
The Attack on St. Nazaire, March 1942	413
The Raid on Dieppe, August 1942	415
CONVOYS TO NORTH RUSSIA 1942–3	417
Medical Organisation Afloat	418
Medical Organisation Ashore in North Russia	429
Arctic Convoy Battles	441
Rescue Organisation	449
Repatriation of Survivors	463
Morale	464
THE OCCUPATION OF NORTH AFRICA: OPERATION 'TORCH'	468
The Plan	468
Medical Organisation	469
Medical Stores and Equipment	475
The Operations	476
Medical Organisation Ashore	481
Commentary	484

CHAPTER 5: MEDICAL ASPECT OF THE CHIEF NAVAL EVENTS 1944–5

MINOR NAVAL OPERATIONS 1944	493
Incidents of Medical Interest	493
Casualties caused by Noxious Fumes	497
The Loss of the Rescue Ship *Pinto*	507
THE NORMANDY LANDINGS	509
The Seaborne Evacuation of Casualties	509
The Naval Off-Shore Force	512
The Evacuation of Casualties by Landing Craft	516
The Medical Organisation of the Port Parties	520
The Naval Medical Organisation for the Reception of Casualties in the United Kingdom	525
The Casualties—Portsmouth Area	529
EVENTS OF SPECIAL INTEREST 1945	535
Landing Craft Infantry (Casualty Clearing Ships)	535
'Kamikaze' Attacks	536
Survival at Sea	539
INDEX	541

LIST OF ILLUSTRATIONS

Plate *Facing page*

I. FRONTISPIECE. Admiral Sir Bruce Fraser, Commander-in-Chief, British Pacific Fleet, during his inspection of the Royal Naval Hospital at Herne Bay, Sydney, Australia.

CHAPTER 1

II. The damaged H.M.H.S. *Somersetshire* in floating dock	32
III. Damaged destroyer, H.M.S. *Quorn*	32
IV. A casualty being transferred from an aircraft carrier to a destroyer in rough weather in the Pacific, to be taken to a Hospital Ship	33
V. H.M.S. *Appledore*. Casualties being lowered down the side of a ship using 2-tier stretchers	48
VI. H.M.S. *Glory* embarks released British prisoners. A stretcher case being hoisted aboard	49
VII. Casualties being transferred at sea by winch	112
VIII. A casualty rescued from sea covered with fuel oil	113
IX. A Fleet Air Arm casualty	113

CHAPTER 2

X. Evacuation of civilians by the Royal Navy during the Japanese Invasion	128
XI. Evacuation of civilians by the Royal Navy during the Japanese Invasion	129

CHAPTER 3

XII. Damage to H.M.S. *Illustrious*	384
XIII. Sinking of H.M.S. *Ark Royal*	385

CHAPTER 4

XIV. Boulogne–Le Touquet area. Raid on June 3, 1942. Wounded Naval and Military personnel being removed from Naval craft on return from the French coast	400
XV. Dieppe. A sick berth attendant stays behind with two British wounded after the raid	401
XVI. Arctic Convoy—thawing out anchor chains and winches by steam on board H.M.S. *Scylla* during a spell of cold weather	480
XVII. Arctic Convoy—conditions on deck in cold weather	481

LIST OF ILLUSTRATIONS

CHAPTER 5

Facing page

XVIII. Normandy Landings, with a Hospital L.S.T. Beach scenes as wounded were being embarked. . . 496

XIX. Off the Invasion Coast. Courseulles Canal scene as wounded were being embarked in a barge for transport to a Hospital Ship 497

CHAPTER 4

Page

Map Convoy Routes to North Russia 419

FOREWORD

By Surgeon Vice Admiral Sir Alexander Ingleby MacKenzie
K.B.E., C.B., B.M., B.Ch., M.R.C.S., L.R.C.P., Q.H.P.
Medical Director-General of the Navy

As stated by Sir Edward Greeson, my predecessor in office, in his admirable Foreword to our Administration Volume, I too regard it as a pleasure and a privilege that I should be required to write a Foreword to this, the Operational Volume of the Official Naval Medical History of the War.

Naturally, being a commitment of my Department, it has been my duty to scrutinise the manuscript of this volume during the course of its production. To begin with I tended to regard this duty as a mere formality. But, as time passed, and as I read more and more of it, I must confess that I found myself becoming enthralled and spellbound by this record of the various activities of the Navy's Medical and Nursing Services during the Second World War.

In compiling this volume, my Editor has, I think wisely, not attempted the impossible task of setting down in monotonous chronological detail all the operational events in which naval medical and nursing personnel were involved. Neither has he given any account of those great naval actions which have no medical interest attached to them and which, in any case, have been adequately publicised elsewhere.

Instead, this volume has been planned as an overall survey of the part played by naval doctors and nurses in every operational sphere of the war, ashore and afloat, with the object of recording, so to speak, a cross-section of their adventures. In addition, attention has been paid to emphasising that impact which can be exerted by medical considerations upon the conduct of modern naval warfare.

The survey begins with a comprehensive chapter which gives a detailed account of the life of a naval medical officer afloat in time of war. Apart from the general historical value of this chapter, its greatest interest is probably gained by the inclusion of notes from a medical officer's journal in which are recorded the day to day problems, reactions, fears and foibles of the average naval doctor on active service at sea.

An account follows of some of the more specialised types of medical organisation for operations ashore which the Navy was called upon to provide. These include the stories of the Naval Tented Hospitals in Crete and the Maldive Islands, the Mobile Landing Craft Advanced Bases which played a part in the later stages of the war against Japan, and the experiences of certain medical officers lent by the Navy for service with guerilla forces in the Balkans and in Malaya.

Next described is a number of selected events which display a common feature in that the medical incidents recorded first arose under the weight of heavy defeat by the enemy, and full accounts could only be collated after the war, from the numerous reports of personnel who survived captivity as prisoners-of-war. The incidents here recorded include the events subsequent to the losses of H.M.S. *Gloucester* and H.M.S. *Exeter*, and the detailed story of the Royal Naval Hospital, Hong Kong, at the time of the Japanese invasion. This latter is of historical importance, being the record of the only naval hospital actually captured by the enemy during the war.

Of outstanding interest is the story of the events which are described following the evacuation of Singapore, and this interest is emphasised by the fact that no medical personnel or nursing staff were actually involved. My personal opinion, and I fear no contradiction, is that this narrative which tells of the impact of tropical disease upon a shipwrecked Service community is one of the most valuable contributions which has ever been made to the study of preventive medicine inside any Fighting Service. Historically it is probably the most important material in this volume, declaring as it does how vitally necessary it is that isolated parties should always contrive to include at least one member with medical experience and training. This particular portion of our narrative will, I feel sure, be studied and fully taken to heart by those who may be called upon to decide the fate of others in the future the world over. If the significance and the lesson of this story are appreciated by Men in Command, that appreciation alone will have made the writing of this volume well worth while.

Our Operational story concludes with an account of the medical aspects of the chief naval events from the years 1939 to 1945.

The result of this survey is that the Operational History of the Naval Medical and Nursing Services is here presented to the public in simple and non-scientific terms, and in a form which is eminently readable. To this extent it should appeal to the layman no less than to the professional reader.

The story tells much of personal suffering and hardship. Above all, it tells of our mistakes and our failures, a necessary factor in any History which purports to be accurate. But the story also tells of great successes and medical achievements of which we feel we have the right to be proud. In this respect my Editor has again avoided technical expressions and has made full allowance for the non-scientific reader, thereby producing a narrative which, to my mind, is historically unique in its very human approach to so many events in which tragedy and tears are so frequently offset by that sense of humour which is characteristic of the sailor.

Once again this volume reveals how much naval medicine owed to the constant assistance and co-operation of our colleagues from the Allies and the other British Medical Services, particularly the Royal

Army Medical Corps whose vast achievements were so much greater than anything which the Navy could ever hope to equal.

Space prevents me from paying individual tribute to all those persons who have been responsible for the preparation of this volume. Our grateful thanks is due to Lieut. Colonel C. L. Dunn, of the Editorial Committee and to Mr. W. Franklin Mellor, Secretary of the Official Medical Histories, as well as to those Admiralty Departments which have come to our aid. In particular we are grateful to the Chief of Naval Information and the Head of the Military Branch of the Admiralty, both of whom have done so much to guide us towards an accurate assessment of those naval events in which our doctors and nurses were mainly involved.

Finally, I must express my thanks to my Civil Assistant, Mr. P. A. Cackett, for the help of his staff, especially Miss Gwendoline Lock and Miss Winifred Dolden, both of whom have worked so hard 'behind the scenes' towards the successful production of this volume.

A. INGLEBY MACKENZIE

1954

CHAPTER 1
THE NAVAL MEDICAL OFFICER AFLOAT IN TIME OF WAR

(i)
The Medical Organisation of H.M. Ships in War

IN THE chapters of this History which describe naval medical administration, repeated mention has been made of that versatility which is necessary in the mental make-up of a naval medical officer. From the administrative viewpoint, such versatility implies that a doctor who enters the Royal Navy must be prepared to undertake clinical duties of any and every kind. He cannot anticipate employment in a particular speciality during his whole period of service. It will be understood, therefore, that wherever versatility has been referred to in the previous pages of this History, the intention has been to employ the word in a clinical sense.

But once a naval medical officer finds himself divorced from a purely medical environment, and absorbed into the routine machinery of naval life afloat, he soon discovers that that versatility which has been constantly impressed upon him during his training extends far beyond the limits of his purely clinical work.

One of the most difficult questions which a naval medical officer may be asked by a civilian doctor is this:

'How do you manage to pass the time?'

The question is difficult because the questioner is asking it in a clinical sense, and this is the sense in which he expects to be answered. The naval medical officer will therefore find that his answer, embracing the odd mild illness or accident on board his ship, is unlikely to impress his civilian colleague. Naturally, an intelligent questioner should be capable of appreciating that the medical officer's professional duties afloat are more concerned with preventive than with curative medicine, and he should also be capable of understanding that in any case, certainly in time of war, a medical organisation afloat must be ever ready to deal with the casualties which may arise in the medical officer's own or other ships as the results of enemy action or some other catastrophe.

Nevertheless, it is only when he himself understands, and is capable of explaining, the true nature of his life afloat, that a naval medical officer can truthfully answer that a day of 24 hours is all too short. The medical officer's efficiency is not judged merely on the clinical skill which he may display in dealing with the sick and wounded, for this is something which he is expected to display and is taken for granted from the beginning. On the other hand, there are various incidents of preventive medicine afloat with which he cannot be expected to be fully conversant at a moment's notice. But it is his duty to acquaint himself with what is required of him as soon as possible, and it is a poor medical officer indeed who, after a few weeks in his ship, does not know the general state of health of his ship's company, their state of vaccination and inoculation, the quality of their food and water, the adequacy of the ventilation of their living and working spaces, the suitability of their clothing, and their knowledge of how best to assist themselves and their fellows to cope with the dangers of wounds in action and to guard against the perils of diseases which may exist in future ports of call.

But, in addition to these professional duties, this same medical officer will be expected to display versatility in many other directions. In the eyes of his commanding officer he will be judged not merely on his professional efficiency, but also on his zeal, leadership, social accomplishments, athletic prowess and those many other attributes which together constitute his 'officer-like qualities'.

Thus, once afloat, the medical officer is expected to fulfil many of the functions of a naval officer as well as those of a doctor.

In time of war, a ship's medical officer will probably find himself acting as chief censor. This means that he will be responsible for seeing that all correspondence which leaves the ship has been efficiently censored, and the delegating of this duty among his brother officers is something which calls for a high degree of organising ability and an infinite display of tact. Occasionally a medical officer has found it convenient to combine the duties of chief censor with those of mail officer, which means that he must acquire a high degree of knowledge of postal regulations. In addition, he must fully appreciate the probable movements of his ship in order that the despatch of outgoing mail and the receipt and distribution of incoming mail may be effected at various ports of call with that frequency and minimum of delay which is so vital to the general well-being and happiness of sailors afloat. Some idea of the responsibility carried by a medical officer who performs this duty may be gained when it is realised that when action is impending, sailors are inclined to send their ready cash away by post rather than run the risk of losing it should the ship be sunk. At such a time, the medical officer acting as mail officer may thus find himself the custodian of several hundred registered letters containing a total of some thousands of pounds.

In some of His Majesty's Ships it became customary, under war-time conditions, for medical officers to take part in the cyphering organisation. This assistance was most valuable, particularly in small ships whose meagre complement of officers had little time for rest, and even in flagships in which a vast amount of signal traffic had constantly to be coded and decoded every hour of the day and night. Nevertheless, this willingness of medical officers to assist with cyphering duties became complicated, as the war progressed, by the fact that in certain ships the commanding officer failed to appreciate the precise status of medical officers in regard to this particular type of employment. The difficulty was concerned with the exact definition of cyphering duties *qua* combatant duties, with the consequent problem of whether such duties could only be performed by a medical officer on a purely voluntary basis, or whether he could be compelled to co-operate.

In most ships the question did not arise, as medical officers were only too willing to assist. But in the occasional ship in which the difficulty did arise, the executive authorities were inclined to rely upon the strict wording of King's Regulations and Admiralty Instructions, which pronounced that 'responsibility for this duty may be delegated to a commissioned officer of the accountant (now supply) or *any other branch*'.

The words 'any other branch' seemed to afford authority for the compulsory employment of medical officers on cyphering duties.

It must not be imagined that this problem was in any way widespread, but a time did arrive when the Medical Director-General of the Navy deemed it advisable to obtain an authoritative ruling in order that the correct status of a medical officer should be fully appreciated wherever he might be serving. The result was the promulgation, in February 1944, of a Fleet Order, which gave the conditions under which medical officers, chaplains and sick berth ratings might be employed on cyphering duties.

In this Order a comprehensive preamble outlined the conditions for entitlement to treatment as protected personnel, and the rights and privileges appertaining to this status as regulated by the 1929 International Convention for the Amelioration of the Condition of the Wounded and Sick in Arms in the Field. Although this Convention did not specifically cover personnel serving afloat, it was considered that all belligerents were likely to regard all protected personnel ashore and afloat as falling within its terms.

The Fleet Order then pointed out that cyphering could not be regarded as strictly consistent with the duties of protected personnel, and that persons known to have carried out cyphering duties, if captured by the enemy, would lose the privileges to which they would normally be entitled, and would be liable to treatment as ordinary prisoners-of-war. But, having expressed the true state of affairs, the Fleet Order then drew attention to the shortage of officers available for cyphering duties, and to the vast and increasing volume of such work which made it most desirable that every suitable qualified officer and rating should render assistance whenever his routine duties should permit.

In conclusion, the Fleet Order considered that medical, dental and wardmaster officers and chaplains might volunteer for cyphering duties, provided that the terms of the Fleet Order had first been brought to their notice, and on the understanding that there should be no interference with the performance of their proper duties. Sick berth ratings were also included under the same provisions.

The position was now clear, with the result that from February 1944 onwards, commanding officers understood that, although King's Regulations and Admiralty Instructions did not expressly exclude medical officers from the delegation of cyphering duties, they could only be employed upon such duties on a voluntary basis. Furthermore, it was the duty of commanding officers to remind them of the reversion to combatant status which would be implied in consequence. Therefore, should a medical officer volunteer for cyphering duties, he understood that he automatically lost the status of a protected person. In any case, his cyphering duties were always subordinate to the requirements of his professional duties in his ship.

It is of some importance to record that this directive regarding cyphering duties by medical officers applied only to those employed afloat or ashore as part of a primarily combatant organisation. Naturally, it would have no application to medical officers serving as part of an exclusively medical organisation. For example, in a hospital ship there would be no question of cyphering duties, for the reason that the signals and communications from such ships must be made in plain language, and all a hospital ship's personnel must conform to the provisions of the Hague Convention of 1907 for the Adaptation to Maritime Warfare of the Principles of the Geneva Convention, 1906.

In addition to these more specific duties, most naval medical officers have always made a point of interesting themselves in the various off duty activities of their ship's companies. Under conditions of war, when shore leave from His Majesty's Ships is necessarily curtailed, it is of the utmost importance that an organisation should exist in every ship which aims at relieving the long periods of monotony afloat. Medical officers have been active in giving lectures on current affairs, and have taken part in the educational and vocational training courses which were provided for the National Serviceman whose scholastic studies had been interrupted. Few ships failed to indulge the sailors' love of concert parties and amateur theatricals, and in these hobbies the doctor was usually to be found playing his part either on the stage or behind the scenes. Many ships made use of their sound reproduction equipment to broadcast their own programmes around the messdecks, and medical officers were usually in great demand as announcers, 'quiz masters' and members of 'brains trusts'.

It will be seen therefore, that a medical officer afloat was expected not only to display professional efficiency, but also to play his part as a 'good citizen' in maintaining the 'municipal morale' of the population with whom he was in such close contact for months or even years on end. After all, the crew of one of His Majesty's Ships afloat differs little in its basic essentials from any community of British people ashore, and, though the Naval Discipline Act is known to exist, it plays but a minor part in the efficient working of a man-of-war. The high standard of conduct which is so obvious in the British Navy can invariably be traced to the domestic harmony and happiness which exists throughout every unit of the Fleet. In such an atmosphere, the medical officer is thus apt to find himself acting rather like a family doctor towards his patients, and a friendly adviser towards his commanding officer on matters of welfare which frequently have little to do with matters medical.

In the Administrative Volume of this History mention was made of the lack of special training in naval medical matters in the case of newly joined medical officers, that the Navy was forced to apply a system of apprenticeship, but that this lack of special training was largely compensated for by the personal initiative, courage in action, and constant devotion to duty which these doctors displayed.

Reference to the first chapter of the Administrative Volume will show the various reasons which brought about these training difficulties. But even if ample facilities for training newly joined medical officers had existed in September 1939, it is doubtful whether up to date instruction in the important subject of medical organisation for action afloat could have been given at all. At that time few serving naval medical officers could be spared for training duties. Of those who could be spared, few had any practical experience of action at sea, and such experience was almost exclusively confined to that of the First World War. It is true that a certain small number of naval medical officers had seen action off the coast of Spain during the Spanish Civil War, but the experience of these few had been very short and confined to local minor incidents. For example, the destroyer H.M.S. *Hunter* had been mined off Almeria in 1937 with the loss of eight lives and some 30 other casualties. The quarter deck of H.M.S. *Royal Oak* had been struck by a bomb splinter. H.M.H.S. *Maine* had spent some 18 months in Spanish waters from 1936 to 1938, and her medical staff had seen the effects of air warfare and had had frequent opportunities of studying the treatment of war wounds in a number of Spanish military hospitals ashore.

One medical officer had been decorated for gallantry in the 'Panai Incident' in China, and another, with a sick berth rating, for outstanding conduct when a train was bombed by Japanese aircraft, an incident of the Sino-Japanese War.

Nevertheless, the knowledge gained by these few was so elementary as to exert little, if any, influence on the existing naval medical policy as regards action afloat. Broadly speaking, although a time was soon to arrive when this policy called for serious revision, the principles of medical organisation for action in September 1939 differed little from the principles which were observed in November 1918. These principles, which were outlined in King's Regulations and Admiralty Instructions, were still founded on the assumption that a Fleet action with the ships of the enemy was the most important incident likely to occur afloat. The potential strength of enemy aircraft against men-of-war had not been fully realised, and the menace of the magnetic mine had yet to be encountered.

King's Regulations and Admiralty Instructions directed that the senior medical officer should take care that every preparation is made for the accommodation and treatment of wounded in his ship. When clearing for action he and the medical officers serving under him should report to their station, where every facility should be provided. Instructions then followed indicating the broad lines on which wounded should be treated on board vessels of war. It was pointed out that, in armoured ships, it might be possible during an action to bring the wounded to the dressing stations, and thus clear the fighting parts. But in other ships, all that was recommended was that the wounded should be placed in a comfortable position near where they had fallen, and out of the way of the combatants.

Sensibly, it was laid down that nothing but first aid should be attempted during action and it was obviously not contemplated that the medical staff should be involved in such first aid, for the regulation goes on to specify, somewhat naively, that opportunities would occur during lulls when the captain of the ship may summon 'by some predetermined bugle call' the whole of the medical officers and their staff to render assistance whenever it might be required!

Great emphasis was, in fact, laid on the importance of protecting the medical officers themselves from danger, it being considered that their lives were of the greatest possible value when regarded from the standpoint of the wounded. For this reason, any action organisation in a man-of-war stipulated that the medical officers should be stationed under the best possible protection, due regard being paid to the possibility of their being incapacitated if retained during a prolonged action under atmospheric or other conditions likely to prostrate them.

To recapitulate at this point, it will be seen that the intention was that, during the course of action afloat, the medical officer was to be kept out of harm's way, so that he should be available to deal with the wounded after the action had ended. The only attention which the wounded could expect during the course of the action was first aid. This first aid would not be given by the medical staff. But that first aid should be applied efficiently was well realised, particularly if those wounded in action were to be kept alive to receive the attention of the medical officer later.

With this in view, King's Regulations directed that it should be the duty of medical officers to arrange for the instruction of officers and men in the principles of first aid to the injured, and to ensure that the necessary appliances for use by those instructed should always be readily available in the parts of the ship where they would be likely to be needed in action. Particular attention was to be paid to the first-aid training of any officers and men told off to assist the medical staff in action and afterwards, and such officers and men were, in addition to first aid, to be given instructions in some of the simple rules of nursing.

It was laid down that a minimum of 10 per cent. of the ship's company in all classes of ships should be qualified in first aid. Officers qualified in first aid had to be given a certificate, and ratings had to have their qualification noted on their Service certificates. Such qualified members of the ship's company were required to re-qualify in first aid every four years.

At this time, a single medical officer was appointed to each destroyer flotilla, and medical duties of an elementary nature were carried out in individual destroyers by the torpedo coxswain of each ship. It was the duty of the medical officer of a destroyer flotilla, not only to qualify 10 per cent. of the personnel of the whole flotilla in first aid every four years, but also to give short revision courses in first aid to each torpedo coxswain at least once a year, and more frequently should opportunity permit.

Other medical measures for action provided for two distributing stations in a man-of-war, which were to be conveniently selected if not already laid down in the vessel's design. Here all medical stores, instruments, etc., were to be placed for their conservation, and for the replenishment of first-aid supplies elsewhere. These stores were to be duplicated as far as possible, so that in the event of one portion being destroyed, the other portion would be available. In addition to these two distributing stations, provision was to be made for the supply of first-aid requisites in other parts of the ship.

Further regulations made recommendations regarding the treatment of wounded after action had ended. It was considered that, in the absence of a hospital ship, the most suitable place for the treatment of wounded after action, probably in all classes of vessels, would be some portion of the upper deck properly screened in, so as to afford some protection against weather, and yet to permit of the freest ventilation. Nevertheless, it was realised that objections to the use of the upper deck for this purpose might at the time be considered paramount, in which case places were to be selected which, it was directed, 'must be the very best the vessel can offer'. In the event of a further action being fought, it was considered essential that the wounded from the previous action should be removed to spaces between decks under whatever protection could be obtained.

In selecting a situation for the performance of pressing operations and other surgical work after action, it was again realised that the choice must be governed by the conditions obtaining at the time. But, for guidance, it was considered probable that the best possible space would be found on the upper deck. Between decks, the Captain's fore cabin, in all larger vessels, was recommended as the most suitable place, taking into consideration the questions of lighting, ventilation, and the fact that its temporary occupation would inconvenience the fewest number of persons.

Broadly speaking, it was on these lines that newly joined naval medical officers were to be trained on the outbreak of the Second World War. The feelings of those few Active Service R.N. medical officers who were available for instructional duties may well be imagined. To instil the rudiments of naval customs, traditions and discipline into the receptive minds of a large number of doctors, who had eagerly volunteered for service, was relatively easy. But to advise them how best to prepare themselves for action afloat was very much like 'the blind leading the blind'. Nobody, not even the Instructor, could have any definite notion of what type of action afloat should be catered for. The only guide laid down in regulations was suspected to be out of date and probably unlikely to meet the requirements of modern sea warfare. Yet it was impossible to forecast these requirements until bitter personal experience had proved their nature.

Such instruction was not without a tinge of pathos, as was recorded in the words of one of the instructors at that time:

'There were 83 of them, all newly joined Surgeon Lieutenants, R.N.V.R. They all stood up when I entered the room, and remained standing until I myself was seated. I looked around at their faces, and saw all types and all ages, stiff and formal in their new uniforms, but obviously thirsting for knowledge and ready to learn.

'My task was to teach them how best to set up a medical organisation for action afloat, and I felt very unfitted for it. One or two were wearing medal ribbons of the First World War, which was ended when I was still a schoolboy. One of these, it later transpired, was a grandfather, who had left a flourishing practice to join the Navy on the day war broke out.

'I did what seemed to be the most sensible thing. I outlined such regulations as did exist and warned them that they would probably be of little help, and I then frankly confessed my own personal ignorance. I told them at such a time it was best for us all to remain mentally elastic, and to avoid hard and fast rules until experience had revealed what was really needed.

'Finally, I pointed out to them how dependent people like myself would be upon the information which would soon be forthcoming from them themselves, and how we instructors would soon be looking to the newcomers to teach us in the light of their experience.

'Within a few weeks most of them were at sea, and many had been "blooded". Some had lost their lives within a matter of months, and the grandfather, after being sunk twice in a year, was forced to admit that prolonged and repeated immersion in sea water was perhaps not the best treatment for the arthritis from which he undoubtedly suffered!'

These were the pioneers, the general practitioners, old and young, who hastened to the assistance of the Royal Naval Medical Service at short notice. Some were peace-time sailors of the regular R.N.V.R., but the rest had mostly no experience at all of Service life. Nevertheless, in the same way as they had been the backbone of the medical profession in civil life, so they rapidly became the backbone of the Navy's medical organisation afloat.

Though it has become customary to speak of the winter of 1939–40 as the 'phoney war' period, this was never so in the Navy. By the end of 1939 much had happened afloat, and it was soon possible to begin to assess some of the new requirements of modern action afloat from the actual experiences of medical officers who survived those first desperate months.

Despite the numerous incidents of enemy action afloat between the outbreak of war and the end of 1939, and which included the sinking of H.M.S. *Courageous* and H.M.S. *Royal Oak*, the mining of H.M.S. *Adventure*, H.M.S. *Belfast* and H.M.S. *Nelson*, and the Battle of the River Plate, the only practical change of medical organisation afloat which resulted involved the overworked destroyer flotillas of the Fleet.

As has been described already, before September 1939, the medical complement of destroyer flotillas consisted of a medical officer and sick berth rating in the flotilla leader, and a coxswain specially qualified in first aid in each of the other ships of the flotilla. During the period of preparation for war, the Medical Director-General of the Navy was not required to allocate more than one medical officer for each destroyer flotilla. Some doubt had been cast upon the suitability of this arrangement, which seemed to presume that in time of war, the destroyer flotillas of the Fleet would continue to act collectively, and that individual destroyers would not be detached from their flotillas for independent employment. However, these general principles of complement which were laid down for the Medical Director-General did not wholly agree with the mobilisation returns which were issued in due course. These returns required a complement of two medical officers for the *Tribal* Class flotillas. Some further confusion arose from a later return which appropriated two medical officers for each of a further eight destroyer flotillas.

The Medical Director-General was in no position to comment on the need for this increase, but he felt entitled to enquire as to the reason for the anomaly which would exist when two medical officers were allocated to some destroyer flotillas while others were left with only one medical officer. His enquiry elicited the explanation that a *Tribal* Flotilla was likely to be split into two groups of ships, and a medical officer would be necessary in each group. As regards the other flotillas, the extra medical officer was required for the depot ship of each flotilla, not truly for the more active and mobile work among the destroyers themselves. Therefore, at this stage, with the exception of the *Tribal* flotillas, the seagoing medical requirements for all other classes of destroyers remained at one medical officer per flotilla. In other words, as far as the Medical Director-General was concerned, the independent use of individual destroyers did not appear to be expected, and even if it were, the fact that it might be advisable to appoint more than one medical officer to every destroyer flotilla did not seem to have been visualised.

Study of the existing records suggests that the conception of any departure from this principle arose more by accident than by design.

On September 13, 1939, it was necessary for the Medical Department, Admiralty, to be informed of the approximate total number of medical officers which should suffice for the various medical duties required to be performed at the R.N. Barracks in each of the three home ports. Accordingly a request was made to the Commanders-in-Chief at Portsmouth, the Nore and Plymouth, that a statement should be given of the minimum number of medical officers considered essential, these numbers to include authorised complements, permanent supernumeraries, and also medical officers for all extra and additional work likely to occur in and around each of the depots.

The replies from the Portsmouth and Nore Commands were of little importance at this point in the story, but the reply of the Commodore, R.N. Barracks, Devonport, was accompanied by forwarding remarks of the Commander-in-Chief, Plymouth, dated October 2, 1939. The substance of these remarks was to draw attention to the fact that the nature of destroyer operations in the Western Approaches indicated that these ships were likely to be almost continually at sea, acting independently, and rarely in company with the flotilla leader in which a medical officer was carried. After less than a month of war, cases had already occurred in the ships where a medical officer was urgently required but was not available. As a temporary measure, the Commander-in-Chief, Plymouth, had already employed a number of supernumerary medical officers from R.N. Barracks, Devonport, in the destroyers concerned. He now represented that he considered it essential for the well-being of their personnel, that a medical officer should be appointed to each destroyer acting independently. He also recommended that in the ships, medical duties should no longer be delegated to coxswains, but that each destroyer should carry a sick berth rating.

This representation, coming as it did without warning, was viewed with some concern by the Medical Director-General, who felt that should he respond without question to all such commitments of individual Commanders-in-Chief, it would not be long before every destroyer in the Navy would be carrying its own medical officer and sick berth rating. Apart from the implied drastic alteration of the policy accepted for medical organisation afloat, it was also necessary for him to consider the grave impact which would result upon the whole medical and nursing man-power situation in the Service. This was something which the Medical Director-General could not contemplate without consulting his own Higher Authority, and he therefore requested that a ruling should be given.

In order to appreciate the full effects of such a change of policy, it is necessary to divorce the elements of morale and well-being from other considerations, which would immediately have to be taken into account, should a medical officer and sick berth rating be appointed to individual destroyers. Much as it might appear to be desirable to approve such appointments, it had to be remarked that a destroyer is by no means a large man-of-war. Accommodation in such ships was always very limited, particularly now that complements had been brought up to war-time strength. The arrival in each destroyer of a medical officer and sick berth rating would mean an extra sleeping berth to be found and mouth to be fed both in the wardroom and on the lower deck.

For each destroyer to carry a doctor and sick berth rating also meant that the very elementary medical chest carried by such ships for first-aid purposes would have to be replaced by an adequate supply of medical stores and equipment, including drugs and instruments, in keeping with the requirements of an official ship's medical officer. For such stores and equipment storage space would have to be found, and already these ships considered themselves to be stored to capacity.

The presence of a medical officer and sick berth rating also meant that, somewhere in the ship, a sick bay would have to be created, or if one already existed, it would have to be made available to the doctor, for experience showed that in many ships advantage had been taken of the absence of a doctor to employ the compartment set aside as a sick bay for some other purpose.

In short, to appoint a medical officer and sick berth rating to a destroyer, meant a reorganisation of the internal domestic economy of the ship by the creation in it of a medical department and all that goes with it.

With all these matters in mind, Their Lordships invited the views of a number of the sea-going Commands likely to be affected by the suggested change of policy. At the same time, the Medical Director-General was able to forecast the probable number of medical officers likely to be required to meet the new commitment, and it seemed that it would be necessary to recruit into the Royal Navy an extra 94 medical officers at an early date.

The views of the sea-going Commands varied. For example, the Vice Admiral Commanding the Second Cruiser Squadron, concurring in the views of the destroyer captains under his Command, considered that a medical officer should be carried in each destroyer with a complement of over 200.

The Commanding Officer of the Fifth Destroyer Flotilla reported that he would propose to await the further experience of his flotilla under war conditions before urging such a serious measure as appointing a medical officer to each ship. At the same time, he pointed out that the complement of each ship in his flotilla numbered 206, and he recommended an immediate increase by one sick berth rating to each destroyer.

The views of the Commander-in-Chief, Home Fleet, were definite, but tended towards compromise in certain directions. It was claimed that the presence of a medical officer in a man-of-war was known to add considerably to the confidence and morale of men going into action. It must be contemplated that individual destroyers or small groups of destroyers would frequently be carrying out detached duty, with no medical officer in any ship of the unit. Even should a sick berth rating be appointed to each ship, it was always likely that casualties might result from an engagement some distance from port, and that this might call for the attendance of a qualified doctor. It was therefore considered essential that a medical officer should be carried in each destroyer. But having established this principle, the Commander-in-Chief neutralised it to some extent by recommending that such a medical officer should be as junior as possible, because the limited accommodation available would necessitate him slinging in a hammock!

After sifting the views forwarded by the sea Commands, the Operations Division of the Admiralty applied the suggested medical changes to the probable involvement in enemy action of the various destroyer flotillas of the Fleet. As a result, it was possible to divide the flotillas into three classes of priority.

Destroyer flotillas of the Home Fleet, Nore Command, and those based on the Humber, were considered to be most liable to enemy attack from the air, mine and surface. It was therefore proposed that a medical officer and sick berth rating should be appointed to each destroyer of these flotillas.

Second priority was given to the flotillas normally employed on assault duties and submarine hunting in the Western Approaches. Somewhat strangely, it was not considered at that time, November 1939, that these flotillas ran the same risk of damage by enemy action as those given first priority. But it was considered that these ships were likely to find themselves long distances away from medical assistance in case of sickness, and for this reason it was considered desirable that they too should each be allocated a medical officer and sick berth rating.

The third priority consisted of destroyer flotillas based at Gibraltar, Portsmouth, Dover and Malta. These would be employed on miscellaneous and comparatively local duty, and it was therefore considered that one medical officer should suffice for each flotilla, as under the peacetime system.

As an overall consideration, however, it was strongly urged that every destroyer at sea should carry a sick berth rating.

The Medical Director-General now took steps to implement the appointments as recommended, and, pending the recruitment of extra medical officers, a temporary reduction was made in the medical staffs of a number of naval medical establishments ashore. By December 28, 1939, a medical officer and sick berth rating had been appointed to each destroyer of the Western Approaches flotillas. On January 8, 1940, the Board of Admiralty approved the appointment of a medical officer and sick berth rating to each destroyer of the Home Fleet. Other appointments followed to all destroyers as medical officers became available.

From the domestic angle it is of some interest to record that, while in most destroyer flotillas the arrival of a medical officer and sick berth rating with their impedimenta was welcomed, in others their presence was an embarrassment as regards space and accommodation. Here and there minor difficulties arose which eventually had to be resolved by official action, and medical officers appointed to individual destroyers were now to be regarded as part of the normal complement, for whom suitable cabin accommodation was to be provided.

This alteration in the medical complement of destroyer flotillas was the first major development of the Second World War which affected the medical organisation for action afloat. The subsequent mortality among medical officers and sick berth ratings in destroyers was high, but their presence was amply justified in the numerous operations in which small ships were engaged throughout the whole course of the war. In addition to destroyers, medical officers and sick berth ratings were later appointed to individual corvettes and frigates whenever possible.

As regards the smaller units of the Fleet, it is of some interest to record that medical officers and sick berth ratings were not carried in H.M. Submarines, neither would it appear from the records that such a suggestion was ever seriously raised, though, towards the end of the war, consideration was given to appointing a sick berth rating to each submarine operating either in tropical or in arctic waters.

One medical officer did lose his life in one of H.M. Submarines, but only while being carried as a passenger between Gibraltar and Malta.

Naturally, the medical requirements for service in submarines constitute a special branch of medicine in which all naval medical officers receive training early in their careers, and an experienced medical staff is always carried in each submarine depot ship.

As time passed, as was expected, large numbers of medical officers afloat became involved in enemy action, and in due course it was possible for the Medical Director-General to assess and evaluate the many recommendations which were placed before him. To the action experiences of the small ships could now be added the experiences of the larger units of the Fleet.

Many changes were obviously necessary in the pre-war regulations which governed Medical Organisation for Action. During 1940 and 1941 a number of these changes had already been implemented either by local arrangements or individual enterprise. But in April 1942, a comprehensive Fleet Order was issued which recognised officially that modern circumstances of war afloat called for modern medical measures.

The Fleet Order stated that before 1941, the organisation for action in H.M. Ships had been centralised in the medical distributing stations. War experience had now proved the necessity for a much greater degree of decentralisation, and for more posts where emergency treatment could be carried out. The Order recognised that considerable latitude must be allowed in its application, having regard to the great variations in size and construction of H.M. Ships. But, while the arrangements recommended were primarily intended for larger ships, it was considered desirable that in smaller types the principles should be followed as far as possible.

The following posts for medical use were recommended in all H.M. Ships, wherever possible:

(a) *A Main Distributing Station*. This position was recommended to be sited either forward or aft, as convenient, in a compartment of the ship under protection. Where possible, it was to be allocated as such in the ship's plans, and appropriated and fitted out solely for medical purposes.

(b) *An Auxiliary Distributing Station*. This position was recommended to be sited towards the end of the ship remote from the main distributing station, in a compartment under protection and of considerable size. Suggested positions were a messdeck, laundry, store room, any space which, although primarily allocated for other purposes, could quickly be converted for use as a medical distributing station. With this in view, it was important that any permanent medical fittings provided should be such as to interfere as little as possible with the primary use of the compartment.

As regards these distributing stations, an important change of policy was based on the great harm which experience has suggested had been done to wounded men by carrying them through a series of narrow passages and man-holes to the treatment centres. It was now considered of primary importance that the distributing stations should not only offer adequate room for treatment, but also should be so sited that there would be easy access for stretcher cases.

(c) *First-Aid Posts*. A number of first-aid posts was recommended to be sited principally on upper decks near to action stations. The types of compartment suggested for consideration were crew spaces, bathrooms, recreation spaces, captain's quarters, gun room, sick bay, wide lobbies and posts in the 'island' on the flight deck in aircraft carriers.

In selecting compartments for use as first-aid posts, the following main requirements had to be observed:

Working space.
Protection from weather, explosive blast, and shell and bomb splinters.
Accessibility from fighting and working parts of the ship.
The easy passage of stretchers.
The minimum of interference with the working and fighting of the ship.
Proximity to hot and cold water supply.
Adequate light and ventilation.
Adequate telephonic communications.
Stowage space for first-aid equipment.

The recommendations contemplated that the number of such first-aid posts could not be defined with accuracy, but must depend upon the local arrangements in each ship. But a broad principle was laid down which aimed at every man-of-war being divided into areas, each area having its own first-aid post as a casualty reception centre.

It was also realised that the number of such first-aid posts which could be established in a particular ship would be affected by the number of personnel available to man them in action. As a general guide, it was considered desirable that each first-aid post should be occupied by a sick berth rating or a specially qualified first-aid worker, together with a less skilled assistant.

If possible, a medical officer was to be in charge of each of the two distributing stations. But should only one medical officer be carried, then he would be in charge of the main distributing station, and the senior sick berth rating would be in charge of the auxiliary station. In addition, a minimum of two competent first-aid assistants was to be allocated to each of the distributing stations, and the ship's master-at-arms was to be allocated to the main distributing station for the important function of recording the designation and particulars of casualties as they should occur.

As regards the suggested principle to be observed in the employment of personnel in the distributing centres and first-aid posts, a short reflection shows that the underlying policy aimed at eliminating some of the disadvantages already observed under action stations at this stage in the war.

In certain ships involved in action with the enemy, a too rigid adherence to the policy of immobilising the medical personnel, though well meant, had in fact resulted in defeating what had been originally intended. The old policy had visualised doctors and sick berth staff being collected together under armoured protection during the course of the action, so that they would be unlikely to come to any harm and would be available to deal with casualties when the action was over. But experience had already proved that in some cases, the whole medical staff had been quickly killed or wounded by isolated damage to that part of the ship in which they had been ordered to remain. It was obviously necessary therefore, that under conditions of modern warfare, medical personnel should be widely distributed and split up during the course of action. It was also considered important that the employment of medical personnel should be fluid and elastic. With this in view, it was considered vital to the working of an efficient medical organisation for action that the senior medical officer should on no account be required to immobilise himself at any one point, but should instead be free to move about as necessary in order to supervise and adjust his medical organisation to meet changes in the situation which were bound to arise during the actual course of the action.

It was necessary to support the new policy of greater decentralisation by taking steps to ensure that a far greater number of personnel of every ship should be qualified in first aid than had been considered necessary in the past. It will be remembered that King's Regulations specified that at least 10 per cent. of personnel should be trained in first aid. The new Fleet Order emphasised the importance of regarding this figure as a minimum number, and that as far as possible all officers and men should receive instruction in first aid. Furthermore, it was now provided that certain selected persons should be given more advanced instruction, which would include the technique of hypodermic injections. Concurrently with this provision, further instructions were issued which concerned the supply of omnopon in the form of tubunic ampoules.

The new Order outlined the broad principles which should be observed in implementing an efficient modern medical organisation for action afloat. It was considered that during the course of the action, casualties occurring in the immediate vicinity of first-aid posts would be able to be dealt with readily, while casualties occurring in situations beyond the easy reach of first-aid posts would be shifted to the nearest cover and would receive simple first aid which would be rendered by the nearest qualified person. Should opportunity offer, sorties would be made from first-aid posts in order to render more skilled assistance to the more serious cases, and from time to time the more serious cases would be moved to the nearest first-aid post where they would be treated and retained until the end of the action.

It is important to note that no attempt was to be made to transport a casualty to any position but a first-aid post during the course of the action. In fact, the Fleet Order emphasised that no attempt should be made to take any casualty to a distant distributing station during the course of an action, except on the instructions of a medical officer.

War experience showed that this latter point might well have been emphasised even further. The reason for the particular emphasis was originally concerned with the harm that might be done to a wounded man should he be transported further than was advisable without his condition first being assessed by a medical officer. But there was more to it than this, because to transport a man to a medical distributing station at a time when a ship was still engaged in action with the enemy might well involve considerations which it is not within the province of the medical officer to judge.

A man-of-war is divided into a number of watertight compartments, which inter-communicate through a system of watertight doors. In time of war, before a ship even leaves harbour, all these doors must be closed and held in place by clips or other mechanical devices.

Also, the approaches to engine and boiler rooms consist of watertight doors with an air lock in between, for the purpose of maintaining the necessary air pressure in the working compartment. This system only permits one door guarding the air lock to be open at a time, because if both doors should be open together, the air lock would fail, and this might result in a serious back-flash from burning oil fuel, with consequent grave danger to engine and boiler room personnel.

As has been stated, in time of war, all watertight doors in a man-of-war must be shut when the ship is at sea. Provided there is no reason to believe that enemy submarines are in the vicinity, or that any other type of action with the enemy is impending, it is permissible for certain watertight doors to be open for the transit of personnel between various parts of the ship in the course of their duties and for the general routine maintenance of the ship's domestic life afloat. But there are other doors which must be kept closed the whole time until the ship returns to harbour. It is usual, in a man-of-war, to paint markings on all watertight doors, in order to show their priority of importance.

Once action with the enemy is impending, however, it may be accepted that, as a general rule, no watertight door should ever be opened at all. Moreover, during the actual course of an action, to open a watertight door would be equivalent to hazarding the safety of the ship itself, and there could be no greater crime at such a time.

It will be seen, therefore, that to state that no attempt should be made to take any casualty to a distant distributing station during the course of an action, except on the instructions of a medical officer, is totally wrong. Such a statement may be justified to the extent that only a medical officer should decide on the clinical fitness of the particular casualty to be transported a certain distance in the difficult circumstances which are present in action. But here, it is submitted, the authority of the professional doctor ends, and the authority of the professional seaman begins.

The distributing station to which it is intended to transport such a casualty may well be some distance away from the place where he received his injury or from the first-aid post to which he has been taken. The route to the distributing station may be obstructed at many points by watertight doors which would have to be opened to get the casualty through. Even if the route to the distributing station should involve the opening of merely one watertight door, and then only for a brief period, a risk would be bound to arise. At the moment when the door was standing open, a torpedo might strike the ship in one of the two compartments which the door is meant to divide. The stricken compartment might be flooded, but should the door be open, then the next compartment might well be flooded too, and the surrounding circumstances might be such that this additional flooding would mean the loss of the whole ship.

To accept this risk for the sake of obtaining better medical attention for a casualty by transporting him to a distributing station is something which a medical officer must not attempt to do on his own initiative. An executive authority must at once be consulted, and this authority alone can weigh up the welfare of the casualty against the safety of the ship and her whole complement.

This particular subject is one which became of even greater importance as the war at sea progressed, when, in the light of experience, each of H.M. Ships developed a most rigid 'damage control organisation'. Broadly speaking, this organisation covered all the various measures to be adopted in order to prevent a man-of-war from sinking, once she had been damaged by enemy attack. The measures included such things as provision of emergency lighting, running repairs, the pumping out of flooded compartments, and the deliberate flooding of other compartments, such 'counter-flooding' being devised to correct the list of the ship occasioned by flooding due to damage elsewhere.

As part of the damage control organisation, a fire-fighting system was developed in every man-of-war. This system naturally embraced the employment of highly-trained teams skilled in the science of fire-fighting, but it also insisted that personal initiative should be paramount in this respect, and that, should an individual find himself in the vicinity of a sudden outbreak of fire, his first duty would be to attempt to extinguish it himself. In association with fire-fighting were the many measures of fire-prevention which were also developed in men-of-war. These measures included the reduction to a bare minimum of every type of inflammable material on board. Wherever possible, wooden furnishings and chattels were replaced by metal, carpets and curtains were removed from living spaces, stores of petrol and even bottles of 'lighter fuel' were dumped into the sea, and even the anaesthetic ether and surgical spirit of the ship's medical department came to be regarded as a dangerous, if necessary, risk.

It was at no time the policy that the medical department of a man-of-war should be involved in the ship's damage control organisation, because it was felt that a small medical staff should not be required to perform anything more than its own specialised duties during the course of action with the enemy. Nevertheless, it was very necessary that each member of the ship's medical staff should be capable of displaying initiative as regards the immediate control of damage, should fire occur inside his place of duty. It was also essential that he should possess a thorough understanding of the general damage control organisation of the ship itself. In fact, the very elasticity of the new type of medical organisation for action afloat made it not merely desirable, but vital, that each member of the medical staff should be thoroughly acquainted with every nook and cranny of his ship. It became the duty of a senior medical officer to train his staff to plot out alternative routes to the various first-aid posts and distributing stations, due allowance being made for possible damage in particular compartments. This training had to take into account the likelihood that these routes would have to be followed in darkness, with the ship on an uneven keel, and in circumstances in which the spoken order would be drowned by the noise of gunfire. Some senior medical officers brought this training to such a peak of efficiency that the members of their medical staffs knew the number of paces between various points in the ship, and the number of steps on every ladder.

This elasticity of organisation also caused senior medical officers to take into account the question of 'gun shyness', both in themselves and in the members of their staffs. To the uninitiated, the noise, concussion and flash which occur when the full armament of a man-of-war is fired, may well be an alarming experience. Added to the explosion of depth charges, torpedoes, or bombs in the vicinity, a veritable wall of sound and blast may be created at the height of an action at sea which may deter even the most stable of persons from performing his duty efficiently unless he has been taught what to expect.

(Plates II and III are included as examples of damage to ships which would adversely affect medical organisation.)

An example may be cited of the unfortunate effects which may accrue when a completely untrained person finds himself suddenly involved in action at sea:

A young doctor, newly qualified, entered the Royal Navy as a Surgeon Lieutenant, R.N.V.R. His civil experience of war on land had been limited to the sound of anti-aircraft gunfire at a distance of some miles. On joining the Navy, he was appointed to a shore establishment where he was given the briefest period of training in Service customs and discipline. The shortage of medical officers was such, that within a period of less than six weeks, he found himself afloat. Within a few days, his ship was involved in heavy action with the enemy, and this unfortunate medical officer found himself on duty in a distributing station, well below the waterline with all the sounds of battle going on around him, and creating a terrifying environment the like of which he had not imagined.

The noise was so deafening, and the movement and vibration of the ship so disturbing, that he felt an uncontrollable impulse to find out for himself what exactly was happening outside his action station. Yielding to this impulse which, it must be admitted, was as much inspired by curiosity as by anxiety, he left his distributing station, set off on a personal tour of the ship, and eventually made his way on to the upper deck. It so happened that his arrival coincided with an attack by enemy torpedo bombers, and he emerged from a man-hole into darkness relieved by gun flashes and streams of tracer bullets. He was stunned by noise and choked by fumes. As the ship heeled to an alteration of course, he was also soaked to the skin by sea water.

Realising that he was exposing himself uselessly, he now set out to grope his way back to the distributing station from which he had started. Unfortunately, he could not remember the way, and he travelled through the whole length of the ship opening watertight doors which he left behind him unclosed.

Fortunately, this ship escaped unscathed after herself inflicting heavy damage upon the enemy. Nevertheless, the personal conduct of this single individual had placed his ship temporarily in such peril, that severe disciplinary measures came under consideration and were only avoided by the representations of his senior medical officer regarding the young man's lack of training.

This story has a happy ending, as in due course this same medical officer displayed conduct of the highest order on numerous occasions in action.

This whole subject of the pre-knowledge of action environment afloat was one of which the importance was well realised and emphasised in the 1942 Fleet Order. It was directed that adequate drills should be conducted frequently in order to ensure that everyone in the ship's company should know the positions of the distributing stations and first-aid posts, and what should be done immediately in the event of casualties. It was also stressed that such drills should visualise the wounding of large numbers of men at the same time, and should be designed to test the organisation for dealing with numerous casualties in one area simultaneously. Some senior medical officers even went so far in their efforts to combat possible 'gun shyness', as to insist that whenever a practice 'shoot' took place, the medical staff should be present in the open, in the vicinity of the guns, in order to become accustomed to the noise, flash and concussion.

By 1942, numerous instances had occurred of failure to use stretchers, and in consequence, much unnecessary injury and suffering to wounded personnel had been caused. The new Fleet Order admitted that it was a natural reaction in times of stress for a man to be taken for medical attention by the quickest, as opposed to the correct method. But it was considered that by efficient drills, it should be possible to impress on a ship's company the understanding that unconscious patients and those whose injuries might not be evident should be man-handled only as a last resort.

The Fleet Order now went on to describe the types of stretcher in use. Three types of stretcher were supplied to H.M. Ships:

(1) Pattern 475. Neil-Robertson type.
(2) War Office type.
(3) P.B. Mk. IX with telescopic handles.

The P.B. Mk. IX was provided for easy decontamination, and consisted of a tubular steel frame with a paper mattress. It had to be inspected frequently, and the parts greased to maintain easy running of the sliding handles. Spare paper mattresses were provided for each stretcher.

This advice regarding the use of stretchers and the avoidance of man-handling, save as a last resort, was indeed sensible and essential. For the rest of the war every effort was made by senior medical officers afloat to see that it was fully understood and put into effect by all members of ships' companies. But among laymen, tradition dies hard and bad habits are always likely to be revived in moments of excitement. Despite adequate drills, it proved impossible to control human tendencies and cases always continued to arise in which the safety of the stretcher was neglected and preference given to the greater speed of man-handling. There were also odd occasions when a carefully planned medical organisation fell to the ground under the stress of enemy action.

An example is seen in the story recorded by a senior medical officer who had spent some months developing a medical organisation for action which, as far as he knew, had allowed for every contingency. His ship was in action on several occasions for prolonged periods, during which his organisation worked according to plan, and appeared to be 'fool-proof'. The numerous casualties which occurred were immediately taken to neighbouring first-aid posts where their immediate needs were dealt with. During lulls in action, casualties were taken from the first-aid posts to the distributing stations. Stretchers were employed and man-handling was unknown.

At dusk one evening, while on convoy duty in the Mediterranean, the ship was suddenly engaged with enemy U-boats, high and low level bombers and torpedo-carrying aircraft, all of which attacked simultaneously. Two ships were hit, and one sank immediately, leaving a large number of survivors struggling in the sea. At the height of this action a member of the ship's company was badly wounded, and fell to the deck, out in the open at his place of duty. For some reason unknown, nobody in the vicinity of the wounded man attempted first aid, neither was any effort made to transfer him to the nearest first-aid post, a matter of a few yards away. The crew of this first-aid post remained stationary. The only positive act was that some individual, who could never be identified, shouted urgently for 'a doctor' over the ship's broadcasting system. Hearing the broadcast, the senior medical officer himself made the mistake of obeying the call personally, instead of trusting in the working of his own medical organisation. Acting on impulse, he climbed to where the casualty lay prone on the deck. He arrested the severe bleeding which was obvious, and then, breaking all his own rules, he proceeded to hoist the casualty on to his shoulder and to slide down several ladders with him to the nearest distributing station, forgetting the resources and shelter of at least two first-aid posts which he passed on the way.

Looking back on the incident later on, this senior medical officer was himself apt to be hazy in his recollection of what he actually did at the time. There is no doubt that, as the ship was being heavily attacked, the story would seem to attribute great courage to this doctor. Nevertheless, the sequence of events derives its main interest from the series of errors and omissions which represented virtually a sudden and inexplicable breakdown in the medical organisation for action. In a moment of excitement, the human element suddenly overcame the fruits of deliberate training. A panic call was made for a qualified doctor. The call was unnecessary, but the doctor's own human instinct urged him to fall into a trap against which he had so frequently warned others. The result was that the doctor exposed himself unnecessarily, a highly trained first-aid organisation was neglected, and though the life of a casualty was saved, he was man-handled in circumstances which probably did him far more harm than good.

The 1942 Fleet Order took steps to consolidate previous Fleet Orders which had been issued in 1940 and 1941, and which concerned the subject of identity discs. It was emphasised that in the past, great laxity had been displayed in the wearing of identity discs, and on several occasions there had been reports of unidentified remains having been buried after an action at sea. The Order directed that all identity discs should be stamped with the wearer's blood group, that the discs should be worn at all times, and that their presence was of great importance in regard to that part of the organisation for dealing with casualties which concerned the sorting and appropriate labelling of cases.

The Fleet Order also incorporated the provision of anti-flash gear as laid down in the Manual of Victualling in 1939, and reiterated by a Fleet Order in 1940. Attention was drawn to the need for wearing anti-flash helmets, gloves and masks, in conjunction with anti-flash goggles as a protection against burns. Some concern was expressed that the protection afforded by avoiding exposure of any portion of the body should have been neglected and ignored in the past, with the result that many cases of burns had occurred on the face and arms which might well have been avoided had anti-flash gear been worn.

The subject of emergency lighting was one which was raised by the new Fleet Order which emphasised that oil lamps were unsuitable, not only on account of their poor light, but because they had already been known to cause fires due to breakage from the shock of explosion. Head lamps were recommended as well as a liberal issue of torches to individual members of medical parties called upon to deal with casualties.

At this point it is necessary to pause a moment, and to study more closely the subject of emergency lighting in a man-of-war, both from a general and a medical point of view.

Since the invention of the 'Ironclad' and the development of the armour-piercing explosive shell, the scuttles or 'port holes' of a man-of-war have obviously represented points of weakness. The number of scuttles was therefore limited, and it was important that in rough weather they should be firmly closed by a thick glass cover, and that in time of war the glass cover should be reinforced by a metal cover or a 'deadlight'. This 'deadlight', lowered and firmly screwed into position, fulfilled the purpose of protection and of aiding the ship's 'blackout' precautions. In the same way, in time of rough weather or of preparing for action, all horizontal square-cut apertures of access to the ship's interior from deck level are covered by a metal plate which is clamped into position, leaving a small man-hole for entrance or exit.

This somewhat elementary description should demonstrate that in very rough weather, or whenever a man-of-war is in a state of readiness at sea, even in broad daylight, all natural light is excluded, and artificial lighting is necessary throughout the whole of the ship's interior.

When new ships were constructed from 1939 onwards, it was considered essential to limit even further the weak spots in the side of a man-of-war, and consequently scuttles were greatly reduced in number, which meant that natural lighting was even more restricted.

The constant vulnerability of the ship's main electrical supply during the course of a sea action is obvious, and shipbuilders have employed a number of secondary lighting systems at various times, all of which have aimed at the constant maintenance of artificial lighting in the essential working compartments should the main lighting fail for any reason. In some cases even a tertiary emergency lighting system has been included. In the case of failure of any of the main or reserve lighting systems, it has been customary to supply all working spaces in the ship's interior with individual sources of light such as battery lamps, with electric torches added for certain individuals. As a last resort oil lamps might be employed.

Before 1939, the emergency lighting system of the compartments used by the ship's Medical Department during action, was frequently a matter for local improvisation. In some men-of-war it was left to the Senior Medical Officer to arrange what system he considered to be most suitable to medical requirements, and he was usually able to fulfil the needs of his department by arrangement with the ship's electricians. But it cannot be claimed that a system so frequently based upon personal relationships was always successful, and it happened occasionally that shortages of such items as electric battery lamps meant that the emergency lighting requirements of the Medical Department had to be subordinated to the claims of other departments in the ship, whose efficient working was considered of greater importance.

The new Fleet Order, while recommending that its terms should be adopted as much as possible in ships already in commission, emphasised that in new ships to be constructed or already under construction or reconstruction, primary and secondary lighting should form part of the permanent fittings to be included in the ship's sick bay and medical distributing stations. This instruction also applied to the dental surgery of certain ships.

It is surprising, however, that in spite of this particular directive, certain men-of-war were constructed and commissioned with sick bay and distributing stations devoid of a secondary lighting system, and senior medical officers found themselves once again dependent upon improvisation and local resources.

The reason for this state of affairs is to be found in the chain of administration and responsibility which existed around the time of the completion of a new man-of-war in a shipbuilding yard and her acceptance and commissioning by the Royal Navy.

When the keel is laid of one of H.M. Ships in a shipbuilding yard, her construction is the responsibility of the shipbuilder. An Admiralty Overseer or representative attends the shipbuilder permanently in an advisory capacity.

During the war, as the building progressed, reports were made to the Admiral Superintendent of Contract Built Ships, and, in due course, 'Key' officers were appointed to stand by during the construction of certain departments of which they would have charge when the ship was finally commissioned. Thus, the ship's senior engineering officers would be appointed early in her building programme, as would her senior electrical officers and those officers who were to take charge of her armament. At a much later date her commanding officer, executive officer, navigator, supply officer and so on would be appointed. Naturally the senior medical officer would be appointed late in the construction period. But during the whole course of her building, the construction of her living spaces, sanitation, ventilation and medical requirements were inspected from time to time by the local Naval Medical Officer of Health of the area.

It will be realised that the whole of this programme of building, fitting out, storing and progressive manning had to be effected in a manner which was consistent with the requirements of war-time security measures.

As soon as building is completed, trials are carried out at sea, and this peace-time procedure was continued under war conditions.

Her company having joined, the ship was taken to sea on a number of successive days, and her engines, technical machinery and armament were all subjected to standard trials. On completion of these trials, a conference was held between the shipbuilder and the ship's commanding officer attended by his heads of departments. At this conference each head of department would report any defects noted during trials, which would mean that they would have to be remedied by the shipbuilder and further trials carried out. But where no defects existed as a result of these acceptance trials, the commanding officer would inform the shipbuilder that his contract had been satisfactorily performed. On behalf of the Admiralty, the commanding officer would then formally accept the ship, which would then cease to be the property of the shipbuilder and would pass to the Royal Navy.

Contractually, the importance of this procedure lay in the fact that once a particular department of the ship had been accepted as satisfactory in all respects, the shipbuilder was considered to have performed his task, and he could not be called upon later to re-open his contract in order to remedy a defect which the acceptor had himself overlooked. Thus, a defect overlooked in such circumstances, if remedied by the shipbuilder, would be regarded as an 'extra' outside the terms of his contract, for which he would be entitled to charge in excess of the agreed price. Therefore, unless such a defect happened to be vital to the very existence of the ship, it was customary practice not to call upon the shipbuilder to supply the remedy. Instead, the defect was usually remedied by local improvisation on board, and this state of affairs would continue until such time as the ship became due for an official refit in dockyard hands, which would probably be many months later.

Medical emergency lighting is an example of the kind of non-vital omission which might be overlooked, the result being that the ship's medical department would have to depend upon improvised emergency lighting until such time as it became possible for a permanent lighting system to be installed during an official refit. In time of war, such a refitting period is impossible to forecast because so many factors have to be taken into account which did not exist in time of peace. Should the ship be damaged in action the damage will probably necessitate placing her in dockyard hands almost immediately. In this case, while the actual damage is being repaired, it may be possible for other defects to receive attention at the same time. On the other hand, a ship may be actively employed at sea indefinitely without ever being damaged. Her official refit may become long overdue, but shortage of shipping may be such that she must carry on as best she can until she can be spared to enter dockyard hands. Even so, her eventual refit may well be curtailed in time of war, and the priority given to her list of defects will depend upon the availability of labour and materials. In this way it is possible that a non-vital defect or omission may never be properly remedied during the whole of the ship's life.'

Where such a defect existed in the ship's medical department at the time of her acceptance, the fault probably was to be found in the administrative system which existed in the case of contract built ships. The actual senior medical officer who was to serve in the ship was unlikely to be appointed to her until such time as sufficient naval personnel had joined her as to make his presence necessary. His date of appointment depended upon the strength of the ship's company, also to some extent on the embarking of medical stores and equipment, but never did his arrival depend upon the state of construction or the fitting out of the medical department of which he was to have charge.

In ships under construction, where more than one medical officer was to be carried on commissioning, it was customary to appoint the junior medical officer to stand by the ship at a date when her sick bay was in course of completion. This procedure thus allowed for supervision of the fitting out of the ship's medical department by a medical officer. But unfortunately, the procedure proved impossible to maintain owing to the medical man-power situation, and the shortage of medical officers was so severe that it was rarely possible to appoint any medical officer to a ship under construction until virtually the last moment. The result was that the senior medical officer, on joining, was more than likely to find himself taking charge of a medical department which was presented to him as a *fait accompli*. He might well have little time in which to become acquainted with his department before the date of acceptance, and therefore defects might be overlooked. He might find also that the medical arrangements had already been certified as satisfactory by some visiting medical officer on behalf of the Admiral Superintendent of Contract Built Ships. This certification, produced by the shipbuilder at the final acceptance conference, was irrefutable. This meant that the medical officer would be required to take charge of and organise the running of a medical department without ever having had the opportunity of supervising or expressing an opinion on its construction and fittings.

Another matter which received attention in the new Fleet Order was the adequacy of the fresh water supply for medical requirements in action.

Mention has already been made in this History that, in a man-of-war, fresh water is at a premium. Also, the fresh water supply which does exist may be quickly interrupted should the ship receive damage.

The Fleet Order emphasised the supreme importance of providing an ample supply of water for wounded persons, such as the insistence of siting dressing stations in positions where fresh water would be readily obtainable. The need was also visualised of fresh water for drinking and for surgical uses. It was recommended that water bottles should be worn, not only by members of medical parties, but also by a proportion of the fighting personnel of the ship.

In view of possible damage to the ship's fresh water mains, it was recommended that should enemy action be imminent, a supply of fresh water should be stored in baths, wash basins and other receptacles in and around the distributing stations and first-aid posts. It is of some interest in this respect, that some medical officers of experience habitually kept one or more baths filled with very hot water, into which they would immerse any survivor taken from the sea, as a rapid method of aiding his recovery after exposure or immersion.

A separate section of the 1942 Fleet Order took the important step of directing that a scheme of medical organisation for action, based on the principles in the Order, was to be prepared for all ships, including the allocation of spaces as distributing stations and first-aid posts, together with a statement of the additional fittings required.

In the case of ships under construction or reconstruction, the scheme was to be prepared by the ship's officers, in consultation with a representative of the Medical Director-General, as soon as possible after the appointment of the ship's executive officer, detailed proposals being submitted.

In the case of ships in commission the scheme was to be prepared by the ship's officers, existing facilities being developed and additional stores demanded as necessary. Work involved was, as far as possible, to be carried out by ship's staff. Should dockyard work be involved, items were to be inserted in the ship's list of alterations and additions, but such work was to be kept to a minimum.

In the light of what has been stated above, it is of some interest to study the efficacy of the schemes which were prepared, and to compare the results in ships under construction or reconstruction and ships already in commission.

Obviously the terms of the Order stood a much better chance of being met in full in ships under construction or reconstruction, because the necessary additional fittings could be added while the ship was actually in the hands of the builder. It was merely a case of the ship's officers being required to prepare a scheme of detailed proposals, in consultation with a representative of the Medical Director-General, as soon as possible after the appointment of the ship's executive officer. But this system pre-supposed that there would be no flaw in the administrative chain.

On the other hand, in the case of ships in commission, although there was not the advantage of drawing up a scheme while the ship was still in the hands of a shipbuilder, the chain of administration was much shorter and more simple. In short, in the case of a ship in commission, her own medical officer was already on board and able to assist in preparing the necessary scheme of proposals. Moreover, his presence gave the added advantage that he was able to supervise the development of these proposals, and was always in a position to make sure that they were implemented in due course and that nothing was overlooked.

The Fleet Order made a number of other recommendations in respect of distributing stations and first-aid posts, particularly as regards permanent fittings and medical stores and equipment.

In the case of a main distributing station, it was stated that the compartment allocated should, where possible, be of a size to provide 120 sq. ft. of floor space for the operating table and its immediate surroundings, and 120 sq. ft. for working and stowage space. Provision was also to be made for seating accommodation for 2 per cent. and slinging accommodation for 2 per cent. of the ship's full complement.

In the case of the first-aid posts, it was stated that the approaches to these centres should be conspicuously marked in a uniform manner with the words 'First-Aid Post', and that a red cross with a directing arrow should point the way.

In order to ensure the minimum of obstruction in the compartment, the locker in a first-aid post was to be of a long narrow shape, and placed vertically against an inboard bulkhead. This locker was to be constructed of metal, and provided with several shelves, and raised on a sanitary base. In order to prevent the locker being opened and used for any other purpose by unauthorised persons, it was to be marked with a red cross and closed by a breakable seal. It was also to bear the words 'First-Aid Stores for use in Action Only'.

But these cautionary words and the presence of a breakable seal did not always prove to be an adequate barrier against plundering tendencies. It was perhaps asking too much to expect a sailor, who happened to cut himself shaving, to go all the way to the sick bay for a piece of cotton wool or adhesive plaster when a supply was ready to hand in a locker alongside him in his wash place! Lockers were repeatedly raided by guns' crews who took cotton wool to plug up their ears. The 'medical comforts' contained in the lockers also proved to be a constant temptation. It was the custom for the contents of first-aid lockers to be inspected once a week, and gradually 'turned over' in order to avoid deterioration and waste. But it was frequently found that replenishments were necessary as well, to make up for what had been plundered during the week before.

In due course, a device was adopted in many ships of ignoring the breakable seal, and instead, the locker was closed with an ordinary lock and key. This key was then exposed alongside the locker in a glass container, which had to be smashed before the key could be obtained. A duplicate key was kept by a medical officer for the purpose of opening the locker for inspection as he wished. This device was found to be a more effective precaution against intrusion by unauthorised persons.

For use in action, medical officers were permitted to exercise their own discretion in equipping the lockers from service afloat stores. The Fleet Order recommended the following as suitable contents:

Adhesive plaster.
Bandages, 1 in., 2 in., 3 in.
Bandages, triangular.
Absorbent cotton wool.
Gauze.
Lint.
Safety pins.
Antiseptics.
Methylated spirit.
Morphia, hypodermic solution in 1 oz. rubber-capped bottles.
Morphine, lamellae.
Splints.
Scissors.
Scalpel.
Dressing and rotary forceps.
Anti-burn jelly.
Tourniquets, and length of rubber tubing for spare tourniquets.
First field dressings, and shell dressings.
Sterile swabs, to be replenished frequently.
Ligatures, sutures, needles.
Identification labels.
Paper and pencil.
Electric torch.
Medical comforts.
Blankets.
Hot-water bottles, goose necks, bowls, cups and buckets.

Medical officers in general were quick to avail themselves of the discretion which they were allowed in storing and equipping these first-aid lockers. It was necessary too, to study the policy of the commanding officer and other heads of departments as regards their contents. For example, the views of the department responsible for damage control and fire precautions would have to be considered before placing inflammable liquids and materials in parts of the ship where they might constitute a risk.

In particular, the storage of poisons and dangerous drugs in a number of places around a man-of-war was a matter which would call for the approval of the commanding officer for whom it was a serious responsibility, because such a procedure had the effect of altering the provisions of King's Regulations and Admiralty Instructions regarding the precautions to be observed in the care of poisons and dangerous drugs. Some commanding officers would not permit morphia to be stored in first-aid lockers, and many medical officers felt that it was more acceptable, and more advisable, that supplies of morphia for use in action should be distributed to trained individuals who would be held responsible for accounting for the drug.

The Fleet Order made a large number of other miscellaneous provisions regarding medical organisation for action. For example, in circumstances where it should become necessary to use an emergency position for the treatment of casualties after action, both distributing stations having been damaged, the necessary medical stores and equipment would be required. It was therefore recommended that, apart from stores which might be salved from the damaged distributing stations, a certain amount of surgical gear in the nature of a mobile unit should always be earmarked for the purpose of equipping such an emergency position. The stores and equipment earmarked should include one or more of the emergency dressing cases, and a valise of surgical instruments.

A general directive emphasised the importance of the adequate distribution of all medical stores throughout the ship, particularly in destroyers. As a further precaution it was arranged that a percentage of the breakable stores supplied for medical purposes would be constructed of bakelite or similar material.

The 1942 Fleet Order ended with a list of permanent fittings which were considered desirable.

List of Permanent Fittings. At 'First Degree of Readiness' items marked * are transferred from sick bay or dental surgery to distributing stations:

Main Distributing Station
  Deck fittings and stowage for operating table.*
  Bench seating, fixed, or hinged (if insufficient room), for wounded.
  Position for X-ray plant.*
  Hot and cold water supply.
  Hammock or stretcher billets in, and adjacent to main distributing station. (In some ships it may be possible to arrange tiered bunking if desired.)
  Hinged table for instruments, etc.
  Cupboards or lockers for surgical dressings and comforts. (In a compartment of irregular shape it may be more convenient to build in cupboards to fit rather than to use a general standard size locker.)
  Rod and curtains to screen cases undergoing treatment.
  Folding lavatory or wash basin fixture.
  Portable latrine. (Elsan closets.)
  Sanitary bins or buckets.
  Lighting, primary and secondary.
  Overhead light fitting for operating table.
  Brackets with non-slip edges for steriliser* and kettle.*
  Sockets for X-ray plant, steriliser and kettle.
  Telephone.
  Ventilation.

Auxiliary Distributing Station
　Deck fitting for operating table.
　Bench seating, if not already provided.
　Hammock or stretcher billets in and adjacent to the station, if not already provided.
　Table, fixed or hinged, if not already provided.
　Cupboards or lockers for surgical dressings and comforts.
　Hot and cold water supply.
　Folding lavatory.
　Portable latrine.
　Sanitary bins or buckets.
　Lighting, primary and secondary.
　Sockets for additional operating lighting.
　Sockets and hinged brackets for steriliser* and kettle.*
　Telephone.
　Ventilation.

First-Aid Posts
　Table and seating (hinged).
　Hot and cold water supply.
　Ready use stowage for Neil-Robertson and other stretchers, and reserve blankets.
　Cupboard or lockers for dressings, etc.

(ii)
The Daily Journal of a Medical Officer Afloat

A record of the day to day problems, reactions, fears and foibles of the average naval medical officer on active service at sea.

As has been outlined, by the middle of 1942, the medical organisation for action afloat had undergone many changes in consequence of those features of war at sea which had not been visualised in time of peace. Far from complaining about monotony, most medical officers afloat found that their commitments continued to increase month after month as the war progressed.

In order to give the reader some idea of these medical commitments in a man-of-war, and also, with a view to preserving for posterity some record of the day to day life of a naval medical officer afloat at this period of the Second World War, the following extracts are set down as being typical of the notes made by a senior medical officer in his daily journal. The notes in question cover a period of some months and these daily 'jottings' were made for incorporation, each quarter, in the Medical Officer's Official Journal, one of many thousands which have been perused for the purpose of compiling the Naval Medical History of the War. The notes themselves are of great value historically, and, including as they do, references to many of the personal problems of this doctor, go far towards refuting the suggestion that a naval medical officer afloat, in time of war, suffers from lack of employment.

The notes, which are chronological, commence towards the end of May 1942, a fortnight after the medical officer had joined a newly constructed man-of-war in a shipbuilder's yard in Scotland:

DAILY JOURNAL

THURSDAY, MAY 28

Ship commissioned at Greenock at 1200 hours. A strenuous 14 days has achieved a reasonable state of organisation in the ship's medical department, though much remains yet to be done.

Action Organisation
  (1) Stores to distribute in first-aid posts.
  (2) Lockers to be sealed.
  (3) Haversacks to be stocked.
  (4) First-aid boxes to be stocked.
  (5) First-aid personnel to be trained.
  (6) Stretchers to be distributed.
  (7) 'Abandon Ship' requirements.
  (8) Copies of Medical Orders for Notice Boards.

Stores and Equipment
  (1) Stores unpacked, packing cases passed to Senior Naval Stores Officer, and acceptance indicated by signal.
      R.N.H., Haslar, informed by letter.
  (2) Final medical store demands awaited from Medical Depot, Dunfermline, as arranged by telephone.
  (3) Medical stationery demanded.
  (4) Rotary converter for X-ray machine smashed in transit and returned. Admiralty informed, and replacement demanded by signal. Signal acknowledged and replacement approved.

Sick Bay
Daily routine provisionally arranged, but unsatisfactory at present.
N.B. Situation and space for C.D.A.* Mess to be reconsidered, owing to lack of slinging billets.

---

* 'C.D.A.' is the Navy's customary way of referring to venereal diseases. The custom has its origin in the Contagious Diseases Acts of 1864 to 1882. The term is used in many senses in relation to venereal diseases in the Senior Service; e.g., a 'C.D.A. Mess' refers to the quarters in which venereal cases are accommodated, 'C.D.A. List' refers to the list of names of men in the ship suffering from venereal disease at the moment, etc.

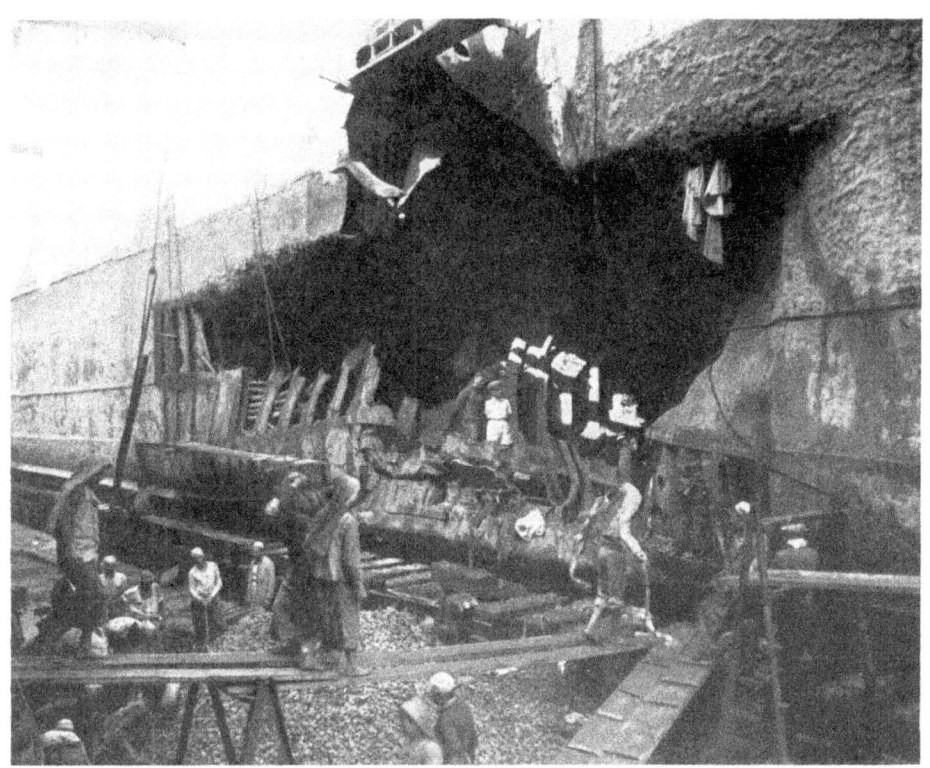

PLATE II. The Damaged Hospital Ship *Somersetshire* in floating dock.

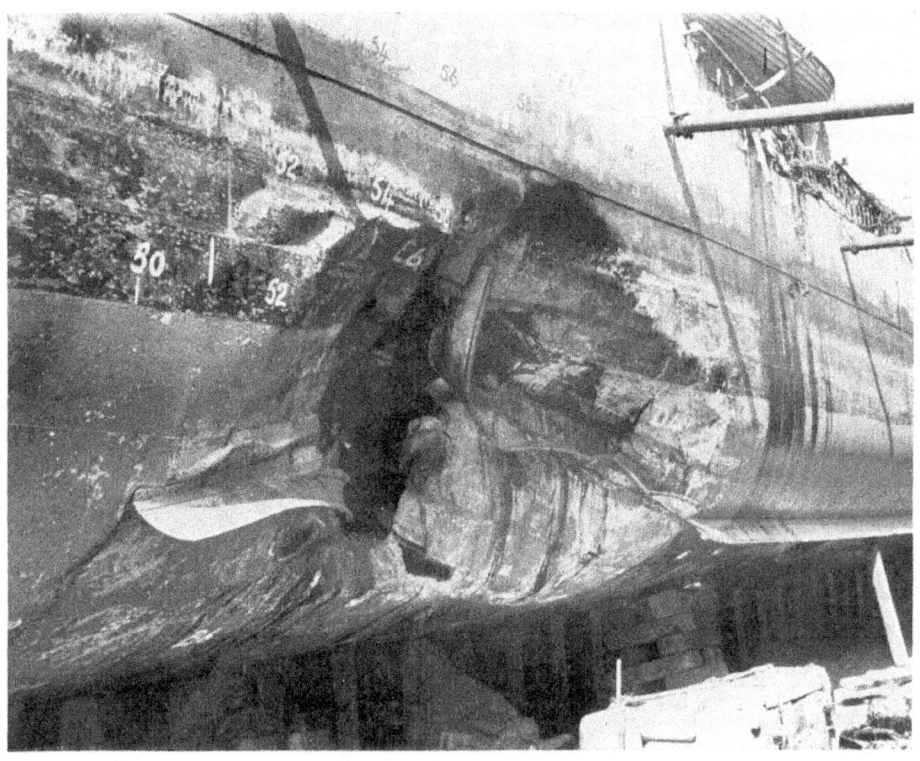

PLATE III. Damage to H.M.S. *Quorn*, a destroyer of the Hunt Class.

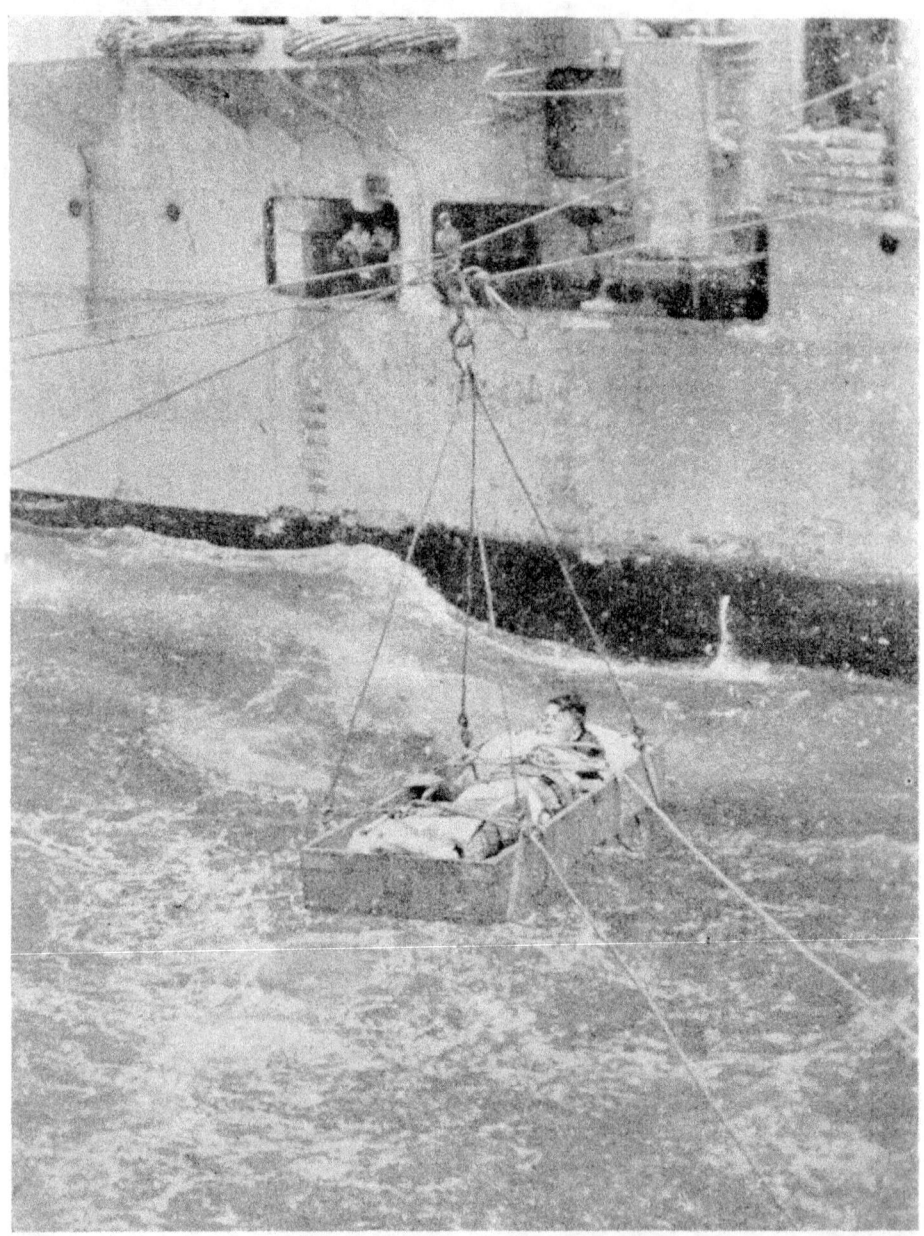

PLATE IV. A casualty being transferred from an aircraft carrier to a destroyer during rough weather in the Pacific, to be taken to a hospital ship.

Immediate Care of Ship's Company
  (1) Daily inspection by Messes.
  (2) Inoculations.
  (3) Vaccinations.
  (4) V.D. continuous treatment cases.
  (5) Study of available Medical History Sheets.
  (6) Health lectures to arrange.

Miscellaneous
  (1) Muster tubular type stretchers and arrange greasing.
  (2) Demand Medical Library from R.N.H., Haslar.
  (3) Instruct Surgeon Lieutenant in record keeping.
  (4) Sick Mess Account.
  (5) Study recent Fleet Orders.
  (6) Study details of water purifier and disinfector.

N.B. (i) Surgeon Lieutenant and self for inoculation.
   (ii) Personal bed linen.
   (iii) Make Will.

Friday, May 29
Ship left Greenock and anchored 'Tail of the Bank' at 1030 hours.

Medical State

Sick	Nil
Excused duty	2
Light duty	Nil
C.D.A.	1

(Acute Gonorrhoea, contracted Portsmouth 4 days before commissioning).

Action Organisation
  (1) Conducted Surgeon Lieutenant round first-aid posts, and instructed him to arrange completion of painting, distribution of instruments, and storing of first-aid boxes. Each to contain iodine, bandages, field dressings, and rubber tourniquet.

N.B. 20 yards rubber tubing demanded from Supply Officer for making tourniquets.
  (2) At 1330 hours talked to men selected for advanced first-aid duties.

Miscellaneous
  (1) Minor injury (Marine, crushed fingers).
  (2) 2100 hours, censored mail for $2\frac{1}{2}$ hours.

SATURDAY, MAY 30
Ship at 'Tail of the Bank', ammunitioning all day.

Medical State

Sick	Nil
Excused duty	3
Light duty	Nil
C.D.A.	2 (both Gonorrhoea)

Action Organisation
(1) Approved Surgeon Lieutenant's proposed distribution of medical stores, and all first-aid boxes and lockers should be stored and sealed within 5 days from now.
(2) Medical Action Organisation typed and delivered to Captain.

Sick Bay
Inspected ledgers and commencement of records.

Miscellaneous
(1) Minor injury (Marine, crushed tooth while ammunitioning. Hurt Certificate to be granted. Emergency treatment by dental officer in *Nelson*).
(2) Interviewed 2 ratings regarding accidental breaches of censorship regulations.

SUNDAY, MAY 31

Ship at 'Tail of the Bank' ammunitioning all day.

Medical State

Sick	Nil
Excused duty	3
Light duty	1
C.D.A.	2

Fresh Water
At 0900 hours water boat arrived alongside, and 40 tons fresh water received. Engineers intended to use water purifiers, but unfortunately the machines could not be employed as there was a fault in the electric equipment, no chlorotex outfit, and no supply of ammonium sulphate. Arranged to charge solution tanks of purifiers before next water boat, and problematical standard flow forecast as 60 tons per hour. Rate of flow to be controlled by testing samples during pumping.

Shore water supply certified as already chlorinated, but found this was not so on testing drinking tanks. Spent rest of forenoon supervising chlorination of main tanks by hand.

Miscellaneous
(1) Elected to Mess Committee.
(2) Meeting of all officers in Captain's cabin at 1600 hours.
(3) 2100 hours, censored mail 3 hours.

MONDAY, JUNE 1

Ship at 'Tail of the Bank', still ammunitioning.

Medical State

Sick	1 (Tonsillitis)
Excused duty	1
Light duty	2
C.D.A.	2

Action Organisation

Practised 'Action Stations' at 0900 hours. Consisted mostly of placing first-aid parties in their right places. 'Abandon Ship Stations' at 1000 hours, carried out in pelting rain.

N.B. Disturbed to find secondary lighting inadequate in the Auxiliary Medical Distributing Station, and completely absent in the Main Medical Distributing Station. Apparently this is no longer a shipbuilder's responsibility, as the medical fittings were certified as adequate by an Inspecting Medical Officer some weeks ago. Am informed by the electricians on board that there are no portable battery lights to be spared for the Medical Department. Have ordered a supply of candles to be stowed in all first-aid posts.

Miscellaneous

(1) S.B.C.P.O. (Sick Berth Chief Petty Officer) reports only one set of keys on board for sick bay and dental departments. Have ordered spare sets.

(2) Distribution of stores by Surgeon Lieutenant continues satisfactorily.

(3) One case of Scabies at 1315 hours. Mess inspected at 1400 hours. Disinfection routine effected.

(4) Ammonium sulphate not yet arrived.

(5) Discussed medical examination of whole ship's company with Captain, who states that there is no time to spare at present for this purpose.

(6) Arranged for neuro-psychiatrist at Southern General Hospital, Glasgow, to examine one officer who is a survivor following his ship sinking only three months ago.

(7) Have arranged to sleep in the sick bay office when the ship is at sea.

From June 2 to 18, the ship remained at the 'Tail of the Bank' while the distribution of equipment and the organisation of the Medical Department continued.

Routine duties were interspersed with periods of trials and training, both in harbour and at sea.

Instruction in rendering first aid and action exercises in varying circumstances were carried out daily. The ship then joined the Fleet at Scapa Flow and the daily journal continues:

FRIDAY, JUNE 19

Ship arrived at Scapa Flow at 1300 hours.

Medical State

Sick	5
Excused duty	5
Light duty	4
C.D.A.	4

Heavy swell during the night, and about 50 per cent. of ship's company very seasick.

Action Organisation
   (1) Night action exercises from 0030 till 0430 hours, effected with some difficulty owing to rolling of ship and seasickness. Nevertheless excellent practice.
   (2) Concentrated mainly on traffic of first-aid parties to first-aid posts and distributing stations.
   (3) Tested out sick berth staff's and Surgeon Lieutenant's knowledge of whereabouts on board in the dark. Found them all literally very much 'at sea', and also very sorry for themselves owing to their seasickness.
   (4) Future programme for first-aid instruction arranged with Commander:
A. Indirect instruction for whole ship's company as part of the seamanship competition, for which prizes are to be awarded.
B. Direct instruction.
   (a) One hour's instruction daily to all guns' crews for 3 days.
   (b) Similar instruction for all engine room ratings.
   (c) One hour's instruction each evening for regular first-aid parties who will also attend the instructional periods of guns' crews and engine room ratings.

Miscellaneous
   (1) Signalled *Victorious* for dental appointments.
   (2) Signalled *Iron Duke* for ophthalmic appointments.
   (3) Sent postman to Flagship to inquire about mails, and to get copies of Scapa Flow General Orders.
   (4) Arranged for mail to close on board at 2000 hours daily while at Scapa Flow, and to be collected by drifter at 0920 hours daily.
   (5) 2100 hours censored mail 3 hours.

SATURDAY, JUNE 20

Ship at Scapa Flow. Weather dull, light rain and mist.

Medical State

Sick	5
Excused duty	5
Light duty	4
C.D.A.	4

Captain's rounds at 1030 hours, and he was impressed with the cleanliness of the medical department.

N.B. I have warned sick berth staff since, that the Captain's satisfaction is no excuse for any possible slackening of their present standard!

Miscellaneous

(1) Ophthalmic appointment for 1 rating in *Iron Duke* at 1000 hours Monday.

(2) Five dental appointments at 1000 hours Sunday in *Victorious*.

N.B. Very tired, and fell asleep during the afternoon. S.M.O., *Curacoa*, came to dinner at 1900 hours. Quite a merry evening.

SUNDAY, JUNE 21

Ship at Scapa Flow. Weather dull and foggy.

Medical State

Sick	5
Excused duty	7
Light duty	3
C.D.A.	4

Divisions at 0915 hours. Church to follow. At 1100 hours visited Flagship and called on Fleet Medical Officer and Fleet Dental Surgeon. Was instructed by F.M.O. that chlorination of water should be by purifier whenever possible. Fleet Dental Surgeon discussed difficulties in arranging regular dental treatment for ships of the Fleet. Returned on board at 1230 hours and got very wet on the way.

N.B. Procedure for discharging patients to hospital ships at Scapa Flow:

(1) Routine cases, signal to hospital ship, and repeat to drifter office and Admiral Commanding Orkneys and Shetlands.

(2) Urgent cases signal hospital ship.

2100 hours censored mail $2\frac{1}{2}$ hours, and studied Scapa Flow General Orders regarding dispatch of telegrams.

MONDAY, JUNE 22

Ship at Scapa Flow. Heavy rain all day.

Medical State

Sick	5
Excused duty	5
Light duty	1
C.D.A.	2

Action Organisation
 (1) Omnopon tubules now ready for distribution.
 (2) Surgeon Lieutenant instructed first-aid parties almost continuously during the day.

Miscellaneous
 (1) Stoker alleged to have miner's nystagmus sent to *Iron Duke* for ophthalmic examination.
 (2) Further signals made for dental appointments with *Kent* and *Victorious*.
 (3) Long discussion with Commander (E) on the subject of fresh water purification and the delegation of responsibility.
 (4) 1600 hours mustered wine stock with navigating officer.
 (5) 2100 hours censored mail 3 hours.

TUESDAY, JUNE 23

Ship at Scapa Flow. Weather slightly improved.

Medical State

Sick	6
Excused duty	5
Light duty	1
C.D.A.	2

Action Organisation
 (1) Captain has issued a standing order regarding the distribution and care of tubunic ampoules of omnopon, and has ordered that the supply shall be mustered and checked every 14 days.
 (2) Surgeon Lieutenant instructed first-aid parties 1400 to 1600 hours.

Miscellaneous
 (1) *Victorious* has arranged dental appointments for 6 officers for Friday next. *Kent* sailed at 0700 hours today. Have therefore signalled *Cumberland* for further dental appointments. Reply received arranging 6 appointments for Friday next.
 (2) Ophthalmic report on stoker states that his alleged nystagmus is voluntary, and that he is considered fit for all duties.
 (3) Another stoker reported at 1130 hours with acute blepharospasm. Considered condition to be acute hysteria, especially as he has recently been granted compassionate leave on account of domestic trouble. Returned him to duty, and discussed the case at length with the Senior Engineer and Commander (E).
 (4) Studied the ship's ventilation with 1st Lieutenant.
 (5) Commenced making a list of officers due for inoculation and vaccination.

(6) Spent 1 hour with S.P.C.P.O., scrutinising Medical History Sheets.

N.B. Most of the ship's company have been painting ship all day. At 1330 hours, all available officers were required to form a painting party, in fancy dress. I wore my old opera hat, and the Padre an old mortarboard. We were given a part of the forward screen to paint. I thought we made a very poor job of it, and felt that the regular ship's painters were very tolerant, considering that they had to do the job again later. Nevertheless, the effect on morale was probably extremely good.

(7) 2100 hours censored mail 3 hours.

From June 24 to August 30 the ship remained at Scapa Flow and continued training and action exercises in harbour and patrolling at sea as a unit of the Tenth Cruiser Squadron. Meanwhile, the Surgeon Lieutenant had been sent to hospital ashore. On August 31 the ship was detailed for duty with a convoy and the journal describes the daily work of the medical department on such duties:

MONDAY, AUGUST 31

Ship at Scapa Flow. Weather very rainy.

Medical State

Sick	1
Excused duty	4
Light duty	1
C.D.A.	1

Miscellaneous
(1) Sick bay visit at 0800 hours.
(2) Omnopon mustered and found correct.
(3) Informed by Commander, on authority of Captain, that owing to ship's movements, 240 second dose inoculations cannot be carried out at present.
(4) Understand that in future, mess traps, i.e., plates, mugs, etc., for feeding personnel while at action stations, will be stored in the mail office and issued from there as required. Am anxious about this, as I have the responsibility for safe custody of mail to consider. Commander is arranging for key of mail office to be held by a responsible person during action.

N.B. Confidential meeting between Captain and all heads of departments at 1015 hours. It would appear that an operation is impending, in which we shall be involved. In view of this, the absence of a Surgeon Lieutenant is now a most serious matter. Captain signalled Commander-in-Chief for immediate temporary Surgeon Lieutenant to be provided. 2100 hours censored mail 4 hours.

N.B. Surgeon Lieutenant on loan arrived on board at midnight.

TUESDAY, SEPTEMBER 1

Ship sailed at 0830 hours. Arrived Loch Ewe at 1530 hours. Weather fine and mild.

Medical State

Sick	3
Excused duty	4
Light duty	Nil
C.D.A.	1

N.B. Spent most of day conducting Surgeon Lieutenant round the ship, and explaining medical organisation for action to him. He seems a very nice lad, and quietly efficient, but very inexperienced, as this is his first time afloat. 2100 hours censored mail 3 hours.

WEDNESDAY, SEPTEMBER 2

Ship at Loch Ewe. Weather fine but windy.

Medical State

Sick	3
Excused duty	1
Light duty	Nil
C.D.A.	1

Action Organisation

(1) Spent whole day instructing Surgeon Lieutenant again.
(2) Tested proposed anti-flash goggles, and found them fairly safe as regards fire.

N.B. Mail received, including letter for stoker who alleged that money order sent to his wife had not been received. Fortunately today's letter from his wife confirms that she has now received it. 2100 hours censored mail 3 hours.

N.B. I note we now have on board a number of strangers, including a Reuter's correspondent and a Gaumont British cameraman.

THURSDAY, SEPTEMBER 3 (14 weeks in commission)

Ship sailed as convoy escort at 0130 hours. Weather extremely rough.

Medical State

Sick	3
Excused duty	1
Light duty	Nil
C.D.A.	1

Very rough night, and a lot of seasickness. Ship's company at night action stations from 0230 hours, after convoy altered course to avoid U-boat alleged to be some 10 miles ahead.

N.B. At 1100 hours Padre broadcast an excellent short Service for 15 minutes, today being the anniversary of the outbreak of the Second World War.

FRIDAY, SEPTEMBER 4

Ship at sea. Weather less rough, but colder.

Medical State

Sick	3
Excused duty	3
Light duty	Nil
C.D.A.	1

Night much calmer, but two alterations of course on account of alleged U-boats.

Action Organisation
(1) Inspected all first-aid boxes and lockers.
(2) Arranged distribution of hot water bottles.
(3) Conducted Surgeon Lieutenant and sick berth staff through most parts of the ship during the day.

N.B. S.B.C.P.O., in conjunction with Canteen Manager and the engine room staff, has had 8 biscuit tins cut down and converted into very good improvised bed pans.

N.B. A rating who recently stated a grievance to the Captain, now reports that he is unfit for duty, having contrived to lose his dentures over the side while being seasick! In the circumstances, I advised him to return to work, and have arranged for him to attend the sick bay for a suitable diet, to include cubes of Oxo for him to chew! I think he thought that it might be possible for him to be landed at our next port of call. There seems to be a legend among the ship's company that a toothless man is not fit for service afloat!

SATURDAY, SEPTEMBER 5

Ship entered harbour at 0900 hours, sailed again at 1100 hours. Weather unsettled, cold very noticeable.

Medical State

Sick	2 (1 stoker with infection of face which might become formidable)
Excused duty	3
Light duty	Nil
C.D.A.	1

Ship's company at second degree of readiness all day.

SUNDAY, SEPTEMBER 6

Ship entered harbour at 0730 hours. Weather much colder during the night, with snow storm around 0130 hours. Sunny and calm today.

Medical State

Sick	3
Excused duty	3
Light duty	Nil
C.D.A.	1

No Sunday divisions. Church at 1015 hours, but was interrupted after 5 minutes by a short sharp air attack by a single Focke Wulfe. By the time we were at first degree of readiness, the aircraft had dropped its bombs and departed. Slight damage ashore only. Further attack by three aircraft at 1400 hours, with similar results.

Miscellaneous
(1) Medical Officer from destroyer called at 1500 hours, and asked advice about a rating who has an attack of hysteria since the air attacks. He wanted to transfer him to us, but I refused.
(2) 4 medical officers from destroyers called on me at various times, and discussed a number of their difficulties. 2100 hours censored mail and landed it at 2330 hours. Incoming mail also arrived at 2400 hours, which speaks well for our organisation. Aurora borealis very clear last night.

MONDAY, SEPTEMBER 7

Ship in harbour. Sailed at 2000 hours. Weather sunny and quite warm in the absence of wind. Much ice and snow ashore. Aurora borealis very distinct again last night.

Medical State

Sick	3
Excused duty	Nil
Light duty	1
C.D.A.	1

N.B. Lunched with Flag Officer and Captain. Both attended performance by ship's concert party between 1600 and 1730 hours.

TUESDAY, SEPTEMBER 8

Ship at sea. Weather foggy, very damp and cold.

Medical State

Sick	3
Excused duty	1
Light duty	1
C.D.A.	1

Spent most of night and whole day patrolling to and fro off harbour entrance. Very monotonous. Played bridge with Flag Officer and two of his staff after supper.

WEDNESDAY, SEPTEMBER 9

Ship at sea, in company with one carrier and several destroyers escorting convoy of merchantmen. Crossed Arctic Circle at 0500 hours. Weather flat calm, brilliant sunshine.

Medical State

Sick	2
Excused duty	1
Light duty	1
C.D.A.	2 (1 case ex-destroyer, for accommodation only)

N.B. Shadowed by one Focke Wulfe early today, but were protected by thick fog for an hour at 1100 hours. 1300 hours alteration of course to avoid U-boats. This brought wind dead ahead, with a most alarming drop in temperature within a few minutes. 1400 hours further alteration of course owing to U-boats. One U-boat attacked by destroyer with depth charges. Result unknown. 1800 hours very much colder. Now being shadowed by two Focke Wulfes.

N.B. Saw a 'white rainbow' today. Looked like a rainbow, but was not coloured. Understand from navigating officer that this is due to the fact that the particles of water in the atmosphere are very minute. The smaller the particles apparently, the lighter the colours of the rainbow. Night very short, about 2 to 3 hours, and almost negatived last night by aurora borealis.

THURSDAY, SEPTEMBER 10 (15 weeks in commission)

Ship at sea in convoy. Weather increasingly cold, squally with showers of sleet.

Medical State

Sick	4
Excused duty	Nil
Light duty	1
C.D.A.	2

N.B. At 1700 hours one destroyer attacked a U-boat and destroyed it. Large amount of oil on surface, and miscellaneous wreckage including green vegetables. No sign of survivors. Shadowed by Focke Wulfes most of the day. Thick fog towards evening and was forced to put on an extra pair of long pants.

FRIDAY, SEPTEMBER 11

Ship at sea in convoy. Weather foggy, calm, visibility poor. Very much warmer.

Medical State

Sick	4
Excused duty	Nil
Light duty	1
C.D.A.	2

N.B. One rating has been sick for 4 days with what appeared to be phlebitis. A single vein appeared to be affected above his right ankle. Today a small black speck appeared at the bottom of the painful area. I made a small nick with a needle, and withdrew what appeared to be a strand of horse hair about $3\frac{1}{2}$ inches long. The patient has no knowledge how it came to be there!

N.B. During the forenoon, one of the 'lookouts' was found drowsing at his post. He was promptly charged by his P.O., and as promptly stated that his eyesight was defective. This cannot be disproved without a specialist opinion, therefore he must be relieved from lookout duties and his case postponed for the time being.

N.B. During last night first degree of readiness was not relaxed at any time, owing to a report that German surface craft are believed to be on the move.

SATURDAY, SEPTEMBER 12

Ship at sea in convoy. Weather calm, but very cold indeed. A certain amount of pack ice about after 1800 hours.

Medical State

Sick	3
Excused duty	Nil
Light duty	1
C.D.A.	2

Action Organisation

Discussed whole organisation with Surgeon Lieutenant and sick berth staff.

N.B. The ship's blacksmith has manufactured us two magnificent bed-pans made of steel. Far larger and more durable than the small china type usually supplied. Not the least of its advantages is that it is large enough to be used by the average sick sailor in comfort!

N.B. Find the inside of my nose and throat very dry, and my skin a bit rough and liable to bleed if rubbed. Have started taking Vitamin 'C' tablets, as it is now some time since we had fresh vegetables or fruit.

*SUNDAY SEPTEMBER 13

Entered harbour at 0100 hours in order to fuel from oilers. Sailed at 0400 hours.

Medical State
                    Unchanged.

When we entered harbour it was quite light, and the surroundings were very beautiful but solitary. Mountains, snow, glaciers and pack ice gave the appearance of a gigantic sugar cake. Weather suddenly terribly cold. Padre broadcast a short service at 0700 hours. Ship's company at first degree of readiness even while in harbour. All guns in action at 0900 hours with a Heinkel 111, and immediately afterwards with two Ju 88's.

N.B. Two merchantmen of convoy were sunk by U-boats during the night. Have had no news of survivors.

N.B. At 1400 hours we rejoined convoy at high speed while it was being heavily attacked by high level bombers. We joined in with all guns firing, but with little success, I think, by either side. The noise was extremely unpleasant, but everybody seemed to stand up to it pretty well. About half an hour later we were heavily attacked by a very large number of torpedo bombers, which were fairly successful. I watched the attack from the back of the bridge, and they approached the convoy in line ahead along the starboard horizon. When level with the convoy they all turned towards it, and attacked in line abreast. Each aircraft flew low over the water, and as the torpedoes were launched, each flew down the whole length of the convoy firing its armament. There is no doubt that the attack was carried out with magnificent courage and precision, and in the face of tremendous gunfire from the whole convoy and its escort. The tanker in the next line abreast of us was hit early on by a torpedo from an aircraft which finished its run-in just above the tanker's funnel. At that second the whole tanker and aircraft were enveloped in a crimson wall of flame which seemed to roll over and over up into the sky until it dissolved

---

* The operation here described is the passage of Convoy P.Q.18 to North Russia, consisting of 40 merchant ships escorted by a naval escort of 16 destroyers led by an A/A cruiser, and accompanied by an escort carrier with 12 fighters and 3 anti-submarine aircraft. The Germans made no attempt on this convoy with surface ships, but aircraft and submarines were formidable. On September 13 approximately 60 enemy torpedo aircraft were in use, of which 13 were destroyed, but they accounted for 8 ships of the convoy. In the words of the official account, they approached in line abreast, like 'a large flight of nightmare locusts', flying 30 or 40 feet above the water, and keeping such good station 100 to 150 yards apart that it was impossible to break them up.

On the next day, however, out of 45 to 50 torpedo aircraft employed, 20 were destroyed, and only one ship was sunk by them.

Convoy P.Q.18 lost 13 of its 40 ships, 10 being sunk by aircraft attacks and 3 by U-boats.

into a vast cloud of black smoke. When I looked down at the sea again, apart from a small occasional flicker of flame on the water, there was no sign of either the tanker or the aircraft, and I realised that they had both blown up. No evidence of any survivors. I also noticed a ship sinking far astern of the convoy. I believe there were others but I did not see them myself. Some of the enemy must have had casualties as well, and we passed very close to a German aircraft with its tail and swastika afloat with two of its crew standing on the debris, but it soon seemed to sink and they disappeared quite quickly.

N.B. After 1600 hours the sky was clear, and we were able to take stock a little. The ship was near-missed several times, but there seems to be no obvious damage and no casualties. I replied to two signals received from merchantmen asking for medical advice. One stated that her master had been hit in the spine and was dying. Spoke to the Captain regarding the possibility of taking them on board, but he was most emphatic in his refusal. At 1730 hours a corvette came alongside and transferred to us some 80 survivors from various merchant ships, including a small number of casualties. The seamanship displayed by both ships, steaming at 12 knots, was excellent, and fortunately the sea was completely calm and free from ice. Most of the survivors were able to jump across on to our deck, while the remainder were man-handled aboard. All the casualties were passed across in Neil-Robertson stretchers, and the Surgeon Lieutenant in the corvette seemed to have done his job well. The organisation for receiving these casualties and survivors on board worked extremely well. Only quite a small number had actually been in the sea, and none had been greatly affected either by oil fuel or exposure. The supply department was able to provide hot soup, clothing and blankets for everybody almost at once.*

N.B. While sorting them out, the convoy was again attacked by a small force of torpedo bombers, but no ship was hit, and I distinctly saw one aircraft pass down our starboard side in flames and later crash into the sea.

N.B. With the exception of three, the casualties boiled down to very little. Of the three, one had fractured a number of ribs, a second had a simple fracture of tibia and fibula, but the third was in a very poor state.

This third man was a naval rating forming part of a short range weapon's crew in a merchant ship. One of the difficulties in dealing with low flying torpedo bombers is that ships in convoy must depress their weapons to a degree which is likely to put neighbouring ships in danger of being hit, but I understand that this is regarded as an acceptable risk. In this case, the magazine of the weapon which this seaman

---

* Plates IV–VII illustrate some of the methods used in transferring casualties from one ship to another at sea.

was firing was apparently hit by a bullet fired from a neighbouring ship, or possibly from an attacking aircraft. In any case the magazine exploded and the man was badly wounded by his own ammunition. Initially he was so shocked that it was impossible to examine him more than superficially. We placed him in a lower cot, and the Surgeon Lieutenant contrived to get a transfusion working with great promptness and skill considering that the ship was constantly altering course and numerous depth charges were being dropped in the vicinity.

This patient had recovered greatly towards midnight, but was obviously dangerously ill.

MONDAY, SEPTEMBER 14

Ship at sea. Weather calm, bitterly cold.

N.B. By 0100 hours, it became obvious that something must be done for our most serious casualty, who, apart from superficial skin lacerations, showed a small penetrating wound over his right iliac fossa. We rigged the sick bay for an emergency operation, which I performed under a continuous pentothal anaesthetic given extremely well by the Surgeon Lieutenant. The S.B.C.P.O. assisted me and looked after the instruments, while the two S.B.As. fetched and carried. Meanwhile the Padre cared for the remainder of the sick.

I excised the abdominal skin wound and underlying muscle, and found a perforation of the peritoneum. Exploration of the peritoneal cavity revealed a large number of small shell splinters which I removed, and seven perforations of the small intestine which I sutured. I then closed the abdomen, after inserting a pelvic drainage tube, and the Surgeon Lieutenant commenced a continuous 'drip'. We strapped the man on to the table and kept him there afterwards, as the 'drip' worked better that way. His condition at the end of operation was fairly good, but I could not seriously hold out very much hope for him. Our nursing facilities are very poor, and the constant circumstances ahead of the ship being repeatedly in action are bound to tell. Also, I am quite sure that there were probably other intestinal perforations which I missed owing to urgency, lack of skill, poor light, etc. There is no doubt that depth charges, alterations of course, and a cold climate do not assist surgical technique.

N.B. The convoy was attacked again, by high level bombers mostly, around noon today. Another heavy torpedo bombing attack followed at about 1400 hours, mostly directed at the carrier. I saw another tanker blow up very near to us, much the same as yesterday. Understand there is one solitary survivor from her, which is surprising. Believe a number of enemy aircraft failed to get home. The carrier must have lost at least one fighter too, as I saw a pilot bale out and end up in the sea.

N.B. Destroyer alongside about 1700 hours, and transferred another 90 odd survivors. A few cases of mild exposure, but nothing severe, and the rescue organisation at the stern of the convoy must be very prompt and efficient.

N.B. During these past two days of activity, the bearing of the ship's company and their morale have been of the highest order. They have been constantly at action stations, and the cold has been intense. Apart from the care of survivors on board, the supply department has excelled itself by contriving to maintain a supply of meals, soup and hot drinks the whole of the day and night.

N.B. The sick bay has been badly shaken about during the day, and the constant noise and general upheaval has been most disturbing to the patients. They became very frightened during the torpedo bombing attack, and I was tempted to quieten everyone down with morphia, but had to bear in mind that should the ship be hit, these patients must be in a state to make an effort to save themselves. The condition of the abdominal case began to deteriorate during the evening, and he became very distressed for a time during a U-boat attack.

TUESDAY, SEPTEMBER 15

Ship at sea in convoy. Weather very cold, but fine and calm.

N.B. Afraid that I could not possibly set down the detailed events of today with any accuracy, as the noise and activity have been so extreme most of the time, that it has been rather a 'blur'. There were certainly some heavy air attacks, but I am not really sure that some of them did not take place yesterday instead of today! I think we have nearly 400 survivors of various nationalities on board. They are all over the place asleep, and it is hard to avoid tripping over them. We have four more casualties, and the Surgeon Lieutenant is looking at them at the moment.

N.B. Outstanding incidents:
(1) During one attack today, I carefully observed a sailor at the back of the bridge, whose job was to telephone the orders of the gunnery officer. I must say the attack was very heavy, and the general noise and confusion were unbelievable. At the height of the attack, the ship was near-missed, and at the same time the safety valve lifted on one of the smoke stacks, and for about 5 minutes there was also the noise of steam escaping under pressure, which was itself deafening. I have never seen anybody quite so terrified as this sailor. His head, body and limbs were trembling, and he transmitted his orders in a voice which was a high pitched squeak. Nevertheless, he continued to do his job, and managed somehow to keep himself from breaking down completely.
(2) The rating 'on approval' from Keilder Camp, who was a member of a guns' crew, was brought to the main distributing station in a state of hysterical collapse some time today. (On second thoughts, it might have been yesterday or even the

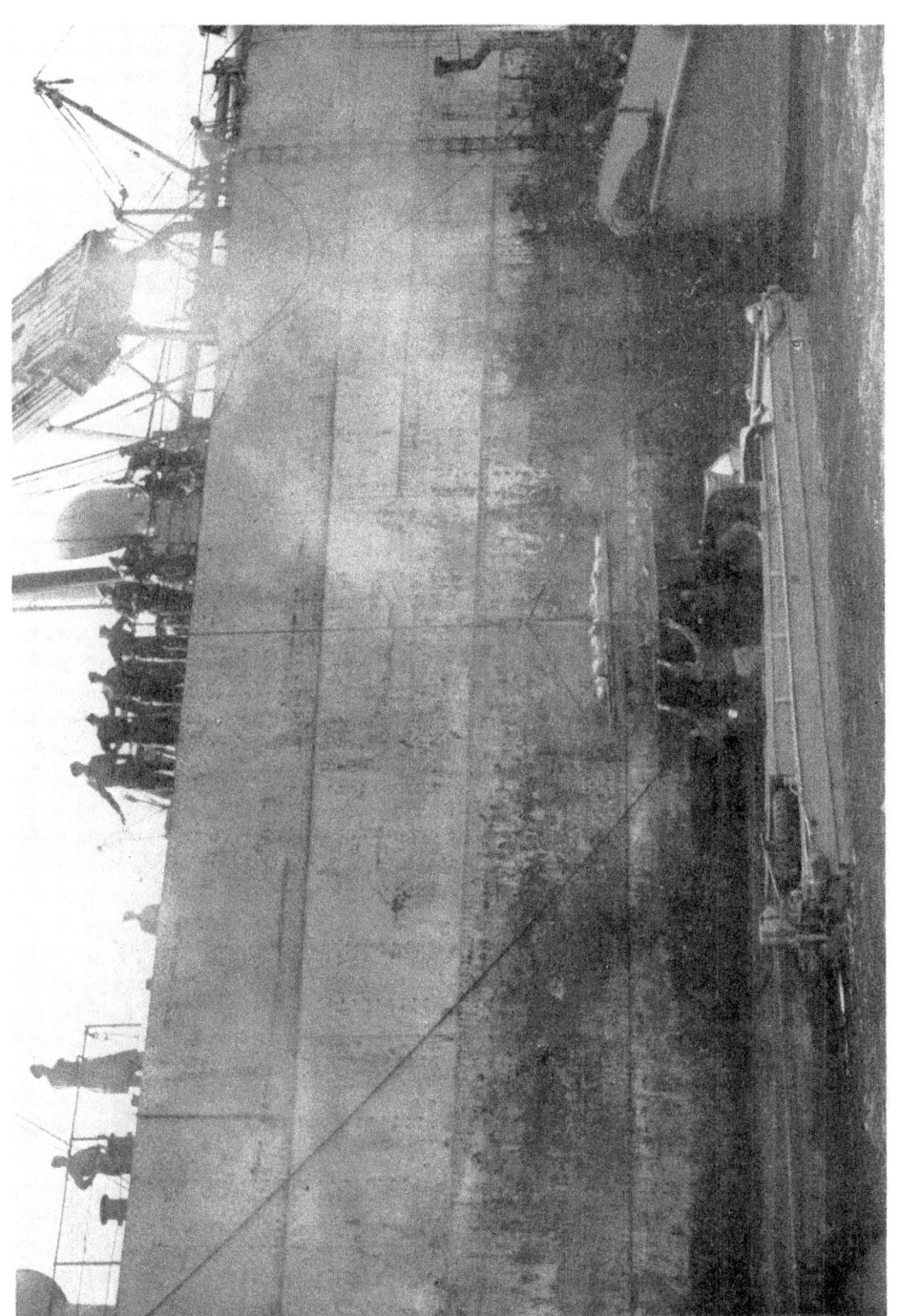

PLATE V. H.M.S. *Appledore*. Casualties being lowered down the side of a ship using 2-tier stretchers.

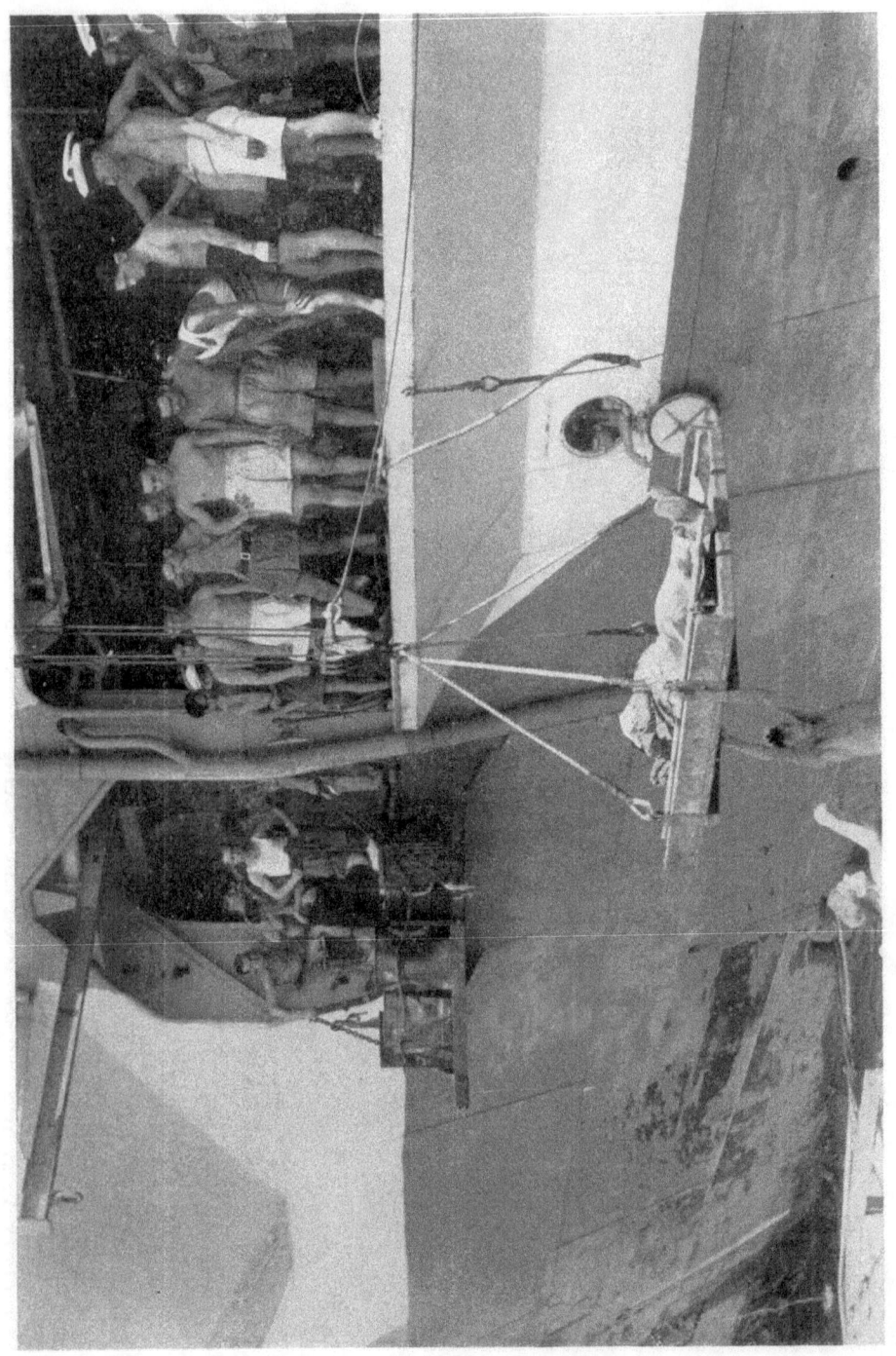

PLATE VI. H.M.S. *Glory* embarks released British prisoners. A stretcher case being hoisted aboard.

day before.) However, the S.B.C.P.O. fetched me, and I told the man to stand up and take a grip on himself. He promptly ran away, and is hiding somewhere on board, and has not been seen since. Nobody has yet had time to look for him.
(3) The abdominal case died during the evening, the Padre attending on him at the time.

WEDNESDAY, SEPTEMBER 16

The night has been fairly quiet, though I believe a merchantman was torpedoed and sunk.

N.B. One of our casualties had a most remarkable escape from death. Something hit him in the chest, with such force that he was knocked over, and received multiple contusions. He is badly bruised all over the front of his chest, but his ribs appear intact and there seems to be no lung damage. In a pocket of his jumper, he was carrying a gunmetal cigarette case full of cigarettes, which had worked itself into a position immediately in front of his cardiac area. There were several perforations in his clothing, and in the front of the cigarette case. The back of the cigarette case was intact. On opening the case, I found a number of bomb splinters inside it and the cigarettes all fragmented! There is no doubt that the cigarette case may well have saved his life.

N.B. At 0400 hours we left the convoy and picked up a homeward bound convoy, and during the day we have started the return journey in dense fog and have not been disturbed by the enemy. We have managed to get things sorted out a little, and most of us have had a short sleep.

THURSDAY, SEPTEMBER 17

Today was clear and calm but very cold, with the ice edge in view all day on our starboard horizon. Everything has been quiet, and we must be almost out of the range of aircraft.

N.B. At 1700 hours, I was at the back of the bridge, and saw a torpedo hit one of the naval escort astern. She began to list and sink immediately, and in less than a minute, was hit by a second torpedo. There was some confusion in the convoy, and a number of heavy depth charge attacks were made where the U-boat was assumed to be. An hour later, we received orders to leave the convoy, and to proceed independently. A destroyer came alongside, to take off our Flag Officer, who will transfer his flag to her and will remain with the convoy. He was 'piped' over the side ceremonially, being transferred from us to the destroyer in a 'bosun's chair' rigged for the purpose. I though he looked very cheerful albeit very tired. We immediately increased speed and parted company with the convoy. As we were doing so, one of the escorting destroyers was hit by a torpedo. She remained afloat, and another destroyer took her in tow.

FRIDAY, SEPTEMBER 18

Spent the night and the whole day under some difficulties, as a gale has started to blow up and the added zigzagging of the ship has made conditions most unpleasant. The weather is intensely cold still. All casualties and survivors appear to be doing well.

N.B. Discovered today that we have a small puppy among the survivors.

N.B. The damaged destroyer in tow was lost this evening.

THURSDAY, SEPTEMBER 24 (17 weeks in commission)

Ship arrived at Scapa Flow at 1030 hours. Weather fair and warm. Weather was appalling during our return journey, and it was literally impossible to make adequate notes. At 1200 hours five casualties discharged to *Amarapoora* by hospital boat. Also all survivors taken off by drifter about the same time. They seemed very grateful for what had been done for them, and cheered us as they left. Captain ordered ship to be got ready for sea again as soon as possible. Fuel and water taken on board, and signal made for replacements of medical stores. Discharge of 'empties' and re-ammunitioning commenced about 1600 hours.

N.B. Discharged Surgeon Lieutenant to shore, thanked him for his assistance.*

From September 25 to October 25 the ship remained based at Scapa re-conditioning and exercising. On October 25 she sailed for Plymouth en route to Gibraltar for duty in the Mediterranean. She arrived at Gibraltar on November 1 where she remained on routine duties till November 5. The journal details another typical period of duty:

FRIDAY, NOVEMBER 6

Ship at sea in Mediterranean. Weather calm and warm.

Medical State

Sick	1
Excused duty	2
Light duty	Nil
C.D.A.	Nil

---

* The various incidents described above refer to Convoy Q.P.14, which left Archangel on September 13 for United Kingdom, and which lost the minesweeper *Leda*, the destroyer *Somali*, and 4 out of a total of 15 merchant ships, all by U-boat attacks.

The above details do not accurately correspond to the official record, which states that the *Leda* was torpedoed and sunk at 0520 hours on September 20 in about 76.30° N., 5° E. The *Somali* was torpedoed at 1900 hours on September 20 in about 75.40° N., 2° W. She was taken in tow by the *Ashanti*, but a gale sprang up on the night of September 23, and the *Somali* broke in two without warning at 0230 hours on September 24. She is recorded as having sunk, after being towed 420 miles in 80 hours, in position 69.11° N., 15.32° W.

N.B. At dawn today we were steaming west, with the Spanish coast close to our starboard side, in company with *Sheffield, Charybdis, Argus* and *Avenger*. At 1000 hours we joined a large convoy of obvious transports, and accompanied it due east for the rest of the day. Query destination Malta.

N.B. U-boat report at 1700 hours.

SATURDAY, NOVEMBER 7

Ship at sea in Mediterranean. Weather calm and warm.

Medical State

Sick	Nil
Excused duty	1
Light duty	Nil
C.D.A.	Nil

Action Organisation

(1) First degree of readiness at 0500 hours, but all quiet.

(2) Italian reconnaissance aircraft reported directly ahead at 0800 hours.

(3) Ship dropped depth charges over alleged U-boat at 1030 hours, but with no result.

(4) Arranged for soda fountain to be left unlocked so as to allow a constant water supply to the first-aid post in the recreation space.

(5) Visited boiler and engine rooms with Commander (E) and Commander (S) during the forenoon. Temperatures were 90° F. in engine room and 93° in boiler rooms. No evidence of fatigue or distress on the part of any man there. Commander (S) arranged to issue gruel and tea during the day. No other precautions considered necessary. At midday specimen temperatures elsewhere were sick bay 76° F., transmitting stations and central communications office 70°. No rating complained of heat, which was interesting considering the fact that these sudden climatic conditions are quite warm for a ship's company which has spent the summer at Scapa Flow, and which was in the Arctic less than 2 months ago. None of the engine room personnel complained of discomfort or distress.

N.B. The result of these observations is that the Commander (S) agrees that there is no reason to consider special diet or 'action messing' as recommended for hot weather in the recent report made by *Kenya* following the last Malta convoy.

N.B. One officer fell down ladder leading to transmitting station. Slight concussion. Confined to bed and observation.

N.B. At 1300 hours today a crisis developed in the sick bay regarding laundry, as the Surgeon Lieutenant was suddenly told by S.B.C.P.O. that we were short of clean bed linen. I investigated this matter and found we have altogether only six clean sheets, and I discovered forty unwashed sheets in a cupboard, where they have been for nearly 2 months. Set the staff to work washing the sheets today.

N.B. Ship continued on an easterly course, in convoy, as if for Malta, until 2000 hours. Then turned south.

SUNDAY, NOVEMBER 8

Ship at sea off Algiers.

Medical State

Sick	1
Excused duty	Nil
Light duty	Nil
C.D.A.	Nil

At about 0030 hours, the ship's company was informed that we are part of a force for the invasion of North Africa. At much the same time, Algiers was visible in the distance brilliantly lighted. Beaches were occupied at 0100 hours, and at about 0200 hours a destroyer, I believe *Malcolm*, tried to ram the boom but retired with a number of casualties, having been hit in the engine room by shore batteries. I believe *Broke* then succeeded in breaking the boom and getting alongside in the docks. Meanwhile we stayed about 4 miles from shore, and were undisturbed till 0300 hours, when a number of aircraft dropped flares over us. Shortly afterwards some more aircraft flew over, and a ship astern opened fire at them. Searchlights from shore immediately turned in our direction, and one of our destroyers was vividly illuminated and engaged by shore batteries. The nearest shell to us was at least a $\frac{1}{4}$ mile away. At daybreak a large number of aircraft passed over towards the shore, bearing American markings. Some landing craft also passed close to us, carrying commandos who, I understand, are actually survivors from a transport torpedoed and sunk nearly 24 hours before!

Ship patrolled up and down the coast during the forenoon and afternoon, and things were very quiet except for odd warnings of U-boats in the vicinity.

N.B. Took this opportunity to blast the first-aid party in the Main Medical Distributing Station for being slow off the mark, and complaining of feeling tired.

N.B. At 1730 hours a most unpleasant torpedo bombing attack was carried out by enemy aircraft. Judged by their perseverance and skill, they were obviously German. The light was very bad, and they were difficult to see, so we put up a heavy barrage and hoped for the best.

Very noisy. The attack lasted ¾ hours, and two destroyers were hit, I think.

MONDAY, NOVEMBER 9

Ship at sea. On patrol off Algiers.

Medical State
>Unchanged.

All quiet during the day, but another torpedo bombing attack at 1730 hours, precisely on the same lines as yesterday.

Miscellaneous
   (1) A certain number of ratings is reporting to the sick bay complaining of blepharitis. Investigation shows that they are all 'lookouts and range takers'. I find that the only ones affected among the lookouts and range takers are those who spend long periods peering through binoculars which have sorbo rubber shields around the eye pieces. Examination shows that in all cases the sorbo rubber has started to perish, and I think it may be causing some irritation. More as a demonstration than as a precaution, I have ordered all the eye pieces of binoculars and range-finders to be swabbed over daily with 5 per cent. Dettol.
   (2) On the Captain's authority at 1200 hours today I broadcast to the ship's company on the question of keeping their bodies covered as much as possible as a precaution against flash. Also warned them that the weather becomes very cold in the afternoon, and the Commander has ordered the wearing of jerseys by all upper deck personnel after 1600 hours daily.

TUESDAY, NOVEMBER 10

Ship at sea. Patrolling off Algiers.

Medical State

Sick	2 (1 case of varicose oedema)
Excused duty	1
Light duty	Nil
C.D.A.	Nil

All quiet today until 1730 hours, when a most vicious torpedo and dive-bombing attack developed at dusk. One bomb exploded a ship's length astern and lifted us a bit. Two aircraft launched their torpedoes at us from each side simultaneously, but we avoided both, one literally by inches. One Heinkel burst into flames during its attack, and crashed on the sea between ourselves and *Avenger*. Another caught fire, and crashed in the far distance.

N.B. I found this attack most trying to the nerves.

WEDNESDAY, NOVEMBER 11

Ship at sea. Patrolling off Bougie.

Medical State
            Unchanged.

Again the day passed quietly until about 1745 hours. We were in company with *Argus*, *Charybdis* and some corvettes, when a most alarming attack was made by medium level bombers and torpedo bombers just after sunset. There was also a U-boat alarm much about the same time. The aircraft, at one time, seemed to come at us from all angles, and we were surrounded by near misses, but only slightly dented aft. I saw *Argus* hit by a bomb, I think towards the edge of her flight deck. Understand she had some casualties, and a number of fighters destroyed. A torpedo hit one of our small escorts on our starboard bow, and she seemed to split open and burst into flames and sank very quickly. We went at high speed, but as soon as it was dark, we turned round and went back. We could see survivors in groups in the water, flashing torches. We could also hear them shouting and singing. *Charybdis* patrolled around us in the far distance, while our Captain stopped the ship, and we lowered boats and let down scrambling nets over the side. Altogether we rescued 102 out of a total complement of 220. We might have stayed longer, but the moon rose and further attacks were anticipated.

All the survivors were covered from head to toe in oil fuel, and some were rather shocked. One rating, a cook, was pulled out of the sea unconscious. The ship's Commanding Officer was in the centre of a large group of survivors, and all were held afloat by their inflated lifebelts. The Commanding Officer was leading the rest in singing and cheering and seemed to be very much alive until the moment he was pulled out of the sea, when he appeared to be unconscious.

N.B. I distinctly noticed this feature in the case of several of these survivors, that they seemed to be full of energy until the moment of clambering on board us, when they immediately gave up. It was therefore necessary for rescue parties to catch hold of them and hoist them on board quickly, before they fell back into the sea and drowned.

The casualty reception organisation on board worked extremely well. All who could walk, or who were not obviously injured, were guided or carried to the seamen's and stokers' bathrooms. Here they were promptly cleansed of oil fuel, given hot showers, and inspected by the Surgeon Lieutenant for any sign of wounding. He also washed out the eyes of each man and dropped in castor oil to prevent further oil fuel irritation. The few who were worse off were carried to the sick bay where they were resuscitated very quickly with the exception of one man with a fractured radius. Injuries were superficial. The ship's Surgeon Lieutenant was among the survivors, and rather shocked and exhausted. We gave him omnopon and wrapped him in blankets, and he went to sleep at once in the sick bay office.

N.B. I did not realise at the time that this was the second sinking for this Surgeon Lieutenant, neither did I know that he had just performed an act of great bravery. It would appear that when his ship was struck, the Surgeon Lieutenant was between decks. Among the wounded quickly brought to him was an engine room rating with a badly burnt arm. The ship was now sinking, so the Surgeon Lieutenant injected morphia, assisted the man on to the upper deck, and then, as the man had no lifebelt, the medical officer put his on him, inflated it, and lowered the man into the water. The Surgeon Lieutenant waited until the man was free of the ship before he himself tried to escape. Consequently he became entangled in the rigging, and was taken down some way before he could free himself and get clear. He then swam for 3 hours without a lifebelt before being rescued.*

N.B. Meanwhile, from the time that the unconscious cook and Commanding Officer had been taken to the sick bay, artificial respiration had been continued on each. In response to a broadcast by the Commander, there was no lack of volunteers to form artificial respiration teams for these two casualties. But in any case we found it impossible to resuscitate them, and life was obviously extinct. I am in some doubt regarding the actual cause of death in these two cases. I did not really have the impression that either had died from drowning. Also, I am quite certain that the Commanding Officer was alive until shortly before he was taken from the sea. The only sign in each case was blood-stained froth at the lips and external nares. I feel that 'immersion blast' must be considered either from underwater explosions from the ship itself, or explosion of depth charges from some other ship. I am assured that there were no explosions from the ship's own depth charges.†

FRIDAY, NOVEMBER 12 (24 weeks in commission)
Ship at sea off Algiers.

---

* This Surgeon Lieutenant R.N.V.R. was subsequently awarded the Albert Medal in Gold 'for gallantry in saving life at sea'. A sick berth attendant of the same ship was also awarded the Albert Medal in Gold (posthumously).

† There is a discrepancy between the account given above and the official record, concerning time and date. The ship referred to is the sloop *Ibis*, which is officially described as having capsized almost immediately after being hit by an aircraft torpedo, at 1002 hours on November 10, in a position 10 miles north of Algiers. She shot down 3 aircraft before being herself hit.
Six officers and 86 ratings from *Ibis* were picked up after dark by one of H.M. cruisers. It is recorded that these survivors included the Commanding Officer of *Ibis*, who died later.

Medical State

Sick	. . . .	2 plus 4 survivors
Excused duty	. . .	Nil
Light duty	. . .	Nil
C.D.A.	. . . .	Nil

N.B. Survivors are recovering remarkably well, particularly the Surgeon Lieutenant, who was up and about early this morning as though nothing very extraordinary had taken place.

N.B. At 1400 hours, the deceased Commanding Officer and cook were buried at sea following a Service on the quarterdeck. Full honours were accorded, with firing party, 'Last Post', etc., and photos taken to be forwarded to the next-of-kin.

N.B. At 1700 hours the ship was attacked by a series of torpedo bombers, and had a very narrow escape. In the course of the attack a gunner on duty aft was hit in the left leg by a bomb splinter, or possibly some metal from a torpedo, as I believe one exploded in the ship's wake. The casualty lost a large amount of blood, but a tourniquet was applied and he was carried to the Main Medical Distributing Station. He was extremely shocked, and the Surgeon Lieutenant transfused him with good effect, so that he was much fitter by 2100 hours. Under a general anaesthetic given by the survivor Surgeon Lieutenant, my own Surgeon Lieutenant and myself explored the wound, which was large and penetrating and had badly disintegrated the left calf muscles and had passed upwards to behind the knee. It was obvious that a large piece of metal was somewhere towards the bottom of the left thigh behind, and was either compressing the popliteal vessels or had severed them, but was acting as a haemostat. We had to decide what to do about it, whether to trace and remove the metal for the sake of restoring the circulation to the lower leg, or whether to play for safety and avoid further haemorrhage in view of his condition which had deteriorated again. Remembering how poor our surgical facilities really were, and bearing in mind that our first job was to save life, we made no attempt to interfere further, but merely packed the wound with sulphonamide powder and vaseline gauze. At the end of operation the man's general condition was bad, and the outlook for his lower leg even worse.

N.B. Two of the officer survivors on board were wearing private non-Service pattern life saving waistcoats when they entered the water. These garments button up in front like an ordinary waistcoat. It would appear, that as soon as the survivor found himself in water bearing a layer of oil fuel, the tendency was for the buttons of the waistcoat to slip through the buttonholes, and consequently the unfortunate survivor 'slipped through his life saving waistcoat'. One officer stated that he was actually 'nearly drowned' by his inflatable waistcoat which ended up over his head. This seems a most important matter. I have informed the Captain officially, and have also advised the officers concerned to complain to the outfitter who supplied the waistcoat. The remedy, which is very obvious and very easy, is to replace the buttons and buttonholes by clamps or hooks.

FRIDAY, NOVEMBER 13
Ship at sea off Algiers.

Medical State
Unchanged.

Day passed in convoy between Algiers and Gibraltar.

N.B. Walked round first-aid posts with Surgeon Lieutenant, and stores all appear quite satisfactory and adequate. Omnopon mustered by Surgeon Lieutenant, and self mustered all dangerous drugs.

N.B. Leg case unchanged, and must be regarded as dangerously ill. Other casualties and survivors satisfactory.

N.B. Unfortunately had to take disciplinary action in respect of one S.B.A. who fell asleep while on watch in the sick bay during the night. Regretted having to do this, but it was a repeated offence. Mail closed on board at 2000 hours and censored at 2100 hours for 3 hours.

SATURDAY, NOVEMBER 14

Ship arrived at Gibraltar 0600 hours. Base Medical Officer was waiting with ambulances, blankets and everything necessary to receive our casualties. He certainly could not have been more helpful and attentive, all of which we greatly appreciated. Casualties discharged, and survivors taken ashore to depot ship.

N.B. We spent the forenoon fuelling and ammunitioning ship. We subsequently secured alongside *Vindictive*, and by 1230 hours, were planning to land during the afternoon for some exercise. However, no leave was granted, and at 1530 hours we were ordered to stand by to sail. Ship eventually sailed at 2030 hours, in brilliant moonlight.

SUNDAY, NOVEMBER 15

Ship at sea off Spanish coast in company with *Nelson*, *Renown*, *Victorious*, *Charybdis* and a number of destroyers. Weather fair and calm. No sick or excused duty on board. Light duty and C.D.A. likewise. First degree of readiness at dawn, but we have passed a very quiet day. Meanwhile the sick berth staff have had a busy day laundering sick bay dirty linen, and a working party has been cleaning off the oil fuel which was left behind in the sick bay by the survivors. 2100 hours censored mail 3 hours.

From November 16 to November 25 the ship was in Gibraltar and then sailed to join Force 'H' at Algiers.

From November 28 till December 21 she was on patrol duty off the North African coast without actually going into action except for a few air attacks during which the ship escaped damage.

On December 30 she returned to Gibraltar and while there received sailing orders for the United Kingdom and left at 1530 hours. The journal continues with a description of the voyage:

THURSDAY, DECEMBER 31 (31 weeks in commission)

Ship at sea *en route* for United Kingdom. Weather very rough and unpleasant, and getting much colder.

Medical State

Sick	2
Excused duty	1
Light duty	3
C.D.A.	2

Miscellaneous

(1) Wrote up continuation notes and discharge papers for all invalids on board.
(2) Italian prisoners-of-war visited, and have no complaints.
(3) Sick mess account completed and audited by Commander (S).
(4) Signal made to Dunfermline, asking for repeated issue of medical stores ordered and reported as transmitted to us last October, but which we have never yet received owing to our varied movements.
(5) At 1400 hours held a long consultation with the Surgeon Lieutenant regarding certain men in the ship's company who we consider need hospital treatment which should not be unduly delayed any longer. In consequence, saw Captain and Commander, and have arranged that on arrival in United Kingdom or as soon as convenient afterwards, 9 ratings shall be discharged to hospital. 2 varicose veins, 2 haemorrhoids, 1 anxiety state, 1 effort syndrome, 2 otitis media, and 1 chronic dermatitis of hands.

FRIDAY, JANUARY 1 (New Year's Day)

Ship at sea. Weather rough and wet, and very much colder.

Medical State
               Unchanged.

N.B. Today we found ourselves unexpectedly in action again, and greatly to our surprise. It would seem that at daybreak this morning, a Coastal Command aircraft sighted an unidentified merchant ship off the Bay of Biscay. A report was made to Admiralty, and we were informed, as being the nearest ship in the vicinity at the time. We increased speed during the forenoon, in response to further reports which confirmed that made earlier. On board, I think our reactions were not particularly enthusiastic about the prospect of a possible engagement with an unknown ship. I must admit that myself, I sincerely hoped that the search would be called off. After all, we are on our way home, and our chief thought is the prospect of leave with our wives and families. Being so near home, we can hardly be blamed for hoping to keep out of trouble and to avoid risks at this time!

However, we made a big alteration of course at noon in response to further reports, and made a further increase in speed. At this point it appeared that at our present course and speed we should meet with the unknown ship at about an hour before dark. But naturally, everything depended upon the accuracy of Coastal Command in reporting her movements. As it turned out, the co-operation between ourselves and Coastal Command could not have been better, which is somewhat surprising in view of the bad weather and the most difficult flying conditions for aircraft.

At 1600 hours we went to action stations and first degree of readiness. At 1700 hours a strange ship was visible on the horizon ahead. I thought she fired twice in our direction, but I may be wrong. We opened fire immediately, and appeared to hit her almost at once. In any case a fire broke out in the first moments on her upper deck amidships. We then proceeded to plaster her until she was burning furiously from end to end. We could see her crew trying to lower boats. We drew very close and fired a torpedo at her, which missed. We then circled around and fired a second torpedo which hit her amidships, and she turned over and sank in about 4 minutes, still burning furiously. We did not attempt to pick up survivors but we left the scene of action at high speed, I believe, on account of warnings of enemy U-boats and aircraft.

N.B. This was certainly a most successful and unexpected start to the New Year, but peculiarly we were all inclined to be a bit depressed in the wardroom afterwards. This reaction was rather queer and hard to account for. Perhaps it might best be explained by remembering that the action was rather a massacre, that there is something depressing about watching a ship sinking in flames, even an enemy, and anyway, we are all a bit tired and not really ourselves these days.

N.B. I myself am most irritated as the gunfire has put my watch out of order again.

N.B. The Captain's signal to Admiralty after to-day's action was very typical of him and very satisfying to us all. It merely consisted of two words 'Enemy sunk'.*

---

* The incident here referred to is the sinking of the blockade runner *Rhakotis*, 6,753 tons, homeward bound to Axis territory and almost at the end of her long journey from Japan and Batavia. According to official records, the *Rhakotis* was reported at 0515 hours on January 1, 1943, in a position about 200 miles north-west of Cape Finisterre. One of H.M. cruisers proceeded to intercept, and eventually sank the *Rhakotis* at 1700 hours, in a position about 140 miles north-west of Cape Finisterre. 75 survivors from the *Rhakotis* reached Corunna in two boatloads, on January 3 and 4. These survivors included 1 Briton, 1 Swede and 8 Norwegian P.o.Ws.

SATURDAY, JANUARY 2

Ship at sea off Scilly Isles. Weather very rough but much warmer than yesterday.

Medical State

Sick	Nil
Excused duty	1
Light duty	3
C.D.A.	2

Miscellaneous

(1) Resuscitation apparatus defective on testing. Added to our demand for stores.

(2) Signal made for reliefs for men considered medically unfit. Instructions from Captain that these men are not to be discharged to hospital until their reliefs have arrived.

N.B. Since daybreak today we have been at first degree of readiness, and constantly anticipating enemy air attack, as our presence must be known since our action of yesterday. But in any case the rough weather would make air attack hazardous, and the whole ship is a shambles, with water and filth everywhere, and 'life lines' rigged in all exposed places on the upper deck.

SUNDAY, JANUARY 3

Ship arrived off the Clyde at daybreak, and proceeded up to Greenock in fine but bitterly cold weather.

Medical State

Unchanged.

Miscellaneous

(1) Mails landed at 0900 hours.

(2) All invalids landed plus two of our own cases, chronic appendix and effort syndrome, and all discharged to E.M.S. Hospital, Mearnskirk.

(3) Landed Italian prisoners-of-war, who were complaining of the cold in spite of the extra clothing and duffle coats provided for them by Commander (S). I think they found the journey more exciting than they had expected, in view of the action on January 1.

N.B. At 1100 hours Commander (E) reported complaining of abdominal pain after meals, and occasional vomiting without relief. Could find nothing on physical examination, but there is no doubt that he looks anaemic and has lost about 1 stone in weight during the last 6 months. I think that he has suppressed his symptoms while the ship was actively engaged, and has now decided that he had better do something about himself. He will certainly need prolonged hospital investigation. Official report in writing to this effect handed to Captain. 2100 hours ship sailed.

MONDAY, JANUARY 4

Ship at sea off West Coast of Scotland. Weather calm, occasional snow, and bitterly cold.

Medical State
    Unchanged.

A quiet day.

TUESDAY, JANUARY 5

Ship arrived at North Shields in thick fog, at 0930 hours.

N.B. Immediate instructions from Flag Officer locally, that all ship's company and officers are to proceed on leave in two halves, 14 days each. As special train had been organised, this meant rapid arrangements by myself.

(1) Am proceeding on first leave myself, with half sick berth staff, and have advised Surgeon Lieutenant and S.B.C.P.O. to bring their wives up to live locally.

(2) Position regarding medical stores is becoming acute, and Dunfermline has again been signalled demanding a complete re-issue of the October supply which has never reached us. Further additions demanded by signal, including 6 electric blankets and 5,000 aspirin tablets. Meanwhile, I have instructed the Surgeon Lieutenant that he is to make friends with all the ships locally with a view to begging, borrowing and stealing all possible medical stores and equipment.

(3) Instructed Surgeon Lieutenant to prepare all statistics for Quarterly Medical Journal during my absence.

(4) Captain approved immediate discharge of Commander (E) to R.N. Hospital, Chatham, this being near his home, for medical investigation regarding fitness for service at sea.

(5) Discussed question of arctic clothing requirements with Captain, Commander, and Commander (S). I have undertaken to visit M.D.G's. Department, Admiralty, to ask advice on this subject while on leave.

(6) Base Medical Officer, North Shields, came on board and was most co-operative and helpful. He has arranged hospital accommodation, dental treatment, specialist appointments locally as required.

N.B. This question of Base Medical Officers is one which might well be represented officially. They can be very good or very bad, depending on the port, and their assistance is of such vital importance to visiting H.M. ships, that the work performed by such Base Medical Officers as North Shields and Gibraltar deserves the highest praise, and even more so as it is not the kind of work which achieves very much 'limelight'.

From January 6 to January 22 the Medical Officer was on leave, and from January 23 the ship remained in dry dock until February 5 with the crew living in uncomfortable conditions with emergency lighting, no heating and all sanitary conveniences on board out of action.

From February 5 the ship was at North Shields preparing for sea and sailed for Scapa on February 8. She remained there carrying out routine duties and exercises until February 15, when she joined a convoy of merchantmen as escort on a voyage to Iceland and North Russia. This voyage and its incidents, some of which are of great interest, are described:

TUESDAY, FEBRUARY 16

Air temperature 41° F., Sea temperature 49° F.
Ship at sea. Weather very rough.

Medical State
    Unchanged.

Weather has continued to be very rough, and it has been impossible to do more than carry on the bare ship's routine. A lot of seasickness, and was very sick myself all night. Managed to get some notes made in preparation for a broadcast talk to the ship's company on the subject of personal precautions in the Arctic.

WEDNESDAY, FEBRUARY 17

Air temperature 44° F., Sea temperature 50° F.
Ship at sea. Weather very rough.

Medical State
    Unchanged.

N.B. We were supposed to have joined a convoy of merchantmen as escort p.m. yesterday, but so far they are a long distance behind time. This terribly rough weather has altered the ship's programme, but it has one advantage in that the temperature has remained warm. Myself, I am still wearing the same clothing as I was in the Mediterranean, and feel quite comfortable.

N.B. We sighted Iceland during the forenoon, and intended entering harbour at 1500 hours, but this proved impossible owing to the rough weather.

N.B. Regret that my own personal programme has been sadly thrown out of gear by seasickness, which I have not yet been able to overcome.

THURSDAY, FEBRUARY 18

Air temperature 24° F., Sea temperature 34° F.

Ship at sea off North Iceland. Weather fine and sunny, but with heavy swell. Have now stopped being seasick.

Medical State

Sick	3 (1 engineer officer with influenza)
Excused duty . . .	1
Light duty . .	Nil
C.D.A.	2

N.B. The ship is really doing little more than go round in circles today, waiting for the merchantmen to catch up.

Miscellaneous
  (1) At 1145 hours, I broadcast to the ship's company regarding personal precautions which they should observe in the Arctic.
  (2) A number of people on board have common colds, and the Captain is anxious about a possible influenza epidemic. More as a demonstration than anything else, I have ordered the whole ship's company to be given quinine sulph. grains X by mouth today and tomorrow. Incidentally, this is contrary to Admiralty instructions, which nowadays insist that all supplies of quinine should be carefully conserved.

N.B. Despite a fall of 20° in temperature, there has been no wind, and conditions on board have remained comfortable.

FRIDAY, FEBRUARY 19

Ship at sea off North Iceland. Nothing more than routine work was possible on board, in conditions which were very bad. The whole of last night and today was spent steaming slowly into a snow blizzard, with visibility reduced almost hourly during the last 24 hours, and temperatures rising as high as 28° F., and falling as low as 13° F.

SATURDAY, FEBRUARY 20

Weather became calmer during the night and we were able to enter harbour at 0900 hours. Ship sailed at 2000 hours, and steered N.E. to join convoy.

SUNDAY, FEBRUARY 21

Air temperature 32° F. all day.
Ship at sea. Weather calm, overcast, with occasional short snow storms.

N.B. Joined convoy at 1900 hours today. Unfortunately, understand that escort has been reduced owing to the single aircraft carrier and one cruiser having been damaged by bad weather during the past 48 hours.

N.B. At 2100 hours, short conference between Captain and heads of departments, and he informed us that from a.m. tomorrow we shall be within the danger zone from enemy aircraft, surface craft and U-boats.

MONDAY, FEBRUARY 22

Air temperature 36° F. all day.

Ship at sea, approximately 68° N. Weather perfect, like a Spring day. Sea calm, sky clear and blue.

Medical State

Sick	1
Excused duty	Nil
Light duty	Nil
C.D.A.	2

N.B. Ship at second degree of readiness for the past 24 hours. Captain addressed the ship's company and gave them a 'pep talk' at 1000 hours today. Later, I myself gave a similar talk to the Surgeon Lieutenant and sick berth staff. Was also able to inspect all first-aid posts, stores, etc.

N.B. Climatic conditions on board are very comfortable today. I am also surprised that we should be getting as much as 8 hours' daylight in each 24 at this time of year. For interest I visited the engine and boiler rooms several times during the day. Found that in the engine rooms, maximum temperatures were 68° F., and minimum 63° F. In the boiler rooms maximums were 80° F., and minimum 66° F.

TUESDAY, FEBRUARY 23

Ship at sea. Weather choppy, sky overcast. Heavy snow during the night.

Medical State
      Unchanged.

N.B. Health and morale of the ship's company extremely good on the whole, and certainly better than at Tyneside.

N.B. During the last 24 hours we have tried out the experimental arctic clothing. I think we are agreed that the suits have much to recommend them, but they give the impression of having been constructed and devised to be worn by a man doing hard manual work in a cold climate, e.g., hauling a sledge. But there is doubt about their suitability as an adequate protection for a seaman sitting on watch in the open on board a ship at sea. Several wearers have also complained that the suits are not proof against heavy sea spray.

N.B. At 1130 hours we were within 250 miles of enemy bases. Soon afterwards we were obviously discovered by two enemy aircraft, which shadowed us for about 2 hours. We recognised their presence as an almost certain forerunner of an attack of some kind. However, at 1400 a heavy snow blizzard started to blow, and continued for the rest of the day. This was most fortunate, and probably protected us for a time.

WEDNESDAY, FEBRUARY 24

Ship at sea, approximately 73° N. Weather very rough, alternating patches of clear and snow.

Medical State
$\qquad$ Unchanged.

N.B. First degree of readiness at 1200 hours. Approximately 60 aircraft reported approaching to attack, but eventually to our surprise only one arrived, and it quickly went away. From 1400 hours onwards the weather improved, the sea became calm, and the sky clear and blue. We were shadowed by aircraft until dark. At 2030 hours, a number of U-boats attacked and were countered by large numbers of depth charges. But none of our ships was hit.

THURSDAY, FEBRUARY 25

Ship at sea. Approximately 73° N., and steering due E. Weather calm, sunny, and sky clear.

Medical State

Sick	1 (Pleurisy)
Excused duty	Nil
Light duty	Nil
C.D.A.	3 (One fresh case (?) Chancre but impossible to investigate under present action conditions)

N.B. We were at action stations all night, countering U-boat attacks. Things were very noisy, but no damage to any of us. Soon after daybreak shadowing aircraft appeared, and were obviously 'homing' in other aircraft. At 1200 hours we were attacked by a large formation of Ju 88s. and Me 109s. They attacked out of the sun in the face of a tremendous barrage from our naval escort. A number of them did not press home their attacks at all. Four bombs fell in our area but none nearer than 200 yards from the ship. There were many near misses on merchant ships, but nothing was actually hit.

N.B. During the attack, I noticed a clinical phenomenon which was new to me. It concerned the rating sick with pleurisy. Early this morning his temperature was 99° and pulse 78. At the beginning of the air attack, his temperature was 102·2° and pulse 84. During the attack he became rather distressed, and at its peak, his temperature was 105° and pulse 162. 2 hours after the attack his temperature was 100° and his pulse steady at 84.

FRIDAY, FEBRUARY 26

Ship at sea.

Medical State
    Unchanged.

N.B. The night was very noisy again with U-boats about, but the convoy remained unharmed. We were at second degree of readiness most of the night but went to first degree of readiness at 0350 hours. It was bitterly cold, and I could not get warm in spite of lots of extra clothing. During the forenoon we steamed through 'pancake ice', with lots of seals about. We were shadowed by aircraft the whole forenoon, and at 1230 hours were attacked by a formation of Ju 88s. In the face of our barrage, their attack was very half-hearted, and they kept at a fairly high altitude, and apart from a near miss on a merchant ship astern of us, all their bombs were completely outside the target area.

N.B. At 1410 hours the *Lord Austin* was instructed to transfer to us a serious casualty from a merchantman astern. But by nightfall the transfer had not been effected.

SATURDAY, FEBRUARY 27

Ship arrived at Kola Inlet, North Russia, at 0900 hours. Weather bitterly cold, ice everywhere, snow ankle deep on upper deck.

Medical State
    Unchanged.

N.B. At 0500 hours, the *Lord Austin* transferred one casualty to us. He was a seaman from U.S.S. *Francis Scott Kay*. He was conscious, with a deep shrapnel wound of head which was already obviously heavily infected.

N.B. As we came into harbour a.m. today there was a fairly heavy air raid, and one merchant ship was set on fire at the harbour entrance. Otherwise the whole convoy arrived unharmed.

N.B. Transferred casualty to R.N. Auxiliary Hospital, Vaenga, at 1100 hours.

SUNDAY, FEBRUARY 28

Ship at Kola Inlet. Weather bitterly cold, but fine.

Medical State
    Unchanged.

N.B. None of us is as rested as we had hoped, as we found it almost too cold to sleep. Called on S.M.O. in *Belfast* at 1100 hours. A routine day followed, chiefly spent trying to keep warm. At 2000 hours heavy air attack developed, and two enemy aircraft were shot down. 2100 hours commenced mail censoring routine again, which has been interrupted now for some days.

MONDAY, MARCH 1

Ship at Kola Inlet. Weather unchanged. Ship sailed with homeward bound convoy at 1500 hours.

Medical State
    Unchanged.

N.B. Steaming into the wind tonight, the weather was colder than we had ever imagined it could be.

TUESDAY, MARCH 2

Ship at sea. Weather a little warmer a.m. Light snow. Passage slow owing to slow speed of convoy.

Medical State

Sick	2
Excused duty	1
Light duty	Nil
C.D.A.	3

N.B. One marine injured left hand in ammunition hoist, resulting in a fracture dislocation of two fingers. Surgeon Lieutenant undertook treatment. Hurt Certificate to be granted.

N.B. A very quiet night, during which we were at second degree of readiness, and most people had some sleep. It is of interest that we have only now been able to prevail upon men to sleep at their action stations when not at first degree of readiness. It has taken time to make them realise that by doing so they avoid expending a lot of energy unnecessarily.

N.B. Since noon today the ship has been running through continuous 'pancake ice', and continuous fine snow has been falling. A slight but keen breeze caused a fall in temperature in about 10 minutes. Air temperature fell to 9° F., and sea temperature to 29° F. Average speed of the convoy during today was only $4\frac{1}{2}$ knots.

N.B. At 1700 hours P.O. reported with giant urticaria. He had a hot bath during the afternoon, went on watch in the open, and the urticaria commenced at once and persisted. He states he has never had such an attack before. 2100 hours censored mail 2 hours, and instructed master-at-arms to post fresh notices regarding censorship regulations and privilege envelopes.

WEDNESDAY, MARCH 3

Ship at sea. Weather still very cold but sea not frozen a.m. today. Air temperature minimum 14° F.

Medical State

Sick	1
Excused duty	2
Light duty	1
C.D.A.	3

N.B. Very noisy night with U-boats, but convoy safe as far as I know. We have been warned to expect air attacks during the day.

N.B. Spent forenoon investigating climatic conditions on board, with some rather curious results. The temperatures in engine and boiler rooms were 61° F., but nevertheless, numerous icicles, several 18 inches long and 2 inches thick, were hanging down from the air-intake fans. The inside of the sick bay scuttles, skylight and bulkheads were coated thickly with a film of ice, nevertheless the atmosphere was pleasant, and temperature 58° F. The unfortunate feature is that the temperature rises and falls so quickly in response to a change of course by the ship, that freezing, thawing, and freezing again is constantly taking place. This makes living conditions extremely uncomfortable, as thawing makes the mess decks wringing wet and subsequent freezing coats them with ice again.

Miscellaneous
(1) Put Surgeon Lieutenant and sick berth staff through a stiff hour's training p.m. today.
(2) Instructed S.B.C.P.O. to commence statistics for Quarterly Journal.
(3) Instructed Surgeon Lieutenant to draw up list of officers and ratings who need dental and specialist appointments at an early date.

2100 hours censored mail 2 hours.

THURSDAY, MARCH 4

Ship at sea. Weather calm and bitterly cold.

Medical State
Unchanged.

N.B. Aurora borealis was very bright all last night, and the night itself was extremely disturbed owing to U-boat attacks which caused no damage.

N.B. Climatic variations have been very wide during today. At 0900 hours the air temperature was 10° F. At noon it was 22° F. Up till then snow had fallen since daybreak, and the decks were well iced up. A film of ice also covered the inside of all living spaces throughout the ship, but the atmosphere was quite pleasant. By 1600 hours the air temperature was 33° F., snow had ceased, and fog was tending to form in streaks across the sea. Between 1600 and 1800 hours the two sides of the ship were different owing to a cross breeze. On the port side a rapid thaw was taking place, while a correspondingly rapid freeze was occurring on the starboard side! By 2000 hours snow was falling again, and the cold had become general, with the air temperature 10° F.

N.B. At 1130 hours signal received from a tanker in convoy, asking advice regarding a seaman sick with primary syphilis, a gland in his groin having burst. Reply made instructing complete rest, repeated foments, and stating the condition need cause no anxiety, and is probably chancroid and bubo, and not syphilis at all. 2100 hours censored mail 2 hours.

FRIDAY, MARCH 5

Ship at sea Arctic Ocean, S.W. of Bear Island. Weather very cold, sky clear.

Medical State

Sick	2
Excused duty	Nil
Light duty	Nil
C.D.A.	3

N.B. One seaman, member of a gun's crew, suddenly found his dentures broken inside his mouth after heavy gunfire today.

N.B. Last night and today life has been very exciting and noisy. During the night navigation was very difficult, owing to icebergs. After midnight a number of U-boats was reported in our area, and numerous depth charge attacks were made. At about 0100 hours, a torpedo track appeared directly ahead, and passed the ship close to its port side. This must have been a very narrow escape for us, as I understand the attack was quite unexpected at that particular moment.

At 1000 hours today, a small number of Ju 88s. appeared on the horizon, some miles ahead of the convoy. We fired at them several times, but without success, and they remained where they were. Shortly afterwards the commodore of the convoy signalled to our captain, suggesting that these aircraft might be launching mines or 'circling torpedoes' ahead of the convoy. Thereupon, ourselves and the convoy made a series of emergency turns to avoid any such possible attacks. Shortly afterwards, I was talking to the Padre on the flag deck, and we both suddenly saw the tracks of two or three torpedoes on the surface, about 200 yards from our starboard side. We also thought we saw a floating mine at the same time, but could not be certain. There is no doubt that the torpedoes were very shallow, and in the choppy sea, were actually breaking surface here and there between waves. At least, that is how it appeared to me. A number of merchant ships opened fire on them with short range weapons. They quickly passed astern of our own ship, but the ship immediately behind us was hit on her starboard side under her bridge. There was a tremendous explosion, and a sheet of flame as high as the top of her masts. She was a large merchantman, and she staggered like a maimed animal, and then started to settle down in the water. More or less simultaneously, the second merchant ship in the next line of the convoy to us on our port side was also hit, and started to heel over. We immediately increased speed and drew ahead of the convoy, and opened fire on the aircraft ahead. We harassed them for about an hour, after which they departed. The whole incident was over by 1300 hours, by which time we had the medical organisation ready for the reception of possible casualties and survivors. At 1315 hours the captain sent for me on the bridge, and asked me if I had seen the torpedo tracks, and if so, how many, etc. I gave him my description of what I thought I saw, and rather gathered that my description did not wholly agree with what other people saw, or thought they saw. However, I understand that the captain was inclined to conclude that the attack was by a salvo of torpedoes from a U-boat, and that they were not launched from aircraft. At 1325 hours I received information that the ship torpedoed astern of us was the U.S.S. *Executive*, and that 9 of her complement were missing. Fifty-three survivors have been picked up astern of the convoy and will be transferred to us later today. Apart from shock and exposure, the known casualties among the survivors are one case with severe injuries to arms, and one fractured ribs.*

At 1415 hours, the convoy was attacked by a formation of Ju 88s., which came in at about 2,000 ft. We put up a terrific barrage but they unloaded their bombs in and around the convoy area. No ship was hit and no aircraft touched either that we could see.

SATURDAY, MARCH 6

Ship at sea between Bear Island and Jan Mayen Island.

Medical State
      Unchanged.

N.B. Weather much warmer and there has been a marked thaw. But since about midnight a gale has been blowing, which has been getting steadily worse. By 1800 hours today the weather had become really bad, with a heavy sea running. In consequence the convoy has reduced speed, and has made poor progress. Nevertheless, this bad weather has favoured us in other ways, and although we were being shadowed by aircraft at 0900 hours today, no further interference has occurred.

---

* The incident here referred to concerns a convoy of 30 ships, including 4 tankers, which left Kola Inlet on March 1. According to the official record, U-boats gained contact the next day, and dogged the convoy all the way to Iceland. On March 5, in a position 72.30° N., 11.30° E., two American ships were attacked. The *Executive*, 4,978 tons, was sunk, and the *Richard Bland*, 7,191 tons, was damaged. The attack was by either circling torpedoes dropped ahead of the convoy by flying boats, or from long range torpedo fire.

SUNDAY, MARCH 7

Ship at sea, still between Bear Island and Jan Mayen Island. Weather continues warm, but gale blowing and very rough indeed.

Medical State

Sick	5 (1 lacerated arms, remainder influenza)
Excused duty	1
Light duty	1
C.D.A.	3

N.B. Quite suddenly today, an outbreak of influenza has started on board. This was endemic when we left Scapa Flow, but I thought it had vanished. The navigating officer is a potential patient, and the gunnery officer had to go sick a.m. today, very much against his will, at a time like this.

N.B. The weather has been abominable all day today, and by this evening the gale had become alarming. In consequence, the convoy has scattered badly, and ships are all over the place. At 1900 hours we were informed that U-boats are again in contact, and also that there is the possibility of interference by German surface craft.

N.B. One merchant ship reported herself leaking and threatening to break up. Another reports herself as icebound, which sounds peculiar, as we are well south of the ice.

N.B. The weather being so rough yesterday, and the ship moving so much, I found it rather difficult to climb up to the bridge with the sick list for the captain, and when I got there, I found he was resting in his sea cabin. As there was nothing of particular importance to tell him, I decided not to disturb him. However, I was wrong, because when I took today's sick list to him, he made no bones about rebuking me very severely for my omission of yesterday!

MONDAY, MARCH 8

Ship at sea south of Jan Mayen Island. Weather continues bad.

Medical State

Sick	7
Excused duty	3
Light duty	1
C.D.A.	1

N.B. The small wave of influenza continues throughout the ship, and a large number of men are complaining of headache and malaise, etc. I suppose it is only to be expected that something like this would occur, considering that we have been transferred from the Mediterranean to the Arctic, *via* Tyneside, in mid-winter. The gunnery officer is a little better, but his temperature is still around 101°. Another officer sick during the forenoon, with temperature 103°. Very difficult to nurse them efficiently under our present conditions of impending action, and rough weather.

N.B. At 1210 hours today two enemy aircraft suddenly appeared out of the haze and passed close down the ship's port side. We were not really at first degree of readiness at the time, and each appeared to ignore the other. Probably the aircraft were as surprised to see us as we were to see them. They were very low over the water. Naturally, this incident caused some excitement and rushing about, and standing at the back of the bridge, I suddenly observed the gunnery officer running up a ladder, and pulling on an arctic suit over his pyjamas! I felt he was unfit to be there, and prevailed on him to return to bed, which he did very much against his will, and obviously most upset at being unfit for his job, which is understandable.

N.B. At 1900 hours the weather was a little calmer, though still extremely rough. We received a report of possible enemy surface craft, and went to first degree of readiness for the night.

N.B. Ship which reported herself as breaking up yesterday, sank today. Fortunately none of her complement was lost.

N.B. There is no doubt that tonight we are all feeling very tired and noticing the strain of this present operation. Frankly we have all nearly had enough, and we shall be glad when it is finished.

TUESDAY, MARCH 9

Ship at sea off North Iceland. Weather a little improved. Air temperature 14° F. all day.

Medical State

Sick	3
Excused duty	3
Light duty	1
C.D.A.	1

N.B. Weather was bitterly cold all night, and the sick bay completely iced over on the inside, but the atmosphere was not uncomfortable.

N.B. Both officers sick with influenza are virtually unchanged, and I am a little anxious about the gunnery officer, who has developed a very bad bronchitis. Meanwhile, the influenza epidemic has not sent anyone else sick, but we are watching everybody carefully, and during the course of the day, the Surgeon Lieutenant and myself have managed to get round the whole ship and cast an eye over every officer and man on board. I don't think we missed anybody.

WEDNESDAY, MARCH 10

Ship entered harbour, North Iceland, at 0930 hours.

Medical State

Sick	4	(One further case of influenza)
Excused duty	3	
Light duty	1	
C.D.A.	2	

N.B. Weather bitterly cold during the night, and still is. Upper deck is knee deep in snow and ice. Our future movements are unknown. We left the convoy during the night, that is to say, the few ships which were still in company. The ship damaged by the torpedo attack the other day was hit again early today and has sunk, I believe. Another ship was also sunk during the night.

There is no doubt that the bad weather has had a very adverse effect on the second stage of this operation.*

N.B. Visited my cabin today for the first time for some days, and found it in an awful mess, with a few things smashed.

N.B. Two cases are causing me some anxiety at the moment:

(a) Stoker reported 5 weeks ago with small, moist, eczematous patch on groin and infected scabies. No evidence of venereal infection. He responded to routine treatment, and cleared up in about 48 hours. Today he has reported with:

(i) Eczema and ulceration of groins and lower abdomen.

(ii) Severe infected scabies

(iii) Generalised maculo-papular eruption on chest and back.

(iv) Generalised adenitis.

There is no faucial congestion, and there has never been any history of exposure, or anything to suggest a venereal lesion. But, at the moment, he looks remarkably like a secondary specific infection.

(b) A seaman with an indolent sore strongly suggestive of primary infection, but dark-ground repeatedly negative. Have instructed Surgeon Lieutenant to commence sulphonamide therapy, and to control observation by repeated blood tests as opportunity arises for getting these done.

---

* The official record states that the weather, which was of full gale force, caused this convoy to drop far behind its scheduled time, and to straggle, which favoured the U-boats in the area.

The above description is not quite accurate as to date, according to the official record, which states that the *Richard Bland* was torpedoed again on March 10, but did not sink until March 11. On March 9, the *Puerto Rican*, 6,076 tons, was torpedoed and sunk in 66.45° N., 10° W. There were therefore three U-boat victims of this convoy, the *Executive*, the *Richard Bland*, and the *Puerto Rican*. A fourth ship, the *J.T.L.M. Curry*, foundered in the gale on March 8. On March 14, 22 out of 30 ships arrived at Loch Ewe, 4 others having proceeded to Iceland.

N.B. One sub-lieutenant reported sick at 1800 hours, with temperature 101°, general malaise, and generalised abdominal pain. No sign of acute abdomen, and probably influenza.

THURSDAY, MARCH 11

Ship sailed from Iceland at 0800 hours. Snowing. Weather bitterly cold.

Medical State

Sick	5 (All influenza)
Excused duty	1
Light duty	Nil
C.D.A.	2

N.B. Sea was calm to start with, but became rough p.m.

N.B. Severe outbreak of pediculosis in four lower deck messes. Treatment commenced, but under our present conditions it is well nigh impossible to adopt the usual cleansing and disinfestation routine. This outbreak, which has involved a large number of men, is mainly due to the fact that few of us on board have been able to bath properly or change into clean clothing for a considerable time. 2100 hours censored mail 3 hours.

FRIDAY, MARCH 12

Ship at sea south of Iceland. Weather much warmer, and all ice and snow has melted. But weather is extremely rough, and the constant rolling and pitching of the ship are making life very irritating on board.

Medical State
Unchanged.

N.B. Sought the Commander's assistance during the day in order to resurrect the routine for censoring mails, which has fallen into abeyance of late. This is very necessary, as the number of letters in the mail to be landed on our arrival, and still uncensored, must run into several thousand.

SATURDAY, MARCH 13

Ship arrived at Scapa Flow at 0700 hours. Calm and sunny weather, and it felt very good to see green fields and to feel warm again.

Medical State

Sick	Nil
Excused duty	Nil
Light duty	Nil
C.D.A.	2 (1 relapsed urethritis)

N.B. Landed mail at 0745 hours, having spent most of the night censoring it.

N.B. Hospital boat alongside at 0900 hours, and 10 cases discharged to *Isle of Jersey*. Included 3 officers with influenza.

N.B. From 1000 hours onwards the usual post-operational routine of ammunitioning, fuelling, storing, and general clearing up of the ship has continued all day. Everybody very worn out and tired, and I have not seen the ship's company and officers so much below par since the ship commissioned.

N.B. Spent the afternoon studying new Fleet Orders and local Medical Orders. Was interested to read that attention is drawn to the efficient chlorination of fresh water in all ships. Was even more interested to discover that there has been a severe generalised epidemic of influenza in the Fleet. The ships most affected have been *Kenya, Belfast, Glasgow* and *Furious*. One cruiser has had cases at the rate of three a day, including her Captain and Commander. Another has reported 300 cases. I understand that the Commanding Officer of one ship developed an acute pneumonia and died after an illness of 8 days. So there is no doubt that we have escaped very lightly. 2100 hours another very heavy mail to censor, the natural result of receiving several long overdue incoming mails.

SUNDAY, MARCH 14

Ship at Scapa Flow. Weather fine and sunny.

Medical State

Sick	Nil
Excused duty	1
Light duty	Nil
C.D.A.	2

The whole day spent ammunitioning and cleaning ship.

MONDAY, MARCH 15

Ship at Scapa Flow. Weather dull and rainy.

Medical State

Sick	2 (Both influenza)
Excused duty	Nil
Light duty	Nil
C.D.A.	2

Miscellaneous

(1) One P.O. to hospital a.m. with phlebitis.
(2) One shipwright to hospital p.m. with renal colic.
(3) One warrant officer with pleurisy.

(4) One officer reported p.m. and confined to bed with bronchitis.
(5) Two specialist appointments made with *Isle of Jersey*, and five ophthalmic appointments with *Iron Duke*.
(6) 24 routine dental appointments made with *King George V*.

N.B. Communication received that a packing case of medical stores has been dispatched to us from Dunfermline *via* Rosyth. Discussed this with S.B.C.P.O., and we agreed that this consignment of stores is rather like 'the Flying Dutchman,' which everybody talks about, but nobody has seen!

N.B. P.m. today part of the ship's company was allowed ashore for recreation, and for some reason or other got itself involved in a private battle with some members of another ship in the local canteen. It probably did everybody good to 'let off steam', but a few blows were struck, and at 2100 hours our sick bay was full of 'casualties', mostly with black eyes. The only serious case was one seaman with a fractured fibula. I gather there are similar 'casualties' in the sick bay of the other ship involved! I have made a report to the Commander, but understand that disciplinary action is unlikely to be taken officially against anybody. Instead, the captains of the two ships concerned will settle the matter amicably, realising that the whole thing is largely a matter of 'high spirits'.

TUESDAY, MARCH 16

Ship at Scapa Flow. Weather sunny and fair.

Medical State

Sick	3 (All influenza)
Excused duty	1
Light duty	Nil
C.D.A.	2

Miscellaneous
(1) Seaman with fractured fibula discharged to *Isle of Jersey*.
(2) One cook to hospital with otitis media.

N.B. A.m. today heads of departments were informed by Captain that a V.I.P. will visit the ship in 48 hours' time. Apparently this Personage is of such importance that we are going to take even more trouble than usual for his reception. General clearing up of ship has been intensified, and we have also started to paint ship as well. Unfortunately, Captain developed a temperature p.m. today, and I was forced to confine him to bed, somewhat against his will.

From March 16 to the end of the daily journal, the ship remained at Scapa.

The Daily Journal of this Medical Officer ceases at this point.

(iii)
Lessons to be learned from the Daily Journal

GENERAL

Study of the above notes recorded by a Naval Medical Officer reveals to some extent the special medical problems and hazards which had to be catered for during the war at sea, and how an efficient medical officer taught himself to cope with these while at the same time contriving to fit himself, his staff and his medical organisation into the general background of a typical naval environment afloat. It must be understood that the term 'environment' is here used in a comprehensive sense, and is intended to embrace the whole pattern of domestic life on board a man-of-war, as well as her working routine which aims at making her an efficient fighting unit of the Fleet.

As has already been described, the notes recorded refer merely to one single ship out of the many whose medical achievements during naval operations would fill many volumes. But the notes concerning this one ship are fairly representative of the gradual development of naval medical life afloat in all men-of-war during the Second World War.

For example, the reader cannot fail to recognise two outstanding features which are evident throughout the ship's career from her date of commissioning. The first feature is the position of responsibility held by the ship's Commanding Officer, and how it is necessary for specialist officers constantly to acquaint him with the state of their departments on board and to seek his guidance, obtain his approval and to postpone, pending his opinion and acquiescence, even minor matters of procedure in the organisation for which a particular head of a department is responsible, but which nevertheless must be viewed from the perspective of the Commanding Officer in relation to the impact on the welfare and efficiency of his command as a whole.

The second feature which is outstanding is, that for every department of the ship, the constant training and exercising of personnel in their duties is paramount. It will be seen, that even when the ship has fought a successful action, the immediate aim is that she shall be got ready to fight again, and that advantage is taken of any interim period of inactivity to continue the constant upward struggle to achieve a peak of perfection through repeated practice.

RECEPTION OF SURVIVORS

It is of some interest to read of the separate organisation which existed in a man-of-war for the reception of survivors from other ships, and in which the Medical Department naturally played a major part.

During the war, the Navy wisely made no attempt to lay down any rigid routine to be observed when survivors were picked up. Each ship was in fact left to work out its own scheme in the light of its experience. It was soon realised that the circumstances in which a man might become a survivor at sea varied so widely that it was impossible to do more than indicate in outline the way in which he should be managed after his rescue.

It came to be realised that the emotions of a survivor might be temporarily unstable. At the time of his rescue his output of nervous energy would have been enormous, and consequently his immediate need would be prolonged rest. The complication to be avoided on his recovery was mainly the tendency of the survivor to become a prey to self pity, and to develop a complex that he was being unfairly treated. Therefore the problem of his best management did present certain difficulties.

The rescue of a man from the sea at any time carries with it an element of sentiment and drama which is likely to affect the rescuer as much as the rescued. But on active service in the Navy, such sentiments must be subordinated to the underlying principle that in time of war, the object of saving a man's life is that he shall be quickly rendered fit to fight again. In this respect the medical department of the rescuing ship plays a most important part, and in all ships it was considered essential that when survivors were picked up, a close liaison should exist between the medical and non-medical departments when decisions had to be taken as regards their management.

Broadly speaking, a system of care had to be devised for a survivor which bore in mind the principle that on the one hand too much sympathy must be avoided at all costs, while on the other hand an apparent lack of sympathy could be equally disastrous to the survivor's future fighting efficiency.

In general, when picked up by a man-of-war, it was found that each batch of survivors, owing to local circumstances, presented its own problems as regards maintenance of morale. The mood of the men varied between either a state of excitability and talkativeness or a state of apathy amounting almost to stupor, even where there was no physical exhaustion.

The immediate burden of care fell upon the medical and supply departments of the rescuing ship. The former was concerned first of all with the treatment of obvious casualties, and later with the general assessment of the medical well-being of the remainder. The supply department, meanwhile, was concerned with the problem of feeding and clothing. Finally, as ever, the Commanding Officer found the ultimate disposal of such unfortunate men yet another addition to his many burdens.

Once the initial shock of their experience had passed it was an important principle that survivors should not be allowed to think that the fight was over. Even the medical officer owed a duty to the Navy to remind each survivor, unless he was obviously incapacitated as a casualty, that the war was still on, and that the ship which had rescued him was still at sea and just another man-of-war as far as he was concerned. From that moment it was customary to treat a survivor not as a passenger, but as an addition to the crew of the rescuing ship, until that ship reached harbour. This was regarded as the first important step in rehabilitation.

The subsequent care and rehabilitation of survivors was the duty of the authorities of Naval depots ashore, and here again close liaison existed between the medical and other service departments.

On arriving in depot each survivor would be subjected to a rigorous medical examination, and in this respect, it was most important that a detailed history should be provided by the medical officer who had first seen him immediately after his rescue. This report was necessary in order that examining medical officers in depot should fully understand the extent of any severe experiences which a particular survivor might have suffered. It was also considered essential that the depot medical officer should not be dependent for his information on personal interrogation of the survivor himself. This was because many survivors were in a highly suggestible state of mind, and any nervous strain would but be exaggerated by further cross-examination about personal experiences, thereby impressing the circumstances even more upon the mind.

It was also necessary for medical officers to remember that officer survivors, although ostensibly calm and under control, in reality might well be suffering even more severe emotional strain than survivor ratings, and it was important that due allowance should be made for this contingency.

FIRST AID

Much has already been written, earlier in this volume, on the subject of first aid in action, and the above notes do little more than to confirm that as regards the immediate treatment of casualties afloat, the damage control and salvage of personnel was designed from the medical point of view to relieve pain, to prevent injuries becoming worse, and to save life by the control of bleeding and shock. But as the war progressed, naval medical officers were quick to appreciate the point of view of the executive in respect of a ship's casualties, the vital object being to maintain the fighting efficiency of a ship by making it necessary for as few wounded as possible to leave their action stations, and to restore highly trained men to duty with the minimum delay.

Even after the war at sea had been in progress for some three years, and even after new Fleet Orders regarding medical action organisation had been produced to supplement the inadequacies of King's Regulations and Admiralty Instructions on the subject, it still continued to be a popular belief that first aid could only be carried out by first-aid parties, and that wounded must be taken to distributing stations at once. It took a long time to teach the Navy that wounded are best treated where they fall not only for their own sakes, in that increase of shock and jeopardy of lives is prevented, but also because the transport of wounded which interferes with ammunition and repair parties and takes fit men away from more important duties, is obviated. Above all, the crowding together of wounded in dressing stations necessitates the centralisation of the medical department, which came to be regarded as a dangerous practice, particularly after the main dressing stations of first a battleship, and later a cruiser, had been obliterated by direct hits and the majority of the ship's medical personnel in each case lost at one blow early in the action.

Quite apart from the Fleet Orders which had a purely medical bearing, the naval damage control handbook which was eventually issued stressed the importance of decentralisation. A policy of decentralisation naturally had to include the dispersed treatment of casualties, and it was necessary to have widely scattered medical damage control in each ship. Clearly, this latter could only be effected to the limit by every individual having the ability to perform simple first-aid measures combined with confidence in the efficiency of those measures. It became essential to instil into every officer and man the idea that first aid had to be done, and done well, by men on the spot. It was even more essential for such officers and men to understand that this first aid was their own responsibility, and one which could not altogether be delegated to the ship's medical department. It had to be noted that whereas there is always a certain number of a ship's company off watch both during and after action, the smallness of the ship's medical branch never permits a watchkeeping routine to be observed while wounded are being treated. Therefore experiences of prolonged action at sea soon showed, that unless ample assistance was available, the strain on a small branch was extremely heavy. It was in fact a constant task of every ship's medical officer to make other departments realise the need to overcome the tendency of sailors to regard wounded messmates as of first importance, and therefore to rush them off to the ship's doctor wherever he might be. This task was one which continued as long as the war itself, and was never wholly successfully achieved.

The above notes confirm that when the oft-repeated principle of the dispersed care of casualties was correctly followed, the senior medical officer, or single medical officer where only one doctor was carried, could not be immobilised in a crowded distributing station. He had to be free to move about to supervise the treatment of casualties wherever they occurred. Only in this way could efficient care be quickly given to a large number of wounded during action.

Preparations for such medical decentralisation included the issue of morphia to officers and the provision of first-aid equipment at many points. But concurrently with the ample supply of first-aid equipment throughout the ship, steps had to be taken to overcome the lack of ability of the bulk of a ship's company to make use of this equipment. This defect was due to the continued observance of an old tradition that first-aid instruction was something which was only given to volunteers, and never during normal working hours. For generations too, first aid in general had been wrongly regarded as a specialist matter far beyond the comprehension of the ordinary individual. Also, certainly as regards sailors, there existed the type of mind which tended to regard first aid with contempt, particularly if it was going to be given by somebody non-medical. Such a man was the type who, when wounded, would continue to man his gun, scorning attention only to die later, whereas a simple tourniquet or dressing might have saved his life and still permitted him to carry on the fight. This kind of attitude was deplorably unfortunate, as such naval ratings were almost always those who were the most devoted to the Service.

Thus the need for a changed perspective came to be recognised, whereby first aid was placed alongside damage control. The aim was that every officer and man should come to be capable of making use of first-aid equipment just as much as he was able to make use of the sextant, compass and other tools of his trade afloat. The necessity for such individual ability was even further stressed when analysis of the early actions of the war at sea showed that 85 medical officers were among the first to be killed, thus leaving the care of the wounded entirely in the hands of laymen in the ships concerned.

To implement this changed perspective in every ship afloat was not easy, and much of its success depended upon the enthusiasm of medical officers coupled with the active co-operation of commanding officers. The co-existence of these two elements was essential. Where either or both elements were absent it was found that the non-observance of orders and instructions concerning medical organisation afloat endangered life just as greatly as the absence of damage control hazarded the ship itself. For instance, when a battleship was badly bombed, very few of the wounded who found their way to the Main Distributing Station had had any first-aid attention at all. Subsequent investigation showed that they not only could, but should have received this attention at their action stations, and should have remained there instead of unnecessarily and dangerously crowding the distributing station.

EFFECTS OF OIL FUEL ON CASUALTIES

In the above journal, a note on Wednesday, November 11, states: 'All the survivors were covered from head to toe in oil fuel'.

Early in the war the Royal Navy and Merchant Navy, including many of their doctors, believed that oil fuel in the sea would certainly add greatly to the hazards of men who abandoned ship. This view gained credence from the many lurid articles in the popular press and gruesome accounts of survivors which were given much publicity.

But in fact, the careful assessment of collected experiences during the war showed the contrary to be true, as a result of which steps were taken to reassure all ships' companies on this subject. This procedure was of the greatest importance, for it was frequently proved that an unreasoning fear might just tip the scales in the wrong direction when an indifferent swimmer had to make up his mind whether or not to abandon a doomed ship.

Of all the dangers likely to confront a man forced to jump into the sea, oil fuel was the one most feared by the sailor for the least reason. Study of the subject showed that, far from constituting a danger, oil fuel on the sea had certain advantages.

The first advantage was the calming effect of the oil upon the sea itself. This was of great assistance to the swimmer, by the diminishing of splashing and spray which tended to get into his nostrils.

By coating the body, oil fuel also exerted a protective action against cold and also to some extent against sunburn in the Tropics. But it is only fair to state that this claim of actual survivors was never supported by scientific experiments.

It was claimed by some observers that in tropical waters oil fuel might afford protection from sharks, which it was thought would be unable to breathe in the fuel.

In most sailors there existed a fear that a film of oil fuel on the surface of the sea might hamper swimming and might even drown survivors by its very depth. This fear was proved to be unfounded. The oil fuel carried by a man-of-war is divided into a number of tanks throughout the ship, and when the ship sinks, the majority of the fuel sinks too. It is only a comparatively small proportion of the fuel carried by the ship which will actually escape on to the sea. For example, some of H.M. cruisers carried 3,000 tons of oil fuel in 43 tanks, and it was therefore most unlikely that whatever damage the ship received, more than about a quarter of this fuel would escape on to the surface of the sea. Once having escaped, the rate of spread of this fuel depended upon the state of disturbance of the sea, but the spread was usually very rapid, and an area of some 300 × 200 yards was usually quickly covered. This meant, that average damage to a sinking man-of-war resulted in a spread of oil fuel on the sea round about which was not thicker than one-third of an inch at any place. This thickness was shown to be the maximum, which might well be reduced by the emulsifying effects of explosions and by disturbances caused when the ship actually sank.

It will be appreciated therefore that such a small depth of oil fuel could have little effect upon a swimmer.

It was finally concluded that although oil fuel undoubtedly had unpleasant effects on the body, yet none of them were likely to be serious, and in any case a negligible number of survivors would be affected. For example, after the sinking of H.M.S. *Hermes*, out of approximately 350 survivors, only 3 could be considered as badly affected by oil fuel. In the case of 850 men from H.M.S. *Prince of Wales*, some 20 only were affected by oil fuel. (Plate VIII illustrates the rescue of a rating from an oil polluted sea.)

The chief effects of oil fuel which were recorded were:

(*a*) Vomiting. This was perhaps the most uncomfortable effect of all, but it very soon passed.

(*b*) Sore Eyes. It was found that if the oil was wiped out of the eyes with clean wool, and the lids smeared with vaseline, the soreness was unlikely to last more than 24 hours. In some quarters there was a belief that permanent eye injury might result, and it was always necessary to reassure survivors on this point.

(*c*) The effect of oil fuel upon wounds was probably one of the most important considerations, and there was reason to believe that there was no harmful action. It was even suggested that oil fuel might act as an antiseptic. Certainly, a large number of wounds which had been deeply permeated with fuel showed no increased tendency to sepsis. When H.M.S. *Adventure* was mined in November 1939, one of the wounded, a stoker, was not discovered until four hours after the explosion. The genuine reason given, and accepted, for this delay was that he and his clothing were so saturated with oil fuel as to make him indistinguishable from his surroundings in a damaged compartment! The man was unconscious and had a severe laceration of the scalp extending from his eyebrows to the back of his head. The whole thickness down to the bone was involved, with the flap of scalp turned back over his ear, thus exposing a long ragged fracture of the vault of his skull. The whole wound was saturated in oil fuel which was also seen to have entered through the fracture itself. The wound was cleaned out as well as possible with potassium permanganate and four rough sutures were inserted to hold the flap in place. These surgical procedures were naturally elementary in view of the conditions under which they were carried out.

The man was sent to hospital, still unconscious, about 14 hours after his injury. Three weeks later, without any further surgical measures, the wound was perfectly healed and the patient suffering from no disability whatsoever.

Here then is a somewhat unique case in which, not only was oil fuel sewn up inside a wound, but the patient literally had oil fuel on the brain! Yet, with nothing more than rudimentary treatment, he recovered as well, or perhaps even better than could have been hoped for in the most advantageous circumstances.

(*d*) No deleterious effect upon the skin was ever recorded, and the theory that death might occur from 'closing the pores' was quite unfounded.

Nevertheless the purely mechanical disadvantage of handling the slippery casualty covered in fuel was a very real one, and undoubtedly added to the hazards of rescue work.

Also, the slippery effects which caused life-saving waistcoats to become unfastened, have been referred to. It is also on record that many a survivor forced to abandon ship in a hurry found that, quite apart from cold or excitement, the valve of his lifebelt was too slippery to screw up tightly after the belt had been inflated.

(e) *Psychological Effects.* These were considered by many observers to have been the most important of all, as having encouraged a hysterical prolongation of his experiences in the survivor. The smell and taste of oil fuel are most persistent, and tend to linger on with the survivor, constantly reminding him of past dangers.

Finally it is of interest to record that many of the grave effects formerly attributed to oil fuel proved, on investigation in hospital, to be due to other causes, such as depth charges exploding under water near to survivors, or blast before abandoning ship, or the inhalation of sea water, or to conditions existing before the event, or to the effects of prolonged exposure.

For example, a survivor from H.M.S. *Royal Oak* complained of repeated vomiting after his ship had been sunk. He attributed this to a quantity of oil fuel he had undoubtedly swallowed at the time. On investigating the history, it was found that he had suffered two further experiences of an unpleasant nature within a week of the *Royal Oak* disaster, and that his nerves had been shaken considerably. He had vomited, chiefly after breakfast, for 8 to 10 days after his rescue. He had then gone home on leave, and had been perfectly well for 3 weeks. But 10 days before he was due to join another ship he started to feel unwell. On joining this ship he vomited repeatedly, and was finally discharged to hospital. In hospital he vomited once only at the time of admission, but not again. Gastric investigation revealed a low acid content. It was finally considered that this case, originally seriously considered to be connected with oil fuel, was in reality the effect of anxiety upon a pre-existing abnormality, and the prospect of going to sea again precipitated a nervous type of vomiting.

A patient from H.M.S. *Jersey* was received in hospital with a persistent cough and blood-stained sputum, believed to be due to oil fuel. Investigation showed that he was a member of a torpedo party of which all members but himself were killed by the explosion when his ship was hit. It was therefore obvious that he himself had met with a considerable degree of blast, which in all probability caused some lung damage.

As regards the procedure to be adopted when a survivor was received covered with oil fuel, it came to be emphasised that what was termed treatment was very secondary in importance, and was merely to be undertaken in the interest of cleanliness after everything else had been done in the shape of treatment of shock and wounds, etc. Various substances were used with success for cleaning oil fuel off the skin. Pyrene fluid and shale oil were recommended. Turkey red oil was considered to be the best cleanser by the end of the war, but shale oil always had the great advantage of being available in bulk from the torpedo department of any of H.M. ships.

BURIAL OF THE DEAD

In the daily journal, a note made on November 12 describes the burial of a deceased officer and rating at sea, following a Service on the quarter-deck. 'Full honours were accorded with firing party, with "Last Post", etc., and photos taken to be forwarded to the next-of-kin'.

This note, brief as it is, represents a procedure for disposal of the dead after a naval action which, at all times during the war, was the subject of grave deliberation. The few words of the note are sufficient to reveal the care that was taken to fulfil spiritual needs as well as due ceremonial respect to the deceased. There was no distinction between the commanding officer and rating. A final example of the thought taken for the bereaved families of the deceased is shown by the taking of photographs.

Numerous instructions are laid down in King's Regulations, Fleet Orders, and local Port or Station Orders throughout the whole Navy which aim at the observance of a regulation burial of the dead with due respect and ceremony in any part of the world and under any type of circumstances which happens to prevail. Nevertheless, as so often happens when an attempt is made to cover every contingency, the procedure which has been laid down frequently proves to be so cumbersome and so unrelated to reality as to fail to meet the needs of the particular case. It must be admitted too that under the urgency of war, such regulations are sometimes unread until the need for them becomes urgent, and they are then found to deal with theory rather than practice.

Naturally, although burial arrangements were an executive commitment, the medical department of a ship could not fail to be involved to a great extent, and few naval doctors were ever likely to deny this implied responsibility.

Where a man-of-war had fatal casualties on board after an action, an immediate problem which had to be decided was how best these men should be disposed of. The alternatives which presented themselves were:

(*a*) Immediate disposal during the course of the action, should the action be prolonged.

(*b*) An early organised committal before returning to harbour after the action.

(*c*) A funeral at sea from another ship after returning to harbour.

(*d*) Burial on shore.

Many commanding officers would consider burial on shore as too obviously the path of least resistance. Also, seafaring men in general, it is believed, regard burial at sea as befitting to a seaman and of course the speed of a ship's movements and the need for early burial in a hot climate at times necessitate burial at sea.

But whether at sea or on shore, in time of war it has always been borne in mind by the authorities that funerals place a considerable strain on ship's personnel, especially during that vital period of mental reaction and rehabilitation after a severe naval engagement.

The many problems which arise in relation to burial are well illustrated in the case of one severely damaged ship which returned to a naval base with over 100 dead on board. The bodies were landed into the care of the local Service Hospital. Within 48 hours the bodies were placed on board two escort vessels from which they were buried at sea.

The labour here involved can be seen at a glance. First of all working parties of the deceased men's messmates had to gather the bodies together on board, convey them ashore and place them in a mortuary improvised by the hospital. In this case it proved difficult even to find material in which to wrap each of these bodies before they were landed. Transport to the hospital also proved difficult in this case, and the few vehicles available locally had to be diverted from essential work elsewhere in the port. The small hospital staff had to be supplemented by men from the ship for the task of sewing up the bodies, work which must be done very thoroughly if great distress is not to result at the funeral later. Finally working parties were again needed, and shore transport and boats' crews in order to reconvey the bodies to the ships which were to take them to their final resting place.

It was later submitted that the labour involved in this particular case might well have been reduced had greater forethought been observed. It was suggested that with such mortality, an effort might have been made to reduce the number of dead to be disposed of on arrival in harbour, even if circumstances did not permit a religious committal.

Death in action on board a man-of-war afloat always has its own dignity, and it is on record that in one ship there was nothing either demoralising or lacking in reverence in the action of a seaman who himself buried 15 members of his gun's crew during a short lull in a heavy action. No matter how sentimental a sailor may be about such matters in time of peace, there can be little doubt as to which course is preferable when very large numbers of casualties occur in action.

Two further reports provide an interesting contrast. In one ship, which was very severely damaged in action early in the war, it was recorded: 'During the forenoon the dead were prepared for burial, and a simple but most impressive Service was held on the forecastle in the afternoon. The dead, consisting of 5 officers, and 56 ratings were committed to the deep'.

But in another ship also badly damaged in the same action, the medical officer himself honestly comments on his own failure to ask the captain to bury the dead immediately after the action: 'Had we done so, it would have been easier on the feelings of the ship's company'.

In general, it was evident during the war that every possible effort should be made to clear a damaged ship of her dead while still far out at sea. It was frequently shown that there might always remain a certain number of bodies which were inaccessible. But these should be reduced to a minimum, and it was always urged that very careful arrangements to deal with them should be anticipated if their presence was not to prove one of the most potent factors in undermining morale later on.

All ships were reminded that their early attention should be given to this work, not only because it is more easily carried out while the exaltation of action endures, but because its details are later more likely to be forgotten if use is made of this temporarily elevated state of mind.

Special recommendations were made to ships in hot climates, where every hour of delay would add greatly to the disagreeable nature of such work. It was recommended that should a ship happen to return to harbour before its dead had been buried, fresh working parties from other sources should be employed, who would be likely to work with much more vigour and detachment. Where bodies were still in inaccessible places acetylene cutters were sometimes required for the work of extricating them from wreckage. In some cases too, it happened that inaccessible bodies could not even be approached for some weeks, until dockyard repairs had been commenced. In such circumstances experience showed that civilian dockyard personnel soon became accustomed to this type of work, and displayed great sympathy and co-operation at all times. This was a feature too in ports overseas where native dockyard labour was employed.

Where burials at sea were possible, experience showed that much could be done to ease the strain on personnel and to carry the ceremony through with simple dignity provided that attention was given to small details which were frequently liable to be overlooked. Naturally, the organisation arranged had to be adapted to the type of ship. The question of adequate weighting was of the very greatest importance, and was something which was shown to have been largely left to trial and error since the days when a round shot or a fire bar was employed for the purpose. In this respect, ships were reminded that on each successive day the buoyancy of a body would increase, and that where bodies were sewn up and weighted for burial at sea, the weight would need to be increased if the actual burial was not carried out on the same day. It was pointed out too that fat men require more ballast than thin men of the same weight, owing to the lower specific gravity of fat.

It was particularly recommended that Neil-Robertson stretchers should not be misused for the purpose of burials at sea, not only because they were in short supply, but also because they did not sufficiently conceal the body and they tended to add to its buoyancy. Neither were hammocks considered to be suitable for men who had died as a result of wounds, being particularly inappropriate for the transport of the body from the position in which it had been found. An important point which many ships' medical officers came to know was that where a canvas shroud was used, pockets of air were likely to form inside it, and that therefore the canvas should be slit in two or three places before committing the body to the sea in order to allow this air to escape.

Finally, it is important to note a number of measures which were recommended to be taken with a view to maintaining morale in a ship carrying deceased casualties. Where the ship or the messdecks became pervaded with the smell of decomposition from bodies which were inaccessible, it was customary to secure alternative sleeping and messing accommodation for her personnel. It was also the practice to deduce the list of the dead from a muster of the living, and where identity discs had been destroyed in action, identification by messmates was not insisted upon.

In the above journal it is described how cleaning of the ship after an action was of paramount importance during the days that followed, and it was generally realised that the rapid and respectful removal of the dead, plus the scrubbing of bloodstains from the decks, was likely to restore happiness to a ship much more satisfactorily than any academic procedure in the conduct of funerals on shore.

Nevertheless, it must not be imagined that the rapid burial of casualties at sea meant that the Navy intended these men to be forgotten. Such recommendations as were made were always mindful that every possible endeavour should be made to hold a Ceremonial Service ashore in memory of the dead, and later, if possible, to construct some memorial in the ship's chapel or in some other appropriate place out of regard for the human instinct which finds comfort in this manner.

MEDICAL ASPECTS OF ENEMY AIR ATTACKS

During the Second World War one of the earliest new features which influenced medical action organisation afloat was enemy air attack. A number of experiences of individual ships is recorded later in this history. But at this point, it is important to give a general impression of what a naval medical officer afloat came to recognise as the effects of this example of modern warfare at sea.

It was soon appreciated, that compared with past naval actions, the surprise of a bombing attack and its frequently long and sustained nature were qualities peculiar to this weapon. As in the First World War, torpedo attacks by U-boats might be unexpected, but were nevertheless brief when they did occur. Also, surface actions between men-of-war had their lulls, and were never really long sustained. But the instances of continuous attacks upon ships by waves of bombers for perhaps 10 hours or more at a time presented special problems in maintaining the nervous and physical endurance of personnel.

It was found that the most important feature of a successful bombing attack upon a ship was the peculiar psychological reaction which was always present in a varying degree, and which was commonly found in communities elsewhere which had been subjected to this form of sudden and destructive assault.

It will be remembered that the note for Tuesday, September 15 in the above journal states: 'Afraid that I could not possibly set down the detailed events of today with any accuracy, as the noise and activity have been so extreme most of the time, that it has been rather a "blur". There were certainly some heavy air attacks, but I am not really sure that some of them did not take place yesterday instead of today!' This brief statement, which represents a factual description of a medical officer's state of mind, was all too common.

In another ship, the medical officer recorded that: 'Following the explosion many men were found on the upper deck sitting about in an apathetic state'. This experienced medical officer had had knowledge of certain peace-time catastrophies which had affected large numbers of persons, and he compared this apathy with the effects of an earthquake in Greece, when the populace could only be roused to action by a ship's band which played through the streets. The fact that this loss of initiative is not a racial characteristic was proved by its being noted frequently during the salvage operations which followed the great earthquake at Napier in New Zealand in 1930. It was noted at that time, and confirmed in men-of-war which had been heavily bombed, that the condition of apathy was apt to be more marked in those with no special duties to perform. On the other hand increased concentration was necessary in those who had definite work to do.

Another ship reported that after a severe bombing attack, the ship's company displayed mental torpor and complete apathy with regard to passing events. These men, although to all outward appearance uninjured physically, and having had no period of unconsciousness, were in a dazed condition. They offered no resistance to outside help, but seemed utterly unable to take any step to help themselves. Numbers of them were found on the lower deck sitting at tables, with their heads in their hands. They were found there some 45 minutes after the explosion occurred, and although there was a perfectly easy avenue of escape for them, they had made no move to take advantage of it. Had the ship gone down during that time, they would undoubtedly have gone down with her, although every man was perfectly capable physically of climbing to the upper deck unaided, merely being guided by the hand of a rescuer. Observers stated that if one of these men got into any particular position, he could not seem to summon the energy to change it, and should one of them trip and fall, he might well drown in a few inches of oil or water because he was too apathetic to rise.

It was found too that this stupor did not depend upon a ship being hit directly. It was found to be associated also with underwater explosions, where a whole ship had been lifted by near misses of bombs.

Once the Navy had appreciated that this type of 'mental concussion' was always likely to occur following heavy bombing attacks afloat, steps were taken to avoid it as much as possible by inculcating a spirit of fearlessness and enthusiasm by giving every man a specific job to do as far as possible.

As regards the purely physical effects of a bombing attack afloat, it was soon found that wounds could be broadly classified into two groups depending upon whether the ship had been hit directly or had suffered a near miss.

In the case of the near miss, though men might be thrown into the air, or might fracture their legs, spines or skulls, the vast majority of casualties was due to splinter wounds. In one ship, of 13 men killed and 32 wounded by a near miss, all were cases of splinter wounds and all the casualties occurred on the upper deck. In general, it was found that bomb splinters tended to follow an inclined upward path. They were likely to cause wounds which were almost invariably above the hips. In one ship 8 out of 9 casualties were wounded in the chest and abdomen, and another ship reported 70 cases of similar wounds. This wound distribution was certainly due to the fact that the lower limbs were protected from a splinter inclining upwards by the ship's deck and side. This was a strong argument in favour of personnel on the upper deck keeping well inboard during bombing attacks. Experience also showed that the incidence of wounds could be largely avoided by lying down, and it was found that those ships which enforced the order 'lie flat with your head inboard during raids if not required for duty', suffered relatively few splinter casualties.

Splinter fragments varied in size, but most of them were little larger than the size of a pea. The track of the wounds caused was usually from below upwards, but though the wound itself might be very small, that was no indication either of the size of the fragment which had entered or of the damage caused to tissues and organs by its penetration. Splinter wounds of the chest or abdomen usually caused intense pain, whereas similar wounds of the limbs were often relatively numb for a period of about an hour. Head wounds were common, with penetration of the skull and brain damage occurring from even tiny fragments. It was found that scalp wounds might occur even when upper deck personnel wore steel helmets, owing to splinters passing either directly, or by ricochet, upwards through the headband. It is of some interest that, on the whole, eye wounds were remarkably rare in the Navy, but the few which did occur were almost all due to bomb splinters.

Although the fact was stressed that bomb splinters were most likely to cause damage among upper deck personnel, this did not mean that personnel between decks were safe from harm when near misses occurred. The near miss was frequently an incident to be dreaded, and in some cases it caused more vital and widespread damage to a particular part of the ship than a direct hit would have done elsewhere. It was frequently found that bomb splinters were capable of passing through the side plating of a destroyer, and though the force of such a splinter might be well spent, so that even a cork life jacket has been known to stop it, this could not be regarded as a general rule. Many severe casualties were caused by splinters passing through a ship's hull, and bomb splinters were even known to cause death after travelling a considerable distance.

An example is seen in the case of a solitary enemy aircraft which dropped a bomb which exploded near to an escort vessel lying at anchor. A splinter passed through the hull of the ship and killed her commander and another officer who were seated in the wardroom at the time. Both suffered severe head wounds.

Another example is seen in the case of the Hospital Ship *Maine*, which was near missed in Alexandria Harbour. Fatal casualties, which included the ship's senior medical officer, were due to bomb splinters which passed through the ship's side, but in this case the size and velocity of the splinters must be considered in relation to the age of the ship and the poor condition of her hull.

'Freak casualties' were always likely to occur from splinters following an explosion of any kind, and could not be guarded against by even the most stringent precautions. An occurrence of this kind is on record, which, though not connected with enemy air attack, nevertheless provides an example of remote and unexpected damage. This instance occurred on March 8, 1941, when a motor torpedo boat caught fire after refuelling in harbour. A petrol tank exploded which seriously injured two of the ship's complement. The fire gained control, and the vessel was towed away from her moorings to avoid damage to other craft in the vicinity. A quarter of an hour later another explosion occurred which was more violent than the first, and which did considerable damage to buildings in neighbouring naval establishments on shore, and also scattered large and small splinters of metal in all directions over a wide area. Among the casualties which occurred was a number of members of the W.R.N.S., employed ashore in the local Coastal Forces base.

One of these casualties was a girl aged 29, who had been working in an office several hundred yards away from the creek in which the motor torpedo boat finally blew up. She was found unconscious after the explosion, and when taken to the nearest first-aid post she was in a collapsed condition, and her pulse was never perceptible. She was removed immediately to the naval hospital nearby, where she was found to be dead. Her death was first of all considered to be due to the effects of blast, but post-mortem examination showed a minute puncture wound of the left chest over the precordium. Post-mortem examination revealed a wound track from this point of entry, which passed through the pericardium and led to a tiny fragment of metal, no larger than a pin's head, firmly embedded deeply in the cardiac muscle.

The consequences of direct hits by bombs on men-of-war were more varied and serious. A certain number of fractures of the limbs or ribs occurred from men being thrown against hatches or bulkheads, and injuries to spine and skull were also added by decks lifting. But these effects were relatively few, and far less devastating than those within the immediate vicinity of the explosion.

It was found that whenever a bomb exploded between decks, the majority of men within 20 ft. would be killed instantly, their bodies being dismembered, eviscerated or even disintegrated. Certainly, men were known to survive at a distance of 20 ft. and even to show no external evidence of injury, but such cases invariably showed nervous manifestations varying from paralysis to 'blast concussion' and death. In the case of the survivors at a distance of over 20 ft., it is curious that their wounds were commonly caused by flying fragments of the ship itself rather than by bomb splinters.

The total mortality from all causes in direct hits was usually about 50 per cent. of those in the space hit or in the path of the blast through an open door. Practically every survivor, whatever his other injuries might be, would be suffering from burns according to the amount of exposed skin surface. These burns were the most characteristic effect of a direct hit. In one ship with 71 casualties, there were 32 dead and the remainder were all cases of burns.

The flash from the explosion usually scorched all naked skin and even travelled up the legs of trousers. As a rule cases of uncomplicated burns confined to the face, hands and legs escaped with their lives, but anything more extensive showed an 80 per cent. mortality. The incidence was greatly reduced following the introduction of Fleet Orders regarding anti-flash gear, which has already been described.

Apart from the flash of an explosion, other sources of fire were always likely to arise in the ship itself, and cordite was likely to ignite. This meant that in addition to the intense heat generated, the factor of irritant and toxic fumes was introduced as a further hazard.

The less serious effects of direct hits included the rupturing of ear drums in personnel without ear protection. As a precaution, all members of every ship's company were provided with rubber ear plugs for use in action. But these were frequently uncomfortable, and needed to be cut down in order to fit the external auditory meatus of the individual, and in any case it is doubtful whether they afforded any better protection than plugs of cotton wool, though they were probably of some psychological value.

It is of interest to note that gas gangrene was an extremely rare complication of wounds in men-of-war. Where it did occur, the wounds were due to bomb splinters, mostly wounds of the thighs. As the splinter had caused a direct wound, it was concluded that the infection must have been carried in from the clothing or skin, a matter of some historical importance if only in justification of the old naval maxim that a sailor was required to bath himself and don clean clothing whenever action was impending.

Gas gangrene was in fact too rare in men-of-war to justify any drastic surgery on board unless the ship was likely to remain at sea for more than thirty hours. Although a naval medical officer was granted wide discretion, and was rarely hampered by directives insisting upon a particular line of treatment for casualties, it was generally recognised that a man-of-war was not a suitable environment for the performance of major surgical procedures. It would probably be true to say that the more experienced the medical officer, the more was this policy observed. A wise senior medical officer would always avoid operative surgery afloat, not only on account of the obvious technical difficulties, but also on account of the many further difficulties which were attached to the nursing and after-care of the patient. Obviously, there were times when operative surgery had to be carried out for reasons of emergency, but it will be realised that action circumstances, with the associated noise, pitching and tossing of the ship, concussion and blast of gunfire and explosions, probable lack of light and vibration of engines, would all reduce the likelihood of surgical success to a minimum. It may perhaps be stated with some truth, that an efficient naval medical officer would never perform 'cold surgery' in a man-of-war, and only emergency surgery when no other course was possible.

As can be imagined, a dictum of this nature was hardly likely to be appreciated by the newly joined medical officer, straight from the teaching hospital, and filled with clinical enthusiasm and surgical ambition. Until he himself had been afloat long enough to understand and realise the true conditions on board a man-of-war, he was apt to feel thwarted and that his skill was wasted.

The reader of this history will probably recall the occasional report in the press of an operation performed at sea, usually a sensational matter, and written in journalese which is careful to include all those details, such as the anaesthetic given by a ship's officer, the young surgeon lashed to a pillar, the patient lashed to the table, and so on, all of which are necessary to maintain the drama of the situation.

But such cases are rare, and the more experienced the medical officer is the more conservative he is likely to be in his surgical outlook.

It may be accepted that major surgical procedures in a man-of-war can only be justified when they are undertaken to save life or to relieve pain, and even in the latter event other less drastic measures would be preferable.

In addition to bombs and torpedoes launched from enemy aircraft against men-of-war, it is on record that a small number of wounds were caused by darts contained in bombs. The record is brief, applied to only one ship, H.M.S. *Sphinx*, and represents little more than a medical curiosity.

Records show that on many occasions machine-gunning of men-of-war and even of survivors in the sea was carried out by enemy aircraft. Nevertheless, the small proportion of casualties from this form of attack, and their relatively minor nature and low mortality were notable features. For instance, an analysis of casualties from machine-gun fire in 13 ships shows that altogether 24 men were hit. Of these, only 2 were killed immediately, while the remainder were chiefly flesh wounds of the limbs. One of the deaths might well have been avoided had the casualty been wearing a steel helmet.

Where bones were struck they were shattered. There were only two cases of penetrating wounds of the chest, both of which survived, and one of the abdomen who died. One of the casualties survived in spite of six separate bullet wounds.

The majority of these 13 ships were small craft presenting a difficult target, and with a small number of exposed personnel. Had the ships been larger, the target might have been less difficult and the number of exposed personnel much greater. But against this must be borne in mind the very limited cover available in the small ship, and the much greater weapon power of the large ship against an attack.

On the whole, the Navy found this form of attack to be ineffective, except for its demoralising and distracting effects on guns' crews and bridge personnel. This was in marked contrast to the effect of bullets aimed by snipers ashore at the bridge personnel of destroyers alongside during the evacuation of France.

The chief medical interest connected with this form of attack was with the special treatment recommended for tracer bullet wounds, neglect of which could result in gross destruction and delayed healing due to retained phosphorus.

MORALE

Study of the short daily details of the above medical officer's journal reveals much of interest in relation to the involved question of the development and maintenance of individual morale afloat. The Royal Navy, no less than the other Fighting Services, accepted the basic principle of war that the newly recruited sailor is not by nature a hero. It was necessary to make him into a fighter by training him to such a pitch that he was able and eager to overcome all instincts of self-preservation and to carry out his task to the limits of his mental and physical capacity. To this end, the Navy relied upon methods based on the power of suggestion, and consisting of rigorous training and discipline, of leadership and confidence in all officers, of an overwhelming pride in the individual's ship possibly out of all proportion to its actual importance, and in traditions of the Service such as saluting the quarterdeck, the ceremony of 'Colours' and the like. The object of the whole training of the man was to create in him such a personal pride that failure to do his duty would become unthinkable.

It was realised that from the time a man joined the Navy in time of war, he might well be in a state of emotional disturbance. The factors likely to bring this about were first of all worry over domestic affairs at home, secondly the strangeness of his new surroundings and new companions, and thirdly the anxiety about the uncertainty of the future. Later on, this anxious state might be more pronounced by the added presence of constant danger at sea.

Probably the most potent of these factors, particularly in the case of the married man, was worry over domestic affairs at home. One medical officer has recorded that 'the vast majority of men who reported to me with minor physical and mental complaints did so immediately after receiving a worrying letter from home'.

The experienced officer would doubtless agree, that although letters from home did much to support the fighting man afloat, there were also times when they could cast him down. That this possibility was well understood elsewhere than in the Navy was shown in the B.B.C. broadcast on this subject, in 1942, which studied the effect of 'the lily-white hand on the bridle'. This broadcast was addressed to the women of the nation, and it advised those whose menfolk were fighting not to worry them with domestic difficulties which would probably be solved anyway by the time the letters were received.

It became the duty of the medical officer afloat to make himself so familiar with the lives and characters of his brother officers and men on board, that he was able to recognise and assess emotional disturbances when they occurred. Symptomatic of unrest of the mind might be irritability with its train of intolerance, petty annoyances and furious arguments among men living in daily close contact. A successful action might well be followed by talkativeness, boasting, with merry drinking and harmless exaggeration when circumstances permitted. Men would tend to laugh at trifling jokes, and to laugh a little longer than normal. Others would give the impression of feeling lonely and inferior. On occasions, members of a ship's company might follow a fight with the enemy with a fight among themselves or with members of another ship's company on shore, as has been described in the journal note above for March 15. All such incidents were typical of the various forms of reaction which a sailor might display following operational duty afloat. This emotional state in the Navy in war-time was recognised as being of immense importance, since it might prepare the mind to accept suggestion. Just as in times of great public anxiety fantastic rumours may be accepted as true, so in this anxious state the mind may be open to suggestion. In this way it would be possible to regard morale as the cumulative effect of suggestion on a personality prepared by the very emergency to receive it.

War-time training in the Navy directed its suggestion towards the idea that 'I am a British sailor. The British sailor has always been the best seaman and the finest fighter, and the hero of the people. Therefore, I am a hero'. The principle of the Service was that nothing in the course of a man's instruction or surroundings must be permitted to arouse counter-suggestions to this conception of himself. Moreover, everything was done to reinforce this conception by insisting on smartness of dress and erect carriage, on rigid discipline, and on personal pride in self, ship, and the Navy. It was rightly considered that the exigencies of war were no excuse for relaxing naval tradition, even as regards minor customs of the Service which the newly entered officer or man might well regard as irksome and even as an absurd waste of time and energy. On the contrary, it was found that the exigencies of war called for an even greater meticulous observation of naval traditions by officers and men newly joined, as this went far towards identifying the modern sailor with the sailor heroes of the past.

Officers were taught that to praise a recruit under training was all important in order to justify his confidence in his own ability, and that where a reprimand was necessary it was essential to couch it in terms which would leave the man's pride and self-respect intact. The principle here observed was that a man without pride could not be expected to fight well. Therefore, should the man commit an offence or make a mistake it was considered infinitely wiser to express surprise that a man of his ability should have so acted, rather than to lash him with words which might imply that he was useless to the Service and the country.

Having once established a man's morale, the next difficult task was to sustain this morale through long periods of tedious and monotonous routine afloat. This brought other factors into play.

As in the case of the soldier and the airman, so in the sailor, the commonest source of conflict in his mind was usually bound up with the fear of failure and the possibility of personal cowardice. Many medical officers recorded evidence which contended that all emotion must have an outlet either in activity or in free discussion, and that should this outlet be denied the results tended to display themselves as a continuous sense of anxious unrest caused by the conflict of three impulses which were denied expression. These three impulses were the natural urge to run away from danger, the disciplined need to fight, and the profound underlying fear of being thought a coward.

From 1941 onwards, it became customary in many ships for medical officers to give explanatory lectures on the reaction of the mind to fear, and there is no doubt that the experienced medical officer could do much in this way to diminish the individual liability of some men to 'nervous breakdown'.

These explanatory lectures adopted the approach that fear must inspire some reaction, the most primitive form being the reaction of flight. Officers responsible for training were taught that this primitive reaction could always be replaced by other action provided that training was thorough. The importance of meticulous instruction was urged, so that every man in the ship would know his exact job under all circumstances. The men themselves came to understand that the essence of the control of fear was to abolish uncertainty. Panic was never likely to occur without uncertainty of what to do or where to go, and such uncertainty could be entirely prevented by training.

Concurrently, the Navy was always able to rely upon the power of example in its officers. This feature of leadership has been described in some quarters as depending on hero worship. Be this as it may, there is little doubt that the power of example remained throughout the war the most important and fundamental element in the mind of the naval rating. Although its psychological machinery would be difficult to explain, and even more difficult to prove, there is probably much to be said for the proposition that each man tended to identify himself with his leader, and within broad limits would be likely to imitate him. The great sea captains of the past owed much of their success to this power of example, and during the Second World War the behaviour of the officers of a man-of-war was again the keystone of the whole structure of the morale of her ship's company.

Naval medical officers afloat came to recognise that the mirror of morale is mood, and that the most dangerous mood is one of boredom and depression and 'bloody-mindedness', predisposing as it does to undesirable emotions and the destruction of the hero idea. To combat this the Navy was always careful that a man should feel that his personal welfare was being considered as much as possible under the prevailing conditions of service. In this respect, as has been described, the organisation of outgoing and incoming mails was considered to be of the greatest importance. Leave and recreation were studied as much as possible. Encouragement, reassurance, praise and example were re-doubled when men were tired, while the feeling of hate too could be instilled with value should the opportunity and need for it ever arise. A further important measure which was encouraged in all men-of-war was that when a ship was in action, a special officer was detailed to stand at a microphone and broadcast what was going on so that men between decks and engineers and stokers in the bowels of the ship should not be left in ignorance of the details and progress of the action.

In some ships, pride of ship and pride of Service were reinforced by pride of racial tradition as well. For example, in one man-of-war, whose officers and ship's company were almost all Scotsmen, pipers were trained, and played at 'Colours' and 'Sunset'. This particular ship had been adopted by the citizens of Aberdeen, was affiliated to the Gordon Highlanders, and had official permission to play on board the musical rendering 'The Cock o' the North'. When engaging the enemy, it was customary for this ship to steam into action with a piper broadcasting by microphone.

The Second World War once again proved that a man-of-war is the finest background possible to foster morale by virtue of two qualities. One is the affectionate, sentimental pride felt alike by officers and men for their ship, and the other the sober fact that in a naval action the safest activity is steady devotion to duty rather than flight.

As regards the maintenance of morale, one of the most important tasks and duties of a ship's medical officer was to observe his brother officers and men constantly from the viewpoint of individual tolerance of active service afloat. The medical officer had to appreciate that people are like different kinds of liquid with different boiling points. By constant daily contact, he had to recognise that each officer and man possessed a 'threshold' of fear which varied between individuals, and which might be low or might be high. Rigorous training and leadership had aimed at increasing the natural 'threshold', but prolonged mental strain and physical hardship endured through months or even years of active service could not fail to reduce the 'threshold'. It was well therefore, to realise that, no matter how high an individual's morale might appear to be, if pushed too far for too long, there must come a time when his 'threshold' would be reached and passed, with the inevitable result that the individual would suddenly collapse.

This sequence of events was always more likely to happen in the case of the senior executive officer who carried on his shoulders the ultimate burden of the ship's welfare and efficiency. What is more, this officer's high sense of duty caused him always to control and hide his personal feelings, as part of his code of setting a good example to his subordinates. He tended to regard evidences of overstrain in himself as personal weakness which he should struggle to overcome, thereby burdening himself even further and establishing the foundations of a vicious circle both mentally and physically. In the struggle to preserve his high sense of duty it would be only natural that he would demand the same from others, and would be quick to regard the normal by-products of mental and physical strain among his subordinates as weaknesses for which they themselves were personally responsible.

It is probably true to state that a final additional factor also existed in the minds of many officers, in that fear of failure was identified with failure of future career. This is not to imply that a naval officer would ever be tempted to place personal interests before the good of his ship and Service. But unfortunately, the very nature of things inside a Fighting Service is such that it is virtually impossible to divorce personal advancement from personal mental and physical stamina. In a Service such as the Royal Navy, which demands the highest possible standard as regards personal example and efficiency, the inherent system which regulates individual careers and advancements to high command rightly looks for characteristics of dogged determination and perseverance which cannot fail to be identified with the axiom that 'only the fittest shall survive'.

In the early stages of the Second World War there is no doubt that many commanding officers were permitted to remain too long in sea commands. This was particularly so in the case of the many overworked destroyers and smaller units of the Fleet. Later, sea commissions were sensibly shortened, and 12 to 18 months of active service afloat at one stretch came to be regarded as the average period during which a commanding officer could be expected to give of his best. To some extent, this principle also came to be observed in the case of all officers and men as the war progressed.

By 1943, the Navy had firmly established a clinical entity honourably labelled 'Fatigue'. This was applied to many officers and men who had fought hard and successfully, and replaced what would formerly have been a diagnosis of 'Anxiety State', thereby avoiding an implied slight upon the man's character and adverse effect upon his Service career. Above all, it enabled a tired officer or man to be rested, and used to fight again later.

A time arrived when it was the duty of every medical officer afloat to anticipate collapse among his companions, and to recognise those symptoms which give warning that the 'threshold' of an individual is being approached. It was the medical officer's duty constantly to keep his commanding officer informed of such matters, in order that men could be rested in time to save them from collapse. Sometimes the evidence of approaching collapse was so slender that great experience on the part of a medical officer was necessary before he could take action, and even then the medical officer himself might be tempted to delay in making the report which it was his duty to make on account of his personal friendship for the officer concerned, and on account of his reluctance to initiate that personal resentment which so frequently was likely to result.

How diffident a medical officer might be in such circumstances is shown in the following report upon a 'key' officer who had conducted himself magnificently in action on numerous occasions, but who, it was now considered, was reaching the stage when he should be rested:

'As a result of prolonged and intimate observation of this officer during recent months, the following considered medical report is submitted for information and for whatever action might be regarded as desirable:

'To understand fully the present state of this officer, insight must be gained of his personal mental make-up. He has a supreme sense of duty, loyalty to his captain, his ship and his department. Added to this is a passionate desire to do well, which is almost pathetic in its intensity. The efficiency of his ship he regards as a personal matter resting on his shoulders alone, and this latter has now become an obsession with him.

'The cumulative results of the mental effort needed to maintain the high standard he has set for himself have been that a vicious circle has been established in his mind, with the result that his sense of proportion has suffered and his brain has become a highly tuned machine which he now feels must be kept running at all costs. The final factor which stimulates him mentally to an ever increasing speed is a fear of failure, which amounts almost to a phobia.

'The evidences of mental fatigue have been obvious for a considerable time, and I do not think it is realised how slender might be the thread which now remains. Among the many manifestations which support my opinion are the following instances:

(1) During and after action he suffers acutely from mental strain, possibly more than the rest of us who are probably less efficient than he is. There is no question of morale or fortitude, both of which are admirable in his case. It is fear of failure or of something going wrong.

After the second attack on our convoy nine months ago he was mentally exhausted, and asked me to give him benzedrine to keep him awake. At that time he came to me one morning, during a lull in action, in a state bordering on mental collapse, when reaction and emotion had almost got the better of him. He was almost at breaking point. After our engagement with the enemy three months ago he was in a similar state.

(2) Should he have the opportunity to rest, he just cannot relax, and his brain must continue to work. During the course of one of our operations, he passed any spare moments he had in turning his mind on to the material for a book of instruction for newly joined officers. Between our two most recent operations, he spent each 48 hour rest period in developing a paper in which he attempted to deal with the complete post-war reconstruction of R.N.V.R. training. The magnitude of such a task did not seem to strike him.

(3) Irritability and impetuosity of speech and action are most noticeable.

(4) When he sleeps he does not really sleep well, and his brain continues to race. His wife has disclosed to me that on leave he is most restless at night and has shouted 'aircraft', etc., during his sleep.

'Physical effects will inevitably follow such a mental state, and it must be understood that the apparently robust bodily build and appearance of this officer are most deceptive. His stamina is not at all in keeping with his appearance, as evidenced by:

A single inoculation of ½ c.c. of T.A.B.T. affected him more than anyone in the ship.

Frequent headaches and insomnia. For some months it has been my impression that he takes more aspirin habitually than is usual in a young man.

A recurrent infection of his gums.

A recent bout of gastritis which confined him to bed.

A recent attack of influenza, he being the only officer on board to have succumbed.

'My experience and professional instinct warn me that at this moment the physical and mental state of this officer are such that two serious questions must be faced:

Can his brain continue to function efficiently in its present state of high pressure? My feeling is that unless given an adequate period of rest, collapse with a consequent error of judgement must occur eventually.

What will be his physical state during the months to come after his recent indispositions? Here again, unless adequate rest is given, he will continue to be a candidate for any epidemic which we might encounter in our travels.

'I have long made the physical and mental fitness of this officer my personal responsibility. He is a personal friend of mine for whom I have great affection. I make this statement that it may be realised how fully aware I am of the serious nature of this report, and it is not one which I would undertake lightly, particularly at this present stage in the officer's career.

'In his present state I would liken him to a highly tuned, supercharged racing car, capable of giving a brilliant performance, but only for a time. A carefully conserved touring car, with a more phlegmatic and slower performance, would probably last longer and would be more reliable in the long run.

'My opinion is therefore that this officer should be employed ashore in a quiet capacity for a period of at least three months. Such a procedure would have an advantageous effect upon his future well-being, and would avert any breakdown in the near future which might have serious repercussions upon the safety of the ship.'

The subsequent events which followed this report are of some interest, and show how careful the Navy had become to make sure that its highly trained personnel were not wasted and worn out.

As a result of this report, the officer concerned was gently persuaded into a co-operative state of mind, and was discharged to hospital. He was given a period of complete rest for some weeks, and was then retained in a quiet and inactive shore appointment for a few months. He was then sent to a sea-going appointment. In his refreshed physical and mental state, it so happened that within a few days his ship was involved in one of the most important and eventful naval actions of the war. In this action, the success of his ship was due in part to the high standard of efficiency of this particular officer and his department on board, and it is fitting that the story should end by recording that the officer was decorated for his gallantry in this action.

Here then, is a single example, one of many, of the way in which an observant medical officer afloat could save an individual from collapse, thereby permitting him to be restored to health and made capable of being of further use to his Service and his country.

In the particular case which has been described, records of the circumstances suggest that there was certain conflict of opinion about the case. But it is of interest to note that such conflict as did arise concerned doctors, and not the executive authorities as might have been expected from the diffident and deferential tone of the medical report which was made.

Analysing the circumstances, it is quite obvious that the medical officer concerned felt that it was his duty to represent a picture which he considered might terminate in calamity unless certain steps were taken in time. But his experience in the Service warned him that the key position held by the officer concerned was such, that any attempt to have him rested might meet with executive criticism, or even opposition. Facts would be called for, and the facts were few enough to substantiate the medical officer's anticipation of a collapse which the lay mind might well feel justified in regarding as unlikely to occur. At the same time the medical officer felt that he could be sure of obtaining the support of his Fleet Medical Officer should any doubts be cast upon his own opinion.

In point of fact the very reverse happened. When consulted, it was the Fleet Medical Officer who doubted the wisdom of suggesting that an efficient officer might be near to collapse on such flimsy evidence. The view of this senior officer was that potential disaster should not be anticipated until proved more definitely by concrete physical facts.

Nevertheless, the executive authorities took a different view, which was that collapse should be averted at all costs. It is of even greater interest to record that these authorities were inclined to go even further and to suggest that the substance of the medical report showed that the medical officer concerned had been aware of the patient's approaching collapse for several months, and that therefore he might almost himself be regarded as having been dilatory in bringing these matters to notice!

Concurrently with these precautions that officers and ratings should not be retained on active service afloat to the point of collapse, steps were also taken in the reverse direction, with a view to making certain that there was no abuse of the new measures which had come into being.

Also, it was considered necessary to record in black and white that the primary duty of medical officers of the Fleet was to render men fit for service, and not to involve themselves in obscure and often academic clinical controversy.

With this in mind a Fleet Order was published and circulated with a view to explaining standards of medical fitness in relation to the present manning situation. The preamble of this Fleet Order conveyed an idea of the present difficulties of the manning situation, which had made it vital that the number of men found medically unfit for sea service should be limited to those whose medical state justified this classification.

It was believed that there was unfortunately a number of men whose only real ailment was an unwillingness to serve at sea. Such cases frequently presented many difficulties, and the authorities felt that it was desirable that the nature of these difficulties should be realised by all concerned.

The Order explained that many medical officers now serving in the Navy had had little Service experience, and that their natural inclination was always to make the presumed well-being of a patient their only consideration. Medical officers were reminded, however, that experience showed that there were other factors which frequently had to be taken into account, and that these other factors involved both the interests of the Navy and fairness to other ratings.

It had frequently happened that a patient who was determined to avoid sea service, sometimes with truly stated and sometimes with untruly stated symptoms, almost invariably succeeded in getting himself discharged to depot or hospital for investigation. Such a man, should his symptoms be false, would be found by a naval hospital to be fit, and would subsequently be redrafted to sea.

On arriving in his new ship, the man would re-state his ailments, adding the information that he had already been in hospital for the same trouble. As likely as not he would now be discharged to hospital or depot for further investigation. The result would be that the man had established for himself a 'hospital history', which eventually made it almost impossible to get him to sea, or to keep him at sea.

The terms of the Fleet Order well appreciated the difficulties which confronted medical officers, in particular sea-going medical officers, when dealing with such men who 'knew the ropes'. It was also fully appreciated that heads of departments in men-of-war under whom such men were employed, could not fail to display a natural desire to get rid of a 'passenger', *via* the medical route if possible, and this natural desire was likely to operate as an additional incentive to send such men into hospital.

The Fleet Order now urged closer co-operation between medical officers on the one hand, and the executive officers, heads of departments, and divisional officers on the other. This co-operation was considered essential in order that suspected malingerers might be adequately and fairly dealt with.

It was also considered essential that ships' officers should take a broad view of the interests of the Service as a whole. No matter how tempting it might be to an individual ship, to get rid of a rating with a long and doubtful medical history, it had to be remembered that this also meant the loss of one more rating to man the Fleet.

The cumulative effect of such action by many ships would be most serious, on account of the total numbers involved, besides clogging the drafting machinery with difficult cases who would continually pass through it with no prospect of finding a more useful billet than that from which they had started. To obviate the serious position which was thus likely to arise, the Fleet Order directed that the following action was to be taken in regard to all future cases suspected of malingering:

(a) An insight into the man's character was to be afforded to the medical officer by the officers under whom the man had been employed. The existing Fleet Order which required an executive officer to render a report on all neuro-psychiatric cases was now to be extended to include all cases suspected of malingering.

(b) If, after frank exchange of opinion with the executive officer, the medical officer still decided to send the case to hospital or depot for investigation, a full statement, including the above report, was to accompany the man.

(c) In the case of any man suspected of substantial malingering, this suspicion was to be noted on his medical history sheet, as well as the result of any investigations, and a record of any disciplinary action already taken.

(d) Suspected malingerers, on discharge from hospital, were to be the subject of special reports in detail, and of thorough investigation by naval depots. Hospital specialists were to be consulted as necessary, and should disciplinary action be applicable, this was to be taken by the depot authorities before the man was redrafted to sea.

DIET

Apart from a passing reference to shortage of fresh vegetables and the use of Vitamin 'C', the above medical officer's journal makes little mention of food or diet in his ship. It certainly seems that food or diet never constituted a problem at any time in that particular ship to the extent of being a subject worthy of comment.

This is as would be expected, because, in contrast to the other Fighting Services, ships of the Royal Navy have advantages in that they carry their supplies so to speak 'under their hat', and even if they wander far they are unlikely to have to wait for their supply column or their field kitchen. Towards the closing stages of the war, any small delays or inconveniences which had been experienced in this respect had been reduced, if not entirely eliminated, by the establishment of the Fleet Train in the Pacific area.

Much has been recorded historically about the development of adequate and suitable diet for seamen engaged on long voyages. But in the present century, times have changed and the average naval rating afloat is not expected to expend the same physical and muscular energy as in days of sail. Most of the heavy work of the past is now done by machines.

The Second World War went far towards proving that the diet of the modern naval rating was not comparable with that required by a navvy, a dock labourer, a coal miner or a soldier engaged in muscular effort in jungle or desert warfare. As regards quantity of food, the Royal Navy was at all times more than amply supplied in its rations, and many medical officers felt that their ships' companies ate too much and got too little physical exercise. There were times too, when the good living on board men-of-war could not fail to be compared to the reduced fare upon which naval families ashore were managing to exist.

The authorities were always mindful that the food required by a naval rating to maintain his fighting efficiency should be of the kind to keep mind and body alert and ready for action, while taking note of the special difficulties to be faced according to where his ship might be serving. On the one hand there was the cold, wet and absence of sun in Northern Waters, and the stifling enervating heat of tropical seas on the other. Clearly, the same diet in the two sets of circumstances, even if correct in all its calories and constituent parts, would be quite wrong in aiding good health and fighting efficiency.

Speaking generally, the Admiralty could only plan that the rations supplied to the Navy were fully adequate in all the known requirements, and the dietary was constantly under the review of experts. Legislation for every type of local condition was impossible, however, and in some cases, a particular ship might have to plan for itself. Naturally, in many ways, the difficulties were greater than in any previous war because the supply of so many things became either severely diminished or cut off. Furthermore, whatever plans were made, it had to be remembered that the sailor, no less than his contemporary in the Army or Air Force, is a creature of habit, who tends to demand steak and kidney pudding and suet pudding and treacle, regardless of whether his ship is in the arctic or in the Tropics. Any departure from what he himself has come to regard as the traditional bulk and quality necessary to his needs he is likely to view with grave suspicion and even resentment. As a rider to this attitude of mind, it is only natural that the professional sailor should be averse to the introduction of 'stunt feeding' into his diet.

During the Second World War the Navy was fortunate to have as its Medical Director-General a doctor of scientific eminence combined with shrewdness and great common sense. Over many years a great amount of scientific work had been performed with a view to establishing the most suitable form of diet for seamen, but in spite of this there was still uncertainty as regards the ideal or optimum amount of any of the essential constituents of a dietary, i.e. proteins, carbohydrates, fats, salts, vitamins and water. Whatever results were achieved scientifically had always to be modified to allow for individual and climatic variations. The essence of the task was always to see that the ration of the sailor should provide a sufficient supply of these essential constituents, and there appeared to be no difficulty in ensuring this with the exception of those elusive vitamins which, while essential for health, could not always be made visible on the plate.

During the period between the wars vitamins had become popular 'news', and even the Royal Navy showed signs of becoming afraid of them. Vitamins were a modern discovery, and although of supreme importance, they were not visible to the eye. They tended therefore to be shrouded in mystery for the ordinary man, to become 'good copy' for the popular newspapers, and commercially they were excellent material with which to exploit the public and even the Fighting Services.

The Medical Director-General of the Navy was not slow to warn the Navy as a whole that it must not be gulled or alarmed by any publicity campaign which aimed at the widespread introduction of synthetic and tablet forms of vitamin into the daily life of the population. A memorandum was circulated to explain that the chief known vitamin which might concern the Navy was ascorbic acid or Vitamin 'C', contained in fruits (especially berries) and vegetables (potatoes and greens). Its absence or deficiency over a long period would give rise to scurvy. Nevertheless, scurvy was essentially a sailor's disease in the days of long, slow voyages without fresh food, and the Service was reminded that the prevention of scurvy by the provision of fruit juice had been discovered in the Navy long before Vitamin 'C' had even been heard of. In the modern Navy there was no reason why there should be any deficiency of Vitamin 'C' in the diet of ships which could obtain and use regular supplies of fruit or potatoes and green vegetables. But in any case, the vitamin was already supplied in jam and in many other simple ways devised by the Navy's food experts. The introduction of dehydrated vegetables marked a considerable and important practical advance.

In spite of this memorandum, occasional alarms of scurvy were received from units of the Fleet, and these received thorough scientific investigation. But it was always found that the sponginess and bleeding of the gums which had been reported was due to Vincent's disease, and had been enthusiastically reported as scurvy by mistake.

Mention must be made of the attention paid by the Navy to the controversial question of vitamin deficiency in connexion with night vision and the power of adapting the eye to see in the dark. It was considered that Vitamin 'A' played a part, its chief source being dairy products such as milk, butter and cheese, fish such as salmon and herrings, and also liver of all kinds. Should this Vitamin 'A' be absent or deficient it was considered that the power to see at night might deteriorate.

There were, however, other causes of poor night vision beside lack of Vitamin 'A', and investigation showed that the faculty of seeing at night varied greatly in different individuals quite apart from any question of diet. The Navy's food experts were able to show that the amount of Vitamin 'A' in the normal Service diet was more than adequate to prevent any deterioration of night vision. The important thing to understand was that, provided there was the usual amount of Vitamin 'A' in a man's food, any further amount of extra Vitamin 'A' given to him could have no power to increase his capacity to see at night. Hence it was futile to give vitamin tablets to night lookouts and aircrews, etc., in the hope of improving their night vision, unless it was known that the food they were getting was already deficient in Vitamin 'A'.

Throughout the whole Navy afloat, medical officers and the experienced supply officers of the Fleet constantly co-operated to keep the sailor suitably and adequately fed. Their task was not easy, because quite apart from difficulties of supplies, they frequently had to combat the popular opinion which existed even among flag officers, that vitamin deficiency must exist unless supplied medicinally in addition to normal diet. Some flag officers became so heavily infected with the wave of 'vitamin publicity' which had swept through the United States, that they came to regard themselves as expert advisers to their doctors and supply officers, a reversal of the procedure normally observed in the Navy. It is recorded that on one occasion, in the Tropics, an experienced senior medical officer was directly and deliberately corrected by an inspecting Commander-in-Chief, who had considered the diet supplied to sailors locally to be unsuitable and inadequate, and in any case certainly needing to be supplemented by 'vitamins' in some proprietary form!

But, as in the case of this particular medical officer, a naval doctor in such circumstances would always be likely to accept such correction in the spirit with which it was conveyed, and he would certainly keep his own counsel and control the irritation he might feel, even if he permitted such irritation to arise. This reaction of an experienced naval medical officer was one which would be natural in him in the light of his long training. Understanding the background of the Navy, he would fully realise at such a time that the attitude of the flag officer concerned would not so much represent criticism of the medical officer's ability, but rather should be regarded as evidence of that interest and consideration which it is the duty and habit of senior naval officers to display as regards the personal welfare of the men under their command. Commanding officers in the Royal Navy have been so trained over the course of years, that the constant well-being of their ships' companies becomes second nature and the subject of continual study. In their constant aim to do what was best for their men, the modern trend induced by 'vitamin publicity' made it most difficult for their lay minds to sum up the situation, and it was at times even more difficult for the medical mentality to convince them that ships of war could depend on obtaining, with a little care in the provision of vegetables and jams, everything which was required for a complete and adequate dietary.

But once commanding officers had been converted to this understanding and belief, medical and supply officers were faced with yet a further task, which was to convince them that even the best diet could still be spoilt both in palatability and vitamin content by bad or prolonged cooking. This was something which no general instructions could provide against. It was something which commanding officers of individual ships had to appreciate and bear in mind. In this respect, quite early in the war, the Admiralty was careful to inform commanding officers that they were expected to accept responsibility in this important matter, and that they must constantly guard against the possibility of good rations and their essential content being reduced in nutritional value by bad cooking, with the inevitable result that fighting efficiency would be impaired.

Following the many scares and rumours which arose from time to time, it was with great satisfaction that the Medical Department of the Admiralty was able to record at the end of the war that there had been no scurvy in the Royal Navy, which had confirmed the view originally expressed that there should never be any need, except in most exceptional circumstances, for the supply of synthetic or tablet Vitamin 'C'.

Though not strictly a medical matter, doctors afloat did find themselves likely to be consulted by officers of the supply department who had the responsibility of organising 'action messing' in men-of-war. 'Action messing' was concerned not so much with the quality, quantity or nutritional value of food as with the manner in which the sailor could best be supplied with his food in an edible form during lulls in action, without being required to leave his place of duty. The Second World War soon showed that enemy action at sea might last for hours or even days on end, and during this time it would be virtually impossible for men to leave their posts. In every ship therefore, it became necessary to build up an organisation whereby food and drink could be prepared and distributed with a minimum of time and trouble. No general directive was issued for this purpose, but individual ships were left to make their own arrangements. These arrangements varied according to the size, type and age of the ship, and according to the size of her company. The organisation also varied according to the climatic conditions, and also the type of operation upon which the ship was being employed.

For example, 'action messing' in Northern waters involved a constant supply of hot soup and tea or cocoa, combined with such items as hot meat pies, which could be eaten by hand. In these waters, it was also necessary for some improvised shelter to be adjacent to a man's action station, and it was also important to remember that china or plastic mugs or cups were to be preferred to metal utensils which might freeze on to the lips or fingers.

In tropical waters different considerations would apply, and though ample fluids needed constantly to be available, it was found, in general, that prolonged action inhibited a man's appetite and he tended not to feel hungry. Engine room personnel needed even greater consideration, although they had already long been catered for to some extent by a Service supply of gruel while on duty. Also, in the Tropics, lime juice had been supplied each day to all members of a ship's company from Service sources for many years.

As regards 'action messing' in the Tropics, attention was paid to the bodily need for water and salt, and this need was also considered generally, quite apart from circumstances of action.

Though always mindful of this need, by May 1943, the Royal Navy had noted with interest the results of investigation carried out by the United States Naval (Medical) Authorities with a view to determining the requirements of water and sodium chloride for men working in high temperatures. On the basis of these findings, the following recommendations were made to all ships:

(a) Water should, if possible, be made available at all times during the day for men working in hot compartments, or in hot climates. They should be strongly encouraged to drink as much as they want whenever they are thirsty. By this means a very striking improvement in efficiency may be gained. Water considerably in excess of the amount required to quench thirst is more beneficial than merely the amount necessary to quench thirst.

(b) When the water supply is limited, men should be taught that a hard day's work may become uncomfortable, but can be tolerated although efficiency decreases progressively throughout the day. They should be encouraged to drink as much as they wish at night and in the morning before starting work, and instructed to consume their limited ration in small sips throughout the day.

(c) Men working in hot environments will need an average of 15 to 20 g. of sodium chloride per day. Since the average diet contains only from 10 to 15 g. a day, from 5 to 10 g. (1 to 2 level teaspoons or 7 to 15 of the 10-g. salt tablets) must be taken in addition. Preferably, this salt should not be administered during the day's work, but with the food and during rest periods, especially in the evening.

Some men may fail to take sufficient salt with meals, and facilities for the ingestion of salt, during or between watches, may therefore be necessary. In this connexion, it should be noted that salt tablets frequently cause irritation of the stomach with pain and nausea, especially when swallowed whole. Therefore, whenever practicable salting the drinking water should be preferred. A level teaspoon of salt per gallon of water is sufficient, and when no more is used a salty taste can barely be noticed.

(d) Excessive amounts of salt should be avoided, since they lead to unpleasant symptoms of thirst, gastric irritation, and occasionally nausea, diarrhoea and vomiting. Excess may therefore result in a measurable decrease in efficiency for work in the heat just as much as may result from a deficiency of salt.

In addition it was directed that all officers and men should have explained to them the fundamentals of this method of meeting the requirements of water and salt when working in hot environments, and the improved physical condition and better performance that might be expected from following out these instructions.

MEDICAL STORES AND EQUIPMENT

In the previous volume of this naval history, the chapter concerned with naval medical stores and equipment explains the vast increase of commitments which arose during the course of the war, and also gives some idea of the many difficulties which had to be overcome. These difficulties covered problems of production, problems of packing, problems of transit, and the recurrent problem of losses by enemy action. The chapter closes, however, with the statement that it was to the credit of naval medical administration and the small and overworked Pharmaceutical Branch of the Royal Navy, that at no time during the Second World War was there anything approaching a major breakdown in the supply of medical stores and equipment, either to the Fleet or to establishments on shore.

This statement is so emphatic, that it is necessary at this point in this volume of the Navy's operational medical history, to confirm its truth, because the frequent and almost day to day references to medical stores' problems in the above medical officer's journal might well be construed as casting some doubt upon its credibility.

There is no doubt that all over the world H.M. ships repeatedly engaged upon operational duties involving action with the enemy, did constantly find themselves short of medical stores and equipment. This was so common an occurrence as to become a subject of jocular comment in the great Fleet anchorages. When a damaged ship entered harbour, in a condition which at first glance made it obvious that she would need repairs at dockyard hands which would put her out of commission for a considerable period, it became customary to point out the various small boats which would be approaching her for various reasons as she came to anchor, with the comment: 'There go the doctors'! The inference was that whenever such a ship appeared over the horizon, there was a race between the doctors from all other ships in the vicinity in order to 'steal' her medical stores.

It is perhaps, only fair to state that this routine was one which was not wholly confined to the Medical Department, because surplus supplies of all kinds, from food and clothing to paint and canvas were also tempting objects to be coveted and acquired either as replacements or as reserve material to be conserved against future shortages. Also, it is perhaps, only fair to admit that the sailor, be he officer or rating, is no less a practised 'scrounger' than his soldier or airman contemporary in the other Fighting Services! Circumstances of war have always led to shortages of all kinds, with the result that the desire and tendency to hoard anything which may be useful is encouraged. This is so even in the case of the civilian ashore, and is therefore doubly so in the case of those individuals whose lives are spent in the isolation of a ship at sea. The urge to hoard becomes paramount, and is evidence not so much of present existing deficiencies as evidence of fear of deficiencies which might arise in the future. This tendency to be acquisitive which becomes evident in every fighting man is a natural symptom of war itself, and really represents another example of 'over insurance'.

With this understanding of the sailor's mentality, it is possible to study with tolerance and even with amusement the devices to which medical officers resorted in order to insure against deficiencies in their supplies, and instances of which have been given in the above journal.

In point of fact, whenever a ship did find itself deficient in medical stores following enemy action, application to the nearest naval medical store for replacements, always and without exception, met with a response which was both prompt and adequate. It is perhaps a legitimate matter for criticism that a permanent medical store depot was not constructed in the area of the vast Fleet anchorage at Scapa Flow until comparatively late in the war. Nevertheless, this question of the supply of medical stores and equipment to ships engaged on active operations at sea was one which involved other considerations, and which would have been in no way solved by extra provision in the Scapa Flow area.

One constant difficulty was that of transport, which usually involved supplies for any individual ship being carried by road, rail, sea and sometimes by air. The other difficulty was the unpredictable movements of units of the Fleet. This was a difficulty which called for almost supernatural intuition if it was to be solved to the satisfaction of everybody.

The above journal gives instances to illustrate this difficulty. A ship found itself short of medical stores at Scapa Flow. Replacements were immediately despatched from a medical store depot in Dunfermline, and so commenced a journey involving transport by road, rail and sea. Before this journey was half over, the ship had left Scapa Flow and had arrived at Plymouth. At Plymouth, stores were obtained locally, and the ship left for Gibraltar and North Africa. In due course the ship arrived at Newcastle and repeated her demand to Dunfermline. The original consignment was still undelivered, but the store depot willingly despatched duplicate replacements. But before this consignment could be wholly received, the ship had again disappeared from the proposed port of delivery.

With such rapid movements multiplying and occurring daily in various parts of the world, it is no wonder that ships' medical officers afloat and medical stores' authorities ashore found themselves almost in despair at times.

To this difficulty occasioned by a ship's sudden and unpredictable movements there can never be a satisfactory answer. The very nature of war at sea demands that a man-of-war should at all times be ready to proceed to any part of the world at short notice. Apart from a ship's preliminary training period and periods of refitting, she must always be in a constant state of readiness. Future movements always tend to be sudden and secret, and whatever other reason may exist, the overall need for security is obvious.

SECURITY

On the subject of security it is suggested that in some units of the Fleet, secrecy and security about future operational movements were carried to an extreme as regards their medical departments, which did not make for all-round efficiency. An instance is seen in the above journal note for October 30. After stating, on October 29, that both himself and other heads of departments are equally in ignorance of the ship's destination, the medical officer repeats that he still has no knowledge of the ship's destination at the moment. His personal anxiety about his own department's capabilities to deal with unknown circumstances ahead is revealed by his further note which he elaborates to the extent of expressing the difficulties of planning ahead. He mentions yellow fever inoculation as a possible omission. He then expresses his view that there is a tendency for doctors to be left out of things until the last moment, or until they are expected to advise without reasonable warning.

On the other hand, the same journal gives numerous instances of the medical department being made well aware of the requirements of future operations.

This whole question is one which arose on occasions during the course of the Second World War. Some medical officers, including those holding staff appointments to flag officers, complained that they were not fully acquainted with impending events. Others did not hold this view. But possibly this lack of unanimity may itself be regarded as evidence of a weakness in the chain of administrative control. It is

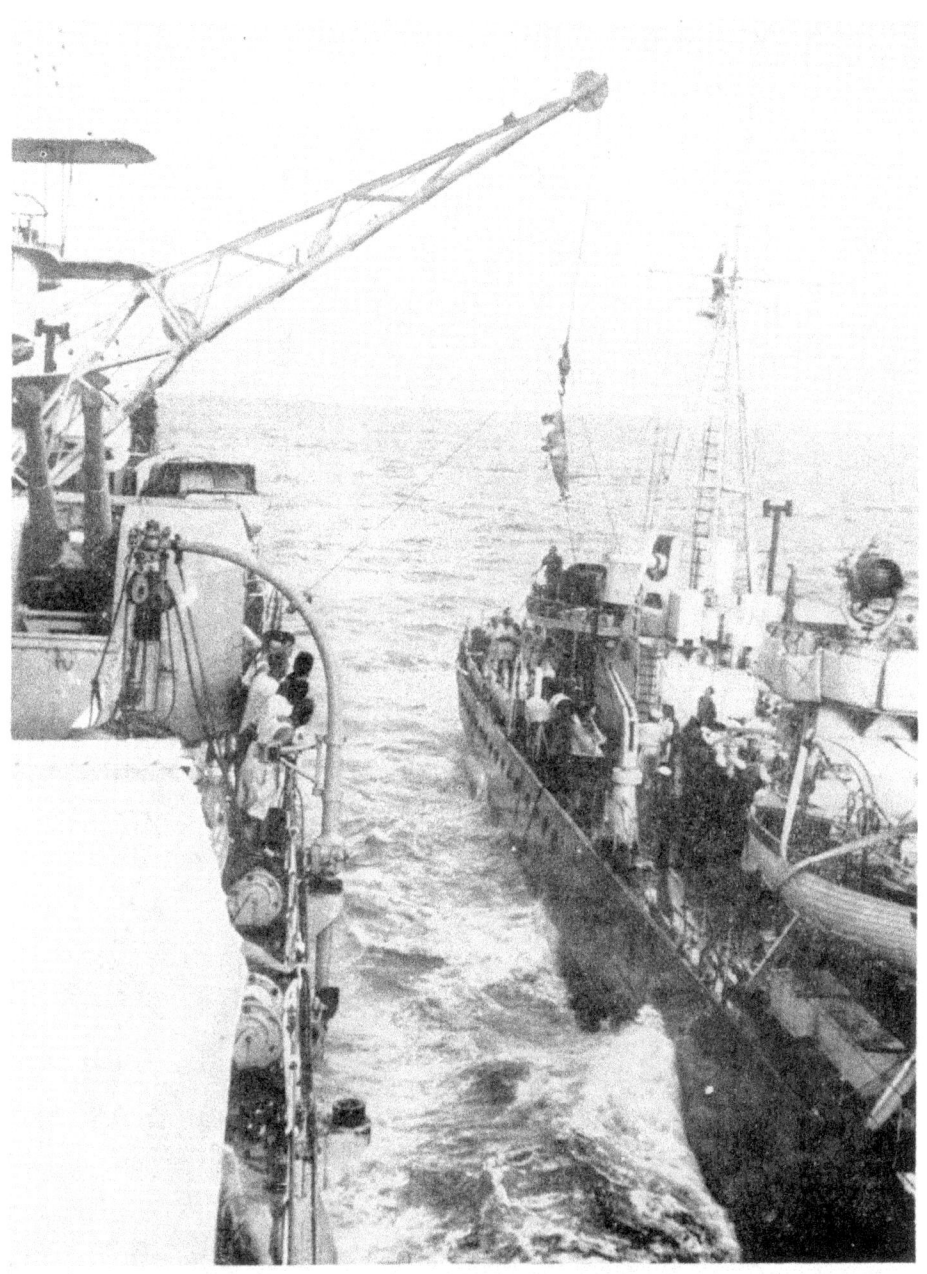

PLATE VII. Casualties being transferred at sea by winch.

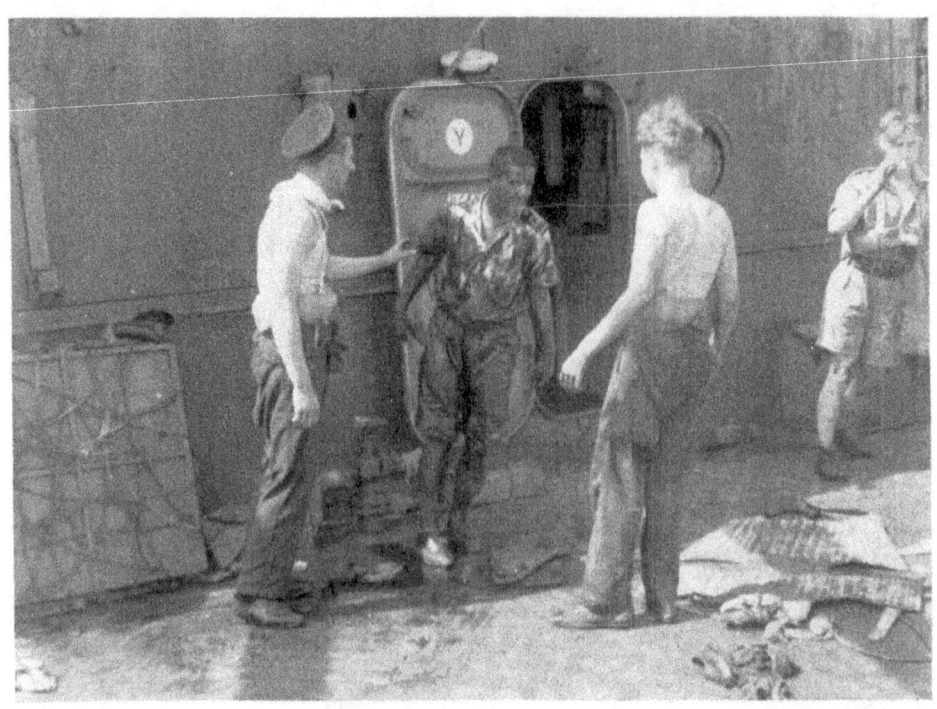

PLATE VIII. A Casualty rescued from sea covered with fuel oil.

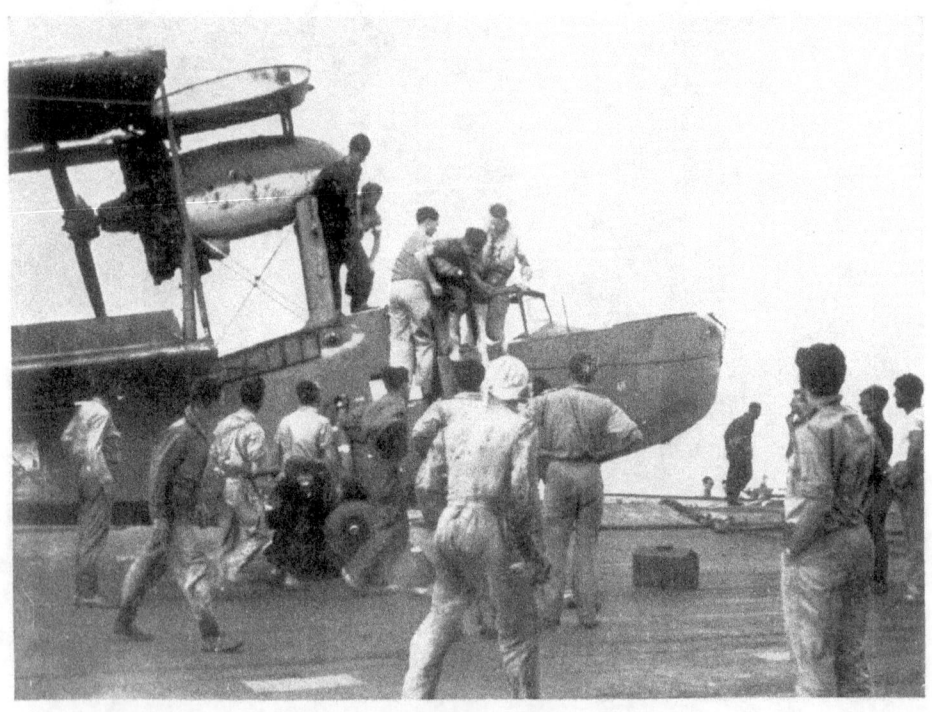

PLATE IX. A Fleet Air Arm Casualty.

probable that there were times when security requirements granted flag officers and commanding officers no discretion. It is probable too, that there were times when flag officers and commanding officers were permitted to exercise discretion and to reveal details of impending operations to members of their staffs and heads of departments most likely to be involved. It is only natural that in these latter circumstances, such discretion would be exercised in a different way by different commanding officers, with the result that in one ship the medical department would be made fully aware of its future commitments, while in another ship, similarly employed, the medical department would be left in complete ignorance.

It is not suggested that failure of the executive to consult the medical department about, or to acquaint it with impending operations afloat, was in any way widespread. Neither, in cases where the omission was evident, could it be claimed that any breakdown occurred in the medical organisation. But the fact that medical officers could complain that they had not been fully informed of certain contingencies, and were therefore forced to improvise at short notice, suggests that from time to time a weakness in liaison did exist in this respect.

RELATIONS BETWEEN THE MEDICAL DEPARTMENT AND THE EXECUTIVE

At the beginning of the first chapter of the Administration Volume of this History it was remarked that in a history devoted to the Medical Branch of a Fighting Service, it is essential to give some idea of the basic principles of relationship involved, and how it has been possible for the Royal Navy and the profession of medicine to combine to the advantage of each.

This statement is of some importance, implying as it does the necessary existence of the naval medical machine as an essential ingredient of a great Fighting Service. Translating this statement into more simple terms, what is meant is that the Royal Navy is very dependent upon its doctors, no less than upon its engineers, its electricians, its supply officers, its instructors, its constructors and its dental surgeons. The system observed, which is both essential and convenient, is that the executive is the responsible branch of the Service, but dependent upon the other subordinate branches which act towards the executive in an advisory capacity.

In the chapter on Preventive Medicine in the Administration Volume some mention is also made of the relationship existing between the executive and their doctors.

The essential observation to be made is that if the full medical commitments of a ship were to be met in the course of an impending operation against the enemy, the medical department must be given sufficient information of the circumstances ahead in order to be able to make the necessary preparations to meet them. In other words, operational planning in the Fleet had to include medical planning as well, and should this point be overlooked, a ship's medical department tended to be hampered and embarrassed.

As regards medical planning it is perhaps most informative to study a difference which existed between the Navy and the Army in the attitude of each of these Services towards its Medical Branch. In the Army, as long ago as 1930, the principle was accepted that a knowledge of staff duties was essential to the medical authorities if they were to be capable of advising on and arranging for future operational requirements. Long before the Second World War, two medical officers were nominated and included in every Army Staff Course. These officers were specially selected, and were not required to sit the competitive examination for the Staff Colleges at Camberley or Quetta. But in the Royal Navy, medical officers received no such training, and although the Army principle was adopted in the Royal Air Force Medical Service at a much later date, doctors in the Navy had to acquire what small knowledge they did gain of planning and staff duties in the light of their own experience as they went along. It was only long after the Second World War had come to an end, and with the example of the Medical Corps of the United States Navy, that the Royal Navy at last conceded the wisdom and necessity which made it desirable to appoint selected naval medical officers to the Royal Naval College, Greenwich, for training in staff duties.

DENTAL SERVICE

The existence of dental difficulties afloat in a man-of-war has been amply illustrated by almost day to day references in the above journal. Reference to the chapter on the dental organisation in the administration volume will show some of the reasons which caused these difficulties. Obviously, unless a dental surgeon could be carried in every man-of-war it would be impossible to give complete satisfaction to everybody demanding dental treatment. Such a course would naturally be impossible and uneconomical. As it was, the few dental surgeons afloat did their best to cope with the vast dental requirements of the Fleet, and could in no way be blamed if they failed to achieve perfection within their restricted limitations.

STRAIN OF ACTIVE SERVICE AFLOAT

Study of the above journal cannot fail to reveal the insidious fatigue and exhaustion, both mental and physical, which would gradually permeate through the being of officers and men after months of active service afloat. Periods of leave ashore were limited, 'organised monotony' was the rule for the most part, with the danger of death or wounding ever present. It is not surprising that there were times when there was disorientation of time and place, as evidenced by small discrepancies which appear between recorded incidents in the journal and the official authentic records of the same events.

Few people on board had much time for personal leisure, and it can be seen that medical officers, no matter how small their medical duties might be, were fully occupied in satisfying the domestic demands of their ships. While combatant officers were busily engaged at their various tasks, non-combatants were no less busy in attending to the welfare of the ship and her complement. The many hours passed in censoring mails show how burdensome this task must have been, and how much of it was borne by doctors and chaplains. That the task was necessary there is no doubt, but that it might have been better effected in central censoring depots on shore is also a question worthy of consideration. Suffice it to say that the bulk of the burden of censoring letters at a speed consistent with the welfare of the sailors who had written them, fell upon the shoulders of the medical officers of the Fleet throughout the whole course of the war.

The close harmony and liaison which existed between chaplains and doctors afloat is something which would be expected, because in the Royal Navy it has always been recognised that the spiritual needs of the sailor should be cared for no less than his physical and mental wellbeing. The stress and strain of war afloat called for much human understanding of men's personal problems, and doctors and padres habitually worked hand in hand in these matters.

REFITTING IN DRY DOCK

A brief reference to a period in dry dock is given in the above journal. The description is one which might be applied to the case of any man-of-war in such circumstances, in the United Kingdom, in winter.

The civilian does not always appreciate that when a ship, which after all is a sailor's home, enters dockyard hands, the home life of the sailor is completely disrupted for the time being. Should a person's house ashore be invaded by decorators, builders and plumbers, the situation is often regarded as desperate, whereas it is really little more than inconvenient to the occupier. But a similar invasion of a ship is much more than inconvenient to the sailor whose home it is. The first of his difficulties is that of hygiene and sanitation. In short, faecal and urinary excretions of individuals on board, which are normally ejected into the sea, cannot be ejected into a dry dock. This means that the sailor must clamber over the side of his ship and visit a dockside lavatory, which might be a considerable distance away, in order to open his bowels or pass urine.

Likewise, water supplies on board will either be restricted, or probably suspended altogether, and the sailor will have to go ashore in order to wash and shave himself.

With the ship's dynamos out of action and her fires damped, lighting on board will be from shore supply, and will be restricted. Heating will be non-existent in all probability, though the odd electric fire may be available.

The naval officer will complain bitterly when his cabin is invaded by dockyard workmen, but it must be remembered that the sailor is in a much worse position, as he does not even possess a cabin. The sailor merely has a space allotted to him on a messdeck where he can sling his hammock. Encroachment upon this space is so easy, that the sailor may find himself 'spaceless' rather than homeless, and forced to sling his hammock wherever he can find room for it, at different places, night after night. In like manner, the facilities which a sailor possesses for storing his clothes and personal belongings are limited, and likely to be restricted or interfered with during a dockyard refit.

The noise inside a ship during refitting is something so intense, that it can only really be adequately appreciated by persons who have experienced it. Suffice it to say that electric riveters alone, without the hundred and one other extraneous noises which are produced by dockyard work, are not conducive to accurate auscultation by the ship's doctor or to accurate accounting by the ship's paymaster.

Added to all the other disagreeable accompaniments of ship life in dockyard hands is the filth which collects on board, and this is something which is probably more foreign to the sailor's nature and sense of cleanliness than anything else.

A final hazard which is mentioned, albeit with regret, is that of theft and petty pilfering on board which must always be guarded against at such times.

So far these remarks have only been applied to ships in dockyard hands in the United Kingdom. But dockyard conditions had to be endured by H.M. ships in ports all over the world. In some ports these conditions were much more pleasant than in the United Kingdom, but dry docking in a tropical port, at the hottest time of the year, created discomforts and hardship for those living on board which were almost unbearable.

For example, records make mention of a ship which underwent a period of refitting in Bombay dockyard, which lasted a month. The average daily temperature on board was 94° F., with pre-monsoon saturation humidity. Prickly heat was universal, and all living spaces were infested by flies.

As was to be expected, there were times when docking periods could be associated with some deterioration in the health of a ship's company, though this deterioration was by no means the general rule. Nevertheless, medical officers had always to be on guard and alert to the fact that much of a ship's immunity to local diseases had automatically been dissolved by placing her in close contact with the shore.

The picture which has been painted of life on board a ship in dockyard hands is no doubt a gloomy one. But it is only fair to remember that many of the disadvantages were more than offset by the shore-going and recreational facilities which existed at such times. In any case, such temporary disorganisation of living conditions in a ship has come to be recognised as a customary burden to be accepted and suffered cheerfully by persons who serve afloat.

CARE OF FLYING PERSONNEL

So far, this account of the life of a naval medical officer afloat under active service conditions, has been a general one, and has not been applied to any particular class of ship. Naturally, medical commitments, action organisation, domestic details and the like would show variations between ships of different classes. Nevertheless, apart from submarines, in which medical officers were not carried, and aircraft carriers, the general medical principles to be observed in men-of-war were basically similar.

But in the case of the aircraft carrier, the duties of a medical officer became more and more specialised as the war progressed. The carrier medical officer had to meet the general active service medical commitments of one of H.M. ships, and on to this general background it was necessary for him to graft the special requirements of aviation medicine, and in particular to play an important part in the operational care of the flying personnel. The supply of trained naval flying personnel was never so far ahead of demand as to warrant complacency with regard to wastage. It was necessary therefore to take every opportunity to reduce the numbers of airmen likely to collapse under operational conditions. This was a problem which demanded the combined attention of executive and medical officers in aircraft carriers.

The prevention of flying fatigue became paramount, and was recognised to be far more effective than the treatment of the actual condition. With this in view, living conditions in carriers received constant supervision, particularly in the case of junior officers and air gunners. Squadron officers tended to be very junior, and unless precautions were taken, were therefore likely to be allotted bunks in double cabins and dormitories which sometimes had to be vacated at sea for an even less comfortable sleeping billets at a time when sleeping was most important to them. Even closer attention had to be paid to the air gunner in this respect, because, as his squadron was only likely to be on board the carrier for relatively short operational periods, there was a tendency for him to be billeted on one of the less desirable messdecks, the more desirable messdecks being already permanently occupied by the carrier's permanent complement.

Noise in aircraft carriers was likely to be much greater than in other ships, chiefly on account of the complexity of duties which made a great deal of broadcasting or 'piping' of instructions unavoidable. But steps were taken to eliminate unnecessary noise, because it was realised how greatly its cumulative effect could undermine the well-being of men in need of undisturbed rest.

The large complement carried by an aircraft carrier frequently called for close scrutiny of existing ventilation, and it was also necessary to make provision for the stowage and drying of flying clothing.

'Action messing' became even more important in aircraft carriers than in other ships. A satisfactory meal had always to be made available for those requiring it before an operation, and the official view was expressed that coffee and sandwiches were inadequate, particularly on a cold dawn, for men who had an operation flight against the enemy before them with the possibility of prolonged immersion in the sea to follow. It was also directed that flying personnel who happened to be on patrol at meal times should receive hot freshly cooked meals at their convenience, and should not be expected to make do with cold meat or something left over.

As experience was gained, it was shown that leave should be given to fully operational squadrons as often as conditions permitted, and also special leave to individuals whenever this was warranted by the circumstances. But when leave was out of the question, or unlikely to benefit the flier because of the lack of facilities locally, steps were taken to change over squadrons from carrier to carrier and from carrier to shore, and it was found that this system of interchanging went far towards mitigating staleness.

As regards recreation on board, flight deck games were organised whenever possible, and it was found advisable to employ flying personnel on ordinary routine ships' duties whenever they were not engaged upon their own specialised task. It was found that such duties made for a more unified wardroom, and eliminated much of the brooding and introspection of waiting periods between flying operations.

In aircraft carriers more than in any other of H.M. ships early experience showed and emphasised that the policy of driving flying officers and men to the point of exhaustion and collapse was too expensive a means of achieving so-called success. Above all, it was urged that squadron personnel should not be allowed to develop operational fatigue, and that leave should be given as a preventive measure and never as a curative.

Ideally, it was realised that after a spell of operational flying, the change should be automatic, and not dependent on illness. But to lay down the exact number of operational hours which a man should be capable of tolerating was impossible, neither could a true parallel be sought from the Royal Air Force, because the conditions of flying in the Navy varied to such an immeasurable extent. The views on this important subject varied, but became more definite as experience of war was gained. For example, it was found that very few men were able to stand up to more than nine months of operational work in the Middle East without the production of a state of anxiety. But this period varied very much with the amount of stress, and in relation to the characteristics of the individual. When a man should be relieved had to be decided ultimately in every case by the commanding officer with the help of the medical officer.

It was particularly important to guard against the overloading of particular individuals. There was a natural tendency for a competent, steady flier to be given more than his fair share to do, particularly after heavy losses. Such a man was always considered to be ready for yet another operation, and he was usually the last to suggest his need for rest. In such cases it was vitally necessary for the medical officer to recognise the danger signals of approaching collapse which such a man might well exhibit in his everyday life on board the carrier. The tendency of such an individual to transfer blame to his colleagues, his aircraft or its instruments, and the development of phobias for flying over the sea or night flying had all to be regarded as manifestations of a general nervous illness. It was wrong to regard them as specific fears which could be treated individually by limitations of category. It is of some interest to note that this group of symptoms was greatly reduced in number consistently with the improved instruction in the use of the dinghy, and in first aid throughout the Navy.

It became necessary for medical officers to realise, and also to explain to the executive, that even the most minor of aircraft crashes must be regarded as a distressing experience for persons involved, and might well inflict mental in addition to physical wounds. The traditional principle that a flier who had crashed and survived should be sent up again as soon as possible, had to be fought against by medical officers. It was preferable to admit such a survivor to the sick bay for at least twenty-four hours as a routine, and a short course of sedatives in such cases became of proved value, and did much to prevent indelible psychological damage.

This short account shows how necessary it was for the medical officer of the aircraft carrier to identify himself with his flying colleagues on board. The welfare of these men represented a continued combined operation by the commanding officer and the medical officer. The medical officer obviously could not always be expected to understand the full extent of operational commitments, neither could the commanding officer be expected to appreciate fully the limitations of a man's physical capabilities and psychological make-up. But it was possible for these two authorities to combine together in order to arrive at a policy of care of the trained airman which resulted in the reduction of avoidable wastage to negligible proportions throughout the whole Fleet Air Arm. (Plate IX illustrates a pilot on the verge of collapse being taken out of his plane.)

CHAPTER 2
THE NAVAL MEDICAL OFFICER ON ACTIVE SERVICE ASHORE

(i)
Some medical operations ashore

A selection from the records of the more important shore units.

OPERATIONAL commitments have frequently required naval medical officers to perform their duties under active service conditions on shore. Historically, these duties seem mostly to have been concerned with landing parties, minor punitive expeditions and the like.

But during the First World War naval personnel saw action on shore for prolonged periods and under more highly organised conditions. Examples were the Naval Division which served on the Western Front, and also those forces which took part in the Gallipoli campaign.

During the period between the wars, the probability of active service on shore by naval forces was always kept in mind, and a number of medical officers had some experience of the medical organisation which would be necessary in such circumstances.

During the Second World War the Navy was called upon to play a very large part in shore operations in company with the combined operational organisations of the other Fighting Services.

It is not the purpose of this chapter to attempt to describe in detail every minor incident in which naval doctors and sick berth ratings were involved, because to do so would be impossible in the space available and little use would be served. Neither is it proposed to give an account of the medical aspects of 'Combined Operations' as a whole, many of which were not primarily a naval medical commitment. The real purpose of this chapter is to hand down to posterity a record of some of the more important types of medical organisation for operations ashore which the Navy was called upon to provide, and of the chief events in which naval medical officers and nursing staff were involved.

THE MOBILE NAVAL BASE DEFENCE ORGANISATION (M.N.B.D.O.)
PRELIMINARY DEVELOPMENTS AND MOVEMENTS

The Mobile Naval Base Defence Organisation was a comparatively modern conception, dating from the 1920's. Consisting mainly of Royal Marines, the proposed function of the organisation was to provide the

Fleet with a shore base in any part of the world, and to maintain and defend such a base once it had been prepared.

From small beginnings, the organisation grew until one complete unit had a strength of about 8,000 men with a major general in command. The complement included engineers and mechanics, transport and crane drivers, armourers and gunners, surveyors and draughtsmen, bricklayers, masons, carpenters, plumbers, painters, decorators, camouflage modellers, miners, blacksmiths, tinsmiths and divers. These expert craftsmen were in addition to the personnel of all kinds necessary to maintain the domestic welfare of the organisation.

The original conception of the M.N.B.D.O. was that it should be carried to the scene of operation in specially equipped merchant vessels. A landing and maintenance group would then be responsible for placing the M.N.B.D.O. ashore in landing craft, and for transporting it once it had been landed. This landing and maintenance group would then complete its function by building wharves or converting existing jetties, by making roadways from the beach, and by erecting such buildings as might be necessary.

The proposed defence side of the organisation was divided into artillery groups with naval coastal guns, anti-aircraft and anti-tank guns, with searchlights to co-operate with all three. There was also a land defence section consisting of rifle companies, machine-gun sections and light artillery batteries.

The Group Headquarters of the M.N.B.D.O. was to have under its control the coastal artillery, the light and heavy anti-aircraft guns, the searchlights, the ordnance and workshop units, and the departments responsible for signals, postal, meteorological, camouflage, provost, decontamination and medical services.

Such early training exercises of the M.N.B.D.O. as are on record, appear to have consisted of transporting and laying boom defences. The full title of 'M.N.B.D.O.' was used in a Conference Report on April 12, 1931, in reference to a full scale exercise which had taken place at Milford Haven in 1930. Local operational exercises were held during 1933 at Portsmouth and Colchester. A further large scale exercise was planned to take place in company with units of the Fleet, at Lamlash during 1935. There is, however, no record that this exercise actually took place.

Following these exercises, it became possible to study some of the medical aspects of the M.N.B.D.O., and it was considered and agreed that reliance should not be placed solely on Fleet hospital ships, but that the medical staff attached to the M.N.B.D.O. must be large enough to permit routine visits to all the included units by medical officers, to establish a sick quarters inside the base to deal with seriously ill cases, to deal with local epidemics and to guard against endemic diseases, and to cope with casualties caused in action.

To meet these commitments the smallest staff was estimated as 3 medical officers, 13 sick berth ratings, and additional domestic staff should a sick quarters be established on shore.

In September 1935, the naval developments in the Mediterranean which followed the outbreak of the Italo-Abyssinian War, resulted not only in an exercise more nearly under active service conditions than had been expected, but also in abandonment of the original idea that the M.N.B.D.O. would be ready not earlier than two months after the outbreak of war.

In this particular crisis, the embarkation of base defences was one of the first measures to be demanded by the Commander-in-Chief, Mediterranean, and one which was promptly undertaken by the Admiralty.

This 1935 Mediterranean expedition of M.N.B.D.O. was under the command of a Brigadier, R.M. It was conveyed to Alexandria in the hired transports *Bellerophon* and *Neuralia*, arriving there in September 1935. The medical staff and stores were carried in these two ships in preparation for a possible move to an advanced base.

On arrival in Alexandria it was soon realised that the maintenance of health and hygiene among the personnel of the M.N.B.D.O. during a long waiting period in a Fleet anchorage was likely to become a large medical commitment. This was perhaps one of the most important results to flow from the experience of the abortive Mediterranean M.N.B.D.O. expedition.

From 1935 onwards the idea of the M.N.B.D.O. continued to be developed. In June 1936, it was reported that allocation of Royal Marine recruits for the M.N.B.D.O. could not be commenced until 1937, and would take about four years to enter, with a further seventeen months for training. This meant that the M.N.B.D.O. could not be manned, completed and in working order until 1941.

During 1937, it was recommended that the medical services of the completed M.N.B.D.O. should include a standard mobile naval field hospital, at a cost of £3,000.

On March 16, 1939, the M.N.B.D.O. was recognised as a future war commitment of the Royal Navy and Royal Marines. It was to be composed of:

(*a*) An underwater unit consisting of booms, indicator loops and a controlled minefield.

(*b*) A Royal Marine Group consisting of:
  (i) An anti-aircraft brigade, including associated searchlights.
  (ii) A coastal defence brigade.
  (iii) A communications company.
  (iv) A landing, transport, maintenance, workshop and administrative unit, with ancillary supply and accounting, meteorological, and comprehensive medical services.

By September 1940, the framework of the M.N.B.D.O. had been constructed, but many of the final details of the organisation remained to be evolved in the light of subsequent experience.

During the war, two of these complex bodies came into existence. The first of them was sent to Alexandria at the beginning of 1941, expecting to be employed with the Mediterranean Fleet. But the speed of local events, including the evacuation of Greece, brought a decision to use this M.N.B.D.O. to provide a naval base in Crete. Unfortunately there was little time for this M.N.B.D.O. to fulfil its complete function, and only the advanced groups arrived in Crete shortly before the Germans invaded that island. These advanced groups were composed of some 2,200 men of whom only about 1,000 returned to Alexandria in due course. As part of these advanced groups was one of the two tented hospitals attached to this first M.N.B.D.O.

This M.N.B.D.O. was re-formed after the return of the survivors from Crete, but subsequently units of it became scattered between India, Ceylon, the Maldive Islands, Suez and Syria. In June 1943, the main body of this M.N.B.D.O. was moved from Egypt to Ceylon, the organisation then being some 6,000 strong. By September 1943, this first M.N.B.D.O. had become known as a 'Royal Marine Group', re-organised into two brigades, with a group headquarters and a base depot. But this re-organisation was short lived, and early in 1944 the Group was recalled to the United Kingdom and disbanded.

Meanwhile, a second M.N.B.D.O. began to be formed at Hayling Island, early in 1941. During that year, it acquired a strength of 7,000 but it had no separate medical unit until August 1, 1942. This second M.N.B.D.O. was shipped to the Middle East early in 1943, and became involved in the Allied invasion of Sicily.

M.N.B.D.O. (1)

Early in 1941, the first and second naval tented hospitals came into existence, as part of the first Mobile Naval Base Defence Organisation (M.N.B.D.O. (1.)).

These tented hospitals were new commitments which involved the definition and collection of much equipment for which there had never previously been any demand. These hospital units had to be both mobile and entirely self-contained. To medical stores were added such items as tents and entrenching tools, ambulances and field latrines. In theory there was every prospect of these units serving a most useful purpose as part of the M.N.B.D.O.

There were, however, certain aspects of these tented hospital units which only time could reveal. For example, the naval medical officer was not familiar with the special training necessary for work ashore in the field as opposed to work in an established hospital, hospital ship or man-of-war. Nor was it fully realised at first that the Navy might find these unfamiliar units difficult to fit in to its general Operational Medical Organisation. This latter problem was aggravated by the tented hospitals being attached to Royal Marine groups which themselves eventually came under military administration when they were later moved to the Middle East.

THE FIRST ROYAL NAVAL TENTED HOSPITAL

The original intention had been that the first tented hospital should be attached to the R.M. Group Section of the first M.N.B.D.O., while the second tented hospital would be attached to the naval staff side of the organisation. So much for the original planning in theory. But what actually happened to these two tented hospital units in subsequent active shore operations proved to be something very different.

The first Royal Naval Tented Hospital was evolved by a surgeon lieutenant commander, R.N., after many months of various experiences. This officer was at sea on the Northern Patrol in the winter of 1939, when he responded to an appeal for volunteers for special service. In April 1940, he was ordered to join a small medical unit at Lee-on-Solent. This unit consisted of 3 surgeon lieutenants and a small number of very inexperienced sick berth ratings.

It was intended that this unit should be a casualty clearing station for the Naval Air Arm which was about to form a landing ground on an island off the coast of Norway. The members of the unit were provided with battledress and other clothing for arctic conditions. One medical officer went on ahead with the main body of Naval Air Arm personnel. The remaining medical officers and staff were to follow in the S.S. *Manelia*, sailing from Glasgow a few days later. At the time of their arrival on board the *Manelia*, they had not yet seen the medical stores provided for their use, and a long and tedious search eventually revealed that these stores had been loaded into another ship. These stores weighed several tons, each pound of which the senior medical officer claims to have remembered personally in his report, because he, with his colleagues, had to take part in the manual labour of unloading them and getting them on to the right ship!

The *Manelia* now put to sea several times, but, to their disappointment, they failed to reach Norway before the organised resistance in that country had collapsed, and orders were received to disband the unit. It is of interest to record that the senior medical officer could obtain no definite instructions about the disposal of his stores on board the *Manelia*, and he loaded them into a pantechnicon and drove them about Glasgow, till he finally got them accommodated in a furniture warehouse where, it was recorded, 'they may be still'!

A few days later the senior medical officer was ordered to join a Royal Marine Brigade which was under canvas near Aldershot. He collected with him his two remaining surgeon lieutenants and his sick berth ratings, and formed a casualty clearing station for the brigade. A large supply of medical stores was available as well as ambulances, water trucks, etc.

In addition to the casualty clearing station, the brigade had its medical officers for its routine requirements, with a surgeon commander, R.N., as senior medical officer of the brigade, and a surgeon lieutenant as unit medical officer to each battalion. The brigade spent some time moving around South Wales and the south west coast of England.

This period of movement was one of some uncertainty for the casualty clearing station, and by July 1940, the Brigadier in command suggested that the casualty clearance duty would be better performed by the Royal Army Medical Corps rather than by an inexperienced naval medical party.

It was therefore decided to detach this small medical unit yet again, but not to disband it. The surgeon lieutenant commander and his party were sent to the Royal Marine Depot at Exmouth, and here, for the first time in their existence, they were able to settle down to a most useful period of training, and were permitted to take part in the general medical work of the depot.

The unit was able to erect its tents and unpack its stores for the first time. Field days and exercises were organised in which the unit constructed latrines, urine pits, etc., and eventually, it was able to pitch or break camp in a minimum of time, at any time of the day or night, and in any kind of weather. As part of the unit's training, all medical officers and sick berth ratings were taught to read maps and to ride motor cycles, measures which were to prove of the greatest value at a later date.

The unit was given valuable assistance by the Commanding Officer of an Army Field Hospital which was being trained in the vicinity, and the personnel of the unit were able to attend the lectures and exercises held by this field hospital. Members of the sick berth staff were sent to a local hotel to acquire a knowledge of cooking, and also to a local civil hospital for practical nursing instruction.

By the end of 1940, this unit had completed its training and was regarded as fit for active service. It was now instructed to join the M.N.B.D.O. (1), for service overseas. The unit now became the first naval tented hospital, and a second tented hospital was already attached to M.N.B.D.O. (1), which, though organised on more established lines, had not yet completed its training or gained experience. Both these tented hospital units travelled to the Middle East at much about the same time, but the fortunes of each were very different.

The first tented hospital sailed from Glasgow on February 8, 1941. Its personnel consisted of 10 medical officers and 26 sick berth staff, who were divided mainly between three merchant ships, with a sick berth attendant also allocated to each of three other cargo vessels.

While this dispersal of personnel was a very wise measure in case the convoy should be attacked and some ships lost, it nevertheless militated against the unit becoming more organised during the long voyage around Africa. This dispersal, in fact, became symbolic of the major difficulty which always lay ahead of the tented hospitals, namely, that of maintaining contact. This difficulty was even aggravated further when the ships in convoy were diverted to different ports on arrival in the Middle East.

For part of the unit, this voyage ended at Suez on April 21, 1941, when the medical personnel were landed and sent to a transit camp at El Tahag, near Qassassin. But the stores of the first tented hospital, and also those of the second tented hospital, were carried on to Haifa. The remainder of the medical personnel arrived at Port Said. At this point therefore the personnel of the first tented hospital were dispersed far apart in Egypt, while the stores of the unit were at a port in Palestine.

In due course, all the medical personnel met at the transit camp, and were together for the first time since leaving the United Kingdom. But the term 'together' must be qualified, because El Tahag consisted of 40 different camps scattered over many miles, with a total accommodation for more than 10,000 men. Each of these camps had a frontage of 400 yards, and extended backwards up to 1,000 yards according to the size of the contained unit. The first tented hospital was in Camp No. 16, but two of its medical officers were detached and accommodated in Camps 22 and 24.

By arrangement with the Army Medical Authorities, a small sick bay was run in each camp, and Army personnel were catered for as well as the Royal Marines of the M.N.B.D.O. The necessary limited medical supplies for this purpose were supplied by the Army, as the only naval medical stores in company at this time were a few field valises.

ACTIVE OPERATIONS ON CRETE

On May 1, 1941, the first tented hospital left Tahag, three medical officers remaining behind with individual units. The medical officers and staff arrived in Port Said the same afternoon, and embarked in the S.S. *City of Canterbury*. This ship sailed from Port Said on May 5, by which time the destination of the first tented hospital was known to be the Island of Crete.

At this time the first naval tented hospital consisted of a surgeon lieutenant commander, R.N., as senior medical officer, 6 surgeon lieutenants, 2 sick berth chief petty officers, 5 sick berth petty officers, 5 leading sick berth attendants, 8 sick berth attendants, 3 cooks, and 4 marines as wardroom attendants. On May 19 the numbers were slightly increased by the addition of 2 extra sick berth attendants, and 1 extra wardroom attendant.

The duties were allocated as follows:

- 2 surgical teams consisted of 1 medical officer and 3 attendants.
- 1 medical officer was an anaesthetist.
- 1 medical officer in charge of casualty reception and resuscitation.
- 1 medical officer as physician.
- 1 chief petty officer for general administration.
- 1 chief petty officer in charge of stores.
- 1 petty officer for reception duties.
- 1 petty officer and 1 S.B.A. for dispensary duties.
- 1 petty officer for baggage and patients' effects.
- 1 L.S.B.A. for laboratory and mortuary.

Additional duties performed by medical officers were hygiene, medical transport, mail and censoring, and paymaster. The remainder of the nursing staff was divided up into sections for duty in two surgical and one medical ward, with a small V.D. section.

The unit landed at Suda in Crete on May 9, and marched at once to a transit camp where it was accommodated under most insanitary conditions. A working party was immediately formed to clear up the area and to dig latrines and urine pits. An incinerator was constructed, and also a field oven, and a ditch was cleared to act as a slit trench.

The senior medical officer had already been informed that for operational and administrative purposes he would take orders from the S.M.O. of the island. He now explained to his medical officers and staff the general situation as he knew it, and he conveyed instructions to all personnel in the transit camp regarding sanitation, meal times, general routine and in particular, emphasised that all drinking water must be boiled.

Meanwhile, a large building was found by the water's edge, which had a red cross on its roof. This building turned out to be a deserted mental hospital, containing semi-looted stores of all kinds, many of which proved to be of great value later on.

On May 10, the senior medical officer accompanied the S.M.O. of the island to Force Headquarters at Canea, where he discussed the prospective site for the first tented hospital. On the same afternoon, he visited the site with his hygiene officer. The site itself was at Mournies, 7 or 8 kms. due south of Canea, and 4 kms. east of Perivolia.

The orders were that the hospital should move in to its new site as soon as possible. Meanwhile the unloading of stores was proceeding at Suda Bay, and serious omissions were soon discovered.

The records are a little confusing at this point. However, it will be remembered that when the personnel of the first and second tented hospitals had arrived in Egypt, the stores and equipment of these hospitals had gone on to the port of Haifa. It would seem that arrangements were now made for the stores of the first tented hospital to be extracted and re-loaded at Haifa, and sent on to Suda. Nevertheless, owing to misunderstandings and conflicting instructions, 36 cases of the stores of the first tented hospital were not sent, while certain stores of the second tented hospital were sent in error. The result was that the first tented hospital in Crete found itself with duplicated stores of some kinds, while its omissions included such important items as knives and forks, 2 X-ray tubes, shovels and tent boards, and 15 beds. But there were compensations. For instance, the hospital had all the latrines which had been supplied to both hospital units. Also, in the light of subsequent events, it was indeed providential that such stores and equipment as did not arrive in Crete were at least saved to be used elsewhere at a later date.

The process of moving into the camp site at Mournies was obviously much slower than had been expected by the senior medical officer. Some delay was occasioned by a sharp air attack on Suda on the night of May 10. On May 11, two surgeon lieutenants and a working party were sent to Mournies to occupy the site, and efforts were made to move the stores and equipment, but under difficult conditions owing to lack of transport and a further air attack that night.

The whole of May 12 was passed in moving the hospital to Mournies, using one ambulance and two lorries. The loading was done by Australians and Cypriots, while the unloading at the camp site 10 kms. distant was done by officers and men of the hospital party. During this busy day, tents were put up as they arrived, trench latrines and urine pits were dug, and a small incinerator was constructed. Lack of tools was a severe handicap, and it is recorded that only two spades and two picks were available. As regards water supply, what there was had to be carried by hand over a distance of 80 yards, but the Royal Engineers had already been approached about piping the supply over the centre of the site.

On May 13, construction of the first tented hospital continued consistently with the arrival of its stores and requirements. The lack of tools continued to be a handicap, and further time was lost through the natural inexperience of the men themselves. Fortunately one sick berth rating had been a coal miner, and was able to give a lead to others. The construction of grease traps caused great difficulty, particularly as the soil was not porous.

On this day the senior medical officer visited the 7th General Hospital, where he found that tented wards had been sunk into the ground, a manoeuvre which gave more head space as well as protection at the sides. Consideration was given to adopting this method in the case of the first tented hospital, but a serious argument against it was the possibility of such tents being set on fire by incendiary bombs, and patients finding difficulty in escaping. By this time certain of the deficiencies in stores had started to make themselves felt. For example, eating utensils were at a premium, and such meagre table instruments as were available had

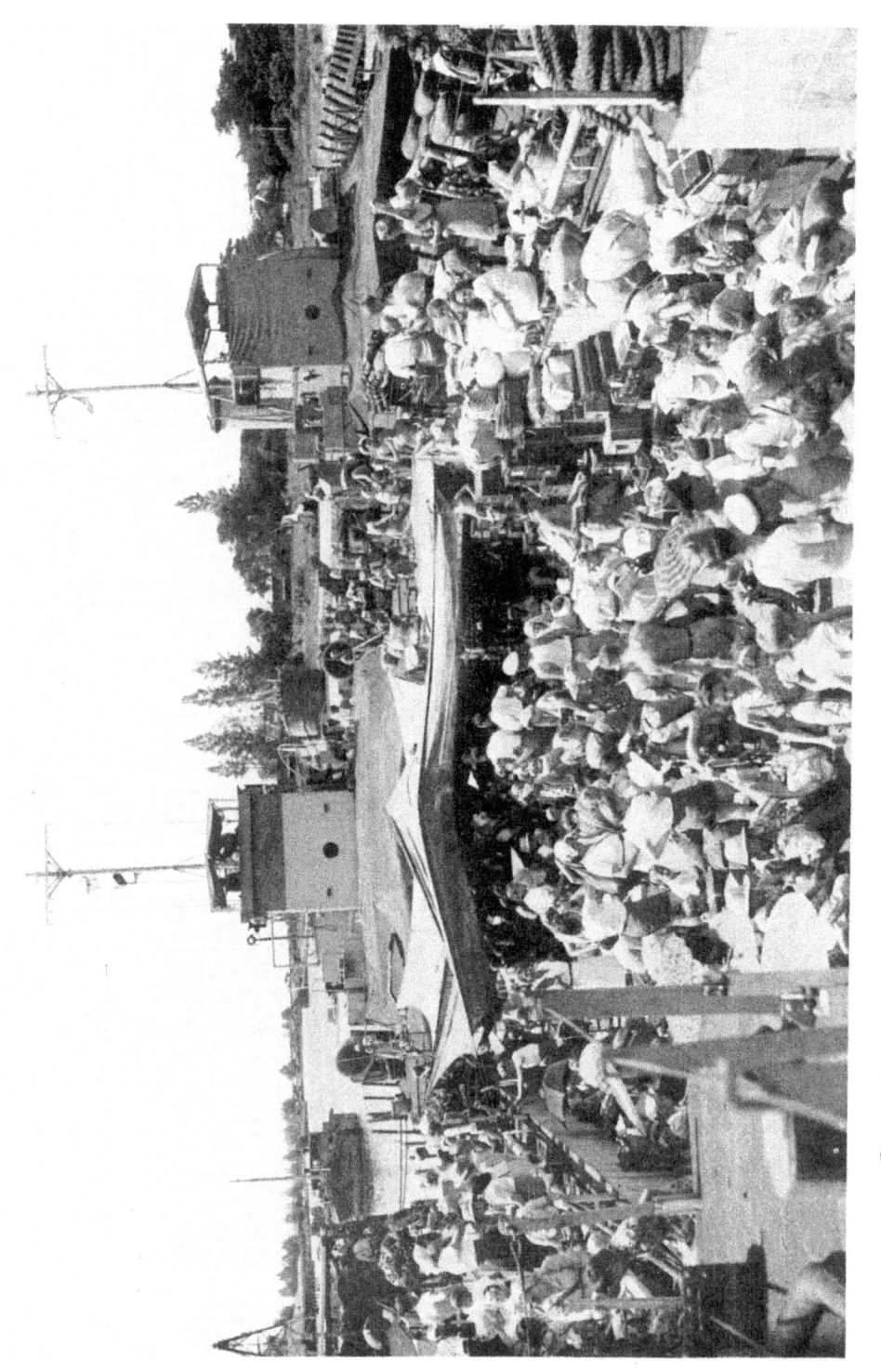

PLATE X. Evacuation of civilians by the Royal Navy during the Japanese Invasion.

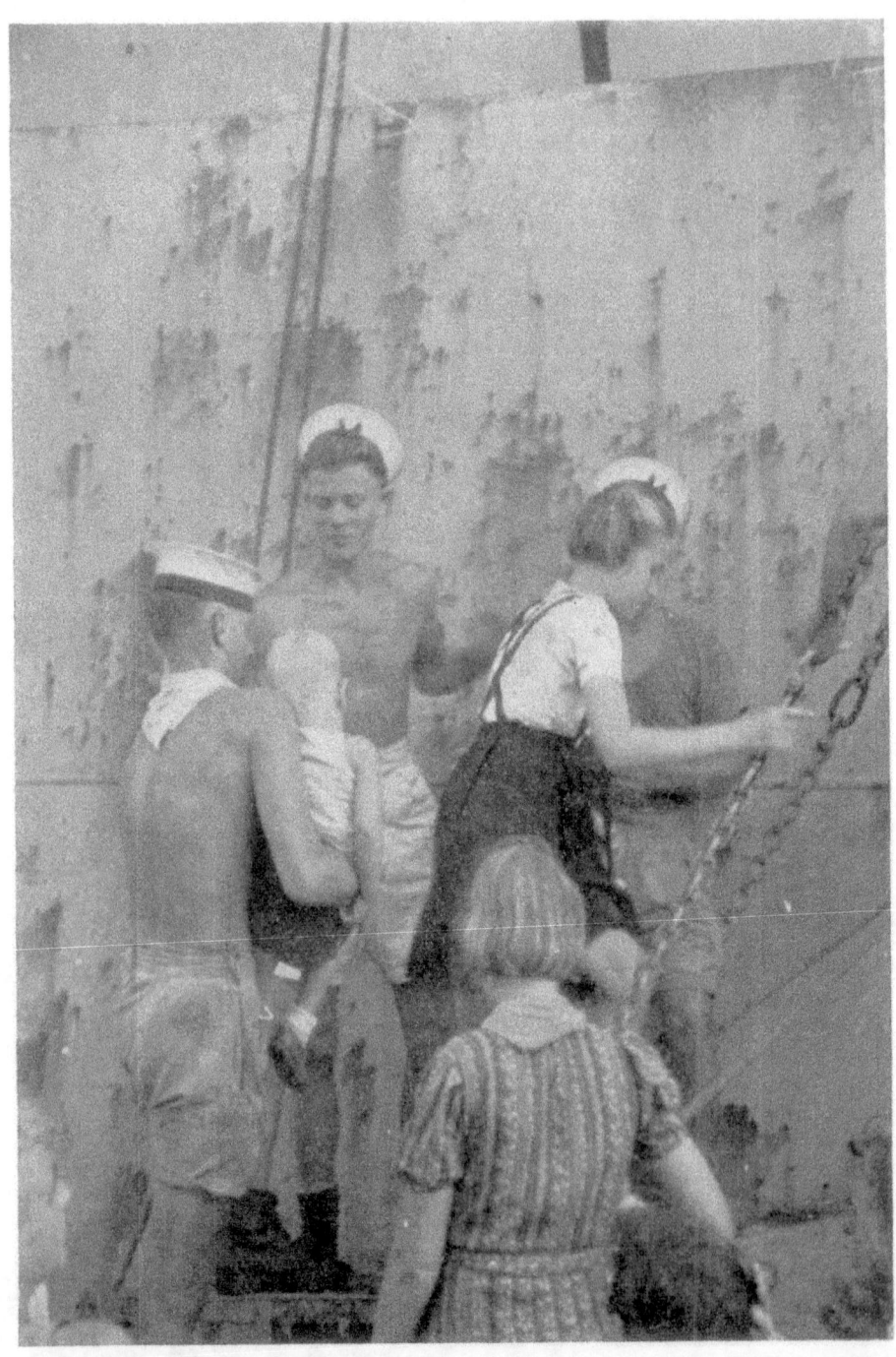

PLATE XI. Evacuation of civilians by the Royal Navy during the Japanese Invasion.

to be set aside for the use of patients and staff. Medical Officers themselves were forced to adopt the system of eating off each other's plates with each other's knives, forks and spoons! Later on, of course, when food became very scarce, fingers became the custom.

Already lack of cigarettes was becoming a great hardship.

The first ward in the first tented hospital was opened in working condition on the evening of May 13, and ironically, its first patient to be admitted was one of its own sick berth attendants suffering from enteritis.

On May 14, work continued which included the difficult task of digging a trench latrine some 9 or 10 ft. deep. Attention was also given to creating an efficient camouflage system. But in this connexion, it was soon found impossible to remain hidden from enemy aircraft flying very low, and camouflage was abandoned, and sheets were painted red and cut up and pegged out on the ground as red crosses. On this day hospital routine was established and Standing Orders were issued. By this time transport had been augmented and now consisted of two ambulances, one 30-cwt. truck and two motor cycles! Steps had been taken to place direction signs on roads in the vicinity, pointing the way to the hospital. But owing to shortage of materials, these signs were rudimentary and written in pen and ink! Meanwhile, the Royal Engineers had expressed some pessimism about the possibility of arranging a piped water supply.

On the morning of May 15, the first tented hospital was officially declared open to receive patients, and all authorities were informed of this in a signal by dispatch rider, which gave a map reference of the hospital's position.

The same evening the first casualty arrived from Suda with a wounded foot after a bombing attack.

From now onwards, the work of the first tented hospital increased almost hourly, and was conducted under the most strenuous and hazardous conditions. Many cases of enteritis were received, and on the evening of May 17 a batch of wounded was admitted, which gave an opportunity of seeing how the surgical arrangements worked.

On May 18 the ambulance was sent to Suda at 1100 hours to collect casualties. That evening it was bombed and machine-gunned while carrying these unfortunate men.

At daybreak on May 20, air bombardment started, and increased in intensity until 0820 hours, when parachute troops were seen landing to the north and west. Red crosses were hurriedly painted on all tents and trees in the perimeter of the hospital in the hope that these would be respected by parachutists. Meanwhile, two Greek soldiers were sent from a neighbouring wireless station to guard the hospital. The senior medical officer sent them back, but one of them returned a few days later as a stretcher case.

There were many Greek patients in the hospital by this time, and an interpreter was provided from a Greek battalion nearby.

In the course of this day a sick berth petty officer and two attendants were sent out to collect wounded from a gun site which had suffered severely all day in action with the crews of two enemy gliders which had landed near to it. At one time during their fight the men of this gun site had actually been taken prisoner, but had been rescued later by a body of Royal Marine reinforcements.

It is of interest to record that the senior medical officer had ordered the bolts of all rifles of personnel entering the hospital to be withdrawn and deposited outside the hospital perimeter.

Early on May 21, the senior medical officer was asked to receive casualties from other hospitals which had to be evacuated as the enemy advanced. But he had to refuse, as the first tented hospital was by now over full.

At 0540 hours on this day a surgeon lieutenant and one S.B.A. drove the ambulance into Canea to try to get food but without very much success. This ambulance brought back a little bread, and some casualties, including a German parachutist with a wound in the leg.

The operating theatre was in constant use throughout the day. By 1600 hours its lighting was causing anxiety, and a surgeon lieutenant and driver went through a heavy bombardment to get a spare battery from the ordnance depot. Meanwhile the X-ray engine was used for lighting until it broke down. After that, one of the ambulance batteries was used.

During the day the senior medical officer decided to bury two men who had died, as no chaplain had arrived. This was the first funeral he had conducted, but was not to be the last. Not having a Book of Common Prayer, he read from the Epistle to the Corinthians, Chapter xv. He has recorded that subsequently his burial services tended to get shorter and shorter, but that he always tried to carry them out with as much dignity as possible.

At 1800 hours on this day a Roman Catholic priest called, having walked from Canea, and was able to bury a patient who had died.

By now, machine-gunning of the hospital from the air had become frequent and usual, and red crosses made of sheets were pegged out on the ground. But the hospital was never actually bombed, although both bombs and bullets were aimed at a road and path round the edge of its perimeter, where troops were frequently on the move.

On the evening of May 21, the S.M.O. of the Island called and gave news of the general position.

Work continued to be strenuous on May 22. Large numbers of wounded were received including some Maoris, one of whom had walked 4 miles with his left buttock missing. Operating teams were working continuously, and their task and the task of those nursing the wounded was made most difficult by the noise of action all around the hospital and the large numbers of enemy aircraft diving low overhead.

In addition to the strenuous surgical and nursing work of the hospital, and its overcrowded state, further hardship was inflicted by minor domestic deficiencies. Rations were in very short supply, and had to be fetched by the limited transport of the hospital, which meant diverting a medical officer and sick berth rating from their proper duties. Also the only time at which rations could be collected was at 0530 hours each day. A good supply of naval tobacco was made available, but the few cigarette papers were soon exhausted, and cigarettes had to be improvised out of toilet paper. To continue the boiling of all drinking water became too heavy a burden with the ever increasing numbers of patients to be catered for, and chlorination had to be resorted to instead. Hot tea was kept in a hay box for administration to patients on first arrival. Fortunately the incinerator worked well and solved all problems of refuse.

As the aerial bombardment was intensified so the work of the hospital increased and became more difficult. Medical officers and staff were constantly being summoned to assist in medical duties outside the hospital, and on one occasion a S.B.A. accompanied a Greek battalion on patrol, and personally tended 50 casualties.

On May 24 news was received that the Suda area headquarters might be forced to move westwards. This news was received with mixed feelings, because though it was some satisfaction to know the retreat of Allied Forces was towards and not away from the hospital, it did mean that the hospital itself was more and more likely to be involved in severe enemy action.

By this time the personnel of the first tented hospital were very tired from lack of sleep. The morale of the staff remained remarkably high, but their efficiency was visibly affected by their physical and mental exhaustion.

On this day a Greek priest was obtained with some difficulty, for the burial of two Greek patients, and a second German patient was admitted. This man was another parachutist with a severe infection of the throat. He was confined in a bell tent with an Australian to guard him. This patient was most truculent, and constantly insisted that the Australians would take his life, despite the fact that his guard armed himself only with a fly whisk!

Early on the morning of May 25, 37 casualties arrived, some on stretchers lent by a Greek Army medical officer who did most skilful work with very limited equipment.

During this day the hospital became so crowded that it was necessary to dig further urine pits and trench latrines, and by arrangement with the priest of a local monastery, two enclosed barns were taken over as additional wards for 60 cases. The last remaining red paint was used to paint crosses on these barns.

On the evening of May 25, six German parachutists landed immediately to the south of the hospital. At 2100 hours a message was received from the Army Medical Authorities offering assistance with the evacuation of approximately 100 patients. A rapid survey of the wards showed that only 83 men were fit to move. However, this message was soon cancelled, but it left behind it the strong feeling that all was not well and that evacuation might prove to be necessary at short notice.

At 0300 hours on May 26, 200 patients arrived without warning, accompanied by 12 orderlies of the Australian Medical Corps. Large numbers of these men were medical cases, complaining of enteritis and 'bomb hysteria'.

Soon after daybreak the air bombardment became heavier than ever, and large quantities of earth and stones were constantly being hurled into the camp. The conditions made it impossible to use the operating theatre, whose staff in any case were far too exhausted to give of their best. One medical officer dealt with minor cases all day, while the rest dressed such wounded as had come into the hospital overnight. Some of these wounds had not had attention since they were received several days before, and the men were in a pitiable state after waiting for attention in the open without food or drink. For example one patient had a shattered right elbow full of maggots.

As well as attending to Service casualties, numerous civilians from a local village received attention.

By this time all patients who were able to move, spent the daylight sheltering in slit trenches in the hospital area. With more than 400 patients, the lack of food and accommodation had become so serious that the senior medical officer suggested, albeit with regret, that it would be of assistance to the rest if patients whose condition was not serious, and who had had a period of rest and treatment, would volunteer to rejoin their units. This appeal met with a good response, and an Australian Army Officer patient marched a number of men away under cover of darkness.

By now, too, the bed patients began to show grave anxiety concerning the general situation and their own future welfare.

During the afternoon, troops to the right and left were withdrawing down the road eastwards, and the sound of small arms fire around the hospital came nearer and nearer during the evening. When darkness fell, German parachutists began to 'crow' and 'catcall' in the vicinity, with the object of injuring the morale of hearers.

The senior medical officer had had no contact with the outside world for some hours, and finally, when a marine with a broken jaw volunteered as dispatch rider, he sent him into Suda on a motor cycle with a message for Naval Headquarters asking for information and instructions.

This dispatch rider returned with a message 'Move what you can eastwards immediately'.

It is important to record in this history that this was the first instruction which the senior medical officer had received from Naval Headquarters for about 40 hours. Naturally, being under the direction of the senior medical officer of the island, the first tented hospital was in no way a responsibility of Naval Headquarters which immediately acted on the hospital's behalf as soon as the senior medical officer took the initiative himself. That he did take this initiative was most fortunate, as the enemy entered the site of the hospital at 0700 hours the next morning.

As soon as this message was received, all patients who felt equal to walking the distance were told to make their way to a point one mile beyond Suda, and there take cover and await instructions. This party was put in charge of the Roman Catholic chaplain, and was accompanied by the sick berth staff with the exception of 1 C.P.O., 2 P.Os. and 7 others who were kept behind.

Ambulances were drawn up and provided with food supplies. These ambulances were loaded with patients, two to each stretcher head to heel, in some cases 10 patients to each ambulance.*

By 0430 hours on May 27, the last of the ambulances had left, and a small medical party remained at the hospital with 11 stretcher cases. Meanwhile the walking patients who had set off earlier, made their way to Suda where some managed to get passage on board a destroyer. The remainder were advised that the enemy was expected at Suda by dawn, and that it would be best to make their way to Kalives, where it was believed a field hospital was being organised. Some of the patients obtained lifts in Bren carriers and trucks belonging to a Highland regiment.

Acting on the same advice, the loaded ambulances took their patients on to Kalives.

The small remainder left behind at the first tented hospital loaded 5 of its stretcher cases into a farm cart which set off with 4 members of the staff. This cart broke down after travelling 3 miles, but the patients were fortunately soon transferred to one of the ambulances which returned.

There were now left 6 patients, but no bearers for one of the stretchers. Various lifting devices were tried without success, and finally the small party moved down the road in relays, the fastest stretcher going ahead for 200 yards, and the bearers then doubling back and picking up the last stretcher. Eventually another ambulance returned, into which all except two of the stretchers were loaded. These two stretchers were now carried by the senior medical officer, a surgeon lieutenant, and two sick berth attendants.

---

* The available records give no indication of the number of ambulances in use at this time, or how they were obtained. It is, however, assumed that the two ambulances described as in use on May 15 were augmented by others.

In this manner the first tented hospital was evacuated, and the only patients left behind were the two German parachutists. Each of these had been given morphia, and a supply of food and water was placed within their reach. The senior medical officer has recorded that had he found it impossible to get all his patients away in time, he had planned to surrender to one of these two German patients.

The senior medical officer, surgeon lieutenant and two sick berth attendants toiled on with their two stretcher cases, and after daybreak they were repeatedly forced to take cover from enemy aircraft. They became so exhausted that they found they could only cover about 15 paces at a time without resting. It was recorded that these two patients, heavily built Maoris, were 'almost unbelievably patient'.

Just outside Suda this small party was picked up by an ambulance, and arrived at Kalives at 0920 hours.

The rest at Kalives was all too short, and even so the staff of the first tented hospital was soon called upon to join in the work of the hospital at Kalives. Meanwhile, the senior medical officer and one surgeon lieutenant made a fruitless search for headquarters, and were machine-gunned so frequently that they spent long periods taking cover in ditches.

During the evening the Kalives area was heavily attacked, and at 2100 hours, orders were received that all patients who could walk 4 miles were to do so at their own risk during the night. Staff and stretcher cases were to be taken by ambulance through Neon Khorion, Vrises, Askifou and Imvros to Sfakia.

Ambulances were packed to capacity, and a nightmare drive followed over tortuous roads crowded with men and vehicles. The ambulance drivers could only stand the strain for a few minutes at a time, and medical officers and staff were completely exhausted. The senior medical officer has recorded that he himself began to have hallucinations.

By dawn the ambulances had arrived in a saucer shaped depression having covered only 18 miles in 9 hours.

The ambulances were now hidden under trees while the drivers rested. At 1100 hours they moved on, and the sea was sighted soon after 1300 hours. Unfortunately, the convoy was attacked by German aircraft on the crest of a hill outside Sfakia, and although their occupants were able to take cover in time, the ambulances were hit by incendiary bullets and burnt out.

The rest of the day was spent taking cover among rocks and crevices. There was little food, but water was obtained from a nearby village. When it was dark, the party, which now included over 100 wounded, approached the village, and then by a precipitous path down the cliff side, made its way to the beach. Here boats were waiting which took patients and casualties off to destroyers anchored off shore.

After surviving an aircraft attack at sea, what remained of the first tented hospital arrived at Alexandria at 1500 hours on May 29. Muster on the quayside showed that the only persons missing were two ambulance drivers, two cooks, and one sick berth rating. But it is pleasing to record that these too were landed in Egypt a few days later.

This brief account of the service of the first naval tented hospital in Crete records a constant sense of striving in the face of ever increasing difficulties, and ending on a note of tragedy and grave hardship, so much being lost which had been so carefully planned and built up in the months before. Nevertheless, in a short time, the hospital performed a valiant and useful task, and the conduct of its personnel was at all times outstanding.*

THE SECOND ROYAL NAVAL TENTED HOSPITAL

The second tented hospital had also sailed from Glasgow on February 8, 1941, as part of M.N.B.D.O.(1), but attached to the Naval Staff (N.S.1) portion of it. Unlike the first tented hospital, it had not seen any of its equipment, and the invoices of its medical stores were, in fact, only received at Capetown while on passage.

On arriving in Egypt, the second tented hospital also went to El Tahag transit camp where it remained till May 15. The unit then left for Palestine, and arrived in Haifa on May 17. Here the first week was spent in checking and mustering its medical stores and equipment. As has already been described above, the stores of the first and second tented hospitals had become intermingled and confused, and they were even further disorganised during the period of sorting at Haifa. But this situation, though it had greatly embarrassed the first tented hospital on active service, was of little importance in the case of the second tented hospital which continued to remain at Haifa unemployed, though at 24 hours' notice for active service.

Originally, the personnel of the second tented hospital had consisted of two surgeon lieutenant commanders, two surgeon lieutenants, one warrant wardmaster and fifty sick berth ratings.

The naval staff to which the hospital was attached consisted of 6 executive officers, an accountant staff, and some 70 ratings. To this unit was appointed a separate base medical officer.

Many of the administrative difficulties experienced by the second tented hospital could be traced to the fact that this small naval staff unit did not require a hospital for itself. Also, not being in operational control, the unit itself was unable to allot any more useful duties to the hospital elsewhere. Then again, M.N.B.D.O.(1) was itself gradually becoming widely dispersed and under the administrative

---

* The senior medical officer of the first tented hospital was subsequently mentioned in despatches. The official record states that 'he carried out his work in a most praiseworthy manner under trying conditions, and his encouragement and coolness gave all who came in contact with him courage and hope'.

command of numerous officers in charge of the various areas in which its components happened to be stationed.

The administrative limitations were immediately illustrated when hostilities broke out on the Syrian border, in connexion with which the medical authorities in Palestine would have been grateful for the assistance of the second tented hospital. But this unit was at that time still under 24 hours' notice for active service in Crete, despite the fact that Crete had been evacuated a week before. Also the Naval Staff (N.S.1) to which it was attached had left Palestine, though it was still the administrative authority of the second tented hospital. Permission was therefore sought from Group Headquarters in Cairo for the second tented hospital to unpack its stores and assist in the local situation in Palestine and Syria. Group Headquarters was, however, unable to grant this authority. Instead, the second tented hospital soon received instructions that it must surrender its own medical stores and equipment to the first tented hospital to replace those lost in Crete.

During its life in Haifa, the second tented hospital occupied itself with occasional stretcher-bearing or non-professional clerical duties. Gradually its staff began to be split up. One medical officer and three sick berth ratings had already been sent to Crete. Another medical officer and four sick berth ratings were transferred for duty at Beirut.

On July 11, disorganised, lacking stores, and suffering from the discouragement of continuous unemployment in a most intensely active theatre of war, the second tented hospital returned to Egypt. The unit tried to attach itself to the 64th General Hospital in Alexandria, but there was neither accommodation nor work for it in this fully staffed and busy establishment. The personnel lived in tents in the grounds of the hospital and took part in a variety of casual work ranging from consultations by the medical officers to the duties of telephone operator and messenger by the sick berth staff.

The official records of this unit end on October 5, 1941, and on this date the second naval tented hospital may be regarded as having been disintegrated after an existence of 10 months during which, in spite of every endeavour and willingness to serve, it can never be claimed to have been put to any useful purpose.

FURTHER MOVEMENTS OF THE FIRST R.N. TENTED HOSPITAL

To return to the activities of the first naval tented hospital. With the close of operations in Greek waters, this unit had now returned to El Tahag, but completely lacking any medical stores or equipment. Since landing at Alexandria after leaving Crete, there had been a period of some nine days during which it had been virtually impossible to find any authority capable of accepting administrative responsibility for the movements or future of this unit. In fact, at this time, a period of military and naval re-organisation was in train in this part of the

Mediterranean area which made the future of M.N.B.D.O.(1) itself somewhat uncertain. Meanwhile, the personnel of the first tented hospital performed general medical duties at El Tahag until the unit was resuscitated concurrently with the dissolution of the second tented hospital and the acquisition of the stores and equipment of the latter.

On July 9, 1941, the senior medical officer visited Haifa with two members of his sick berth staff, and arranged to take over all the stores and equipment of the tented hospital units which were available there. These stores eventually arrived at the Bitter Lakes in September.

The first tented hospital was now once more responsible for 5,500 men, but these men were scattered over the whole of Egypt in large and small groups. For example, one searchlight unit was dispersed over 400 square miles in 35 parties of 10.

The larger groups of the M.N.B.D.O. had their own medical officers allotted to them. The smaller groups each had a sick berth rating. The very smallest had two Marines qualified in first aid. There were in all some 8 sick bays deployed over a large area, the largest with 25 beds, and the smallest with 4 beds.

The senior medical officer had his own sick bay at headquarters, and spent much of his time travelling about to visit the others.

The general pattern in which these sick bays were dispersed aimed at preserving them all as part of the whole tented hospital unit, which could re-assemble its personnel into a single organised unit within a minimum of time.

At this time a constant difficulty, as always, was that of transport. The senior medical officer had no personal transport to begin with, and had to depend on what he could borrow from other units. Eventually he was given a 2-ton truck by the British Red Cross Society, but he would seem to have found difficulty in obtaining petrol for it.

Eight ambulances had been promised to the tented hospital, and these had actually been despatched from the United States, but they were unfortunately sunk in transit.

During this period, the senior medical officer expressed much anxiety about the general hygiene of M.N.B.D.O.(1). In his opinion both officers and men of the Royal Marines had much to learn about camp sanitation in hot climates. The correct use of latrines and the disposal of refuse was ill-understood. Flies were numerous. Garbage bins were almost unobtainable. A rule was also in force which permitted urination at a distance of 25 ft. from a tent. Within a few weeks this distance had been reduced habitually to 5 ft. or even less.

A hygiene drive was commenced with the object of improving camp sanitation. Bucket latrines were replaced by deep trench latrines built out of two or three tar barrels sunk into the ground one on top of the other. 'Squatter type' latrines were recommended, and there was no prejudice against these among the men. Urine buckets were installed.

Officers and men were constantly reminded and educated in their hygiene and sanitation responsibilities.

A dog belonging to a rating fell sick, went mad and died of rabies within a few days. In consequence, 5 ratings had to attend hospital daily for two weeks for preventive treatment. This incident had the effect of reminding officers and men of the dangers of at least one of the diseases endemic in the country in which they were now living.

The most valuable function performed by this tented hospital at this time was to reduce the number of possible hospital admissions through the institution of its satellite sick bays. It was estimated that the existence of these sick bays, each with its small number of beds, had saved some 70 per cent. of the usual admissions to hospital. This was a matter of some importance under the system existing at that time, particularly as a satisfactory liaison between the Service Medical Authorities had not yet been fully developed. Naval patients who found their way into local Army hospitals were likely to be absorbed into an inflexible system of evacuation. For example, one rating of M.N.B.D.O.(1) who was discharged to hospital with a minor ailment was rapidly transferred to another hospital, and as rapidly evacuated to a convalescent establishment in India!

Another difficulty was that men from isolated units were liable to be sent into an Army hospital without the senior medical officer of M.N.B.D.O.(1) being informed. Also, when Army Form B.117 (the equivalent of a Naval Hurt Certificate) was rendered to Royal Marine Group Headquarters by any military hospital, the senior medical officer was frequently not informed of its existence. Such matters as this were also complicated by the fact that the loss of all medical records in Crete had necessitated the preparation of some 6,000 new Medical History Sheets for M.N.B.D.O. personnel, and from then on, a record office was attached to the first tented hospital.

In the light of the experiences in Crete, some attention was given to the question of accommodation inside the hospital. Sandbagging of tents up to 6 ft. was the rule rather than sinking them, to which practice objections have already been set down above. However, the most successful of the sick bays constructed consisted of three tents joined together and sunk 3 ft. into the ground, the sunken portion being concreted. This structure contained a ward of 12 beds, an office, a dispensary, a galley, dressing room, and a small stores space. The work of construction was undertaken by Italian prisoners-of-war.

In addition to his routine duties and responsibilities, the senior medical officer was involved in the medical planning for two impending operations.

In the first of these, a medical officer, sick berth staff and stores were required for the care of 500 marines for an indefinite period. This party eventually left at two hours' notice in the middle of one night, but it is not clear from available records which particular operation was involved.

The second operation was one in which about 1,500 men were to leave on detached duties for about three months. These 1,500 men were to be divided into two parties, and there were to be personnel and stores for two sick bays. The casualties in this operation were expected to be wholly medical ones, and the exploit is fully described later.

A further task was the medical organisation for the whole of the first Royal Marine Group, which had been warned to be ready to take up an operational rôle oversea in a few weeks. As part of this organisation a 200-bedded tent hospital had to be planned. With this in view, extra medical stores and equipment were collected from all over the Middle East, and were sent to a central depot at Geneifa.

At this point in the history of the M.N.B.D.O., the available records become both confusing and conflicting, and it has been difficult for historians to trace a continuous narrative. Nevertheless, it would seem that the proposed 200-bedded tent hospital mentioned above resulted in the eventual production of two separate tented hospital units, which left Egypt for a destination overseas. One of these units undoubtedly saw service in the Maldive Islands, but the other does not seem to have performed any recorded function. It is on record that the original senior medical officer of the first tented hospital fell sick in Egypt. It is also on record that one of the surgeon lieutenants of the first tented hospital was taken prisoner-of-war in the neighbourhood of Tobruk, while others served with isolated units in the Middle East, India and Burma.

A final record also states that the stores for a tented hospital were shipped from Egypt to Madras, and from there to Colombo. But there is no record of personnel being together in numbers sufficient to establish a tented hospital with these stores.

OPERATIONS IN THE MALDIVE ISLANDS

The specific operation involving M.N.B.D.O.(1), which is referred to above, was carried out by Royal Marine Operational Unit T, known as Force 'Piledriver'.

This operation was to be carried out on Addu Atoll in the Maldive Islands, the object being to provide a resting and refuelling base for the Eastern Fleet.

Operational Unit T was embarked from Egypt in one of H.M. ships on September 20, 1941, and arrived at Addu Atoll on September 30. General disembarkation took place on October 8, by which time it had been decided that a second operational force, Unit W, would assist in the first stages of the operation. The total personnel disembarked numbered 1,100.

The medical personnel of Unit T consisted of 3 medical officers and 9 sick berth staff, and that of Unit W consisted of 2 medical officers and

6 sick berth staff. The medical organisation included the setting up of a tented hospital of 20 beds, and the usual medical facilities and hygiene measures.

The area occupied on Addu Atoll had no white inhabitants, and the only information available from previous medical surveys was that cases of elephantiasis had been observed among the islanders, and that malaria was suspected. The Atoll itself consisted of a number of small coral islands, each of which had a fringe of coconut palms and a small central plantation. Undergrowth between the palms was mainly very thick, but at no place impenetrable. The climate was uniformly damp and warm. Heavy rain storms were a typical and frequent feature, ten days being the longest rain-free period. The temperature varied between 75° and 95° F. Mosquitoes were soon found to be common as were tree rats and flies.

The personnel were split up between three of the islands, a hundred men landing on Islands designated as I and II, and the remainder on Island V where the tented hospital was established. Sick bays were set up on Islands I and II, each with one medical officer and one sick berth rating.

The medical story of this expedition was indeed a gloomy one, and has been partly described in the chapter on Preventive Medicine in the Administration Volume of this History. An increasing sick list made it necessary for the tented hospital to be expanded to 90 beds, and even to be reinforced by H.M.H.S. *Vita* between November 20 and December 20.

At one time more than 15 per cent. of the total personnel were on the sick list, and this figure was an underestimate of the number of men unfit for duty, because many were merely excused duty in their tents while unwell, instead of being placed sick officially.

The following diseases were responsible for the high incidence of sickness:

(1) Diphtheria, of which there were 5 cases.
(2) Bacillary dysentery, of which there was a large unspecified number of cases.
(3) Malaria. The records show some 90 first infections of malaria of all types, but with benign tertian predominating.
(4) A major outbreak of scrub typhus, a detailed account of which has been given in the Administration Volume of this History.
(5) Chronic skin ulcerations.
(6) Gastro-enteritis, the largest outbreak being traced to the consump- of food from 'blown' tins.

Apart from specific and identifiable organisms, climate, a diet poor in fruit and vegetables, coral abrasions, mosquitoes, jungle clearing and night work were all considered to have played a part in the poor health of personnel. There seems no doubt, that at this stage of the war, naval hygiene ashore and anti-malarial precautions left much to be desired. As regards malaria, there was no prophylactic medication, and few personal precautions were observed other than sleeping under mosquito nets. The breeding of mosquitoes was little reduced by the spraying of pools in the camp areas, and it was obvious that large scale engineering measures were really necessary to be of real use.

The stores of the unit provided latrine buckets only, so that latrines were improvised and never fully fly-proof. Measures which aimed at covering excrement with coral sand are recorded as having been insufficiently carried out.

The necessary operational duties at Addu Atoll were completed on January 8, 1942, and Force 'Piledriver' ceased to exist as such on January 19. Its personnel were now distributed between three camps in Colombo. Some of these men returned to Addu Atoll in a party numbering 459, and whose function was that of a maintenance unit. A small number was detached for duty at the Island of Diego Garcia. The health of those who remained at Addu Atoll on this occasion was very different from that of the original unit which landed there. The later maintenance unit was accommodated in transports anchored half a mile off shore, and among them there was not one case of primary malaria.

The medical story of operations on Addu Atoll is continued in records of what would appear to be, at all events in part, a resurrection of the second tented hospital, which was established on the Atoll in September 1942. It is not precisely clear how this hospital was assembled, but its purpose was to serve units of M.N.B.D.O.(1) and Royal Marine engineers who were stationed at Addu Atoll with no medical officers of their own.

The site chosen for the hospital was entirely new, and jungle had to be cleared for the purpose.

The hospital had an unfortunate beginning owing to a severe outbreak of gastro-enteritis among its own staff, which affected two medical officers and 38 sick berth ratings. This hospital consisted of 9 tents and a number of wooden huts, the latter containing operating theatre, X-ray room and store, laboratory and galleys.

Rats were very prevalent in the vicinity of the hospital, apparently living in coconuts in tree-tops whence they made sorties to the ground, finding their way into huts and even on to occupied beds. Breakback traps were not satisfactory for dealing with these pests, nor was poisoning, for it was likely that mites would leave the dead bodies of the rats and stray on to human bodies, carrying scrub typhus. The method adopted was to catch the rats in caged traps, and drown them in kerosene or some other liquid lethal to the parasites.

At this time it was possible to study more closely a number of the factors concerned with the prevalence of malaria on Addu Atoll. One difficulty was that it was not feasible to oil the wells of the native villages. Each house in a village would have two wells, a smaller one for drinking and cooking water, and a larger one for bathing. Some of the villages had to be evacuated for a time, and this allowed the smaller wells to be sealed with concrete tops. But such evacuation usually meant that mosquitoes had to find new feeding grounds among Indian and white troops on the Atoll. The Indian troops frequently provided a ready-made reservoir of malarial infection.

In due course an entomological party from Colombo visited the Atoll and carried out investigations. In their opinion the carrier of malaria was *Anopheles Tessellatus*, and in consequence of the rigid observance of many measures which were recommended, by September 1943 anophelenes were greatly reduced in number with a falling off in the incidence of malaria.

Culicines remained as an annoyance, and flies were abundant. But amoebic dysentery is not recorded as having caused many medical casualties on Addu Atoll, though there was a small outbreak in one camp of Royal Marine engineers, which was traced to carriers among food-handlers.

This last tented hospital on Addu Atoll was augmented by the presence of H.M.H.S. *Ophir* in the early part of 1943. In September of the same year, a more permanent sick quarters replaced the tented hospital. This sick quarters was on a more luxurious scale, but it is interesting to record that its daily average complement of patients was only 15, a remarkable contrast with the primitive conditions of twelve months before when a tented hospital was dealing with almost six times that number of sick.

OPERATIONS IN BURMA

Concurrently with the operation involving Force 'Piledriver' on Addu Atoll, early in 1942, units of M.N.B.D.O.(1) in Colombo were asked to find volunteers for 'special service of a hazardous nature'. This service was concerned with the closing stages of the Japanese invasion of Malaya, when the threat to Burma was becoming increasingly grave.

The response of volunteers was immediate, and a party of 4 officers and 102 marines was selected. This party was known as Force 'Viper', and it included a surgeon lieutenant and a leading sick berth attendant. The surgeon lieutenant had already seen active service with the first tented hospital in Crete.

Force 'Viper' left Colombo in H.M.S. *Enterprise* on February 8, 1942, and arrived at Rangoon on February 11. Unfortunately the Japanese advance had made it no longer possible to carry out the duties for which this force had been intended, and instead it took over the task of patrolling the rivers Irawadi and Chindwin in a variety of craft which included motor launches, paddle steamers and small boats.

These craft worked at considerable distances from each other, and it was impossible to organise immediate medical attention for all members of the party.

The boats were all very small, and there was no opportunity for officers or men to get exercise. Consequently when the party finally was forced to take to the land and march in retreat on foot, many suffered with badly blistered feet.

Until Force 'Viper' reached a railhead in India on its retreat, food was very monotonous and nearly all from tins. Fresh vegetables were unobtainable, but plantains were a plentiful fruit. Bread was a rare luxury. Drinking water was obtained from the rivers and boiled.

Unfortunately such medical records as were kept of Force 'Viper' were lost when one of the vessels capsized in the Irawadi river. However, there were few ill-effects of the circumstances in which this party carried out its duties. There was no special accommodation for casualties in the river boats, but fortunately the bulk of any sickness which did result from the expeditions did not occur until the return to civilisation when adequate hospital facilities were available. There were a few cases of enteritis during the retreat, but it is of interest that there were no cases of malaria in Force 'Viper' during the whole six weeks which it spent in Burma.

Two marines were missing after an encounter with the enemy, and only two patients were sent to hospital during the patrol period, one to a river hospital ship in the Irawadi, and the other to an Army field ambulance at Kalewa.

In March 1944 M.N.B.D.O.(1), as such, was recalled to the United Kingdom and disbanded, apart from certain residual units which were merged with the second M.N.B.D.O.

COMMENTARY

At this point it is expedient to study the views which were expressed by naval medical opinion in September 1943, in the light of the experience gained to date of the use of tented hospitals. The senior medical officer of a Royal Marine Group stated in his Medical Officer's Journal:

'There is no place for a tented hospital as part of a military formation. It should be an entirely separate organisation. In effect this was how the first naval tented hospital was used in Crete for all its medical officers worked inside the hospital, and none with outside units. But after Crete, all the medical officers of the hospital were detached to work with outside units, and it would not have been possible to reconstruct the hospital without withdrawing these medical officers from their unit duties.

'It is clear that enough medical officers must be supplied to look after outside units themselves. If by reason of action or epidemic further medical services are needed, then a tented hospital, complete with staff, could be added as a separate unit in exactly the same way as a field ambulance is attached to an Army brigade.

'This would be the rational method of using a tented hospital. But, as regards the Navy, it is for consideration whether a tented hospital is worth having at all in relation to an active service group. It is an isolated organisation, and it has nothing behind it. Inevitably, it must find itself becoming part of an Army organisation which is not designed to accommodate it and into which it does not fit.

'One is forced to the conclusion that the medical organisation of casualties incurred on land is far better dealt with by the Army Medical Services, and this point is made for consideration should the question of employment in land operations again arise.

'However, it does seem that there may be a place for a naval tented hospital in a static rôle, where patients can stay in hospital until they are better, and where the need for rapid evacuation does not arise.'

Many other authoritative opinions were given concerning the value of naval tented hospitals. Many views were also expressed as regards the better practical working and maintenance of such hospitals. Among the latter, were strong recommendations that any future tented hospital should include large numbers of non-medical personnel for the purpose of maintenance, refuse disposal, mechanical repairs and the like.

In the light of these comments, it is of some interest to review the medical arrangements for M.N.B.D.O.(2), and particularly, the development of the medical organisation of the Mobile Landing Craft Advanced Bases which were formed later in the war.

M.N.B.D.O.(2)

The second Mobile Naval Base Defence Organisation (M.N.B.D.O.(2)) began to be built up in the first quarter of 1941. The Group Headquarters of M.N.B.D.O.(2) was at Alton, in Hampshire. To start with, the various components of this organisation were scattered between Hayling Island, Portland, the Plymouth area, Wales and Scotland.

The medical arrangements were in charge of a surgeon commander, R.N.V.R., and by the end of March he had 4,058 officers and men under his care; 1,700 were on Hayling Island, while the remainder were undergoing various kinds of specialised training in other places.

By the end of June 1941, M.N.B.D.O.(2) consisted of 7,500 persons. Its medical personnel consisted of 10 medical officers, 3 dental officers and 82 sick berth ratings.

The medical organisation of M.N.B.D.O.(2) visualised the formation of a base tented hospital, and this came into being on October 7, 1941. During the latter half of 1941, the medical staff as a whole gained valuable experience and training under canvas, and as it was by now realised that the function of M.N.B.D.O.(2) would be in the nature of a combined operation, it was decided to employ Army titles for the various appointments and supply units within the medical organisation, for purposes of convenience. The establishment was worked out on a scale of 1 medical officer per 1,000 men (regimental aid post) supported by 1 sick quarters per 2,000 men (forward field section) supported by a hospital capable of dealing with all major surgical and medical cases (casualty clearing station).

There were also to be a beach embarkation staff for the evacuation of casualties from shore to hospital ship, a dental section and a field hygiene section.

This medical organisation, with its stores and equipment, took some time to build up, but finally became a separate entity on August 1, 1942. It had attached to it an executive Royal Marine officer with a staff for administrative purposes.

From September 1 to November 19, 1942, operational training took place in the Bordon area, and during this period the medical personnel underwent training in such matters as landing drill, deployment, map reading and field hygiene.

The beginning of 1943 found M.N.B.D.O.(2) mobilised, with a strength of 8,000, and on January 14 the organisation was conveyed by sea to Egypt, arriving on March 21.

Training was continued for the next three months under local conditions, and by the end of June 1943, M.N.B.D.O.(2) had been allotted its rôle in the anticipated invasion of Sicily, and its medical organisation was fully equipped and well acquainted with the part it was likely to be called upon to play. The senior medical officer had co-operated closely with the D.D.M.S. 8th Army, to which the Group now belonged. For the purpose of this operation, this M.N.B.D.O. had necessarily been split up into various detachments spread over the Nile Delta, Tripoli and Malta. Likewise, the medical organisation was also divided so as to be able to deal with various stages of the operation. Convoys of troops were timed to reach Sicily about every fourteen days, and each convoy was to carry a medical detachment. It was planned to land the field hygiene section, including a malaria specialist, early in the operation.

In broad outline, the medical organisation of M.N.B.D.O.(2) worked smoothly and satisfactorily in the invasion of Sicily. The first medical detachment, which had been waiting in Malta, landed at Augusta on July 13, within a few hours of that base having been captured. This detachment consisted of 7 medical officers and 18 sick berth ratings, with 16 marines for miscellaneous non-medical duties. The medical transport of this detachment consisted of five ambulances, five 15-cwt. trucks and nine motor cycles. This medical detachment was accompanied by part of the field hygiene section.

The field surgical unit, with full staff and equipment for an operating theatre, landed at Augusta on July 14, in company with the 151st Light Field Ambulance R.A.M.C. This field surgical unit became responsible for all the surgery of the Augusta area.

On July 24, one forward field section and two regimental aid posts arrived at Augusta, as well as the remainder of the field hygiene section and two anti-malarial control units.

A further forward field section arrived in Augusta on August 3.

The casualty clearing station which had been in Tripoli arrived in Sicily on August 6.

This casualty clearing station began its life in Sicily by being temporarily accommodated on a site 7 miles south-west of the port of Augusta. Three days later a new location was chosen in the vicinity, and, after some slight delay while waiting for the arrival of stores, tents and accessories, 4 wards were ready to receive patients on August 11. These wards contained 38 beds, but extra accommodation had to be improvised rapidly, as 52 patients were admitted in the first 24 hours.

On August 14 the number of beds was increased to 112, and by the end of the month to 185. All these beds were fully occupied during this period, and between August 25 and September 8, the daily admissions to this tented hospital averaged 100.

The mobile laboratory arrived on September 22, and was put into use immediately. This vehicle had a 3-ton Albion chassis mounted on six wheels with the two pairs of rear wheels coupled. The whole vehicle was 22 ft. long by 10 ft. high by 7 ft. broad. The laboratory portion of the vehicle was 15 ft. by 7 ft. by 7 ft., and divided into two compartments. One compartment contained an incubator, water bath, hot air oven and steam sterilisers, all of which stood on slating. The other compartment contained two benches with drawers and cupboards beneath, a sink, space for media containers, and racks for bottles. Towards the back of the vehicle was a refrigerator.

The laboratory vehicle had four large windows which could be lowered, and which were provided with sliding anti-fly curtains and blackout blinds.

This vehicle was well sprung and easy to maintain. It had a 12-volt battery for internal lighting and for microscopy, and there was a transformer of 100–270 volts which enabled mains electric current to be used should it be available. The vehicle contained a water pump for supplying water to a 60-gallon tank in the roof.

The staff of this mobile laboratory consisted of 1 medical officer, 1 L.S.B.A.(L), and a marine driver who looked after the maintenance of the vehicle. During the Sicily campaign this mobile laboratory more than justified its existence, and performed most valuable work for all the medical services in the area. Its apparatus proved to be most satisfactory, although mainly operated by paraffin or primus stove.

It will be remembered that the tented hospital unit of M.N.B.D.O.(2) had previously applied to itself the title of casualty clearing station, with a view to its more convenient working in company with the Army Medical Services. Soon after its arrival in Sicily, co-operation with the Army Medical Authorities went further, and, on August 12, 1943, the General Officer Commanding in Sicily ordered the medical services of M.N.B.D.O. (2) to be reorganised on Army lines. This reorganisation went so far as to include a complete alteration of the constitution and medical documentation of the Group.

Whether such a wide departure from naval routine by a naval organisation was really intended is not clear. That it was justified is certain, on the grounds that the whole operation in Sicily was a combined one, and that the Naval Medical Services were but a small component of the far larger Army Medical Organisation. Nevertheless, the fact remains that the reorganisation ordered on August 12 resulted in a system of medical documentation being evolved which made it impossible to render proper returns to the Medical Director-General of the Navy. Also only a partial Medical Officer's Journal was rendered to the Admiralty for this particular period, and such Journal as was rendered was very incomplete and provided only scanty information.

Study of such poor records as are available suggests the possibility that the Naval Medical Authorities in Sicily assumed that the Army Medical Authorities would return statistics and details of all Navy patients. It is also possible that the Army authorities assumed that this would be carried out by the Navy.

But a far more probable reason for the scanty details of patients treated by the casualty clearing station of M.N.B.D.O.(2) might well be that on August 28, a shell exploded in the officers' lines, and wounded the senior medical officer twice in the right forearm. A nerve lesion was involved and he was transferred to the 11th General Hospital, Catania. On September 20 he was evacuated from Sicily. It seems likely that the absence of this officer at a crucial moment in the administration of the clearing station may have led to a breakdown in its system of medical records for purely naval purposes.

But, whatever the true reason, the full details of the work of this casualty clearing station in the course of an important combined operation are not available for inclusion in the Naval Medical History of the War.

Although figures are not available, it would seem that medical cases predominated in this casualty clearing station. A resuscitation unit was formed, but was not brought into use after September 15, 1943. Also it would seem that a large amount of the work done by this unit was not confined to casualties, because a note states that 'Transfusions were given in the acute surgical and medical wards as required'. This statement suggests that the resuscitation unit was called upon whenever routine intravenous therapy of some kind was required.

Of the medical cases, malaria and enteritis were the main diseases to come under treatment.

Malaria figures are not available; also, a note states that during August large numbers of patients had to be evacuated elsewhere undiagnosed. Confirmed diagnosis of malaria by microscopy were not made until early September. Of the proved cases of malaria, three only were malignant, but two of these three were cerebral in type.

On November 1, 1943, the casualty clearing station moved into winter quarters inside the Royal Naval Base, Augusta, where a unit of 170 beds was established. At the same time, part of the casualty clearing station was divided from the rest as a small operational hospital unit of 75 beds, which left Sicily for duties elsewhere on December 8.

On December 26, 1943, all patients of the casualty clearing station were evacuated to the 33rd General Hospital, Syracuse. Evacuation was completed by December 29. The casualty clearing station re-opened for a matter of a few days on December 31, in order to deal with casualties from a severe air raid, but there is no further record of its existence after January 5, 1944.

At the time when M.N.B.D.O.(2) arrived in Augusta, the town was empty, bombed, looted and desolate. The local inhabitants had mostly fled at the beginning of the invasion of Sicily, and those who had remained lived in isolated farms and villages, or in caves around the coast in conditions of the utmost squalor. Two Italian doctors had remained in the region, but they had no transport and very few trucks. But these doctors were of some value in dealing with a rising incidence of sickness in the civil population. It was soon found that enteric fever was already present, and considerable care was necessary to prevent an epidemic.

Within a few days the medical officers of the regimental aid posts found that they were seeing large numbers of civilians each day, in addition to an average of 120 attending patients from the Services. Civilian sick needing hospital treatment were sent to an Italian hospital in Melilli.

Meanwhile, the field hygiene section of M.N.B.D.O.(2) performed valuable services. During August 1943 camps were sited, local water was purified and investigations were carried out in relation to all the local endemic diseases. The anti-malarial control units tested and sprayed all accessible breeding grounds of anophelenes. The institution of these public health measures in the area of Augusta was highly organised, and carried out with dispatch, and, by the end of September 1943, the return of the civil population and the coming rainy season were regarded with confidence in regard to the control of epidemic diseases.

In addition to measures to control the breeding of mosquitoes, other anti-malarial measures of a more personal nature were prophylaxis with mepacrine for all personnel, dress discipline after dusk, the use of anti-mosquito cream, and mosquito nets or mosquito-proof bivouac tents.

It is of interest to note a short record which puts the number of cases of malaria among naval personnel in Sicily at 212, of which 28 cases were malignant in type and the remainder benign. Unfortunately, it is not clear whether these cases occurred in August and September 1943, or during the last quarter of the same year. Neither is it made clear whether the figures refer to naval personnel in the Augusta area or throughout the whole of the Island of Sicily. But, in any case, it seems likely that the cases occurred during the last quarter of 1943, after the rainy season had commenced. In each case, the figures might imply that the anti-malarial precautions taken were not effective. However, the short record has taken this implication into account by emphasising that the figures compared most favourably with those for other troops in Sicily.

From the beginning of 1944, the medical records of M.N.B.D.O.(2) are so scanty as to be of little value. Already, as early as the end of August 1943, much of the medical organisation had begun to be split up and absorbed into the Army Medical Services in this campaign in Sicily. The R.N. Field Ambulance was soon broken up, some of the regimental aid posts advanced into Italy, and at least one forward field section was detached for duty in Sardinia.

The subsequent history of the medical organisation of M.N.B.D.O.(2) became more and more the history of individual units scattered over a vast area, and appearing at times in the most unexpected places. For example, one regimental aid post seems to have made its way to North Wales, where it became static and reorganised itself as the Royal Naval Sick Quarters, Towyn.*

Another example is that of the regimental aid post which accompanied Royal Marine Detachment 375. This detachment consisted of 100 Royal Marines and 760 Royal Marine Engineers. Its function was to repair and maintain naval ports as the invasion of Southern Europe progressed. It had its headquarters on San Vincenzo Mole, Naples. From here it sent parties to Leghorn, San Giorgio, Ancona and Cesenatico. Each of these parties created problems of accommodation, hygiene and medical and surgical treatment.

As time passed, some of the ancillary units were recalled while others became attached to and absorbed into new military or naval organisations set up in their neighbourhood.

M.N.B.D.O.(2) ceased to exist as such on July 27, 1944.

---

* This is an example of the type of naval sick quarters which came into being sporadically, described in Volume I, Chapter 14.

MOBILE LANDING CRAFT ADVANCED BASES (MOLCAB)

It is appropriate to recount here the history of the medical aspects of the Mobile Landing Craft Advanced Bases of the Navy, organisations which came into being late in the war, and which were in essence natural and direct descendants of the Mobile Naval Base Defence Organisations.

During the invasion of Europe by the Allied Liberating Armies in the years 1943-5, it transpired that there were times when no provision was made for the crews of minor landing craft once the initial stages of an assault were completed. Such craft as were not attached to Landing Ships (Infantry), were abandoned on the beaches, and their crews lived on the land and their wits until they could be relieved or absorbed into other units.

In preparation for the liberation of South East Asia from the Japanese, MOLCABs. were designed to accommodate the crews of landing craft, and to repair the craft as necessary for further assaults.

It was evident that these crews, as well as the personnel manning the MOLCAB organisation, would need medical attention, and since the officers and men concerned were to be drawn from the Royal Navy and Royal Marines, the medical personnel would consist of naval medical officers and sick berth staff. There was already a precedent for this in the medical organisation of M.N.B.D.Os. and there was also a great deal of operational experience gained from the M.N.B.D.Os. which had revealed errors and omissions of medical organisation which it was intended should be rectified and guarded against in the case of MOLCABs.

In broad outline, the intended commitments of a MOLCAB were laid down early in 1945 as follows:

(a) To accommodate, in tents or such other buildings as might be available locally, 1,500 officers and men, over and above the permanent complement of the MOLCAB itself.
(b) To provide first aid, hull, electrical and engine repairs to landing craft, and to supplement the existing repair facilities afloat.
(c) To provide radio and radar maintenance facilities for landing craft.
(d) To provide naval stores replenishment for landing craft.
(e) To provide a 100-bedded hospital ashore for landing craft personnel.
(f) To provide recreational facilities and amenities to include laundering, tailoring, canteens, and the like.

As mobility was to be the essential characteristic of any MOLCAB, the limiting factor in its design was that no structure or item of equipment should be included which would take longer than one month concurrently with the whole, to erect or dismantle. The part to be played by a MOLCAB in the course of an operation indicated that it would follow an assault at about D-day+3, and would establish itself with a view to providing the above services and to assisting the build up for the next assault.

MOLCABs. were to be provided on the principle of two for each assault force, in order to permit them to 'leap-frog' forward as an amphibious campaign developed.

Each MOLCAB was to be commissioned as an independent command on its disembarkation, and they were allocated the ship names of H.M.Ss. *Landswell, Landlock, Landseer, Landline, Landmark* and *Land Breeze.*

The commanding officer of a MOLCAB held the rank of colonel, Royal Marines, and his MOLCAB was divided into two units each commanded by a lieutenant colonel, Royal Marines. The whole MOLCAB was under naval discipline, and the personnel included two naval staff officers to represent naval interests.

The medical team of a MOLCAB was planned to consist of a surgeon commander or surgeon lieutenant commander, R.N., as senior medical officer, a surgeon lieutenant commander or surgeon lieutenant, R.N., as deputy senior medical officer, and 6 surgeon lieutenants, with a sick berth staff of 33 ratings. This medical complement would man the hospital and at least one separate sick bay.

It was considered that the senior medical officer should have experience in tropical medicine, and that the remaining medical officers should include one with surgical experience and one with a knowledge of anaesthetics.

Each MOLCAB was to have its own dental department, with two dental surgeons and two sick berth ratings (D).

Only two of the planned MOLCABs. came fully into being before the end of the war. These were H.M.S. *Landswell* and H.M.S. *Landlock.* Each of these performed valuable service in the East Indies. Part of H.M.S. *Landline* came into being, and was employed in the crossing of the Rhine, after which the bulk of its medical stores and equipment was sent to augment those of H.M.S. *Landswell* and H.M.S. *Landlock.*

H.M.S. LANDSWELL (MOLCAB I)

Officers and men of the Royal Navy and Royal Marines who were required for H.M.S. *Landswell* assembled at Hayling Island in November and December 1944. The total complement was 43 officers and 525 men. There were 8 medical officers and 35 sick berth ratings. There were also 2 dental officers and 2 sick berth ratings (D). The complement included a trained anti-malarial section of 1 officer and 14 men.

The senior medical officer was a surgeon commander, R.N. His deputy was a surgeon lieutenant commander, R.N., who was also surgical specialist. The remaining medical officers were surgeon lieutenants, R.N.V.R.

The sick berth staff included specialist ratings, qualified as operating room assistant, dispenser, laboratory technician, radiographer and physiotherapist.

H.M.S. *Landswell* was accommodated on Hayling Island in a building which had been a school, and overflowed into billets in nearby houses.

As it was known that the party was intended to take part in operations in the Far East, the first steps taken medically were to examine and grade all ranks and ratings with a view to excluding any who might prove unfit for strenuous tropical commitments. Vaccinations were brought up to date, as were inoculations against the typhoid group of infections.

A number of officers and men was detached for duty at Southampton. These latter were accommodated in Southampton Docks, and were employed to unload the stores as they arrived by rail, and in sorting them out and loading them into 5 Landing Ships Tanks (L.S.T.). The stores which arrived at Southampton included a tent hospital unit which had been constructed at the Naval Medical Store Depot, Wellingborough. This consisted of no less than 1,300 cases and bundles. It was impossible to inspect these stores in detail at this stage, so attention was merely concentrated on the loading lists, and suggestions made for any additions which were considered desirable. For example, it was considered that some convenient form of anæsthetic apparatus should have been included, and this was, in fact, added within a few days.

Advantage was taken of the period of assembly at Hayling Island to detach certain personnel for special training. Certain medical officers attended the London School of Tropical Medicine, as did the Royal Marine officer carried for anti-malarial duties. The senior medical officer made frequent visits to the Hygiene Department at the Admiralty and the Royal Army Medical College at Millbank. All medical officers attended a course in tropical medicine at Millbank, and also received training at the Army School of Hygiene, Mytchett. Unfortunately, it proved impossible for any of the sick berth staff to be so trained at Mytchett.

The 5 L.S.Ts. were loaded at Southampton Docks during the latter part of January 1945, and the personnel embarked on the last day of the month, with the exception of 8 officers for whom there was no room, and who had to wait for passage by troopship. The L.S.Ts. concerned were:

 No. 410, carrying the senior officer of the L.S.T. Flotilla and his staff, which included a surgeon lieutenant;

 No. 538, which served as headquarters ship, and which carried the commanding officer of the MOLCAB and his staff, including the surgeon commander;

 Nos. 368, 427 and 413, each of which carried a surgeon lieutenant among its passengers.

At the last moment L.S.T. 368 was delayed by engine trouble, but the remainder moved out to Spithead on January 31, and the following day, sailed on the first stage of their journey to the East. It was understood that, although their ultimate commitment would be connected with an operational assault, there would be a period of training and acclimatisation at some port before actually coming in contact with the enemy.

The journey was broken at Dartmouth on February 2 and Falmouth on February 4–7, after which a convoy was joined which included L.S.T. 368 and a newcomer, 421. Heavy weather was encountered all the way to Gibraltar, in the course of which certain features of L.S.Ts. were revealed to those on board. These craft have a lateral roll which is very quick, and their elasticity makes them bounce repeatedly after meeting a heavy sea. Each of the ships was carrying MOLCAB stores and vehicles on the tank deck, and as there were no scuppers on the upper deck, water collected there and tended to find its way through some of the hatches to the detriment of materials stored below.

Passage through the Mediterranean was more comfortable. L.S.T. 538 was detached at Malta for repairs to her wireless generators, while the others went on to Port Said. Up to this point, the only medical event of the voyage was the development of a dental root abscess by the commanding officer. Unfortunately, he happened to be in one of the craft which had no dental officer and no dental forceps on board!

The ships stopped at Port Said and Port Tewfik from February 28 until March 8. They then continued their journey down the Red Sea and across the Indian Ocean, and on March 25, 1945 arrived at Cochin, Southern India.

H.M.S. *Landswell* now disembarked and was accommodated in Anson Camp, on Willingdon Island, in Cochin Harbour. This camp was originally designed for the Royal Indian Navy, and had been built by engineers of the Indian Army. Like the many adjacent camps on Willingdon Island, it consisted mainly of long single-storied huts with concrete floors, walls of brickwork surmounted by rush work, and tiled double roofs. The dining halls, galleys, and annexes such as latrines and washhouses were of white-washed bricks. Unfortunately, having been built to accommodate Indian personnel, the bulk of the latrines had native style 'squat' pans, and the greater number depended on bucket flushing by hand.

Electricity and water mains were laid on.

At the time of the arrival of the unit, Anson Camp was not really ready for occupation, also, to personnel freshly trained in camp hygiene, the public health aspect of the camp broke every rule. Nevertheless, the purpose of the pause in Cochin was that of training and acclimatisation, and in retrospect, it was perhaps to the advantage of the personnel that they should realise so soon that the maintenance of health in the East calls for active and positive measures.

From the outset, the difficulties presented by Anson Camp were legion. The latrines had no lids to render them fly-proof, and even bucket flushing could not be effected because of lack of labour. The entrances to septic tanks were blocked by builder's rubble and refuse, so that overflow and seepage into the surrounding ground was common. The effluent from the tanks was emptied on to the foreshore, because instead of the usual metal pipes running 20 ft. beyond low tide, there were merely broken pottery pipes projecting a foot or two from the bank. The water was too shallow to wash away this effluent, and consequently there was a constant smell and breeding ground for flies.

The floors of washhouses were uneven, so that water collected in pools, while outside the gutters were inadequate, so that the water drained on to the ground.

In the main cookhouse, the outlets of sinks were merely holes in the walls, so that sullage ran down the outside of the wall on to the grass. On one side of this cookhouse was a ditch, constantly full of foul stagnant fluid, and this ditch was so inclined that the fluid was thwarted in its attempts to reach the harbour a few yards away.

The storm drainage of the camp presented no recognisable plan, and most of the ill-constructed ditches were half finished. Also, as the camp was at no point more than 8 ft. above mean sea level, underground pipes had to start near the surface if they were to carry any distance, and these pipes were therefore liable to be broken by vehicles passing over the ground.

The water supply was a cause of grave anxiety, and was never solved during the stay of H.M.S. *Landswell* in Cochin. Although water mains existed from a modern water works some miles away, automatic chlorination was unreliable, and consequently all the water used for drinking had to be boiled.*

All these conditions were favourable to the spread of disease, but early and rapid improvements were effected by the personal energy of the senior medical officer. Within a few weeks, concrete drains had been constructed around the cookhouse, and concrete standing had been provided outside it. Aldershot stoves were installed inside. All cookhouses and food stores were fly-proofed. The latrine drains were cleared and proper metal effluent pipes run out under the surface of the shallow water, and protected by breakwaters of loosely packed boulders. Adequate monsoon drains were constructed throughout the entire camp. Finally, large numbers of natives were employed to keep the latrines in good condition and constantly flushed.

It is of some interest that in spite of the favourable conditions for their breeding, flies did not appear in the numbers expected. This was

---

* Reference is made to this type of difficulty in Volume I, Chapter 12.

considered to be due to the fact that as Willingdon Island had been built up of reclaimed soil, the salt in the ground was possibly inhibitory in effect.

As regards medical arrangements inside Anson Camp, a permanent building was in course of construction as a sick bay, but meanwhile, the medical department was accommodated in a small temporary building. This building consisted of five rooms and a verandah, badly situated adjacent to a parking ground for transport vehicles.

Instructions were that during this period of training and acclimatisation, medical stores were to be kept intact for use in future operations. Such stores and equipment as were needed at this time were drawn, therefore, from the medical department of H.M.S. *Chinkara*, the local Naval Base in Cochin.

A further hut was made into a small temporary sick quarters. Here a dental surgery was constructed and a minor operating theatre, laboratory and ward with accommodation for 12 patients. Patients likely to be ill for more than a few days were discharged to hospital.

Hospital facilities were provided by the Combined Military Hospital, Ernakulam, on the eastern side of Cochin Harbour. For a short time in April 1945, the Hospital Ship *Vita* was at Cochin, being later replaced by an Army hospital carrier, but the latter had few facilities for long term treatment.*

Storage space for permanent medical stores was not available in the docks in Cochin, so for a few weeks these stores were unloaded on a hockey pitch inside Anson Camp. Nevertheless, this was of value, as it became possible to unpack and inspect many of the items of equipment for the first time since they had been packed at Wellingborough. It was also possible to pick out and test and use some of the permanent equipment. An opportunity was also made to train the staff in the erection of some of the hospital tents on ground inside the camp.

As regards general health, the complement of the ship fared well, in spite of the initial apprehension which had been expressed on its arrival in view of the apparently poor local hygienic conditions. Apart from some 30 cases of unexplained pyrexia during April and May 1945, there was little sickness of note.

Cochin is not a malarious area, but for training purposes, and as personal protection against other than malarial vectors, a mosquito curfew was observed in company with all the various camps on Willingdon Island. This meant that mosquito nets must be in position over all beds, and long sleeves and trousers worn from half an hour before sunset until half an hour after sunrise.

---

* A description of the general medical organisation and hospital facilities in the Cochin area is given in Volume I, Chapter 15.

Early after H.M.S. *Landswell* arrived in Cochin, its anti-malarial section was sent to Ceylon for further training, which its personnel received at the Royal Naval School of Tropical Medicine and Hygiene in Colombo. On the return of this section, it performed much useful anti-mosquito prophylaxis on behalf of all the Services accommodated on Willingdon Island, with the result that even during the monsoon period, the local camps were rendered almost entirely mosquito free. This valuable service not only reduced the mosquito as a nuisance, but it also provided the anti-malarial section with further useful training and experience. This clearance also exerted a certain moral effect among the British Services in the area, most of which well realised that the filariasis endemic in the local native population was spread by a mosquito vector, though the incidence of Europeans suffering from this disease was historically negligible.

As the weeks lengthened into months, and as the trend of war in the East changed so rapidly, perhaps the biggest problem with which the senior medical officer had to contend at this time was that of fending off monotony and finding sufficient work for his medical officers. Five of them he sent to Colombo for a course of training in the Royal Naval School of Tropical Medicine and Hygiene. At times, medical officers and staff were lent to other establishments in the neighbourhood to assist in the general medical organisation in the Cochin area. Two medical officers were sent to survey the medical arrangements and facilities at Tuticorin, on the south-east tip of the Indian peninsula. The surgical specialist and his specialised ratings worked both in the Hospital Ship *Vita* and also in the Civil Hospital at Ernakulam.

But in spite of these diversions, monotony was hard to avoid, particularly after the breaking of the monsoon in June, which virtually brought to a standstill such recreations as sailing, gardening, football, cricket and hockey.

In 1945, the rains began in the second week of June and conditions in Anson Camp became very trying. However, all officers and men received 14 days' leave, and the majority went to rest camps at Wellington and Ootacamund in the Nilgiri Hills.

During July suppressive mepacrine was started, as it was anticipated that the unit would be moving into an operational area within a short time.

At the time of its arrival in India, in March 1945, it was planned to employ H.M.S. *Landswell* as part of Operation 'Roger'. This operation was a proposed invasion of the Malayan Peninsula, and it was intended that the unit should establish itself on Puket Island, off the south-west tip of Thailand before the breaking of the monsoon.

Operation 'Roger' did not materialise, and the unit was not employed in the amphibious operations in the Rangoon area. Instead, this MOLCAB unit was instructed to be prepared to take part in Operation 'Zipper'. This operation was also connected with the proposed invasion of Malaya, and in the course of it, H.M.S.*Landswell* was to establish itself on a rubber estate on Carey Island near Port Swettenham.

When the Japanese capitulated in August 1945, Operation 'Zipper' was not cancelled, but was carried out in a modified form.

On August 27, 240 men and most of the officers embarked in the S.S. *Barpeta*. The numbers included all but one of the medical officers and sick berth staff.

The S.S. *Barpeta* sailed from Cochin on August 30, and arrived off the Morib beaches on September 9 but, after waiting for three days, the personnel were transferred into 2 L.S.Ts. and carried to Singapore, arriving on September 14.

On September 15, the commanding officer and his staff went ashore to investigate possible sites on Singapore Island for the establishment of a landing craft base. They selected the former Boom Defence Base at Loyang, on the north-east corner of the Island.

Meanwhile, the senior medical officer had been informed that there was urgent need of doctors and medical stores at the naval base on the northern side of Singapore Island. This area was the former district permanently occupied by the Royal Navy in Singapore. Here, the legacy of Nippon was evident in the crowds of sick and dying who were imploring medical assistance from the doctors of three destroyers which had just arrived.

The senior medical officer carried out a rapid survey of the area, and he at once realised that there was a need for medical assistance on a vast scale, and that the arrival of a tented hospital unit could hardly have been more opportune.

On September 17, the commanding officer took charge of the Boom Defence Base at Loyang, his L.S.Ts. came alongside the concrete jetty there, and the unloading of stores commenced. The concrete jetty led to a 'hard' on which were offices and workshops, and from here the ground sloped up steeply to a plateau on which were several wooden bungalows built on piles. The ground then rose again to a second plateau on which were more wooden buildings. These buildings were all suitable for offices, messes and general accommodation. One building was fitted out as a commodious sick quarters, containing a ward with room for 16 beds, a tiled operating theatre, a dispensary and X-ray department.

For the first 48 hours, personnel continued to eat and sleep on board the L.S.Ts. Meanwhile, the local hygiene conditions were surveyed.

Except on the roadways which were in good condition, tall *lalang* grass covered the ground. The Japanese had torn out all electric fittings and bare points remained. Water in a gravity tank containing 130,000 gallons was cloudy and harboured frogs. Drinking water was therefore obtained from the L.S.Ts., until a local power pump was repaired and chlorination of the local supply carried out.

For purposes of personal protection, it was assumed from the outset that the worst possible sanitary conditions prevailed at Loyang, and full precautions were taken as regards mepacrine prophylaxis and the institution of a 'mosquito curfew'.

The local sanitary arrangements were in poor condition. Dumps of rotting rice were stored beneath nearly all the buildings, garbage lay about everywhere, and flies and rats abounded. The concrete monsoon drains were overgrown by *lalang*, but fortunately once this grass had been removed, the drains themselves were found to be in good condition on the whole.

Loyang was very near Changi Gaol, in which a large number of British had been confined as prisoners-of-war during the Japanese occupation. From some of these released men much local intelligence was gleaned. The prisoners themselves had been carrying out extensive drainage work which had cleared large areas of local swamp. Among the prisoners was an Army officer in charge of a field laboratory. This officer had been a prisoner in the gaol for 3½ years, and he had contrived to continue a certain amount of anti-malarial work. It appeared that the incidence of malaria among the natives locally was quite low. This tribute to the preventive work of pre-war years was confirmed by a low-spleen-rate among natives in the villages around Loyang. But it seemed that among the prisoners inside Changi Gaol, the position had been very different. No less than 30,000 cases of malaria, including relapses, had been recorded. At one time the Japanese had temporarily forbidden control measures, and within a period of one month 10,000 first infections were recorded. The majority of these cases were benign tertian in type, and the source appeared to be prisoners brought back to Changi after working on the Burma-Siam railway project.

When H.M.S. *Landswell* arrived at Loyang, the population of Changi Gaol had dwindled from 50,000 to 10,000 awaiting repatriation. Active steps were being taken to diminish the danger of this huge malarial reservoir to incoming British troops.

It was learned too that scrub typhus had occurred among Allied prisoners at Sime Road Camp, Singapore. But the disease was apparently unknown in the Loyang area.

The anti-malarial unit carried out an immediate mosquito survey over an area of a radius of 1½ miles around Loyang. There was found to be little breeding in the immediate vicinity, and no anophelenes were found. But in the Pasir Ris area there was a large culicine population, and extensive breeding of several anophelene species, including *maculatus, leucosphyrus, subpictus, hyrcanus, kochi* and *ramsayi*. Breeding places were seepage pools, fish tanks, tidal swamps, freshwater pools and hill streams. Anti-malarial work was commenced immediately, and included anti-larval spraying, anti-adult spraying of 5 per cent. D.D.T. in kerosene, clearance of drains, cutting down scrub, filling in holes, etc. The unit worked in close co-operation with anti-malarial squads of the Army and Civil Administration, and the work performed was most effective.

During this disembarkation at Loyang, the medical party was fully employed in devising local arrangements in Loyang itself, and in attending to the far greater medical commitments at the Naval Base 24 miles away. Two medical officers and 7 sick berth ratings were retained in Loyang with such equipment as they needed for emergencies and short term cases. They were provided with one ambulance, and a jeep for their personal transport. It was arranged that long term cases from Loyang should be sent either to the naval base or to the military hospitals which had already been set up on Singapore Island. These last were the 47th B.G.H. and 75th I.G.H., both accommodated in the buildings of Singapore General Hospital, the 69th I.G.H. and 93rd I.G.H.

Little more remains to be written about the unit. Once the surrounding area of Loyang had been cleared and reconstructed, the purpose of this MOLCAB had really ceased to exist, and the establishment was finally paid off at the end of March 1946. The health of its personnel remained good during their time in Singapore, and apart from one case of scrub typhus and a small number of cases of malaria, only minor ailments are on record.

THE ASIATIC HOSPITAL AT THE ROYAL NAVAL BASE

While the ship's service as a MOLCAB was relatively short, its medical organisation had a far longer life and found itself immersed in commitments so extensive as to justify beyond doubt the care which had attended its original conception.*

While H.M.S. *Landswell* was being established at Loyang, medical officers, sick berth staff, stores and equipment were being transported by road to the Royal Naval Base. Here, the commitments to be met were firstly to deal with the immediate requirements of the hordes of Asiatics who were demanding treatment at the Base's Asiatic Hospital, secondly to prepare the hospital for the reception of in-patients, and thirdly to prepare a sick quarters for Europeans. Concurrently with these activities there were large scale hygiene and sanitary problems to be dealt with.

The Asiatic Hospital of Singapore Naval Base had been used as such by the Japanese during their occupation. But most of the Japanese non-consumable stores were found to be unserviceable, and most of the drugs were unidentifiable.

---

* The reader is referred to the brief account of the medical organisation of Singapore Naval Base which is given in the chapter on Medical Establishments Abroad in Volume I.

A number of the hospital's 70 beds was furnished with MOLCAB pillows and blankets. The naval sick berth staff were daily reinforced by Asiatic dressers employed at this hospital before the war. Indian and Chinese clerks also re-appeared very quickly, as well as two Asiatic midwives. These were followed by a number of Asiatic nurses who had been engaged during the Japanese occupation, and others who had heard that nurses were needed at this hospital.

Before the war, the purpose of the small, but well equipped Asiatic Hospital inside Singapore Naval Base, had been to serve the needs of the large number of Asiatic dockyard employees. The pre-war policy had been only to admit dockyard employees to the hospital. Their dependents, although resident inside the Naval Base boundary, were sent to civil hospitals in Singapore and Johore.

But now, following the Japanese capitulation, the civilian hospitals had virtually ceased to exist, and even where they had been able to receive patients, were crowded to capacity. It was therefore obvious that, for the time being, the Navy must accept all persons inside the Naval Base district who needed medical attention. This undertaking was a vast one which included men, women and children resident locally, as well as squatters and immigrants of all kinds.

The four wards of the Asiatic Hospital were soon filled, and beds were set up in every available piece of space on the verandahs and covered ways.

Fortunately this overcrowding was able to be relieved by overflowing into four blocks of two-storey buildings, which the Japanese had used as a hospital in the Asiatic residential quarter of the naval base. These blocks were within $\frac{1}{4}$ mile from the Asiatic Hospital itself, and were capable of accommodating at least 200 patients. Into them were received Asiatic women and children, cases of chronic malnutrition, and one floor was set aside for tuberculous patients.

Pulmonary tuberculosis was perhaps the greatest legacy left behind by the Japanese occupation of this area, and some months later it was necessary to accept the fact that responsibility for the care of these patients was one which the Naval Medical Authorities had to undertake indefinitely, because of the lack of accommodation for Asiatic tuberculous patients anywhere else in Singapore.

A further commitment undertaken during the next few months was that of building up a maternity and child welfare unit.

The feeding of all these patients was a separate problem, and arrangements were made for them to be catered for by a Chinese contractor who provided Indian and Chinese cooking, and whose accounts were met by the dockyard cashier.

Having begun to solve the Asiatic problem for the time being, the senior medical officer established a naval sick quarters in the local naval barracks, more correctly described as 'The Fleet Shore Accommodation'.

For this purpose, a pleasantly situated building was employed, commodious enough to accommodate 30–50 patients in medical and surgical wards. It was also possible here to establish the Central Medical Administrative Offices.

The medical organisation built up in the Singapore Naval Base by the senior medical officer of H.M.S. *Landswell* was a going concern by the beginning of October 1945. During the next few weeks he was able to undertake the resuscitation of the local dockyard surgery and a number of outlying naval medical commitments on other parts of Singapore Island.

The senior medical officer has recorded that during these early weeks fresh commitments were always coming to light. For example there was discovered a camp full of Javanese coolies, whose condition was deplorable. The Japanese had not informed the British about these unfortunate people, who had been left to die of disease and starvation in the utmost squalor and filth. These Javanese had been imported from Java as volunteers for coolie service under the Japanese in Singapore. Their original agreement had been to remain three months, but no steps had ever been taken to return them to Java, and as they fell sick replacements were obtained from the source of supply.

At the end of the occupation, the Japanese had moved their former Naval Hospital to a barracks in the Sembawang area of Singapore Island. They were told to give attention to these Javanese until the senior medical officer was able to make arrangements for them to be dealt with by his own organisation. The more seriously ill were moved to the Japanese Hospital, but the arrangement was unsatisfactory as the Japanese were found to be adept at avoiding their obligations, and the few British doctors were too busy to supervise them closely. But fortunately, some Dutch medical officers became available, who willingly agreed to take charge of these sick Javanese. The survivors were now moved from the Japanese Hospital and accommodated in a Dutch camp nearby, but unfortunately 64 Javanese patients had died before this transfer could be effected.

As regards professional relationship with the Japanese, the senior medical officer of H.M.S. *Landswell* has recorded that he found their attitude embarrassingly obsequious. Several Japanese labour gangs were housed in camps within the Naval Base area, and their health was looked after by Japanese naval medical officers who were found to be reasonably co-operative with the senior medical officer.

In the years immediately before the war, Singapore Naval Base was a model of anti-malarial work and of the sanitary control of a large Asiatic population. Mosquitoes and flies were a rarity. A high standard of cleanliness was observed everywhere, and the occasional employee found to be suffering from tuberculosis or chronic malaria was quickly removed from the district.

To persons who had known the Naval Base under these pre-war conditions, the post-war state of affairs was most distressing. It was easy enough to accept as the natural sequence of war the 150 bomb craters in and around the dockyard, with the associated ruins of buildings, ships and docks. But the Japanese had so advertised themselves as being meticulously health-conscious as a nation, that the neglected drains, blocked sewers, fouled latrines, indiscriminate dumping of refuse and the overall carpet of tall *lalang* grass were as surprising as they were disturbing.

Investigation of this state of affairs revealed that the Japanese had carried out no anti-malarial work during the year 1942. Then the increasing incidence of malaria prompted the formation of a health department which commenced a half-hearted oiling routine, which did at least reduce the sickness rate from this disease during 1943. But meanwhile the dysenteric diseases progressively increased on account of the poor general state of hygiene of the district. In 1944, an intensive food-growing campaign was begun by the Japanese, and anti-malarial squads were not allowed to enter areas under cultivation. Also, during this year there was heavy Allied bombing, which, with the rains, aggravated a sanitary state of affairs which was already deteriorating. The Asiatic occupants of the coolie lines, numbering several thousands, had been made responsible for the cleanliness of their own quarters, but if supervised at all, the standard achieved had only been that considered adequate by Japanese, and it fell far short of what had been considered desirable by Europeans. Heaps of garbage sprang up on all sides, sewer man-holes were purposely blocked and used as cess pits, from which excrement was collected and spread over the vegetable gardens in its raw state as manure. Livestock had been prohibited by the British, but was permitted by the Japanese, so that poultry, pigs and cattle wandered freely about the district.

The rest of this story is told eloquently enough by the admissions to the Asiatic Hospital in the early weeks after it was re-opened by the British. The immediate admissions to hospital on September 19 numbered 149, and by the end of October had increased to 534. The diseases predominating were malaria, pulmonary tuberculosis, dysentery and beriberi.

These figures unfortunately represented merely those Asiatics who were ill enough to be admitted to hospital. Concurrently, the out-patient attendances grew to enormous proportions, and the whole picture provided a grave warning of the constant threat of serious disease in a tropical community when hygiene and sanitary vigilance are relaxed. Neither did the known figures themselves, which could be gleaned from the hospital records, represent anything approaching an accurate index of sickness among the local Asiatic population. Countless numbers of men, women and children knew they were ill, but did not consider that they were ill enough for treatment, or else were prevented by religious or superstitious scruples from seeking medical assistance. But, in addition to these cases of unreported illness, there was reason to believe that much of the reduced efficiency which was noticeable in both manual and clerical workers was due to unsuspected illness. That this suspicion was true soon became obvious from the routine examinations of police, hospital staff, etc., and it was feared, and later confirmed, that routine chest radiography would disclose a tuberculosis problem of gigantic proportions.

The commodore in charge of Singapore Naval Base made it clear from the start that health problems were to be regarded as of high priority, and that every possible assistance was to be given to the senior medical officer and his staff. At the same time the commodore pointed out that on occasions it would be necessary to accept certain medical risks in order to clear up the naval dockyard and to get it in working order to receive shipping. For example, debris and rubble from the dockyard had to be dumped in open spaces for the time being, which meant that vast deposits sprang up throughout the district which were not only an eyesore but provided a constant refuge for flies and mosquitoes. Similarly work on the main water pipes and sewers could not properly be undertaken until qualified technicians had arrived from the United Kingdom, and it was impossible to receive them in Singapore until some kind of dwelling houses had been constructed for them to live in.

The most urgent medical problem was the prevention of intestinal disease, and here the fresh water supply to the Naval Base caused constant anxiety. Part only of this supply was purified water from a reservoir at Johore. The remaining supply came from a reservoir on Singapore Island, and its chlorination at source was known to be inadequate. Ultimately, satisfactory chlorination of this latter supply was effected at source, but there remained a danger from seepage through fractures in the water mains, and from contamination through damaged sewers. It was realised that these defects would have to be accepted for many months pending their repair. Meanwhile, the immediate precaution of boiling all drinking water was undertaken.

A concurrent problem was the disposal of faeces, and home-made destructors or 'coprocausts' were designed for use where the drains were not satisfactory.

A mosquito survey of the Naval Base showed that culicines and *Aedes Aegypti* were abundant. The anophelenes *kochi*, *karwari* and *vagus* were found about the perimeter of the base.

Anti-malarial work was quickly reorganised on the same plan as in pre-war days, with the additional heavy work of clearing thousands of yards of overgrown drains. Craters and casual pools existed in vast numbers, and pending their obliteration, were sprayed with oil or treated with D.D.T. bricks.

As a result of the strenuous measures adopted by the medical department, the newly returned European community of H.M. Naval Base, Singapore, was little troubled by disease during the early weeks after the Japanese capitulation. But there could be no relaxation of vigilance in the months which followed, and it was soon realised that the struggle against potential diseases was one which must be maintained indefinitely. Sporadic illnesses occurred from time to time, but fortunately never achieved epidemic proportions. Of these, the most important were Bornholm disease, among naval ratings, and amoebic dysentery, among the local British civilian community.* The source of the amoebic infection was traced to one of the Japanese camps inside the Naval Base area. It proved impossible to persuade the Japanese medical authorities that faeces and urine, though excellent fertilisers for their vegetable allotments, were also a breeding ground for fly-borne diseases. Eventually, after repeated warnings, this particular Japanese camp was evacuated, and the buildings were burnt down and the whole area soaked in petrol and oil and scorched.

As regards other diseases, an outbreak of poliomyelitis on Singapore Island fortunately by-passed the Naval Base except for two naval ratings, one of whom died.

One severe case of malignant malaria was seen in a naval rating.

One fatal case of smallpox was seen in another naval rating who was shown to have been re-vaccinated on board his ship, and with a negative result, three weeks previously. Against this ever present danger of smallpox, mass vaccination of the European and Asiatic communities was carried out at an early date, as part of the general medical precautions of the area.

H.M.S. LANDLOCK (MOLCAB 2)

H.M.S. *Landlock*, the second MOLCAB, started to assemble at Hayling Island in December 1944.

Its hospital unit was in charge of a surgeon lieutenant commander, R.N., as senior medical officer. The deputy senior medical officer was also a surgeon lieutenant commander, R.N., and the remaining medical officers were six surgeon lieutenants, R.N.V.R., one of whom had had considerable surgical experience. A dental unit was manned by a surgeon lieutenant commander (D), a surgeon lieutenant (D) and two S.B.As.(D).

With one exception, all these medical officers had attended the Army Camp Hygiene Course at Mytchett, and all had received a course in Tropical Medicine. Ten sick berth ratings and eight Royal Marines had also attended the course at Mytchett.

---

* An account of this outbreak of Bornholm Disease appears in the Volume on Medicine and Pathology in this series.

As in the case of H.M.S. *Landswell*, medical stores and equipment had been collected, sorted and loaded at Southampton Docks, and on April 1, 1945, the MOLCAB embarked in L.S.Ts. 331, 336 and 280, and its first destination was also Southern India, but the journey from the United Kingdom was not uneventful. L.S.Ts. 336 and 280 suffered continuous engine trouble, and the former was eventually abandoned at Port Tewfik as beyond repair.

At Port Tewfik, L.S.Ts. 280 and 331 were joined by L.S.Ts. 373 and 371. The latter two craft carried part of the MOLCAB stores and personnel left behind in the United Kingdom till a later date, in order that the whole unit might be dispersed on passage.

Personnel and equipment, including vehicles, from L.S.T. 336 were distributed between the other four craft. This resulted in some overcrowding of the troop-deck spaces which was not a favourable start to passage of the Red Sea and Indian Ocean in hot weather. L.S.T. 280 had engine trouble again in the Red Sea, and had to be diverted to Massawa for repairs. The remaining craft arrived at Cochin on May 30, 1945, but L.S.T. 280 was delayed until the beginning of July.

The senior medical officer has recorded the following interesting remarks regarding the living conditions on board L.S.Ts. over long distances in very hot weather:*

'Naval ratings and Royal Marines were accommodated in messes running the length of the tank space on port and starboard sides of the ship, and entered by the fore and aft companion ways and escape hatches. The ship's company of each L.S.T. itself was accommodated in the large after messdeck. These messes had folding canvas bunks in three tiers on both sides of the centre gangway. There were from 9 to 24 bunks per mess. The messes were ventilated by a single air vent, but unfortunately the air pressure was poor, and the volume of air supplied was quite inadequate. These ships had escape hatches fitted in each mess, and leading to the upper deck. But these hatches had to be closed at night, or in rough weather, or when in dangerous waters. Wash places and lavatories were inboard compartments just aft of the messdecks, and the exhaust fans fitted in these were virtually useless. No other ventilation was available. The tank spaces were also supplied with fans, but these were of little use in practice as an aid to troop space ventilation.

'East of Suez the iron decks became too hot for bare feet and despite constant flooding of the decks by fire hoses, conditions below during the day were intolerable. The deckheads and bulkheads had been insulated against heat, and were merely warm to the touch. But the strengthening beams had not been insulated, so that these became too hot to touch with the bare hand. Also, as the combined surface area of the strengthening beams

---

* The opinion expressed by this medical officer does not take into account the exigencies of war at a time when speed of construction and simplicity of design were paramount and offered little scope for meeting every climatic requirement.

was considerable, they tended to act as radiators of heat and so added to the general discomfort.

'The sick bays of these L.S.Ts. were small, very hot, and quite unsuitable for any bed case while in the hotter climates. Ventilation was by one louvre only and the air pressure poor. The next compartment forward contained the engine room exhaust in these Diesel-driven ships. The sick bay store room was considered to be the hottest compartment in the ship, and on several days in the Red Sea and Indian Ocean, it was impossible to remain in it for more than ten seconds at a time.

'Food was good on the whole. It was served on the cafeteria system, which proved satisfactory in fair weather but very unsatisfactory in wet or rough weather.

'Fresh water was rationed to certain hours of the day for washing, and for shower baths on two days a week. But drinking water was always plentiful, and salt water showers could be obtained each day.'

In spite of the above conditions, the general health of the crew remained good at this period, apart from superficial skin conditions and a few cases of diarrhoea. On leaving Port Tewfik, mepacrine was administered daily as it had not been definitely ascertained whether or not the port of disembarkation would be free from malaria.

On arriving at Cochin, Anson Camp on Willingdon Island was shared with H.M.S. *Landswell*. Here its problems and progress much resembled those described above in the case of the latter unit. The senior medical officer and three of his staff went to Colombo for a course at the Royal Naval School of Tropical Medicine and Hygiene. Twelve sick berth ratings and the anti-malarial unit also received a course at the school in anti-malarial work and tropical hygiene. By arrangement with the Adviser in Anaesthetics, Southern Army, 2 medical officers were able to take a course in anaesthetics at 127 I.B.G.H., Trimulgherry, Secunderabad.

It is of some interest to record that during June and July 1945, a special study was made of skin diseases affecting personnel. It was found that 39 per cent. were septic conditions, 25 per cent. fungoid infections, 21 per cent. prickly heat, and the remaining 15 per cent. miscellaneous in type.

At the beginning of September 1945, the medical organisation began to be split up into groups, and it cannot be said that the organisation ever really existed again as a separate unit.

On September 4, 11 sick berth ratings and a mobile dental unit were sent to a transit camp in Ceylon for temporary duties with a naval party about to proceed to Singapore Naval Base. This group was actually established in the Asiatic Hospital of Singapore Naval Base when the medical party of H.M.S. *Landswell* arrived there later in the month.

On September 7, an advance party consisting of headquarters staff, a surgeon lieutenant with surgical experience and 4 sick berth ratings with a quantity of medical stores, left for Singapore in L.S.T. 237. On arrival, this party was detailed to make provisional arrangements for the sick in a barracks on Blakang Mati Island in Keppel Harbour, Singapore.

The main body sailed for Singapore in L.S.Ts. 3504 and 3508. This party disembarked at Loyang, on Singapore Island, and the bulk of its medical personnel was transferred to Blakang Mati Island. This Island had formerly been occupied by the Royal Artillery as part of the defences of Singapore, and the main barracks was in reasonable repair. The combined efforts of the medical party, anti-malarial and hygiene unit and of Royal Marine engineers quickly restored order out of chaos on Blakang Mati Island.

A small number of bungalows and buildings was reconditioned as a sick quarters with a space for 90 beds.

On December 15, 1945, H.M.S. *Landlock* paid off, but its medical organisation remained on Blakang Mati Island which was taken over as a naval barracks and transit camp, under the name of H.M.S. *Sultan I*.

During the next few months the medical organisation became responsible for all the naval medical commitments on the southern side of Singapore Island, which included the transit camp which accommodated up to 2,000 personnel. In addition a local Chinese, Indian and Malay population had to be catered for on Blakang Mati Island.

This state of affairs continued until well into the post-war period, when the whole medical organisation was centralised under Singapore Naval Base itself.

The details given of the MOLCAB medical organisations in the case of H.M.S. *Landswell* and H.M.S. *Landlock* have told in outline the development of mobile shore naval medical, surgical and hygiene facilities intended for use at short notice in any part of the world. The story has demonstrated how the more organised MOLCAB medical units were natural followers of the less definite medical units of the original M.N.B.D.Os. But the reader will doubtless appreciate that the basic medical idea had always been present in the minds of the Authorities since as far back as the year 1930. What had perhaps not been foreseen so clearly was the operational use to which such a mobile medical organisation might be put in the way of post-war local relief and reconstruction of areas formerly occupied by the enemy. In the case of H.M.S. *Landswell* and H.M.S. *Landlock*, their attached medical organisations were maintained for long periods after the MOLCABs. themselves had ceased to exist. It would be impossible to exaggerate the valuable part which these organisations played in the rehabilitation of a part of Malaya, and their medical personnel may well be regarded as pioneers in work of this nature under conditions of modern warfare. The reverence with which the medical and nursing staffs of these MOLCABs. were regarded by the local Asiatic population was alone evidence of their worth.

ACTIVITIES WITH SPECIAL OPERATIONS EXECUTIVE

It has already been pointed out that space does not permit mention to be made in this History of the many minor incidents on shore in which naval doctors and sick berth ratings were involved; but some of the more important operational commitments of naval medical officers ashore should be recorded. An account is therefore included in this Chapter of how the Medical Branch of the Navy came to be involved with Special Operations Executive between January 1943 and January 1946, albeit that this involvement was to some extent accidental, and that only two naval medical officers are known to have been concerned.

Towards the end of 1942, the Admiralty was requested by the Headquarters of Special Operations Executive to lend a naval medical officer for special duties. A particular medical officer was designated in this request, who was known to have a knowledge of Yugoslavia, and who was at that time serving as a surgeon lieutenant commander, R.N.V.R.

Early in January 1943, the Admiralty granted this request, and the medical officer concerned was appointed to H.M.S. *President*.

He was placed under the instructions of the 'Naval Liaison Officer with Special Operations Executive', and was sent to the West Highlands for a course of para-military training. At the beginning of March he sailed from Liverpool, and arrived in Lagos a month later and travelled on to Cairo by air.

On his arrival in the Middle East, this medical officer gained further knowledge of his future duties and of the organisation with which he was to play so valuable a part. It appeared that although plans were being made to supply military equipment to the Guerrilla Forces in the Balkans, no plans for the supply of medical equipment had yet been made. To date the amounts required had been small, and no great difficulty had arisen, but it was clear that much larger quantities would soon be required and that plans would have to be made for their supply and delivery. It also appeared that there was need for a further medical officer for service in Greece. As this matter was somewhat urgent, the Fleet Medical Officer of the Mediterranean Fleet was consulted, with the result that a second naval medical officer volunteered for special service. This second medical officer was a surgeon lieutenant, R.N.V.R., who had been serving in a Greek destroyer, and arrangements were quickly made for him to join the organisation.

In May 1943, the surgeon lieutenant commander was transferred to Palestine for parachute training. Unfortunately, during his first jump, he had the misfortune to sustain a crush fracture of the second lumbar vertebra, due to falling on a road with backward swing. This accident meant that he was unable to take an active part in projected operations for several months. However, he was fit enough to perform valuable staff duties in Cairo.

Early in 1944, this medical officer was passed as medically fit for parachuting, and in March he arrived in Italy with Yugoslavia as his ultimate destination.

SERVICE IN YUGOSLAVIA

In April 1944 he successfully completed his parachute training, but by then the medical requirements in Yugoslavia had decreased, and it was suggested that he should work with the British Mission in Serbia instead.

It was understood that guerrilla warfare in Serbia had only recently begun, but it was expected to expand rapidly. This expansion was expected to involve heavy fighting with numerous casualties, and it was anticipated that such medical services as did exist would be extremely primitive. There seemed no doubt that the assistance of a number of British medical officers would be welcomed, whose chief function would be to report on medical conditions and the requirements of medical stores and equipment.

South Serbia is a mountainous country, the mountains themselves being covered with forest and the valleys between fertile and thickly populated. The conditions which existed were ideal for guerrilla warfare. An ample supply of recruits was available, the armies could live off the land and could take refuge in the forests when hard pressed. At that time, the enemy troops in South Serbia consisted of two Bulgarian Divisions and one German Division.

The surgeon lieutenant commander, in company with a corporal, R.A.M.C., parachuted into South Serbia at the beginning of May 1944. The couple dropped near the village of Vuyanovo in the upper part of the Yavlanitsa valley. Supplies had been arriving by air in this area for less than a month, usually from groups of three aircraft per night. But on this particular night there were twelve aircraft, and the naval medical officer and his companion were dropped from the tenth. There was bright moonlight, and the local inhabitants on the ground began to cheer them vigorously as soon as their parachutes opened, and they were given a rousing reception when they landed.

The following morning the medical officer was taken to the local Guerrilla Commander and his medical adviser who requested the help of the naval doctor at his hospital a few miles away.

This hospital was established in and around a farmhouse. In the words of the medical officer: 'The condition of the wounded was appalling, most of the beds had two occupants, many wounded were lying on straw. Medical necessities of all sorts were almost completely lacking, and many operations were being performed without anaesthetics. The ingenuity of the Serbian doctors was beyond all praise. Unfortunately, they had come to accept a high mortality rate and considerable suffering among the patients as inevitable ...'

The medical officer had brought with him two Halifax bomber loads of medical supplies, and these were rapidly brought into use to help get the wounded into proper condition.

At about this time, it appeared that the Germans were seriously perturbed by the growing strength and opposition in this part of Serbia. Typically they used terror as an effective weapon, and this hospital was bombed or machine-gunned almost every day. Fortunately casualties were few, but it soon became necessary to disperse the wounded through the surrounding woods in the day time. This tended to interfere with the work of the hospital, and the necessarily rough movement of the wounded resulted in the deaths of many patients whose lives might otherwise have been saved.

Very soon there was a rapid enemy advance up the Yavlanitsa valley, and at short notice, with mortar bombs already falling uncomfortably close, it became necessary to evacuate the hospital of its patients, medical personnel and stores. For a few days they took refuge in the dense forests which cover the mountain Radan, well realising that a feature of the fighting in this part of the world was that no quarter was given or expected, and that it was customary never to allow wounded to fall into the hands of an enemy. But soon the enemy pressure eased, and it was possible to set up the hospital once more in rather more comfortable surroundings. About this time, news was received that some members of the 15th American Air Force had been shot down some distance away, and that three of them were seriously wounded and unable to be moved. The naval medical officer and his medical orderly at once set off to help these three casualties. Their journey took them five days through enemy held territory, and for the most part they travelled by night and hid by day. They had an escort as guides, and from time to time they encountered enemy troops most of whom fired a few wild shots and then retreated.

They found the three wounded Americans being cared for by the women of a small village in a remote corner of the Lisats Planina. The medical officer did what he could for them on the spot, the most important measure being to render them fit for transport. This involved carrying them by ox wagon over rough roads or frequently no roads at all. Of the actual journey no details are recorded, the medical officer merely stating that he found that plaster-of-paris and the Thomas splint proved invaluable, and 'we got back to headquarters without further incident although there were a few scares'.

A few days after this, a large scale movement was undertaken which involved the transfer of some 3,000 troops in this area across the Toplitsa river into the Yastrebats mountains. It was planned to undertake this journey at night, leaving existing wounded dispersed among the remoter farms in the Radan area. But it was arranged to transfer the three American wounded with the main Army, as it was believed likely that an opportunity would arise to fly them to Italy from a point north of Toplitsa.

These American wounded were again carried by ox wagon, but these were so much slower than the men on the march that the medical party fell behind, and could not cross the Toplitsa valley until two nights after the main body. Forty-eight hours later, two Dakota aircraft landed near the village of Velika Plana and the wounded were safely evacuated to Italy.*

The next task which this medical officer was requested to perform, was to establish his own hospital in the woods of Yastrebats. This hospital consisted of brushwood shelters, and was staffed by Serbian girls, few of whom had any experience of nursing. Casualties soon began to arrive, and were usually admitted during the hours of darkness. This was necessary for reasons of secrecy, and this and the remote position of the hospital made transport to it rather complicated. On the journey to hospital the wounded were carried as far as possible by ox wagon, and they then had to be carried by hand for the last part of the journey. This meant inevitable banging and shaking of these casualties, and the medical officer found it essential to meet them personally each evening in order to render them fit to tolerate man-handling over rough ground. He has recorded that the courage of these wounded under appalling conditions was unbelievable. He has also remarked upon the happiness which existed in his hospital in spite of the hardships which were endured, and how surprising it was that so many lives could be saved even by simple measures in such circumstances.

Early in July 1944, heavy raids began, carried out by German aircraft, mostly Me. 109s, and very soon orders were received to evacuate the area.

At this time there were some 80 wounded in the hospital. The ambulant wounded were disposed of by dispersing them among outlying farmhouses. But there remained 24 wounded whose condition was such that it was obvious that they would not survive a long journey, neither could they do without daily skilled medical attention. To accommodate these wounded, two camouflaged dugouts were prepared about half a mile apart. When the area was evacuated, these wounded men were placed in these dugouts, and the naval medical officer and the R.A.M.C. corporal remained behind to care for them.

---

* For the rescue and evacuation of these American wounded, this naval medical officer was personally commended by the General Commanding the 15th United States Air Force in a citation which reads: 'On May 31, together with two American SBS officers, he proceeded to the aid of three wounded 15th Air Force officers and men who had evaded capture in enemy occupied territory. At great personal risk, he worked tirelessly to aid these wounded men. When the obstacles seemed insurmountable, he refused to abandon the party and finally aided in successfully evacuating them to Italy on June 16, 1944. His determination, perseverance, bravery and coolness in the face of danger won the lasting respect and admiration of the officers and men he aided. His achievements are a credit to him and the Armed Forces of the United Kingdom.'

This tiny medical party quartered itself, with 14 of the wounded, in a dugout which was of such dimensions that there were not more than 1 or 2 sq. ft. of floor unoccupied. It was impossible to stand upright or even to kneel upright in places.

Conditions became worse as the days passed. Lighting was a problem, because torch batteries were soon exhausted and the wounded had to be attended to by light provided by parachute cord dipped in a tin of fat. Washing was impossible, and everybody soon became lice infected. The weather became bad with copious rainfall, and the dugout leaked so badly that nobody ever had a chance of keeping dry.

Food consisted of bread, hard biscuits and cheese. But after the first few days these were all mildewed, and in any case, supplies were only sufficient to last a week.

The medical party had attached to it two guards whose duty it was to hide themselves in the woods in the day time and then at night to inform the medical officer when the way was clear for him to visit the other dugout in which the remainder of the wounded were lodged. In practice, it happened that these guards were only able to do this once, on the fourth day after starting this strange mode of existence.

Altogether fourteen days were spent in this way, and the medical officer has recorded that: 'I recall with ungrateful vividness the stink of sour sweat, pus and faeces that we inhaled with every breath. For something to do, we kept count of the lice we killed on our persons, and towards the end of our stay we averaged over 200 a day each. All conversation had to be in whispers as we had no way of knowing how far away the enemy was. Conditions were bad enough for us who were in good health, but the suffering of the wounded was appalling. But only one of them ever made the slightest complaint, and the bearing of the rest was beyond all praise.'

Several times the sounds of firing were heard nearby, and on the last day but one Bulgarian soldiers passed on the run only a few yards away.

On the morning of the last day enemy troops were obviously increasing in numbers in the district, and the same evening, footsteps were heard overhead with the noise of digging over the roof of the dugout.

Realising that discovery was now certain and fearing that the digging might well be followed by the throwing of hand grenades into the dugout, the naval medical officer felt that the best thing to do was to come out into the open. He therefore shouted that he was a British doctor who had nobody with him underground except sick and wounded, and that there were no arms except for two pistols. A hole quickly appeared in the roof of the dugout, through which the medical officer pushed his head, and found himself confronted by a young soldier brandishing a 'tommy-gun' and a young enemy officer. The medical officer now emerged from the dugout, and the two pistols were handed over to his captors who he arranged to accompany to their headquarters, having requested that the wounded in the dugout should receive proper attention.

Reaching headquarters, two or three miles away, the medical officer and his orderly were placed under guard for the night. The next morning the Headquarters Medical Authorities reported that the wounded from the dugouts would be well cared for, and it is understood that they were subsequently conveyed into a hospital.

The following day the medical party was conducted through the village of Velika Plana and arrived at Aleksandrovats where they were to await disposal. The medical officer records that this journey was a distressing business, because: 'Many houses were burned and charred bodies lay in the ashes. One house where we had waited for convoys of wounded, lay in ashes, and I saw the burned bodies of children we had played with.'

At Aleksandrovats the medical officer and orderly were closely guarded but otherwise treated as honoured guests rather than prisoners-of-war. Orders were soon received about their disposal, and under an escort of local soldiers they set off walking for five days through territory occupied by the Germans. They crossed the Western Morava near Krushevatz, and then passed along the north side of this valley to a point some 50 miles north west of Chachak.

Here orders were given that this naval medical officer and the corporal, R.A.M.C. were to be released unconditionally and permitted to return to Italy. They left by an aircraft brought in by the American Mission engaged on repatriating shot down aircrews, and arrived in Italy at the beginning of September 1944.

By November this medical officer had arrived in Corfu where his duty was to survey the medical requirements for the interim period between the German retreat and the functioning of the Allied Military Government.

SERVICE IN MALAYA

By the end of 1944, this surgeon lieutenant commander, R.N.V.R., who had been selected for special medical duties in the Balkans, was informed that he was not likely to be required for any further operations in Europe. At the same time he was told that medical officers were urgently required for similar operations in the Far East. He at once volunteered for further special duties.

Following a visit to Delhi by air from Italy, and a further air journey to Kandy in Ceylon, the medical officer was given the immediate task of organising medical stores for special operations in Malaya. April 1945 found him undergoing a course of jungle training in Ceylon, and he was also taught the rudiments of the Malayan language. In May 1945 he flew to Calcutta to make further arrangements for medical stores requirements, and at the beginning of June arrived back in Ceylon where he was joined by a sergeant, R.A.M.C. as his medical orderly.*

At the end of June 1945 these two, medical officer and orderly, flew from Minneriya airfield in Ceylon to a dropping zone in Northern Malaya. Unfortunately visibility was bad and their target could not be found. Therefore, they had to return to Ceylon after 20 hours' flying over a distance of 3,000 miles. It was also unfortunate on this occasion, that owing to the fuel endurance of the aircraft it was necessary to throw out all medical stores and equipment on the return journey.

A week later, re-equipped with fresh stores, the medical officer and orderly parachuted successfully into Northern Malaya under much better flying conditions.

At this time in Malaya the Guerrilla Forces consisted mostly of Chinese troops. The medical officer's instruction was to organise the medical requirements of this guerrilla army which, at the moment, was being trained to engage the Japanese concurrently with the projected assault on Malaya by the Allied Forces.

The medical officer and orderly were dropped near the village of Belum in the extreme north of the state of Perak. From the landing point they were instructed to make their way into the adjoining state of Kelantan, and to report to the headquarters maintained by a member of the Malay Civil Service who had been engaged in organising guerrilla warfare in the jungle since the early days of the Japanese invasion of Malaya.

The country was extremely difficult, consisting of steep limestone hills covered with dense jungle, with marshy valleys between. At this time of year it rained almost every day. To cover five miles on foot in a day was considered to be good progress under these conditions. The medical officer and orderly reached their destination, and after a short stay were instructed to make their way to medical headquarters which were in process of being set up in the district of Lenggong. The senior medical officer of these headquarters was a lieutenant colonel.

While on its journey to Lenggong from Batu Melintang, this small medical party with its escort received a message from headquarters that its personnel should disperse into the jungle forthwith because the Japanese had started a drive in their direction. They were also instructed to take precautions against any of their stores falling into Japanese hands. The naval medical officer blew up a dump of medical stores, and then made his way in retreat through Siam in the direction of Kelantan. Unfortunately, while crossing a jungle bridge, the bridge broke and he was precipitated into the river below. He sustained a

---

* This particular Sergeant R.A.M.C. was selected as he had lived in Hong Kong as a child, and could speak fluent Cantonese.

rupture of the internal miniscus of the right knee but, as he remarked laconically in his report: 'I could not, of course, stop, as running away from the Japanese is rather an important matter'!

Fortunately, it was only a little later that news of the Japanese surrender was received. This medical officer then accompanied other officers of the Guerrilla Forces into Kota Bharu in order to take charge of the town and to disarm the Japanese Brigade which was stationed there. The medical officer found that conditions were extremely bad in the local civil hospital, where a Chinese and Indian doctor were doing their best to alleviate sickness among the Asiatic population. This hospital had practically nothing in the way of equipment, so the medical officer commandeered medical stores belonging to the Japanese and handed them over to the Civil Hospital Authorities. He then prepared a report on local medical conditions and requirements which he presented to the principal medical officer of the British Military Government at Kuala Lumpar. Shortly afterwards he returned to Ceylon, sick with his injured knee and amoebic dysentery as legacies of his arduous task which was now completed.*

CONCLUSIONS

Of interest both as part of this History, and as a guide and reference for future planning, are the views of the surgeon lieutenant commander, R.N.V.R. who was engaged on the special operations described, regarding the selection of persons for the dangerous type of work involved.

The medical officer concerned has recorded his remarks with great diffidence, pointing out that he is well aware that the Royal Navy has been doing this kind of selection with admirable success for many generations.

Nevertheless, in his opinion, the operations involved stress factors which he considers were due not so much to physical danger, as to prolonged discomfort and hardship. This discomfort and hardship were aggravated by enforced idleness, loneliness, uncertainty and frustration, and the feeling of being out of touch with the world. Often he and his companions had to wait on the dropping zone night after night for aircraft which never arrived. Their orders from headquarters, which had to be obeyed without question, were frequently incomprehensible when viewed from within the narrow limits of their vision. They had to deal with impatience, suspicion and resentment on the part of local guerrilla troops who like all troops on the periphery in time of war, were only too willing to believe that High Command knew

---

* This surgeon lieutenant commander, R.N.V.R., was subsequently decorated for the part he played in special operations. The citation states that: 'He behaved throughout with the utmost courage, and his example to all those who came in contact with him did a great deal to inspire them and to enhance British prestige.'

nothing of their difficulties and cared even less. He says: 'When frustration had reached a certain point, there was always a great temptation to start a private war of one's own.'

In circumstances such as these it was always necessary to preserve personal balance, to remain loyal to superiors, and above all, to try to be an adequate representative of Great Britain to people, many of whom had never seen a British officer before.

The medical officer urges that in selection, it should be remembered that the impulsive, aggressive 'daredevil' type of individual is not likely to prove suitable. In his experience, the most successful men in this kind of work were those of superior intelligence, inner resourcefulness and imagination.

In this respect two matters of interest arise from the available record. The first is the large number of distinguished professional men who volunteered for this kind of work, and it has been stated that if need be, 'the cream of the medical profession in the Middle East could have been recruited.'

The second matter of interest as regards selection is the subsequent careers, after the war had ended, of each of the medical officers recruited for these special operations. One went to America to study with the Rockefeller Foundation, one is a Professor of Surgery, one is a University Lecturer of Surgery, and four are on the permanent staffs of London Teaching Hospitals.

(ii)

Some Medical Events of Special Interest

Selected narratives of certain naval medical personnel captured by the enemy.

In this section, a small number of operational events has been selected from the abundance of material which is available, but the publication of which would unfortunately occupy more than the space available in this History.

Each of the events selected displays the common feature that the medical incidents first arose under the weight of heavy defeat by the enemy, and the full accounts could only be collated, after the war, from the numerous reports of personnel who survived captivity as prisoners-of-war.

It will be noted that in the case of one of the events, the escape of naval personnel from Singapore, no medical or nursing staff were actually involved. Nevertheless, the later impact of tropical disease was in this case so severe that it is considered of great importance that the sequence of events should be recorded historically for the purpose of emphasising how vitally necessary it is that isolated parties should always contrive, where possible, to include at least one member with medical experience and training.

THE LOSS OF H.M.S. *GLOUCESTER* AND SUBSEQUENT EVENTS*

At dawn on May 22, 1941, H.M.S. *Gloucester* was steaming in company with H.M.S. *Fiji* to the north-west of Crete. The squadron to which these cruisers belonged had been engaged with the interception of a German seaborne invasion force during the previous night.

Soon after daybreak, H.M.S. *Gloucester* was attacked by enemy aircraft which she continued to engage, apart from short lulls, until she was finally sunk later in the day.

During the forenoon the two ships passed through the Elephantos Channel between Kythera and Crete, and at about 1100 hours they joined the main Fleet, taking station on the port side of the battle squadron inside the destroyer screen.

At 1230 hours one of the destroyers was heavily hit and sank, and at 1300 hours H.M.S. *Warspite* was damaged.

By this time the anti-aircraft ammunition of *Gloucester* and *Fiji* had been reduced to about 20 rounds per gun, and at about 1400 hours both ships were detached from the Fleet and sent back into the Aegean. Air attacks on the two ships continued at fairly regular intervals, and they suffered the disadvantage of being isolated targets. The 4 in. gunfire of *Gloucester* was by now only spasmodic. Her pom-poms maintained a brisk fire, but they were insufficient to cope with whole squadrons of dive-bombers whose concerted attacks became bolder.

Soon after 1500 hours she was heavily attacked, and the Medical Officer states that: 'Almost immediately the ship shook violently and all the lights went out. Again there was a dull explosion and the ship heaved, throwing me into the air. I switched on my torch and got to my feet, but the ship was shaken again by several more explosions.'

At 1527 hours, she was hit by at least two bombs. One bomb exploded in the ship's gunroom flat and damaged 'B' boiler room and compressor room and the main wireless office. Another bomb exploded and blew into the sea the after high-angle director and the main topmast. At 1540 hours a bomb exploded on the 4 in. gun deck between the first and second groups of portside torpedo tubes. Most fortunately, all the port torpedoes had been fired before the explosion, for there is no doubt that otherwise the warheads of these torpedoes would have themselves exploded with a far greater loss of life. Yet another bomb penetrated

---

* This narrative has been prepared from the notes made by the Junior Medical Officer of H.M.S. *Gloucester* while a prisoner-of-war. This medical officer is now deceased.

the port pom-pom platform, passed through the port hangar and exploded in the canteen flat.

Up to this time *Gloucester* had been able to steam on her forward engine, but now she lost steam altogether and rapidly began to lose way.

At 1545 hours the ship is believed to have been hit on her port side by possibly three torpedoes launched from enemy aircraft. The main transmitting station and the second wireless office were now flooded and the ship began to list to port.

During the course of this action, all the medical parties, with the exception of one rating on the telephone in each of the distributing stations, had been kept within the ship's armoured belt. In the event of casualties, either the forward or the after distributing station, or both, were manned according to the needs of the situation. The Senior Medical Officer kept his own medical party in a bathroom on the starboard side, and his distributing station was the sick bay. The Junior Medical Officer kept his medical party in a bathroom on the port side, and his distributing station was in the ship's gunroom.

When hit the first time, the immediate concern of the Junior Medical Officer was to conduct his medical party to the gunroom. The party reached as far as an armoured door on the port side, but found it had been jammed. They managed to open it a few inches, but their combined efforts failed to open it further. Large quantities of smoke began to pour out from the Marines' after messdeck, and it became impossible to reach the after part of the ship by this route. At this stage all hands were ordered on to the upper deck.

Meanwhile, the Senior Medical Officer with his medical party, had been able to get forward into the sick bay.*

When the Junior Medical Officer reached the upper deck, the order to abandon ship had already been given and the ship was listing heavily to port. The starboard whaler had been lowered, but was so damaged that it had immediately sunk. The port whaler was also unseaworthy. Many men were leaving the ship *via* the falls of these boats. At the same time H.M.S. *Fiji* was steaming past dropping her Carley floats in the water for the use of *Gloucester's* survivors. After performing this task of mercy, H.M.S. *Fiji* left the scene.†

The Junior Medical Officer established an emergency dressing station on the starboard side of the well-deck, against the bakehouse. There he and his party were sheltered from the stray splinters of pom-pom shells

---

* The reader will observe that the revised medical organisation for action afloat, promulgated in 1942, had not yet come into existence. Reference should be made to the first Chapter of this Volume. Nevertheless, it is obvious that in H.M.S. *Gloucester*, although medical parties tended to be concentrated and retained under cover, the policy of mobility during the course of an action was beginning to develop.

† H.M.S. *Fiji* was herself sunk later.

which were exploding at intervals as a result of a fire which had taken hold around the port pom-pom magazine.

The medical party attended a few casualties, mostly from the guns' crews. The two most seriously injured were placed in Neil-Robertson stretchers and passed into a Carley float which was kept alongside the port side of the ship for this purpose. No more than first aid could be attempted as speed was essential. Dressings were applied and fractures splinted. Those not too gravely wounded were given gr. $\frac{1}{4}$ of morphine only in order that they might help themselves as much as possible. Those who were obviously dangerously wounded were given a minimum of morphia gr. $\frac{1}{2}$, as their survival under these conditions seemed highly unlikely and there seemed no point in allowing them to suffer unnecessarily.*

While these casualties were receiving attention, the Senior Medical Officer arrived aft, and, having assured himself that the medical party needed no assistance, he went forward again, having reminded his junior and the senior sick berth rating not to delay abandoning ship very much longer and also to take off their shoes before doing so.†

Shortly afterwards a number of German aircraft flew over the ship and bombs fell among the survivors who were swimming near the starboard side. Meanwhile, the Junior Medical Officer and his small medical party completed their work on the immediate casualties in that part of the ship, and placed the last one on the Carley float. The Medical Officer then conducted his party along the deck to see if it was possible to reach the after part of the ship, but he found his way obstructed by a fire which was not under control. He returned to the waist of the ship where he found a small party of officers who were throwing loose wood into the sea for the benefit of survivors. At this moment, another casualty was brought to the Junior Medical Officer. This man had a badly wounded leg which the medical officer splinted, after which he managed to lower him into the Carley float which was just about to leave the ship. By now this Carley float was full to capacity, and the wounded in it were up to their chests in water and some of them were already in a critical condition.

The Medical Officer mentions the valuable assistance which he received from the ship's chaplain in tending these casualties. At

---

* By the end of the war, a number of experienced naval medical officers had expressed some criticism of the routine administration of morphia to casualties in action afloat. The opinion was that the sole criterion should be the existence of pain, and that morphia should not be used in cases of shock where there was no pain. The feeling was that a wounded man who had received morphia might consequently lose the will to make an effort to save himself should his ship start to sink. Also, a school of thought arose which considered that morphia was always likely to increase shock in the case of casualties suffering from exposure at sea. This was particularly so in the case of wounds and shock accompanied by exposure in Arctic waters.

† The Senior Medical Officer and senior sick berth rating both lost their lives in the sinking of H.M.S. *Gloucester*.

1715 hours he could find no more wounded needing attention, so doctor and chaplain abandoned ship together. This was simply a matter of stepping down into the sea, as by this time the port gunwales were awash. Shortly afterwards H.M.S. *Gloucester* slowly turned turtle and sank by the stern.

The Medical Officer's first impression on entering the water was that it was agreeably warm. After swimming about a hundred yards so as to get clear of the sinking ship, he came across the blowing head of a torpedo which he thought would be as good a support as he was likely to find. But as soon as he made any attempt to climb on to it, it began to spin and he was forced to swim away from it. Further on he came across a group of swimmers around some floating wreckage which consisted of two 'fenders' loosely connected with a wire rope, and there were also two floating oars. There were far too many swimmers for everyone to benefit from this scanty support, nevertheless, by common consent, swimming survivors began to regard this group as a good collecting point.*

As the ship sank, these survivors were apprehensive about the possibility of depth charges exploding, but these had previously been rendered 'safe', so that the risk of 'immersion blast' did not arise.

The feelings of seamen at such a time are revealed in the pathetic words written by this Medical Officer: 'It felt very lonely in the water after the ship had gone.'

The visibility was still very good and land was in sight at three points in the far distance which could be recognised as Crete, Kythera and the mountains of the Peloponnese. Kythera seemed to be reasonably close, so close in fact, that the Medical Officer decided to swim there. But after swimming for some time, he realised he was getting no nearer. He therefore thought it safer to swim back to the group of swimmers round the fenders, and he rejoined them just before dark.†

After *Gloucester* had sunk, large numbers of German aircraft passed overhead. They then returned and several aircraft dived and machine-gunned the survivors. The Medical Officer mentions how unpleasant it was to see aircraft diving in this manner with bullets from them splashing into the water. He considers that a number of survivors must have been killed at this time, and he himself swam to a raft where he found a man who had been hit.‡

By nightfall, there were approximately 20 survivors left together round the fenders, and support had been augmented by a floating chest of drawers.

---

* Survivors at sea were always instructed to keep together in large groups whenever possible, in order to facilitate rescue.

† Kythera was, in fact, 15 miles distant.

‡ These aircraft were probably on their way to attack H.M.S. *Fiji*.

One by one this party of 20 dwindled in spite of the efforts of the fitter men to maintain the strength of the weaker.* Soon the number was sufficiently reduced to allow everybody to get a hand on one of the fenders. But even so, caution had to be observed as any alteration of weight on the support was likely to make it turn turtle.

Throughout the night their hopes were falsely raised many times. For instance, they saw searchlights shining on Crete, but mistook them for the lights of a ship. Consequently, they shouted for help. Some distance away, in a Carley float, other survivors heard the shouts and mistook them for hails from a rescue ship. A whistle was blown, and the group in the water assumed that they were about to be picked up, and shouted harder than ever. So began a vicious circle which was only broken when they became too tired to shout any more.

At one stage during the night a rubber dinghy passed the group, but though they hailed it, it ignored them and continued on its course.†

This group went on getting smaller as the night passed, and the sky became overcast and a breeze sprang up which added to their discomfort. The Medical Officer found that he was becoming cold and cramped, so from time to time he left the party for a short sharp swim in order to loosen his cramped muscles and to try and get warm. He remarks: 'I discovered that it is not as difficult as it sounds to vomit while swimming. I imagine it was the swallowing of some fuel oil earlier in the day which made me sick.'

When daylight came there were only six left in the group, three hanging on to each fender. Soon after dawn one of the six died. He had become completely exhausted and the others had held him on to the fender. But when the fenders capsized, which they did frequently, it at last became too much for him and he could not regain his hold.

The sun rose, but the sea remained choppy. The Medical Officer still thought that Kythera was very close, and as by now the fenders were adequate to hold the weight of the five remaining, he thought it should be possible to paddle to the land. There was quite a lot of wreckage strewn over the sea, so he swam about and collected two pieces of wood suitable for paddles.

Full of optimism, the Medical Officer and a rating started to paddle, but they found that the other fender would not follow in tow, but

---

* Medical officers with experience of survivors after a disaster at sea, have frequently observed the ease with which some men will give up the struggle for existence and allow themselves to drown without apparently making any effort at all. The inflatable Service lifebelt which was always worn at sea gave valuable support, and was effective if the swimmer helped himself a little. But the lifebelt alone was not sufficient assistance to combat the dangerous lethargy which always became evident as time passed.

One medical officer, recording his experiences after some hours in the sea, stated: 'At times I had an almost overwhelming urge to let down my lifebelt and give up what seemed an unending and pointless struggle'.

† This dinghy is believed to have contained German paratroops, themselves survivors, who were making for Kythera.

merely acted as a sea anchor. So the Medical Officer obtained pieces of wood for each of them and an attempt was made to paddle in unison. Only four of them could take part, as the fifth was too exhausted. The paddling soon became irregular, and the combination tended to move through the sea in circles. Nevertheless, the Medical Officer managed to convince himself that they were getting nearer to the land, though he failed to convince his companions of this. In fact, being seamen, they did not hesitate to express their poor opinion of the doctor as a navigator!

About what happened later on this day, this Medical Officer is uncertain and was only able to recall odd incidents. Occasionally he had a renewed burst of energy and started paddling again. They might have been machine-gunned once more by aircraft, but he could not be sure of this.

Early in the afternoon, one of the five suddenly started to swim away by himself despite the efforts of the others to restrain him, and he quickly drowned.

Finally, later in the afternoon, the remaining four sighted a small ship cruising about and stopping at intervals, presumably picking up survivors. This ship drew closer, and eventually altered course towards these four men and lifted them on board.

This rescue ship was a small Greek vessel with a German crew. Once on board, the Medical Officer and his three companions were stripped of their wet clothing, given a dry blanket apiece, and fresh water to drink. They were then taken to a large cabin below deck where they found other survivors from *Gloucester*. They fell asleep at once and awoke in the evening to find the ship in the small harbour of Kythera. They were mustered on deck and some, but not all, of their clothing was returned to them. For example, the Medical Officer records that he himself was only given his reefer. From the ship all the survivors were taken ashore by dinghy, a few at a time. Eventually they were again mustered on the shore, and now realised that they were prisoners-of-war.

From the landing place, these men were marched along the sea front of Kythera to a deserted house which was to be their quarters. This house was in a very dilapidated state, with long gaps between the floor boards and no glass in the windows. There was one large room with a smaller room leading from it on either side. Adjoining the main building was an outhouse, in bad repair, but containing a large open fireplace. At the back of the house there was a small piece of waste ground which the prisoners were allowed to use.

Altogether there were approximately 70 prisoners-of-war in this house. All were survivors from H.M.S. *Gloucester* with the exception of four from H.M.S. *Greyhound* and four soldiers of the A.I.F. These four soldiers had been captured two days earlier while trying to escape in a small boat from Greece. Among the seventy was one naval rating who had been seriously wounded by a machine-gun bullet from an aircraft, which had passed through the right iliac fossa. This man had bad diarrhoea and incontinence. Another rating had two black eyes of a distribution which strongly suggested a fracture of the anterior fossa of the skull. The remainder suffered from exhaustion and minor injuries.

The Medical Officer converted one of the smaller rooms into a sick bay. Unfortunately there were no sick berth ratings among these survivors, but a seaman petty officer volunteered to undertake nursing duties, and though inexperienced, performed good work.

Greek civilians offered to provide a small amount of clothing, and the medical officer considered himself fortunate to be provided with a pair of well patched trousers which were several sizes too small.

There was a good supply of wood lying about on the ground so that a good fire was made up in the outhouse, and it was possible to keep warm and dry. The whole party slept on the floor that night.

The following morning they were mustered and counted, and then conducted in groups of five to wash at a tap on the foreshore. They had no soap and therefore found it impossible to rid themselves of the mixture of salt and oil fuel with which their hair was caked. However, they managed to cleanse themselves a little and felt much fresher.

Later in the forenoon they were given a little of the German Army dried black bread to eat. They did not find this very appetising, but the local Greek civilians were most generous and brought these prisoners cigarettes, hard boiled eggs and bread. The Medical Officer took charge of this supply and only distributed what was left after the seriously wounded rating had been provided for.

On the following day, which was May 25, the Medical Officer was told that the seriously wounded rating would be flown to hospital, and that the Medical Officer himself, together with the senior naval rating, was to be taken by boat to the mainland. Early in the afternoon the Medical Officer and a chief petty officer were taken on board a small boat flying the Italian Ensign. They were put in the engine room where they were given a meal of bread and cheese, and some cigarettes by an Italian engineer. Two hours later, it proved impossible to make the engines work, so the two prisoners-of-war were taken ashore and marched back to the house.

Later that evening, an ambulance plane arrived, but the German medical officer who came with it decided that there was not room for the wounded rating. He did however arrange instead for this casualty, and the man with the suspected fracture of the skull, to accompany the Medical Officer and senior rating to the mainland by boat the following day.

So on May 26, the Medical Officer took these two wounded on board the Italian vessel the engines of which were now working. The abdominal case was placed in the bed of an Italian officer and quite well cared for. But unfortunately, conditions on board deteriorated with the arrival of about 100 German paratroops who were inclined to be arrogant and aggressive. Once this vessel had put to sea, the Italian skipper gave the Medical Officer a meal of soused cod and onions and, while eating it, the Medical Officer would seem to have derived some pleasure from the seasick state of the German paratroops!

The voyage lasted about four hours, and they arrived alongside a jetty in the harbour of Gythion in the extreme south of the Peloponnese.

They were taken at once by ambulance to a large building in which was a German regimental aid post, commanded by a young German unterarzt. This doctor was most helpful. He provided a camp bed for the abdominal case, and he and the British Medical Officer together changed the man's dressings.

The Medical Officer and senior rating were put into a room where there were two beds and told to rest for a while. After an hour, the unterarzt produced a small book containing extracts of the Geneva Convention, and the two medical officers, British and German, discussed the details of treatment of prisoners-of-war and protected personnel. In consequence, a ration issue was made on the standard of that issued to a German soldier, together with packets of cigarettes. Later in the evening, the two medical officers had a long and earnest talk on the loyalties of medical officers in time of war between nations, and the German medical officer lectured the British on the merits of National Socialism. The conversation was conducted in a mixture of French, English and German. *Gloucester's* Medical Officer emphasises the kindness which was shown towards himself, the senior rating and the two wounded by this unterarzt although, he states: 'We did not manage to reach agreement on all points!'*

The next morning, the abdominal and skull cases, accompanied by the Medical Officer and senior rating, were driven to Tripolis by ambulance. The abdominal case still had diarrhoea and incontinence, but the problem of nursing him was simplified by the provision of a bedpan by the unterarzt.

The party arrived at Tripolis at midday on May 27. The abdominal case was admitted at once to a German Military Hospital, and the Medical Officer regrets that he never had further news of his progress.†

The skull casualty appeared perfectly well and was not admitted to hospital. He, the senior rating and Medical Officer were taken to the local Greek Police Station and handed over to the Police Commissioner for

---

* This unterarzt was the only German the Medical Officer met, during his time of captivity, who appeared to have any knowledge of the requirements of the Geneva Convention.

† This abdominal casualty recovered, and was repatriated as an 'exchange' prisoner-of-war in 1943.

safe custody. As soon as the German guard had left, kindness and luxury became the lot of these three men for a brief period. The commissioner's wife prepared a meal of fried eggs for each of them, and neighbours gave them shoes to wear for the first time since their rescue. They were then taken to a flat where they were given beds with clean linen, a bathroom with hot water, soap and towels, and even a barber was in attendance! The commissioner's wife produced clean underwear, shirts and pairs of socks.

At six in the evening they were entertained to an enormous meal, with brandy to drink, by the local Greek Police Force.

The following morning, they were awakened soon after daybreak and taken to the local railway station to take train for Corinth. While waiting for the train local Greek civilians provided them with bread, butter, cheese, hard boiled eggs and two cold roast chickens. The enthusiasm of the Greeks was so great as to tend to become a riot, and eventually extra German soldiers had to be sent for to clear one end of the station platform!

This small party of three travelled to Corinth in the guard's van and at every station at which the train stopped the platform was crowded with Greeks waiting to welcome them.

On arrival at Corinth, however, their circumstances changed for the worse. After being interrogated at the local administrative headquarters, they were taken to a large transit camp about which there was an atmosphere of finality. For the first time since their rescue the Medical Officer found himself behind barbed wire and surrounded with machine-guns. He states: 'I was now but one among thousands of other persons, and I felt that I had surrendered my individuality!'

The camp at Corinth held approximately 8,500 British, and 700 Yugoslav prisoners-of-war. The camp itself was centred around a former Greek Army Barracks, consisting mainly of three-storied concrete buildings.

Three days after his arrival the Medical Officer was joined by 7 more survivors from *Gloucester*, including the only other surviving officer.

On June 4, warning was given that this camp was to be evacuated. As a preliminary to this evacuation, the camp authorities organised the delousing of the prisoners-of-war. This meant that the clothing of prisoners was removed and placed in a disinfector. Meanwhile, in a naked state, the prisoners had to walk a distance of two miles in bare feet in order to bathe themselves in the sea. As a consequence, large numbers of men cut their feet and suffered severe sunburn, disabilities which proved to be most severe on the long march which was soon to follow.

At 0400 hours on June 5, *Gloucester's* Medical Officer was attached to a group of 1,500 prisoners-of-war who were to be transferred from Corinth to Salonika.

The journey started with a march for some three hours to a railhead on the other side of the Corinth Canal, where the party entrained for Athens. At Athens, they were transferred to a second train which carried them to Gravia, at the foot of the Brallos Pass, where the train stopped until dawn.

The Brallos Pass verges upon a range of mountains, through which, in ordinary times, there was a railway tunnel. But this tunnel had been blown up, and it was therefore necessary for these 1,500 prisoners-of-war to march over the mountains to the next railhead at Lamia, 25 miles distant.

The column of men was drawn up at daybreak on June 6, and the Medical Officer was ordered to select 30 men only whom he considered unfit to make the journey on foot, and for whom limited transport was available. He found over 100 men whose feet were so cut and blistered, and whose backs were so burnt as to make it almost impossible for them to get along at all. He states that: 'I presented this state of affairs to the German lieutenant in charge of our guard. He started to rave and shout at me, and threatened to make everybody march unless I myself nominated 30 from among the 100 odd unfit men. Fortunately my task was eased by all the unfit officers in the party volunteering to try to make the journey on foot.'

The march began, and soon after the second hour the first officers began to fall out by the wayside. Throughout the day the Medical Officer was kept busy collecting these stragglers together, attending to their wants, and putting them into any passing transport he could persuade to take them. His own feet were badly cut and blistered, and he was eventually forced to abandon the very heavy box of medical supplies which he had managed to get together in the camp at Corinth.

By the time the column reached the railhead at Lamia, one officer was moribund from general inanition and heatstroke. The Medical Officer, with two volunteer stretcher-bearers, was permitted to take this patient to a village $2\frac{1}{2}$ miles away, which was reached by a local train, and where there was a hospital. But the Medical Officer states: 'The last straw was that we had to walk back'.

The same evening these prisoners-of-war entrained in cattle trucks, and they arrived at Salonika on the afternoon of the following day.

The P.o.W. Camp at Salonika was finally reached after another 4 miles' march from the railway station, and this march was relieved by the kindness of the Greeks who lined the roadside and showered gifts of food and cigarettes upon the prisoners-of-war. 'But', remarks the Medical Officer, 'I saw two old women struck with rifle butts for trying to give me something'.

At Salonika, these survivors of *Gloucester* were confined in Dulag 183. After the war, the Medical Officer immediately recorded, long before any of his other experiences, his vivid description of the three

Germans in charge of the administration of Dulag 183, whose characters had obviously left a permanent impression in his mind. He has described these three Germans in the following words:

The Oberleutnant. 'A middle-aged man, with greying hair, cold eyes and a weak chin, who took a sadistic pleasure in the misery which he created inside the camp.'

The Oberfeldwebel. 'A born bully. He revelled in the almost unlimited authority he had in the camp, and was at his happiest when he was bawling and shouting at some incomprehending prisoner. He obviously enjoyed an opportunity of using his boot on some defenceless man, a thing I saw him do more than once.'

The Oberstabsarzt. 'It was natural that I should come into frequent contact with this German senior medical officer of the camp, and at no time did I enjoy our meetings. He was a gross, bull-necked man with a shaven head and an enormous paunch. So far as I could judge, his knowledge of medicine was negligible.

'I first met him on the day after my arrival. I was summoned, together with some Yugoslav doctors, to listen to his statement on how the hospital would be run now that large numbers of prisoners-of-war were to be expected. He was very pompous and talked a good deal about the Geneva Convention. But two days later, when I met him with some complaints, he at once lost his temper and told me that the Geneva Convention could go to hell! He also told me that I was British, that I was in no position to demand anything, and that we could take what was coming to us!

'In all matters medical this man's word was law. We could do nothing to alter the arrangements and dispositions which he had made. We could make our requests and recommendations, but they were greeted with abuse. On his periodical tours of the camp he could always be heard screaming and shouting at some unfortunate prisoner who had no idea what it was all about.'

On the other hand, he is unstinting in his admiration of the junior medical officer of the camp. 'The Assistenzarzt stood out as a good deed shines in a bad world. He was genuinely appalled by the existing state of affairs, and he was at all times most sympathetic. He tried to do what he could to help us, but was terrified of everyone in authority over him.'

In his official report of Dulag 183, this Medical Officer has recorded a detailed account of the general health, hygiene and medical arrangements of the camp. The report can only be regarded as adverse in every way, with some defects more glaring than others. For example, the camp is described as having more bed bugs than could possibly be imagined. Newcomers were often bitten so much during the night that on the following morning they were almost unrecognisable! Lice too were greatly in evidence, but the camp remained free from typhus.

Despite the fact that in Salonika there were fabulous stores of British medical equipment and drugs captured during the Greek campaign, the camp was constantly kept short of almost every medical requirement. But the Germans would seem to have taken an interest in malaria at that time, and atebrin was lavish in supply.

Between June and August, there were a great many minor ailments such as colds, coughs, septic scratches, infected blisters and so on. But these minor ailments soon began to be replaced by a steady deterioration in the general health of the community, and several major diseases began to become epidemic. The most important were bacillary dysentery, typhoid, epidemic catarrhal jaundice, sandfly fever, diphtheria and beriberi.

The first cases of diphtheria occurred in July 1941. By the middle of August there were some 30 cases of this disease, which were characterised by extensive pareses. Treatment had to be confined to nursing only, and no anti-diphtheritic serum was available.

That beriberi should appear in the camp was in itself a sufficient indictment of the German camp authorities, and this indictment was aggravated by the fact that the disease was permitted to continue and flourish even after it had been recognised.

It is of interest that the first cases of beriberi to appear were all among men who had been captured in Crete. Not a single case appeared at the beginning among men taken prisoner in Greece.

In the course of his report, details are given of acts of war and violence inside the camp, many of which could not fail to come to the notice of camp medical officers. He states: 'At night it was quite the usual thing to hear the guards firing their rifles and throwing hand grenades. I imagine the fire was mostly directed at Greeks who were unwise enough to be in the vicinity of the camp after dark. But, all too often, this fire was directed into the camp itself, and it is surprising that many more men were not killed.'

One difficulty connected with this tendency of the German guards to shoot first and ask questions afterwards was that there was only one lavatory inside the compound of the camp hospital. Should that lavatory happen to be occupied at night, other patients had to go to the outside latrines, and were then liable to be shot at for being out after dark. Naturally, the men most affected by this menace were those suffering from dysentery, and patients could not be blamed if they sometimes soiled the entrance to the ward rather than face rifle fire outside. Repeated complaints to the camp authorities brought no satisfaction.

The Medical Officer states: 'One morning when I got up there was a corpse on the parade ground. The man had been shot during the night, and his body deliberately left there as a deterrent to potential escapees.'

It is obvious from the report that there was complete confusion and conflict between the various sets of orders issued by the German camp administrators. For example, although no lights were permitted to be shown inside the camp after dark, limited lighting was permitted inside the camp hospital as even the Oberleutnant and Oberstabsarzt were forced to admit, albeit with reluctance, that light was essential if very sick patients were to be properly cared for. Nevertheless, not once but many times, shots were fired at the hospital lights and bullets went ricocheting round the walls. Once again, protests were of no avail, and by good fortune no one was killed.

One forenoon a British R.A.M.C. officer was standing at an upstairs window of the hospital talking to a companion. From outside the camp the Oberfeldwebel fired his revolver at this doctor. The bullet fell short, whereupon the Feldwebel took a rifle from one of the camp guards and fired again. This time the bullet passed very close to the Medical Officer, pierced the door of the hospital dental surgery and narrowly missed an Army dental surgeon who was working there. When asked for an explanation, the Feldwebel merely laughed and said that he had presumed that the Medical Officer was signalling to someone outside the camp.

The two following incidents, specially reported by the Medical Officer, are here recorded in his own words:*

(1) 'One forenoon, about the middle of July, a private of the New Zealand Medical Corps was standing outside the camp hospital. For no apparent reason and without any warning he was shot by a guard. The bullet used was of small calibre and explosive in type, and it caused a very extensive wound of the arm with a shattering of the humerus.†

'Less than an hour later two other hospital orderlies were also shot and wounded by a single bullet fired by the same guard.‡

'The senior Army medical officer and myself protested most strongly to the Oberleutnant, but we were told that an order had been issued that no one might approach to within five yards of the perimeter wire of the camp. We denied that this order had ever been communicated to us. After some discussion the Oberleutnant lost his temper and literally frothed at the mouth. He informed us that we British must realise that the Germans were the bosses now, and that if we did not like it we could do the other thing.

'The following day, the camp guard company was paraded, and the Oberleutnant personally congratulated the guard who had done the shooting.'

(2) 'This incident occurred at night. Two soldiers went to the latrine at the end of the hospital block. While they were urinating, a guard outside threw a hand grenade into the latrine. Both were wounded.§

---

* Both these incidents subsequently became the subject of charges at War Crimes Trials.

† The wounded arm of this private was later amputated in a local Greek hospital.

‡ Both these orderlies died of their wounds.

§ One of these men died of his wounds, and the other lost his right eye.

'Again we protested most energetically to the Oberleutnant. This time we were told that the two soldiers were reported to have been signalling to someone outside the wire, by coughing! Therefore, the Oberleutnant considered that the guard had carried out his duty in a most satisfactory manner.'

The period of captivity of the Medical Officer of H.M.S. *Gloucester* in Dulag 183, Salonika, ended on August 28, 1941, when he was transferred to Germany.*

On August 28, 1941, he and an Army medical officer were put in charge of a party of sick and wounded for transfer into Germany.

The contrast between the conditions in the prison camp and those in the hospital train in which they travelled from Salonika to Germany was almost unbelievable. In fact, they found it hard to understand why the Germans should have reduced them to such a deplorable state only to provide them with facilities for travel which amounted to luxury.

The carriages of the train were extremely well fitted out, with two tiers of bunks down each side and a corridor down the middle. The bunks themselves were most comfortable, well sprung, with good mattresses and clean bed linen.

What appealed most to the British party was the food. The soup was abundant and of good quality, and bread was unlimited.

The German senior medical officer of the train is described as a humourless and rather pompous individual, but he was scrupulously correct in his treatment of prisoners-of-war and eager to supply everything necessary in the way of drugs and dressings for the sick and wounded.

The journey into Europe took five days. On the fifth morning the train passed through Munich, and during the same afternoon the Army medical officer and sitting patients were taken off the train at Ehingen and admitted to hospital there. That night the train arrived at Rottweil where it was met by ambulances, which took the Medical Officer and his patients to the Allied Prisoner-of-War Hospital at Rottenmünster.

The Reserve Lazarett, Rottenmünster, Stalag VB, was one of the detached prisoner-of-war hospitals the chief function of which was to receive sick from the surrounding working camps. This hospital was housed in part of an old mental hospital. There was accommodation for about 400 patients of all Allied nationalities, with French predominating.

---

* In a special report, this Medical Officer paid tribute to the work performed in this camp by officers of the Royal Army Medical Corps and Royal Army Dental Corps. Regarding the Senior British Army Medical Officer in the camp, his report read: 'He was absolutely untiring in his efforts on behalf of the sick, especially those suffering from beriberi. He interpreted at all the more unpleasant interviews with the camp authorities, and put forward our complaints with courage and emphasis. Although tired out at the end of the day, he was still able to enliven our small mess with his keen sense of humour.'

In addition to the Medical Officer of H.M.S. *Gloucester*, there were two British Army medical officers one of whom acted as senior medical officer of the hospital.*

There were also six French medical officers and one very competent Polish medical student.

Nursing duties were performed by a team of British R.A.M.C., French Army and Polish and Serb orderlies.

As far as possible and for purposes of convenience, the wards and special departments of the hospital were cared for by separate nationalities. British and French wards were staffed by orderlies of their own nationality. Yugoslavs were cared for by Polish and Serb orderlies. The theatre staff was all British, while the French administered the laboratory, dispensary and galley.

In this History, there is little point in describing the bulk of the details of medical supplies, hospital routine, etc., which have been recorded by this Medical Officer during the three months which he spent at Rottenmünster. In general, his remarks might well be applicable to all such prison hospitals in Germany at that time. But he has stressed certain matters of outstanding importance and interest.

He found himself busily employed in dealing with large numbers of surgical cases presenting unhealed wounds. His operative surgery was limited to re-amputations where necessary, the removal of foreign bodies and the draining of infected bones. All the amputations needed artificial limbs and, as a result of representations made through the Protecting Power, at that time the United States of America, the Germans provided a supply of wooden 'pegs' and plaster-of-paris. The Medical Officer then set out to teach himself the rudiments of prostheses, and after a period of trial and error, he finally managed to produce some quite reasonably good artificial legs.

As in the case of Salonika, beriberi continued to present a problem at Rottenmünster, and the cases took a long time to show signs of recovery. These facts were reported to the Protecting Power, with the result that the hospital was visited by the Oberstabsarzt of all the Prisoner-of-War Medical Establishments in the area. This German medical officer announced that he wished to examine all cases from Salonika suffering from either beriberi or malaria. But *Gloucester's* M.O. records that: 'He had obviously read up both conditions just before he came, and he appeared to have got them a trifle mixed. For example, he spent a lot of time palpating for the spleens of beriberi patients and testing the knee jerks of those with malaria!'

There were numerous deaths among the prisoners-of-war in Rottenmünster between September and the end of 1941. The fatal

---

* These two medical officers were Captains, R.A.M.C., captured in France in 1940.

diseases were chiefly advanced phthisis and diphtheria. The Germans were most punctilious about the obsequies.*

The hospital at Rottenmünster was visited from time to time by the Mixed Medical Commission. This was a touring Medical Board consisting of two Swiss and two German doctors whose task was to decide which cases were suitable to be repatriated under the Annexe to the Geneva Convention. Theoretically any man had the right to present himself before this Board, but in practice, there was usually a preliminary boarding by the local German senior medical officer. Generally speaking, at Rottenmünster, any case recommended by a British medical officer was permitted to appear before the Mixed Medical Commission without further question.

The Mixed Medical Commission was meticulously fair and impartial on its visits to Rottenmünster, and every patient was considered fully before his application for repatriation was rejected. Unfortunately, it was often necessary to produce specialist's reports, X-rays, etc., in order that diagnoses might be confirmed, and in Rottenmünster several patients failed to pass for repatriation because there were no facilities for carrying out such special investigations.

The Medical Officer's report contains a long account of the many measures which were adopted to provide recreation and to relieve monotony among patients and staff, which ends by describing how the evening brew of cocoa (Red Cross) played such an important part in the social life of the hospital.†

On Boxing night 1941, the British medical officers at Rottenmünster were suddenly informed that they were to be moved with their patients. This move took place by train on December 28 under conditions of extreme cold which approached hardship in the case of prisoners-of-war, many of whom were still inadequately clad in little more than they possessed at the time of their capture in Greece and Crete. Fortunately the journey only lasted a few hours and ended at Nagold.

The Reserve Lazarett, Nagold, still in the Stalag VB area, was housed in an old school. But this building had been used as an emergency German civil hospital for a considerable time, and so it proved to be much better equipped and more competently staffed than was usual for any prisoner-of-war medical establishment.

---

* A funeral party of 30 was permitted, and the 3 British medical officers took it in turn to march the party about 2½ miles to the local cemetery and there to read the burial service. On two occasions the Germans provided an official firing party.

† In all their reports, naval medical officers who were prisoners-of-war have consistently referred to the difference to their well-being which was brought about by Red Cross supplies.

One medical officer has also paid tribute to visits made by a representative of the Y.M.C.A. His report states: 'I do not think that the help given to us by this body is generally realised'.

The patients in Nagold were all British, and the object of the move from Rottenmünster seems to have been to collect together in one place all the sick British prisoners-of-war in that part of Germany.

But, though the entire complement of patients was British, the hospital continued to be administered strictly on German lines. The British medical officers with their orderlies were relegated to a status of little more than ward 'dressers', and found themselves under the direct orders of German doctors and nursing staff.

Accommodation was reasonable and food was fairly adequate and well prepared by an experienced German cook.*

At Nagold, medical and surgical treatment was of a high standard, drugs and equipment were in good supply, and Red Cross parcels were regularly received and fairly distributed.

Gloucester's Medical Officer has commented at length upon the strictness of the rigid discipline which the German medical officers imposed upon both staff and patients at Nagold. It would appear that this attitude was greatly resented by many of the patients, who disliked the constant supervision and lack of freedom of movement. However, the Medical Officer considered that, from the purely medical point of view, the sick thrived at Nagold and were very much better off than in other prisoner-of-war medical establishments. In fact, it was his opinion that correct professional treatment combined with rigid discipline was greatly to the advantage of the sick, difficult though it was to make the patients realise this fact.

Unfortunately, on March 12, 1942, the hospital at Nagold was closed and all British patients and medical and nursing staffs were sent back to Rottenmünster by train. Once again the journey was conducted under conditions of extreme cold with many inches of snow on the ground, but it was eventful in that two medical orderlies made a very good escape while the train was passing through a tunnel.†

His second period of confinement in Rottenmünster lasted from March until October 1942. During this time he continued to improve his knowledge of artificial limb construction. The hospital itself had changed little, but a large consignment of Red Cross stores had been received which made it possible to clothe the patients properly as they recovered.

---

* It is of some interest that the Medical Officer took the trouble to analyse the various systems employed in cooking for the sick in the prisoner-of-war medical establishments in which he served. He considered that the best cooking he encountered in Germany was that of chefs of the British Merchant Navy, which was far superior to that of Army cooks, both British and French!

† These two orderlies were disguised as man and wife, and they walked quite openly into Switzerland. Unfortunately, the frontier was irregular, so that having walked into Switzerland they had the misfortune to re-cross the border back into Germany where they were arrested.

Earlier, a convalescent patient of the Seaforth Highlanders had escaped from the hospital at Rottenmünster. He shaved his head and dressed in blue overalls. Carrying a paint pot and smoking a cigar, he walked through the gate unchallenged by the sentries. He too was recaptured at the Swiss frontier.

In September 1942, he found himself with almost no work to do, so he applied to the authorities for transfer to some naval prisoner-of-war camp. His transfer from Rottenmünster was approved but, instead of being sent to a naval camp, he was sent to a camp for civilian internees at Biberach. He has described this move as 'a typical example of German perversity'.

Biberach is a small town on the river Riss. Ilag Biberach was a camp, situated on a hill above the town, and newly opened to receive civilian internees from the Channel Islands.

On arrival he was immediately interviewed by the Camp Commandant, an Oberst. This interview is described as being rather pointless, though the Oberst put on full uniform and medals for the occasion! The Medical Officer states: 'He told me he didn't like the Royal Navy, chiefly because he was a *bon viveur* and the blockade was interfering with his gastronomic pleasures. He told me that if I found that the food in the camp was inadequate, I must blame the Royal Navy for it and it would be useless complaining to him about it. He also attributed for my benefit, the shortage of coal to the blockade of the Royal Navy, thus accounting for lack of fuel inside the camp. When I pointed out that it was geographically impossible to blockade the Ruhr from the sea, he warned me to behave myself or I would soon be placed in cells!'

On the other hand, the German senior medical officer, though a pompous individual with no sense of humour, was most correct in his professional attitude. *Gloucester's* Medical Officer, who by now could speak German fluently, found that most of his difficulties in dealing with this Oberstabsarzt were due to a speech defect from which the latter suffered. 'He had an imposing array of gold crown and bridge dentures. Occasionally he used to get an abscess under one of the crowns which made him rather irritable and gave his diction a most fascinating impediment!'

The medical staff of the camp included two German nursing sisters, one of whom cared for sick children.*

Camp administration and discipline were in the hands of a Feldwebel who had been invalided from the front suffering from 'shell shock' which made him get hysterical at times. 'But', says the Medical Officer, ever just in his outlook, 'he did us no harm in his lucid intervals!'

The large number of internees in Ilag Biberach consisted of men, women and children from all classes of society and age groups extending from septuagenarians to sucklings. There were about 1,500 persons in all including some expectant mothers.

The Medical Officer soon found that his duties extended far beyond the realms of doctoring. By this time, he was an experienced prisoner-

---

* The report states that child internees in this camp were well cared for, and the Germans produced special rations for the young children.

of-war with knowledge of how best a camp should be conducted to the advantage of those confined in it. He was also one of the few in this camp who could speak German.

The main disadvantage of this camp was its situation on a hillside, exposed to cold winds off the Alps. This, together with shortage of fuel, meant inevitable hardships during the winter months.

The camp hospital consisted of two huts, one for women and the other for men. A British civilian doctor looked after women and children patients while he dealt with the men. The civilian doctor was professionally the senior of the two, but the German authorities insisted that the Naval Medical Officer should be medically responsible to them.

Unfortunately, the civilian doctor was soon transferred, and he found himself involved in problems of gynaecology, infant feeding and ante-natal care, matters with which he had long ceased to be familiar in the course of his naval service. Neither was this burden eased by the arrival of further internees from the Channel Islands, including two more civilian doctors, as one of these men was a public health expert and the other a medical administrator belonging to the Colonial Medical Service. But fortunately a British nursing sister arrived with these internees who was able to render great assistance in caring for sick women and children.

His versatility is exhibited in that passage from his report which reads: 'At 1630 hours everybody was locked up until the following morning. This made it a very long night, but I usually managed to fill in the time. First I started with the evening ward round. Then I cooked supper for the patients on my small stove.* Later there were the usual clothes to be washed and a number of the day's medical problems to be read about.'†

On November 25, 1942, Ilag Biberach was taken over by the German Civil Police, and he was transferred back to Rottenmünster.

This Medical Officer's third period in Rottenmünster was his longest, lasting some 14 months. The principal difference which he found at Rottenmünster at this time was that part of the hospital had been set aside for sick Russian prisoners-of-war, and he was given charge of some of these men.

These Russian patients were confined in a small separate building containing about 200 beds. The building was kept locked, and he held one key and the Germans the other. The Russian sick were not permitted to have any contact with the other prisoners-of-war, and though they

---

* This Medical Officer acted as custodian of the Red Cross medical comfort parcels. He instituted a routine of collecting food left over at the midday meal, and this he augmented from the parcels and re-cooked at night so as to provide extra nourishment for the sick. Hence his personal supervision even to the extent of preparing and cooking this meal himself.

† Realising this Medical Officer's difficulties in the treatment of women and children, the German medical authorities obtained English medical textbooks for him from Rottenmünster.

were allowed Russian medical orderlies, who were described as well trained, efficient and intelligent, Russian medical officers were not permitted to care for them.*

The beds for the Russian sick were in two-tier bunks in rows, side by side, and could only be approached from the foot. It was thus impossible to examine a patient from the bedside. The actual bedding consisted of palliasses stuffed with wood shavings. The whole hospital was infested with fleas and bed bugs. The Medical Officer's first introduction to these Russians was to be taken into a small room where four or five emaciated, naked bodies were lying on the floor. He was required to decide whether one of them was perhaps still alive. He confirmed that they were all dead, whereupon they were wrapped up in brown paper in preparation for being dumped into a communal pit.

His first two living Russian patients had both walked $2\frac{1}{2}$ miles from the local station, each carrying his possessions. One of them appeared little more than a skeleton, with an empyema filling the whole of the right side of his chest. The other case had rheumatic fever with effusions into both knee joints.

A large number of these Russian patients suffered from famine oedema, and pulmonary tuberculosis was very common. More than anything else they needed food, but very little could be done for them. The death rate was high.

The situation of Russian surgical cases was a little better, because the Medical Officer was frequently able to convince the German authorities that operation was necessary. By this means he was able to transfer the Russian patient to the British section of the hospital for 'pre-operative therapy'. As he says, 'this gave me the chance to feed the man up for a week or two on Red Cross food.'

The report dwells at length on the brutality displayed by the German authorities towards these Russian sick. 'The German in charge of a sick fatigue party, frequently made up of patients who should have been in bed, always carried a stick which he did not hesitate to use. It was not unknown, either, for a German orderly to strike a patient in bed.'

But perhaps the most revealing portion of the report is that which describes how these sick Russian prisoners-of-war found their living conditions in this hospital virtually luxurious compared with those of the working camps from which they had come!

His third period of confinement in Rottenmünster ended on January 16, 1943, when he was subjected to a term of solitary confinement in gaol as punishment for a disciplinary offence. The story of the circumstances is best related in his own words:

---

* The report states : 'No Russian doctors were, at that time, allowed to work among heir own sick. Most of them were quarrying stone'.

'When I returned to Rottenmünster from Biberach, I heard that in the German administrative office there was a very good wireless set. This office was empty after 2030 hours each day.

'It was not difficult to obtain a key to fit the lock of the door of this office. In fact, an Australian corporal made three for me in two days.

'At my first attempt everything went perfectly. Taking with me a sergeant of the New Zealand Army Medical Corps, I entered the office after dark. The sergeant stayed in the doorway to keep guard, while I operated the wireless set. I put a towel over the set to keep out any light, as a sentry passed close to the window from time to time. I kept the volume turned right down and got the midnight broadcast from England.

'We continued this routine nightly for some time, and were able to pass reliable news around the camp each day.

'But, one night at the beginning of January, just when the news bulletin was ending, I heard a slight scuffle behind me. I thought it was the sergeant, and told him not to make so much noise. The next thing I knew was that I was in the beam of an electric torch and that a revolver was being pointed at me. The lights went on, and I found that my captor was the Feldwebel, who had been hiding under a bed in the corner of the office. I was glad to see that the sergeant had disappeared, and in order to give him a chance to cover his tracks, I wasted a lot of time by refusing to admit to the Feldwebel that anyone else was in the office with me.

'Unfortunately the sergeant had left his slippers behind, and the Feldwebel found them on the floor.

'After placing me under arrest, the Germans set off to find the owner of the slippers. But meanwhile, all the British medical orderlies had quickly changed from slippers into boots, and the sergeant had in any case obtained for himself a spare pair of slippers. This confused the Germans so much that they were quite unable to trace their "Cinderella".

'But my own future was not long left in doubt. On January 16, 1943 I was removed, under an armed guard, to the gaol in the main camp at Villingen.'

The next twelve days were spent in Stalag VB Gaol, Villingen. This gaol was intended for other ranks only, and the commandant was rather worried about having to accommodate a British officer, this being the first occasion on which he had been confronted with such a problem. Accordingly, special arrangements were made for the comfort of the medical officer who was given a palliasse and two extra blankets. He also had a small table put in his cell, and the commandant visited him personally each day to study his welfare.

The cells were separated from each other by brick partitions which did not quite reach the ceiling. The gap at the top of the partitions was covered with barbed wire netting.

Talking was not allowed, but this Medical Officer soon found himself in communication with the inhabitants of neighbouring cells. He says: 'I found that my brother lags were Polish, Serbian, Russian and French, and we all talked to each other in a kind of *lingua franca* common among prisoners-of-war.'

The food was sufficient in quantity, but so unappetising that it was difficult to swallow. Also, if there was any delay in eating it, it was soon likely to be set on by rats and mice which also inhabited the cells.

Each forenoon this Medical Officer underwent interrogation by the German authorities, who seemed to attach immense importance to the illicit reception of foreign broadcasts. Each afternoon he was allowed two hours' exercise in the prison yard. The rest of the day he passed gossiping through the wall to his neighbours, washing his clothes, and hunting bugs and fleas.

Strange as it may sound, the days are described as passing agreeably enough, and the stay at Villingen as most enjoyable. The report states: 'Unfortunately, this happy state of affairs did not continue, and after twelve days I was moved, under armed escort, to Ludwigsburg.'

The prisoner and his escort arrived at Ludwigsburg late in the evening. Their destination was the Militarhaftanstalt, but the Medical Officer seems to have rebuked his escort who 'with characteristic Teutonic stupidity took me to the wrong gaol, so we were walking for another hour before we finally found the right one!'

The Militarhaftanstalt was a German Military Gaol used for the detention of those awaiting courts-martial. *Gloucester's* Medical Officer was the only prisoner-of-war inmate, the remainder all being German officers and other ranks who had committed various disciplinary offences.

On the morning after his arrival, the Medical Officer was conducted before the German authorities. He was charged with 'breaking and entering', and with 'listening to foreign broadcasts'. He was informed that he would be court-martialled on March 9. He was told that he would be given an opportunity to prepare his defence, and in this respect, the German authorities did in fact inform the Protecting Power of the impending court-martial and a lawyer was appointed for his assistance.

For the next six weeks this Medical Officer was confined in a clean and airy cell.* He was allowed out for five minutes each morning and five minutes each evening in order to draw fresh water. He was not allowed any exercise. Nevertheless, he suffered no discomfort. The food was good though scanty, and he was surprised at being given sheets for his bed. To relieve the monotony he had a pack of cards and a copy of 'The Pickwick Papers'.

Inevitably, although they were Germans, he soon established contact with his brother prisoners. A 'peep hole' soon appeared to communicate with the next cell and it was possible then to obtain information

---

* The cell which this Medical Officer occupied at Ludwigsburg was indeed larger than most, extremely clean and had double doors. It was, in fact, the 'condemned cell'!

about local conditions. It appeared that courts-martial sat in the prison every day, and one of the most alarming features was the severity of the sentences. The soldier in the next cell was soon sentenced to death and executed. His offence had been that of leave-breaking. Learning of this, the Medical Officer became apprehensive about his own ultimate fate, particularly as he realised that, under German law, it was a capital offence to listen to B.B.C. broadcasts.

On March 8 he was suddenly taken before the President of the German Court who informed him that his trial had been cancelled, but that he had been summarily sentenced to one month's solitary confinement and that this meant his immediate release.

He was immediately discharged from the gaol and sent to the nearby prisoner-of-war hospital at Stalag VA.

At Stalag VA, he found himself rather in disgrace with the authorities, being now a man with a 'prison record'. However, on March 29 he was moved again, this time into Silesia. His destination was Lamsdorf, and the journey took 48 hours during which he stood the whole time in the corridor of a train.

He arrived at Stalag VIIIB, Lamsdorf, at 0700 hours on April 1, 1943. He describes the pleasures he felt at finding himself at once in a British atmosphere which he had missed for so long. As he was marched through the main gate, a working party was just moving off, and they gave him a very smart 'eyes right'. Once inside the camp, he was approached by a British sergeant, who saluted smartly and relieved him of his kit bag. 'With great joy', he says, 'I spoke English again for the first time since my arrest in January.'

His report gives a detailed description of the prisoner-of-war camp at Lamsdorf, including its administration and medical arrangements. It is not proposed, however, to record more than two matters considered to be of importance.

The first is the opinion expressed of the camp. At that time, Lamsdorf had the reputation of being the worst prison camp in Germany. But he states emphatically:'What I saw of it during my two months' stay did not justify this description. But probably I saw the camp at its best, when the weather was warm, and when it was not so overcrowded as it had been or as I believe it subsequently became.'*

The second item of interest, particularly from the viewpoint of the Royal Navy, was that the Commandant of Lamsdorf was an old, retired Austrian Naval Captain. This fact made a great difference to his welfare as he found that he was the only Royal Naval officer whom the Commandant had so far met in captivity. Observing that intangible

---

* In April 1943 Stalag VIIIB had some 35,000 prisoners-of-war on its books. But this number included all the working Commandos attached to it. At the time of the arrival of *Gloucester's* Medical Officer, only about 8,000 prisoners-of-war were actually accommodated in the main camp itself.

link which binds seamen together, regardless of race or international relations, the Camp Commandant showed him great kindness. The Commandant even went so far as to suggest that he must find it very trying to be the lone naval prisoner-of-war among so many soldiers! Taking the Medical Officer's agreement for granted, the Commandant went on the reveal that, in any case, he personally had had 'just about enough of the German Army!'

On June 1, 1943, in company with two officers of the Royal Army Medical Corps, he was transferred from Lamsdorf to the prisoner-of-war camp at Marlag, where he arrived on June 3. This move was sudden, as ever, but was a most pleasant surprise as it fulfilled his hope of at last making his way to a naval prisoner-of-war camp.

That this Naval Medical Officer achieved great popularity among all his companions at Lamsdorf is obvious, and there seems to be no doubt that the valuable friendship which he was able to establish with the Austrian Naval Commandant reacted greatly to the advantage of all the other prisoners-of-war. Naturally, in his official report, he is silent regarding the influence which he personally was able to exert. But one short sentence suffices to reveal the esteem with which this young naval doctor must have been regarded at Lamsdorf:

'We had a great send off, and marched from the centre of the camp to the main gate behind the pipe band!'

It is unfortunate that he was prevented by ill-health from completing his report on the last phases of his captivity, particularly as he ultimately became involved in the battle for North-west Germany. There is no doubt that the travels of this Medical Officer were alone sufficient to make his experiences unique as a prisoner-of-war.

Enough has here been extracted from the available records to show that the way in which he conducted himself was at all times in accordance with the highest traditions of his Service and his profession. His official report, based on a diary which he contrived to maintain, was a model of documentary clearness and accuracy. The reader cannot have failed to note his constant fairness in his comments, and his readiness to give credit to his captors whenever it was merited. Perhaps paramount, was his 'puckish' sense of humour which obviously was never far absent during his captivity, and which he could never quite conceal even in his official report. He seems never to have lost an opportunity to ridicule his captors, and he trained others to do the same.

Regarding the rare visits of the German senior medical officer to the Russian wards in Rottenmünster he says: 'Dr. Essig would not stand very near to the Russians for fear of catching something. One of our trivial pastimes was to catch fleas in the ward, put them in a matchbox and later transfer them to Dr. Essig's pocket when he was visiting!'

At Ludwigsburg, when informed that he had been summarily sentenced to one month's solitary confinement, the Medical Officer had already been confined for approximately two months. Thereupon, he officially demanded that the German authorities should credit him with a balance of one month, and he asked if he might commit some crime at his discretion to offset this balance! However, he settled this account on the same day, because on his arrival at Stalag VA, his first act was to walk into the commandant's office, tune in to London on the commandant's wireless set, listen to the news and walk out again!

Regarding his journey to Lamsdorf, he says: 'My guard was a peasant with a low intelligence quotient. If I had not been able to read the timetables and show him which trains to catch and where to change, we might still have been travelling now!'

At Lamsdorf, the German Army guards had little experience of the German Navy, and they frequently failed to recognise the uniform of the Naval Camp Commandant. In spite of his tattered uniform monkey jacket, *Gloucester's* Medical Officer was sometimes mistaken for the Commandant himself. On one occasion a German sentry sprang to attention before the Medical Officer and reported the state of the guard to him. Promptly the Medical Officer rebuked the sentry for his untidiness and ordered him to fasten his top button, which he immediately did!

But by no means insignificant were many of his professional and scientific observations, which at times showed a shrewd insight rare in a young doctor suffering extreme hardship.

Among his many observations, he recorded a memorandum on the subject of 'barbed-wire neurosis' which reads:

'I am in considerable doubt as to whether there is any such condition as "barbed-wire neurosis". But, in fairness, I should point out that I know very little about psychiatry.

'I am convinced that no man between the ages of 20 and 40 who was physically and mentally fit at the time of his capture, developed any neurosis or psychosis merely as the result of his confinement. But equally, there is no doubt that some men of congenitally unstable temperament did find the conditions of life too much for them, and unsuspected weaknesses were revealed. I think it possible, too, that certain cases of psychosis, schizophrenia, paranoia, etc., may have had their onset accelerated by imprisonment.

'Though I do not agree that any actual neurosis developed in healthy subjects, I am sure that we were all under rather more constant mental stress than we realised at the time.

'But moving as I did from one place to another, I realised that, viewed sensibly, the circumstances which I encountered were not all that different from the circumstances encountered when moving from ship to ship in the Royal Navy.

'This view may sound peculiar, but what I mean to express is that as in the case of H.M. Ships, so the morale of individual prisoners-of-war depended largely on the morale of the prison camp as a whole.

Where the discipline, though rigid, was understandable and correct, there the camp morale was high. But, where the discipline was sporadic, haphazard and unreasonable, there the morale tended to sag.'

THE LOSS OF H.M.S. *EXETER* AND SUBSEQUENT EVENTS*

Between January 1 and February 13, 1942, H.M.S. *Exeter* escorted thirteen convoys of troops and war materials to Singapore, in the course of which operations the ship, though heavily attacked from the air, escaped damage. On February 15, 1942, in the Jasper Straits, the ship was attacked by waves of Japanese aircraft from 0900 hours until 1700 hours. She was near missed many times, but there were only a few minor casualties on board. At about 1600 hours on February 27, 1942, an Allied Combined Striking Force engaged a much superior Japanese Naval Force off Sourabaya, Java, N.E.I. As part of this Combined Striking Force, which was commanded by Rear Admiral K. W. F. M. Doorman, Royal Netherlands Navy, *Exeter* was in company with 4 cruisers and 9 destroyers. The 9 destroyers included H.M.Ss. *Encounter*, *Jupiter* and *Electra*. Besides H.M.S. *Exeter*, the cruisers were H.M.A.S. *Perth*, U.S.S. *Housten*, and *Java* and *De Ruyter* of the Royal Netherlands Navy, the latter flying the Flag of the Dutch Commander-in-Chief.

After being in action one hour, H.M.S. *Exeter* received a direct hit.† The shell passed through the 4-in. A.A. mounting, killing six of the guns' crew. It then continued through No. 1 boiler room ventilator, through the boiler room, destroying the main steam pipe and putting two of four boilers out of action. The shell next passed through a superheater and boiler in No. 2 boiler room and exploded in the bottom of the ship, killing 8 stokers. The ship's speed was immediately reduced to 6 knots. In No. 2 boiler room, only one boiler was completely out of action, but there were no stokers available to keep steam on in the other three boilers. At 1714 hours, *Exeter* reported herself stopped.

---

* The account here given has been compiled with some difficulty from a number of reports forwarded after the war by surviving officers and men. In the end, these reports had to be made largely from memory for reasons such as that given by the Senior Medical Officer of H.M.S. *Exeter* whose report begins: 'All my medical records, notes and general information which I religiously kept up-to-date from day to day during my prisoner-of-war period, were forcibly taken from me on searches by the Japanese on no less than seven occasions. I did succeed in holding on to some, which I buried at Macassar, N.E.I., Batavia, and others which I had sewn into various garments. Some of my records were buried at Pamalaa, and Bandoeng, which I hope will be forwarded to me later by some of my Dutch friends.'

The sick berth petty officer of H.M.S. *Exeter* contrived to maintain a most meticulous and detailed record of sickness of prisoners-of-war from H.M.Ss. *Exeter*, *Encounter* and *Stronghold* while in captivity in the notorious Fukuoka Camp at Nagasaki. This record consists of a number of pages from a Japanese exercise book, cut into strips and bound into a brown paper cover with elastoplast. This recording was done always at night and at great personal risk.

† The *Exeter* was hit by an 8-in. shell from the *Nachi* at 1708 hours.

Soon afterwards, *Exeter* was able to proceed at 15 knots screened by smoke from H.M.A.S. *Perth* and protected against torpedo attacks from enemy destroyers by *Jupiter*, *Encounter* and *Electra*. *Electra* was sunk at 1800 hours. But already at 1740 hours, *Exeter* could no longer keep up with the Fleet, and she was ordered to retire from the action escorted by the Dutch destroyer *Witte de With*. *Exeter* reached the entrance of Sourabaya minefield at 2000 hours, and limped into Sourabaya at 2330 hours.

The situation of H.M.S. *Exeter* was now not to be envied, hemmed in as she was, in a disabled state, with only a remote prospect of escape through narrow seas everywhere patrolled by units of the Japanese Fleet.*

At 1930 on February 28, with a maximum speed of 16 knots, *Exeter* left Sourabaya in company with H.M.S. *Encounter* and U.S.S. *Pope*. Her orders were to proceed to Colombo *via* Sunda Strait. Unfortunately, soon after leaving Sourabaya, this small force was discovered by an enemy reconnaissance plane. In consequence, at 1000 hours, on March 1, *Exeter* reported that three enemy cruisers were approaching. In fact, *Exeter* was intercepted by four 7·8 in. cruisers and three destroyers and the ensuing action was a gun duel against overwhelming odds.† *Exeter* was stopped by 1126 hours and subsequently sunk by a torpedo from the Japanese destroyer *Inazuma*. *Encounter* and *Pope* were also sunk.

Describing this action, *Exeter's* Senior Medical Officer, a surgeon commander, R.N., wrote: 'Japanese warships began popping up all over the place. We returned their fire, but at about 1100 hours we were hit in No. 1 boiler room. Somehow, a smoke float on the forward end of the quarterdeck got ignited, and I found the after medical distributing station filled with smoke and I could not see my hand in front of me. I telephoned the Damage Control Officer to shut off the fan, but with no success. I gave orders to my staff to lie on the deck and remain perfectly still.‡ About then we received orders to abandon ship.'

After searching round the after cabin flat for any casualties, the Senior Medical Officer now made his way on to the upper deck. He joined a party who were busy throwing Carley floats, rafts, etc., into the sea, and he then went to his abandon ship station. He found that most of the boats were unserviceable owing to damage by shellfire. He then left the ship by the port side and jumped into the sea.

---

* *Exeter's* position has been described as somewhat similar to that of the *Graf Spee* when the latter took refuge in Montevideo during the Battle of the River Plate in December 1939. However, there the similarity ends, as the *Graf Spee* was scuttled, whereas H.M.S. *Exeter* put to sea and engaged the enemy yet again!

† The Japanese report states that the two heavy cruisers *Myoko* and *Haguro* fired 8,000 rounds in 1½ hours!

‡ This fan supplied air to the distributing station through an 'intake' on the quarterdeck. Hence the fact that the smoke was sucked through the ventilation trunk and discharged into the distributing station.

He says, 'as I abandoned ship, a shell came inboard on the starboard side and helped me on my way!'

When he abandoned ship, the Senior Medical Officer was wearing a pair of flannel trousers, shirt with long sleeves, a uniform cap, long stockings and shoes. He had on him a waterproof bag containing morphia, a hypodermic syringe, iodine, two pairs of artery forceps, scissors, some bandages and cotton wool. He also carried his post office savings book. He was wearing his lifebelt, but did not inflate it until he got into the water. When he got into the sea, he removed his shoes, 'But,' he says, 'I regretted this afterwards, as they would have been very useful to collect rain water.'

The Senior Medical Officer was soon covered in oil fuel, and, after some twenty minutes he heard someone shout for help. He found that this was a marine who was on the point of drowning. In spite of the oil fuel, the Senior Medical Officer managed to swim with this man and to pull him on to a raft.*

Meanwhile, one of the junior medical officers† of H.M.S. *Exeter*, a surgeon lieutenant, R.N., had also not been idle. When the order came to abandon ship, he left his action station and controlled the press of ratings who were clustered around the foot of ladders leading on to the upper deck. When he was satisfied that the lower positions and messdecks were cleared, he went to the upper deck where he concentrated the sick and wounded. He assisted each casualty over the side after making sure that his lifebelt was inflated. As there were enemy ships on both sides of *Exeter*, there was no side of the ship disengaged, so he placed the wounded in the water as far aft as possible. The Surgeon Lieutenant then searched the upper deck for any more casualties, and came across one of the sick berth attendants who was mortally wounded in the abdomen. Having satisfied himself that there was nothing further he could do, and as he could see only one other officer left besides himself, he decided to take to the water. Almost immediately after he abandoned ship, the *Exeter* rolled over to starboard and sank.‡

The Commanding Officer, 44 officers and 607 ratings of H.M.S. *Exeter* were rescued by the Japanese and made prisoners-of-war.

---

* This marine was rescued the next day, but he died as a prisoner-of-war on September 3, 1943. Before his death, he wrote a letter which eventually found its way to the Admiralty after the war. In this letter, the man wrote : 'I was covered with oil fuel and vomited a lot, and my eyes were very burned by the oil. A heavy sea was running and I was just about to give up hope when the Surgeon Commander rescued me and brought me to a raft. The Surgeon Commander swam over 200 yards and saved my life, despite the danger of the Japanese shells which were falling all round us.'

For this act, the Senior Medical Officer of H.M.S. *Exeter* was subsequently recommended for the medal of the Royal Humane Society and was mentioned in dispatches.

† The junior medical officers of H.M.S. *Exeter* were a surgeon lieutenant, R.N., and a surgeon lieutenant, R.N.V.R.

‡ This junior medical officer of H.M.S. *Exeter* was subsequently decorated for outstanding services while a prisoner-of-war in the Far East.

The period which the survivors spent in the water varied. For instance, *Exeter's* Surgeon Lieutenant was picked up after two hours by a Japanese destroyer. This destroyer rescued 380 survivors, all of whom were transferred to an oil tanker at Bandjer Massin, Borneo, on the morning of March 2. Casualties underwent hardship during this day for lack of medical stores of any kind. The Surgeon Lieutenant did manage to obtain a mattress for one badly scalded stoker, and he contrived to immobilise with box-wood the leg of another rating who had a compound fracture. On the evening of the same day, these casualties and the Surgeon Lieutenant were moved to the Dutch Hospital Ship *Op Ten Noort*,* whose staff gave valuable assistance.

Meanwhile, *Exeter's* Senior Medical Officer was one of many survivors who were rescued by a Japanese destroyer on March 2, after being in the water for twenty-five hours.†

On board this destroyer, a Japanese medical officer gave *Exeter's* Surgeon Commander every assistance in dealing with his casualties. Particular attention was paid to a seaman with a compound fracture of tibia and fibula‡ and to the Medical Officer of H.M.S. *Encounter* who was suffering from exhaustion and the effects of prolonged immersion. The Commanding Officer of the Japanese destroyer supplied the survivors with ample water, bully beef and ships' biscuits. The destroyer's medical officer made the Surgeon Commander a present of ten packets of cigarettes. §

The Surgeon Commander and casualties were transferred to the Hospital Ship *Op Ten Noort* on the afternoon of March 3.

All the survivors were well cared for on board the Dutch hospital ship, though all the reports have recorded the fact that the food supplied was inadequate in quantity and poor in quality.‖

These survivors remained on board the *Op Ten Noort* until March 10. On March 10, with the exception of 19 casualties who were unfit to be moved, they were landed at Macassar, in the Celebes. On landing,

---

* This hospital ship was captured by two Japanese destroyers while at sea on February 28.

† The Senior Medical Officer's report states : 'This humane act of the Japanese, coming back the next day to pick up the remainder of us, was a very wonderful gesture for which I give them the highest praise.'

‡ This seaman died during the following night and was buried at sea.

§ This is another example of the 'intangible link which binds seamen together', and which has already been referred to earlier in this Chapter in the case of the Medical Officer of H.M.S. *Gloucester*.

‖ In fairness to the Dutch authorities, it must be remembered that a sudden influx of something in the region of 800 survivors from *Exeter* and *Encounter* would be likely to strain the resources of any hospital ship even under ideal conditions. But the conditions under which the *Op Ten Noort* was working at this time could have been anything but ideal. The problem of resuscitating and caring for this large number of survivors, several of whom were badly wounded, was complicated by the fact that the hospital ship itself had just been captured by the enemy and had a Japanese armed guard on board.

these naval survivors were marched four miles to a prisoner-of-war camp in the local barracks. To say that these men 'marched' would be a flattering description of the straggling procession which they formed, as the vast majority were barefoot, having abandoned their footwear in the sea.

The Barracks at Macassar was at least 100 years old and quite inadequate to accommodate the number of prisoners. Dutch prisoners-of-war numbered about 1,800, Americans 167 and British 868. The British prisoners were composed as follows:

Ship	Officers	Ratings	Totals
H.M.S. *Exeter* . . .	45	607	652
H.M.S. *Encounter* . .	7	143	150
H.M.S. *Stronghold* . .	1	47	48
H.M.S. *Anking* . .	—	2	2
R.F.A. *Francol* . .	5	3	8
Miscellaneous . . .	2	6	8
	60	808	868

One Australian Air Force officer joined the British group a few days later. On April 2, the Commanding Officer of H.M.S. *Exeter*, 12 other British naval officers and 4 naval ratings were transferred to Japan.

The arrival of these prisoners-of-war in the camp at Macassar was followed by an immediate period of confusion which lasted about three weeks, by which time various ailments were firmly established and proved impossible to eradicate completely ever again.

There was no bedding or furniture of any description, and these men had to sleep on a bare, concrete floor exposed to cold and mosquitoes.

The diet consisted of a small cake each in the morning with a half cup of coffee, and a rice ball each evening.

The sanitary arrangements in the camp were appalling and the latrines took several days to clear of filth and obstructions. This work was performed by a hygiene squad organised by the Surgeon Commander whose next difficult task was to train all the prisoners-of-war to use the Asiatic-type latrines and to cleanse themselves with water in the absence of toilet paper. But in any case, it was only possible for these latrines to be flushed every two hours, and as no covers were available, excrement was soon wide open to the millions of flies in the camp.

A further domestic difficulty which had an adverse affect upon health and hygiene was, that for the first three weeks, no prisoner-of-war was permitted to use the latrines without permission of the Japanese. It would seem that even so, permission was not readily granted and such requests were discouraged. The Surgeon Commander records that: 'When you asked permission, you were invariably beaten up by the guard, either with his fist, his rifle, or a pick, bamboo stick, iron bar or whatever weapon he happened to be carrying. It was therefore very common among us not to open our bowels for several days. I myself did not go for eleven days, and one American officer did not go for twenty-eight days.'

These sanitary difficulties persisted for about three weeks, and, combined with the purchase of food through the fence from local inhabitants in order to supplement the meagre prison fare, soon led to a fairly generalised outbreak of bacillary dysentery. Fortunately, most of the cases were fairly mild and responded to sulphaguanidine of which a small stock was held in reserve for this disease by the doctors. The severe cases were evacuated to the *Op Ten Noort* where a small number died.

Meanwhile numerous men were suffering from wounds of the feet, contracted during the march to the camp, which had become infected with ulcer formation. Most of these cases were treated effectively with iodoform and cod liver oil ointment.

During the first three weeks at Macassar, however, medical treatment of the sick was greatly hampered by the fact that the Japanese would not permit the medical officers to have free access to the men's quarters.

After April 1, 1942, conditions at Macassar improved, and the daily ration was augmented by a supply of rice, germinated beans, one duck egg, and a small quantity of pork. This diet, though monotonous, was perfectly sufficient to keep the men in health. Small improvements were also made in accommodation, but the Japanese still did not supply any mosquito nets, and sporadic cases of benign tertian malaria had begun to appear. At this time, it was possible to treat these cases with quinine bihydrochloride.

It is of interest to note that these improvements at Macassar coincided with the arrival of a Japanese First Class Petty Officer* as Commandant. It is also revealing to note, in correct perspective, the true influence and effect which this man exerted upon the camp of which he had charge.†

Exeter's Surgeon Commander describes this Camp Commandant in the following terms: 'A man, aged about 32, of untiring energy, excellent powers of command and outstanding efficiency. Superimposed on these excellent qualities were an uncontrollable temper and every bad characteristic which could be imagined. He became to us the embodiment of everything that was evil and everything that we had been fighting against in this war—sadistic brutality, cruelty, dishonesty, untruthfulness, roguery and tyranny. It was not long before everything connected with the camp revolved around this fiend and his despotic rule. To men always hungry, in most cases suffering from some form of sickness, ill-clothed, and herded in quarters like animals, the addition of this nervous tension to the drabness and monotony of prison life had very exhausting effects upon the mental health of us all.'

---

* Petty Officer Yoshide.

† The reader is referred to the observations which give the view of *Gloucester's* Medical Officer on discipline and morale in German prisoner-of-war camps, p. 201.

On the other hand, *Exeter's* Surgeon Lieutenant, while agreeing in principle with the ill effects occasioned by the constant mental strain of living under the control of 'this terrible person', does attempt to weigh the balance more evenly and to attribute to the commandant certain advantages which flowed from the severe discipline which was maintained inside the camp at Macassar. Also, it is only fair to note that when he was transferred to other areas later where he fared worse, he was later able to assess the camp at Macassar more favourably in retrospect. For example, he has recorded: 'The nineteen months which I spent in Macassar under the Japanese Navy were the best I ever had as a prisoner-of-war. Once the camp was properly organised, living conditions for both officers and men were good. The food was adequate after the first two months, in fact, 40 pigs were raised on the leavings. The water supply was good and came from the main reservoir through the usual mains system. The general health of personnel who were retained at Macassar did not deteriorate very much, and when I left, except for those who had recently returned from labour camps elsewhere the general standard of health was high.'

The Japanese Petty Officer in charge of this prisoner-of-war camp at Macassar soon took steps to make sure that the camp accommodated itself to his ideas of rigid discipline, and certain of his measures added to the burdens of the camp doctors. He issued an order that outside trading with the local inhabitants was to cease.* This order was broken by 27 British, 4 Dutch and 3 American prisoners-of-war. As punishment these men were publicly beaten. The weapons used were a knotted rope's end dipped in water, a baseball bat and a bamboo pole. The parts of the body beaten were the back and buttocks, head, arms and legs.†

Shortly afterwards, 3 Dutch prisoners-of-war escaped from the camp but were recaptured after a few days. They were publicly executed by decapitation.

To accord with the discipline and general humiliation of the prisoners-of-war, all heads had to be shaved.‡

It soon became obvious, however, that the improved conditions in food and accommodation were not aimed merely at increasing the personal comfort of the prisoners-of-war, but that the Japanese authorities were setting out towards some particular purpose. What this purpose was, was revealed in the middle of April 1942 when working parties commenced in the local docks, and every man physically fit was forced to take part.

---

* All the camp medical officers were agreed that such trading was almost certainly the chief cause of the bacillary dysentery which prevailed in the camp.

† During this punishment, one Marine sustained a fractured right radius and ulna.

‡ The camp medical officers were unanimous in their opinion that this shaving of heads, although it was greatly resented, was an excellent measure in a community which tended to become lice infested.

From the start of the working parties, it was noted that the number of skin wounds and tropical ulcers steadily increased, and these became more difficult to treat as the scanty medical supplies were exhausted.*

The working parties were employed mostly upon demolition, and one advantage which accrued was contact and wholesale trading with the local population. The Surgeon Commander records that: 'Anything from a needle to an anchor could be procured as well as clothes, food of every description, razor blades, and pencils.'

At the same time, as a reward for hard work, conditions inside the camp were further improved during the months which followed, and mattresses were provided, and a canteen and library were formed.

Early in October 1942, the Japanese removed 400 of the British prisoners-of-war from the Macassar Camp and sent them to work on an aerodrome some 20 kilometres away. These men continued to be fed from Macassar, but they lived under terrible conditions of overcrowding, bad sanitation and poor water supply. Their work consisted of jungle clearance for the most part, they had no mosquito nets, and the number of cases of malaria now showed a rapid increase.

On October 14, 1942, the Japanese transferred to Formosa all the naval prisoners-of-war who were artificer ratings together with the engineer officers. This party numbered 265, and included the Surgeon Lieutenant of H.M.S. *Encounter*.

During the early days at Macassar, the prisoner-of-war camp contained 31 doctors, 4 of whom were British and the remainder Dutch. As has been described, hospital facilities inside the camp were virtually non-existent. However, the Dutch Hospital Ship *Op Ten Noort* was still in harbour locally and could receive emergency surgical cases. But the Japanese would only permit three types of medical disease to be discharged to the *Op Ten Noort*, viz. pneumonia, diphtheria and pulmonary tuberculosis.

In consequence of the transfer of the various working parties of prisoners-of-war from Macassar, the numbers remaining in the camp had been greatly reduced by the end of October 1942. In November, the Japanese Authorities instructed *Exeter's* Surgeon Commander that no more patients were to be sent to the *Op Ten Noort*. Instead, he was to establish inside the camp itself a small hospital, complete with operating theatre. Water supply, lighting arrangements, sterilisation, stores and equipment now presented themselves as problems to be solved. The *Op Ten Noort* was able to supply a certain amount of stores and equipment, but practically all the surgical instruments were manufactured inside the camp. It would seem too, that the Japanese

---

* *Exeter's* Surgeon Lieutenant states: 'In one case I had to excise the ulcer completely, and put the patient's leg up in plaster. On removing the plaster six weeks later, the ulcer had healed solidly, but unfortunately, owing to the shortage of plaster, it was impossible to repeat this treatment.'

Authorities themselves co-operated towards making this hospital something of a success.* Finally the hospital, though primitive and lacking such luxuries as an X-ray apparatus, was completed and able to perform a useful function. All patients from the *Op Ten Noort* were now transferred to the camp hospital, and the *Op Ten Noort* herself left for duty elsewhere.

By the end of 1942, there were five deaths among the British prisoners-of-war at Macassar, the causes being tuberculous peritonitis, cerebral malaria, bacillary dysentery and two cases of diphtheria.

On January 15, 1943, the remaining prisoners-of-war in Macassar Camp underwent inspection by a Japanese medical officer,† and the following morning, 26 naval officers, 3 merchant navy officers and 170 naval ratings were informed that they were fit for transfer from Macassar and were warned to be ready to leave the camp the same afternoon.

A Captain, Royal Marines, was the senior executive officer of this party of prisoners-of-war which included *Exeter's* Surgeon Commander and Surgeon Lieutenant, R.N.V.R. The Surgeon Commander tried to get permission to take some sick berth staff with the party, but with no success.

At 1500 hours on January 16, the party was marched to the local docks where, after a wait of two hours, they were taken on board a merchant ship and confined in her hold. This ship sailed at 1900 hours and arrived at Kendari, Celebes, N.E.I., the next evening.

After a march of four miles, these men arrived at a prisoner-of-war camp at Pamalaa.

This camp was situated alongside virgin jungle and surrounded by swamps. The camp itself consisted of four fairly large native huts and four smaller huts, all made of rattan and wood. Sleeping billets were wooden planks raised 18 in. off the ground which consisted of red, muddy soil. There was no trench of any description, and shallow trenches had to be dug for latrines. There were no cooking facilities, and cooking utensils had to be fashioned from old petrol and oil drums. The only water supply for all purposes was a single 1½ in. pipe outside the camp.

The Surgeon Commander commandeered one of the huts as a camp hospital. His small stock of medical supplies and equipment consisted of 1,000 tablets of quinine, 2 oz. of iodine, 3 oz. of potassium permanganate, 6 Dover's powders, 15 aspirin tablets, a small quantity of lint and

---

* *Exeter's* Surgeon Commander states: 'Our face fitted with the Japanese Petty Officer, and he helped us quite a lot.'

† *Exeter's* Surgeon Commander emphasises that visits by the Japanese Medical Authorities were almost unknown. He describes this particular medical inspection as being ludicrous. 'He sat on a chair, and while we paraded past him, he gesticulated with his hands or made noises like a pig. After about 200 had passed him, he got up and walked away. Never once did he make the slightest pretence at examining anyone, even though there were obviously some sick men among us. Five were suffering from severe tropical ulcers and two had inguinal hernias. I did my best to get these sick men released from this draft, but my effort was of no avail.'

1 lb. of cotton wool. The only surgical instruments were two artery forceps and two scalpels.*

To assist in the camp hospital, the Surgeon Commander recruited a petty officer† of H.M.S. *Encounter* and the bandmaster‡ of H.M.S. *Exeter*, both of whom possessed an excellent knowledge of first aid.

For the first fortnight prisoners-of-war worked to make the camp habitable. Trench latrines were deepened and attempts were made to render them fly-proof, but no matter what was done, the bottom of the latrines soon became a moving mass of maggots. Arrangements were made for all drinking water to be boiled, though this was difficult owing to lack of suitable receptacles. To attempt to augment the inadequate supply of fresh water, two wells were dug inside the camp, but the water proved to be foul and unfit even for washing. The wells soon acted as a breeding place for mosquitoes, so the Surgeon Commander ordered them to be filled in.

This camp was under Japanese civilian supervision, though with military guards. In consequence of this divided control it was possible for both civil and military authorities to disclaim responsibility for such matters as food and sanitary equipment. The result was that food supplies were always scanty, there was no protection from mosquitoes, no literature was permitted and letters were not allowed to be written or received. Soap was not supplied during the whole period of confinement in this camp.

To augment the meagre rations, and as a desperate measure to render these men fit to perform manual work, the Japanese did allow five buffaloes to be killed in the camp at intervals in the course of the next eight months. These carcasses were immediately cut up and boiled, and provided a meat supply for the whole camp for the next three or four days. The liver and heart were set aside for the sick who were also given soup made from the bones.

Following repeated medical representations, the Japanese did at last supply two large mosquito nets and three small single nets. The two large nets were used in the hospital hut, and were capable of protecting 17 patients apiece.

A fortnight after arriving at Pamalaa, these prisoners-of-war began to be employed as working parties outside the camp, and their task was to reclaim land and fill in mosquito swamps. This work was carried out

---

* One of these scalpels had been fashioned from the steel rib of a woman's corset!

† This petty officer was subsequently awarded the British Empire Medal for outstanding services while a prisoner-of-war. The citation states that: 'He cared for the sick with entire self-effacement. He was always unselfish and thorough, and was ready to attend anyone day or night. Even when his own health had declined and his eyesight had become so bad that he could only read the largest capitals, he insisted on continuing his job.'

‡ This man subsequently died at Macassar from malnutrition and beriberi.

each and every day from early in the morning until late at night, under a tropical sun with no protection by way of shade or clothing.

The end result was never in doubt and, after some two months, it became obvious to the Surgeon Commander that there was a generalised deterioration in health. Cases of malaria and dysentery increased daily, and symptoms and signs of malnutrition and deficiency diseases were apparent. Pellagra rashes of the feet and scrotum, ulceration of the mouth and lips and burning feet were very common. Corneal ulcers and amblyopia also made their appearance.

At this time the Surgeon Commander reported the adverse state of affairs to the Japanese military guard, and he also wrote to the Japanese Medical Authorities, pointing out the need for an increased vitamin content in the food supplied and the state of affairs regarding the scarcity of drugs with which to treat the sick.

By now there did not remain a single tablet of quinine, and the psychological effect of this alone was obvious among patients suffering from malaria. The Surgeon Commander records: 'At this time, everybody became quinine and vitamin conscious, and this complex made our job even more difficult. I did manage to collect some papaya leaves, which I made into an infusion which I found did have some diaphoretic action. To pacify my patients, I told them that this infusion was a native cure for malaria. Thereafter this medicine became known as "jungle juice". But unfortunately, the Japanese very soon refused to allow me to collect any more leaves, as the process was likely to kill their fruit trees.'

Describing the state of those suffering from malaria, the Surgeon Commander continues: 'It was a dreadful experience to see men having these malarial attacks, and not being able to do anything about it. The patient knew when the attack was starting, and would immediately take to his bed. By the time I saw him, he would be "bouncing the boards", and covered with all the available clothing which his friends could find for him.'

One lieutenant, R.N., had twenty-five relapses of malaria in about three months, and there were other similar cases. Naturally, with no form of treatment, there were fatalities, and here the Surgeon Commander has described the peculiar attitude of the Japanese Medical Authorities whenever death was imminent. 'When a man was dying, I used to send for a Japanese doctor, and he would send me 20 c.cm. of glucose, or would bring and give it himself. I tried to explain to him time and time again that this was only a very temporary measure, which could do little more than keep the man alive for another few hours. At such times I always made an appeal for better food for us, for more medicines, mosquito nets and clothing. But my appeals never seemed to make any impression.'

In May 1943 an acute surgical emergency arose in the camp when a rating from H.M.S. *Exeter* developed acute appendicitis. It was with some difficulty that the Surgeon Commander was able to persuade the Japanese Medical Authorities of the need for immediate surgical treatment. Finally they did remove the man by road to Kendari, where he was admitted to hospital and his appendix was removed under a local anaesthetic. Happily, he made a complete recovery.

After six months at Pamalaa, the health of the camp was becoming desperate. There had been six deaths, 144 men had malaria, 64 had amoebic dysentery and everyone showed signs of deficiency diseases. *Exeter's* Surgeon Commander and Surgeon Lieutenant, R.N.V.R., both had had several attacks of malaria and dysentery, and both were suffering from pellagra.

The Surgeon Commander again wrote to the Japanese Medical Authorities and he explained that, in his opinion, unless the food, medical supplies and living conditions were quickly improved, all the prisoners-of-war at Pamalaa would die within a few weeks. The Surgeon Commander suggested that the best procedure now would be to return the party to Macassar, or to some place where hospital facilities could be offered.

As a result of this appeal, a medical inspection of the camp was carried out by a Japanese Surgeon Commander and Surgeon Lieutenant. The Surgeon Lieutenant spoke a little English, and he explained that the best would be done to improve living conditions in the camp. After this visit conditions did improve, but for little more than a week, after which things became much as they had been before.

As the health of these prisoners-of-war deteriorated, they became less capable of conducting with efficiency the internal organisation of the camp at Pamalaa. They were, in fact, too weak and ill to keep either themselves or their surroundings properly clean. Rats now became an added menace, and the camp was overrun with them. The Surgeon Commander records that: 'If you left your rice unattended for a minute the rats would start helping themselves. Septic dressings were actually eaten off two men in the hospital hut while they were asleep.'

After five more deaths had occurred, the Surgeon Commander appealed in writing yet again to the Japanese Authorities, explaining that conditions had now reached a stage inside the camp when men were unable to do any more work and there was no doubt that all would soon be beyond any human aid.

The only relief from monotony around this time was an air attack on Pamalaa by 9 U.S. Liberators, on August 25, 1943. A few stray machine-gun bullets came into the camp, but there were no casualties among the prisoners-of-war.

Finally, on September 15, 1943, this party of naval prisoners-of-war was transferred from Pamalaa back to Macassar.

The report of *Exeter's* Surgeon Commander states: 'Our departure from Pamalaa was a terrible sight for anyone to witness. Thirteen dangerously ill men were carried the four miles to the jetty on improvised bamboo stretchers. Some were taken by lorry. I myself managed the journey on foot, but my Surgeon Lieutenant, R.N.V.R., was a very sick man and had to be carried. But on the way the Japanese guards were very decent to us, and they gave us many rest periods'.

The party was embarked in a Japanese merchant ship, and the Surgeon Commander was now allowed to keep those very sick on the hatches of the upper deck, while the remainder were confined below in the holds which they shared with a cargo of nickel ore.

Immediately on its return to Macassar, this party of prisoners-of-war from Pamalaa was isolated and regarded by the Japanese as a sick unit. Special food and medical attention were now provided, and the Surgeon Commander was able to assess the medical state of these men after their eight months of hardship.

Sixteen men had died at Pamalaa. Thirteen were dangerously ill. Seventy-five were unable to walk. All suffered from malaria, dysentery and deficiency diseases.*

The medical observations of the Surgeon Commander are of great interest. The average loss of weight among these men was three stone. The Surgeon Commander's own weight was reduced from 10 st. 4 lb. to 7 st. 4 lb. while at Pamalaa.

The chief signs and symptoms of deficiency diseases were ophthalmic in nature, and included retrobulbar neuritis, keratitis, amblyopia and corneal ulcers.†

On the other hand, the Surgeon Commander remarks on the remarkable absence of skin diseases among the party from Pamalaa, apart from sunburn and pellagra rashes. He also emphasises the fact that although infected wounds of the feet had to be dealt with from time to time, there were no cases of epidermophytosis.‡ He considers this low incidence the more remarkable in the absence of soap for a period of eight months, and also the scanty facilities for washing in fresh water. In an attempt

---

* A further 40 of these prisoners-of-war from Pamalaa failed to recover, and died during the subsequent months.

† An ophthalmic specialist's report on these men, after the war, stated that practically all showed some degree of defective vision, with abnormalities which included loss of muscle balance, and optic atrophy of a patchy type affecting the central and temporal regions of the discs.

The Surgeon Commander states: 'During the last two weeks at Pamalaa, I could not see the markings on playing cards.'

‡ It is of interest to study this low incidence of skin diseases among these men undergoing hardship, in relation to a statistical survey of skin diseases among naval personnel under normal conditions of service on tropical stations.

In the year 1914, on the East Indies Station, out of a total complement of 3,060, the ratio of cases of skin diseases was 125·16 per 1,000, with an invaliding rate of 0·65 per 1,000.

For the five years 1926–1930, on the East Indies Station, where the average complement was 2,420, the average ratio per 1,000 per annum was 92·11 with an invaliding rate of 1·23 per 1,000. On the China Station for the same period, where the average complement per annum was 7,950, the average annual incidence was 58·85 per 1,000 with an invaliding rate of ·49.

to explain this absence of skin infections he suggests that scanty clothing and the wearing of clogs may have played a part, and the probability that, under normal circumstances, skin lesions suffer from over treatment.*

Meanwhile, during the absence of *Exeter's* Surgeon Commander and Surgeon Lieutenant, R.N.V.R., at Pamalaa, her Surgeon Lieutenant, R.N. had remained in the camp at Macassar. His report of the period describes an increase in the number of surgical conditions which had to be dealt with at Macassar, including the amputation of the leg of a naval rating for sarcoma.† He also mentions the great number of cases of appendicitis, which he attributes to changes in diet and the large increase in the carbohydrate intake. He remarks too, on the improvement in morale which was brought about by the appearance of the first Allied bomber, on January 17, 1943. In the following months Allied air attacks became more frequent, and they were welcomed by the prisoners-of-war at Macassar, despite the discomfort of having to spend many nights in slit trenches during July and August 1943.

On October 2, 1943 an officers' draft was transferred from Macassar to Batavia, Java, N.E.I. The party numbered 350, of whom all were Dutch with the exception of 26 British Naval officers, 2 British Merchant Navy officers, 5 American and 1 Australian Air Force officer. The party included all three medical officers from H.M.S. *Exeter*.‡

During the period 1931–1935, on the China Station, with an average complement of 8,190, the average annual ratio of skin diseases was 44·67 per 1,000 with an invaliding rate of ·73. For the same period, the East Indies Station, with an average complement of 3,260, showed an average annual ratio of skin diseases of 80·03 per 1,000 with an invaliding rate of ·61.

N.B.—During the year 1942, based on a total naval complement of 516,000, the ratio of skin diseases in the whole of the Navy was 35·6 per 1,000 with an invaliding rate of 0·31.

* The reader is referred to the remarks on skin diseases and tropical clothing in Volume I, Chapter 12.

† This man died a few days later.

‡ There was now no naval medical officer left at Macassar, but Admiralty records show that naval prisoners-of-war there continued to be treated by a leading sick berth attendant aided by a naval petty officer. This petty officer was subsequently mentioned in dispatches for his outstanding conduct as a prisoner-of-war. On his release, he described the work carried out by the L.S.B.A., and stated that on one occasion he assisted him to remove the appendix of a Dutch prisoner-of-war. He was able to describe this operation in detail and the subsequent recovery of the patient. He stated that the only instruments available were 'a small surgeon's knife, a pair of forceps, and a needle which bent when we tried to temper it in a fire in our hut. We also tried, unsuccessfully, to improvise skin clips from a piece of chromium wire'.

The petty officer was not able to give the name of the L.S.B.A., as he had only known him by a nickname, but he understood that he was the son of a doctor. Lengthy enquiries were made after the war with a view to establishing the identity of this L.S.B.A. who had never made any reports himself. However, according to Admiralty records no L.S.B.A. was ever identified with the particular medical events described, though a leading sick berth attendant, from H.M.S. *Encounter*, was subsequently mentioned in dispatches 'for efficiency and devotion to duty while tending the sick under difficult conditions'. But it would seem that this latter citation referred to medical care of a detached party of prisoners-of-war who had been transferred from Macassar to work on the airfield some miles distant.

The sea journey to Java was made in a well equipped Japanese troopship in which accommodation was fair though ventilation and overcrowding made conditions difficult to endure.

On arrival at Batavia, the party was marched ten miles to a prisoner-of-war camp known as the 10th Infantry Barracks or 'Cycle Camp'. This camp was under Army administration, and rigid discipline was ruthlessly enforced by a Japanese lieutenant.* As an initiation into the routine of this camp the party of prisoners-of-war was paraded before this lieutenant on arrival, and a number of officers was struck about the face and kicked on the shins for not standing to attention properly. The doctors and medical personnel in the party came in for special scrutiny and interrogation. Those who were wearing Red Cross arm bands had them torn off, and eight members were put into solitary confinement at once because their hair was too long.†

Exeter's Surgeon Commander was now asked to produce his diploma to prove that he was a proper doctor. When he was unable to do so, he was promptly accused of being an impostor, and was beaten on the head and face and kicked on the shins by way of punishment.‡

It was a few weeks before the medical officers were recognised as such by the Japanese, and even then all the doctors were not employed on medical duties, but only a number considered sufficient by the Japanese Authorities to maintain efficiently the medical organisation of the camp.§

Exeter's Surgeon Commander has described this medical organisation as excellent‖ and the supply of drugs and food and the camp sanitation as adequate. During the twelve months which he spent in this camp he found the general health of personnel fairly good considering the conditions. Bacillary and amoebic dysentery were always endemic, and evidence of malnutrition was seen from time to time. But there were comparatively few cases of malaria, and all prisoners-of-war were equipped with a mosquito net, protective clothing and with boots or shoes. There was never any great shortage of food¶

There were no deaths among the naval personnel in this camp.

---

* Lieutenant Sonie.

† *Exeter's* Surgeon Lieutenant, R.N.V.R., was one of these.

‡ The Japanese Authorities later gave as their reason for this attitude the fact that in some areas, red crosses had been worn by such a large number of Allied prisoners-of-war as to arouse suspicion, and on investigation the Japanese claimed to have shown that only 30 per cent. of the alleged medical personnel were truly entitled to that status.

§ There was probably something to be said for this ruling of the Japanese Authorities, as records show that at this time there were no less than 12 British and 260 Dutch doctors in 'Cycle Camp'.

‖ The medical organisation was under the direction of a medical officer of the Indian Medical Service.

¶ The Surgeon Commander regarded this camp as 'a pleasure resort after Pamalaa and Macassar'.

From the twelve months October 1943 to October 1944, 'Cycle Camp' at Batavia became virtually a central prisoner-of-war pool from which these British naval officers were transferred elsewhere as necessity arose. Five drafts left Batavia during this period, carrying men for labour in Japan, Sumatra, Singapore, Siam and Burma. Not all these drafts reached their destination in safety, and three are alleged to have involved loss of life at sea by the sinking of Japanese transports by Allied submarines.*

One feature of this drafting system from Batavia which was regretted by the three medical officers of H.M.S. *Exeter* was that they soon became separated from each other and were never again reunited during the remainder of the war.†

Exeter's Surgeon Lieutenant, R.N., has given an outline of the 'building up' system which was instituted by the Japanese Authorities at Batavia in order to render men fit for hard manual work when their time came to be transferred elsewhere. Early in 1944 a 'fitness test' was introduced for all prisoners-of-war. This consisted of running 100 metres in under 17 seconds. The next feat to be attempted was that of carrying a 40-kg. sack of sand 50 metres in 12 seconds. The Surgeon Lieutenant says that nearly all the prisoners accomplished these exercises successfully but, regarding the feat of carrying the load of sand a distance of 50 metres in 12 seconds, he states: 'I did this myself in $9\frac{1}{2}$ seconds, so it cannot have been very difficult.'

In the middle of April 1944 the Surgeon Lieutenant was included in a party of 2,000 prisoners-of-war who were selected to leave Batavia as a working party in due course. This draft consisted of 300 British officers and men from the various Services, while the remainder were all Dutch.

For the next six weeks this party was placed on double rations and given a course of physical training in order to prepare them for the hard manual labour which they were warned lay ahead.

On May 24, they embarked in a 4,000-ton Japanese merchant ship and, after five days, arrived at Emmerhaven, the harbour of Padang, Sumatra. Their voyage was spent down in the holds of the ship in intolerable heat.

At Padang, these 2,000 prisoners-of-war spent their first day in the local gaol, which they shared with some 5,000 coolies already billeted

---

* Figures of these losses are only approximate and have been difficult to obtain. *Exeter's* Surgeon Commander states that in one Japanese transport which was sunk after leaving Batavia, there were only 34 survivors out of 1,000 prisoners-of-war on board. Those lost are alleged to have included some 40 medical officers of whom 6 were British. The latter are believed to have been 2 Army, 3 R.A.F. and 1 R.N.V.R. doctors.

† *Exeter's* Surgeon Lieutenant, R.N.V.R., was lost at sea in a Japanese transport which was torpedoed off Japan by an Allied submarine on January 25, 1944. This officer was subsequently mentioned in dispatches posthumously for his outstanding conduct while a prisoner-of-war.

there, and large numbers of whom appeared to be suffering from dysentery with no chance of receiving any attention or treatment.*

During the following night, a party of 500 prisoners-of-war, including all the British, were moved by train to Piaja Comdo, and then from Piaja Comdo in lorries they were carried 120 miles to Pakan Baroe. Their journey ended with a march of half a mile to their new camp.

This camp consisted of a number of rattan huts, each 40 yd. long by 5 yd. wide; 100 men were accommodated in each hut, with boards on which to sleep. The previous occupants of this camp had been coolies, and it was overgrown by lalang grass and soiled by piles of refuse left by the former tenants.

Three days' grace were granted in which to clear up the camp, dig latrines and improvise a water supply. Drains also had to be dug on account of the large areas of stagnant, surface water in the camp. During these three days, the Japanese food supplies broke down, and these prisoners-of-war were only given a small amount of rice and salt.

On the fourth day work began on railway construction. The prisoners-of-war were divided into groups for carrying sleepers and metal rails, while 100 were employed on knocking in spikes. Two men were required to carry one sleeper and fourteen for a length of rail. The quota of work for a day was set at 1,500 metres of track, and at the beginning the party found it possible to complete this quota by 1500 hours each day. The food supplied was dried fish with miscellaneous green leaves as vegetables. The doctor was permanently on duty on the track during working hours, but his medical supplies were almost non-existent.

At the end of the first week, this party marched 4 kilometres to another camp further inland. This new camp was the headquarters of all the prisoners-of-war employed upon railway construction. Here a large hut had already been converted into a camp hospital.

Working parties set off each morning to the railway track, and the work became harder as the Japanese Authorities increased its pace. The work was largely manual and unskilled, and was carried out during the heat of the day, neither were any labour-saving devices available which might have eased the burden of manual labour. The method of working which the Japanese employed was at all times crude in the extreme.†

In order to maintain the quota of daily work, the Japanese themselves had instituted a dietary which they intended should consist of rice 400 g., crude tapioca flour 200 g., tapioca leaves 300 g., oil 25 g., and meat or fish 50 g., together with a little salt, pepper and sugar.

---

* The Surgeon Lieutenant has recorded that to his knowledge at least sixteen of these coolies died during that particular day.

† For example, trucks loaded with a ton of sand had to be pushed a distance of 2 km. But at no time was grease or oil available for lubricating the axles of these trucks.

The Surgeon Lieutenant considered that the quota of work could have been met with ease and would have been consistent with reasonable health had this standard of diet been maintained, but quite apart from their usual casual attitude in such matters, the Japanese Authorities soon found themselves faced with the problem of supply and transport difficulties. Food supplies had to be carried over crude roads a distance of some 100 km., and rations were issued to the prisoners-of-war twice weekly. But this road service was badly administered, and these difficulties of supply became progressively worse as more and more railway track was laid and as the prison camp was gradually moved further and further away from the supply base.

The result was that the rations were subject to shortages of about 10 per cent. from the very start, and within a few weeks were 30 per cent. below the amount which had been anticipated. These figures refer to the overall shortages in the bulk rations, but the reduction in some individual items of food was even more severe. For example, of the proposed weekly ration per head of 350 g. of meat or fish, the maximum ever supplied was 150 g.

As was to be expected, and as was so customary in all Japanese undertakings which visualised the employment of prisoners-of-war on manual labour, the inevitable ravages of ill-health soon appeared. Once they had appeared, they multiplied daily because medical supplies were so short and so little could be done for the sick. From the beginning, malaria and dysentery became endemic and gradually increased to epidemic proportions to such an extent that even nursing became impossible to maintain.

Describing this period, he writes: 'The hospital beggared description. There were about 150 patients lying on their mats on the planks and very close together, each man occupying about 60 cm. The dysentery patients were at one end, none of them had been washed, and there was one bed pan and one urinal. One of the patients had pneumonia.

'I managed to get some volunteers, to carry water, after they had returned from their day's work. I had a small amount of sulphaguanidine, but as I had to give it in small doses it was not very effective. The pneumonia patient soon died as he was unable to eat the food obtainable, and in any case, I had so very little sulphapyridine.

'The number of dysentery cases steadily increased. The only food I could give them was rice porridge, with chopped meat when it was obtainable. On this diet, coupled with almost continuous motions, they literally just starved to death, and soon we were having at least three deaths a week.'

Soon the Surgeon Lieutenant had to compete with yet another burden in the form of diphtheria cases, one of whom died of cardiac failure. Of another of these cases he writes: 'As I had no antitoxin, I kept him strictly at rest and gave him sulphapyridine 1 gm. four hourly for three doses. He recovered, but for a long time he had a paralysed palate, and he was still very weak one year later.'

In August 1944 more prisoners were brought from Singapore and elsewhere to Sumatra, and the activities of Allied submarines inadvertently led to the deaths of many at sea.*

This influx of large numbers of prisoners-of-war for work on the railway meant that other camps quickly began to spring up, and eventually the headquarter camp was turned into a prisoner-of-war hospital for the area, consistently with the increase in the incidence of sickness. The shortage of medical supplies continued, there was no emetine to be obtained, and the relapse rate for malaria was 100 per cent. with intervals of ten to thirty days.

Deficiency diseases were by now on the increase, with pellagra predominating.

Operation was successfully performed upon one British officer for a perforated gastric ulcer, and he made a good recovery. In due course, the Surgeon Lieutenant was transferred from this hospital to one of the advanced working camps in which there were 300 British and 400 Dutch prisoners-of-war. Here he found his ingenuity taxed to the utmost in order to try and provide some form of treatment for the illnesses which were suffered by everybody. This camp was in the heart of the jungle and there was the usual shortage of food added to the generalised infection with malaria, dysentery and unhealed septic wounds. Many men were suffering from ascariasis which could not be treated, and relapsing fever now made its appearance. Cases suffering from the latter disease invariably refused to eat even what there was, and this meant that many of them died literally of starvation.

As regards the treatment of wounds, material for dressings was very difficult to obtain and the Surgeon Lieutenant even went to the length of cutting up some of his own clothes. All the used dressings were washed and boiled and used again.†

In December 1944, after the prisoners-of-war of this camp had laid another 25 kilometres of railway track, they were moved on to yet another camp further on. The pressure of work was now greatly increased, and the Japanese insisted that instead of the usual 1,500 metres a day, $2\frac{1}{4}$ kilometres of railway should be constructed each day, including the levelling of the track bed. This meant that the men would go out at daybreak and would return late at night. This work was carried out during the rainy season, and the Surgeon Lieutenant used to light fires in the

---

* One ship carrying prisoners-of-war was lost, about this time, with 60 per cent. of her prisoners including one sub-lieutenant, Royal Canadian Naval Reserve. Another Japanese transport was lost in the Malacca Straits with 1 officer and 24 Royal Naval ratings on board.

† The only ointment available was red palm oil. Fortunately there were rubber trees in the vicinity of these camps, and one device was to dress wounds with small squares of bandage stuck on to the skin with raw latex.

huts between the bed boards in order to give the men a chance to get warm and dry before setting off into the jungle again.

The sickness rate was now enormous and, no matter what his disease, every man was forced to carry on working as long as he could manage to crawl from his bed.

This monotonous procedure continued until the end of June 1945, when the Japanese announced that, come what may, the railway must be finished within a month. A period of literal slave-driving followed, and as the track was now being laid through a narrow channel in rising ground, some hundreds of prisoners-of-war were kept at work in a confined space with the Japanese guards beating them with sticks most of the time. Food was almost forgotten by the Japanese at this time and everything was sacrificed in the interest of speed of construction. Naturally, the sickness and death rate now increased and burials are recorded at approximately ten per day in this region.

On the final stage of this drive, these men were forced to work for three days and the two intervening nights without any rest at all except for brief spells for what scanty food there was. Finally, the railway was completed on August 17, 1945.*

Immediately, the war with Japan now being over, the Japanese Authorities trebled the rations of these prisoners-of-war. Medical supplies were increased, and stores and equipment were also dropped by Allied aircraft. But the work of the Surgeon Lieutenant was by no means finished for, all too tragically, in so many cases the outside aid had arrived too late and many patients were beyond assistance. The Surgeon Lieutenant writes: 'On August 27 I moved all the British down the line to the headquarter hospital and began treating them in the hope that some might recover. But they were still dying at the rate of two a day.'†

After the departure of his two surgeon lieutenants, *Exeter's* Surgeon Commander had remained at 'Cycle Camp' in Batavia. Between October 1944 and the end of the war with Japan the Surgeon Commander had moved to two other prisoner-of-war camps in Java for varying periods. On August 21, 1945 he was transferred back to Batavia, and his period of captivity ended with the arrival there of H.M.S. *Cumberland*.

As in the case of the Medical Officer of H.M.S. *Gloucester* while a prisoner-of-war in German hands, so has the Surgeon Commander of H.M.S. *Exeter* included in his report a number of shrewd medical observations on the conduct and mentality of his captors, the Japanese.

---

* Hostilities with Japan had ended two days before.

† The Surgeon Lieutenant records the case of one American prisoner-of-war, suffering from deficiency disease, who complained of anuria and massive generalised œdema. Several gallons of fluid were tapped from his scrotum but with no improvement, and he died within a few days.

Speaking of the Japanese medical services he describes them as non-existent in a European sense. The few alleged Japanese medical officers who he did meet on rare occasions neither acted nor behaved as doctors. The Japanese guards themselves seemed to recognise the limitation of their own medical officers, because they would sometimes visit the doctors among the prisoners-of-war in secret, seeking treatment for their own ailments, and bringing with them stolen medical supplies in payment. In particular, any Japanese guard suffering from venereal disease would always seek treatment from one of the prisoners-of-war doctors, bringing with him his own syringe and supply of N.A.B., bismuth, etc.*

It proved impossible ever to explain to a Japanese doctor that a man with an internal complaint, unless it was tuberculosis or appendicitis, was unfit for manual labour. Cardiac disease was apparently unrecognised, and visual evidence of a complaint seemed to be the criterion which was accepted. It was often necessary to bandage the leg of a man with cardiac disease in order to save him from having to work!

Preventive medicine was a subject which the Japanese Medical Authorities ignored, certainly in relation to prisoners-of-war. After the death of one prisoner-of-war from anthrax, the Japanese obtained anti-anthrax serum for pigs and horses in the neighbourhood, but none for future use by prisoners-of-war should the need arise. A further precaution in relation to animal life, which brought Japanese doctors locally into ridicule, was a refusal to permit prisoners-of-war to build latrines over the sea. The reason given was that the fish might become infected with dysentery.

In each of these examples it must be observed that the precautions of the Japanese, on their own admission, were aimed at protection of animals themselves, not the protection of persons who might eat them subsequently.

Of psychological interest are the following examples of the Japanese mental attitude to which the prisoners-of-war had to adapt themselves:

(1) A local inhabitant, not a prisoner-of-war, stole some articles from a prisoner-of-war. The Japanese guards punished him by beating him until he was insensible. They then tied him to some railings and set fire to the hair on the various parts of his body. He was then left for the night. In the morning the guards asked for iodine, which the surgeon commander imagined was to be used upon the man's wounds. But instead, the iodine solution was poured up his nose, after which he was sentenced to solitary confinement for one month.

---

* It is possible that lack of faith in their own medical officers was not the only reason for seeking the medical assistance of a prisoner-of-war doctor. To fall sick might mean serious 'loss of face', and venereal disease in a Japanese soldier might well be regarded as a disciplinary offence by his own authorities.

(2) Seeds sown in camp gardens were recommended to have the sprouted tips pointing towards Tokyo, in order to ensure good results!*

Space does not permit more than the transient survey which has been extracted from these naval medical officers who endured three years and seven months of hardship after the Battle of the Java Seas. It is possible that their reports in the hands of the Admiralty reveal their personal courage more by what they have left unsaid than by the words which they have actually written. But as an example to posterity, it is necessary to record in this History the words with which the Surgeon Commander of H.M.S. *Exeter* concluded his final report of his experiences:

'Nothing has impressed me more than the wonderful adaptability, cheerfulness and indefatigable spirit of the British sailor in adversity. We all regret that we were unable to assist the national effort during our time as prisoners-of-war. But I would like to state on behalf of all of us that we are now once again ready for service.'

ESCAPE FROM SINGAPORE†

THE ESCAPE

The chief object of the military defence of Malaya and Singapore Island against the Japanese was the protection of the Singapore Naval Base. So long as it was certain that a strong and balanced British Fleet could, when required, be despatched to the Far East and that it would be able on arrival there to control the sea communications leading to Malaya, the task of the local defence was to ensure the safety of the Naval Base, but for a limited period only.

The loss of H.M. Ships *Prince of Wales* and *Repulse* meant loss of this control of sea communications. The subsequent inability to muster a strong British Fleet in the Far East meant that the Japanese could, without incurring undue risk, establish bases in North Malaya and in South Thailand from which operations by land, sea and air could be developed.

On January 5, 1942, the Commander-in-Chief, Eastern Fleet, moved his headquarters from Singapore to Batavia.

There were two reasons for this move. In the first place, close co-

---

* One Royal Naval officer from the same prisoner-of-war camp reports that a sow which escaped from its sty was given corporal punishment and put on three day's low diet 'for disobeying Japanese orders'. Also, a monkey which made rude gestures at the Japanese Commandant had its swing taken away!

† To gain acquaintance with the background and events which led up to the evacuation of naval personnel from Singapore in February 1942, the reader is referred to the section which concerns Medical Organisation, Singapore Naval Base, in Volume I, Chapter 15.

Reference should also be made to the Second Supplement to the *London Gazette*, No. 38215, of February 20, 1948 (Operations of Malaya Command, from December 8, 1941, to February 15, 1942).

operation with the American and Dutch Commanders could only be achieved at Batavia, and was necessary to ensure the safe and timely arrival of troop convoys at Singapore. Secondly, by this date, it had become apparent that Singapore would shortly be exposed to heavy air attack, and, therefore, would be of little value in the immediate future as a base for heavy surface ships.

The Rear Admiral, Malaya, now became Senior Naval Officer at Singapore, and assumed responsibility for the whole of the local naval defence of Malaya.

By January 15, 1942, the local situation had deteriorated following rapid withdrawals from North and Central Malaya. The need for increased hospital accommodation now began to make itself felt, and sick and wounded not likely soon to be fit for duty were evacuated to the United Kingdom and India, accompanied by a certain number of medical and nursing personnel. To augment troopship services for this purpose, with the help of the Naval Authorities, a Yangtze river boat had been obtained and re-designed as a hospital ship.* She was not considered capable of making an ocean voyage, though later on she did so.

By January 30, 1942, it was known that it was not intended to send any additional naval forces to Malayan waters. It was also known that a small British Fleet was assembling in Ceylon for operations in the eastern waters of the Indian Ocean, and that a strong American Fleet was assembling in the South Pacific. Some British, Australian and American ships were concentrating with the Dutch Fleet for the defence of Java, which was already being threatened by a Japanese thrust south of Borneo.†

The Navy was, however, able to give some military assistance through detachments of Royal Marine survivors from H.M.Ss. *Prince of Wales* and *Repulse* who had joined up with the Argyll and Sutherland Highlanders.

By this date, too, practically all ships returning to destinations within the British Empire had carried their complement of women and children in accordance with the policy of evacuation, and comparatively few women and children remained on Singapore Island.‡ (Plates X and XI illustrate the evacuation of civilians from Singapore.)

By January 31, Singapore Naval Base was under observed artillery and small arms fire and within close range of enemy aircraft. It was therefore obvious that the base could no longer be protected. It was also obvious that Singapore Naval Base had now ceased to be of use.

---

* The *Wu Sueh*, 3,400 tons.
† This is the force which was defeated in the Battle of the Java Seas.
‡ *London Gazette* No. 38215, Section XLIII, para. 417. Some 300 European women were eventually interned in Singapore. The majority of these had remained to perform important war work.

Accommodation for all hospitals withdrawn from the mainland had by now been found in the Singapore town area, where there was naturally much congestion. The Alexandra Military Hospital remained the main hospital for British troops, as did the Tyersall Park Hospital for Indian troops. The Australian Base Hospital, evacuated from Malacca, was accommodated in a school on the northern outskirts of Singapore town. Temporary Service Hospitals were formed in St. Patrick's School, in the Secretariat, the Municipal Offices, the Singapore Club and the Cricket Club. There was an ample reserve of medical stores at Tanglin. At the Naval Base, there were also large quantities of stores of all descriptions including medical stores.

With the Naval Base no longer tenable, the existing Naval Medical Organisation in Singapore rapidly dissolved; and as soon as the inevitable capitulation became obvious, the policy of the Navy was to evacuate its key personnel. In any event, the Naval Medical Organisation was essentially subsidiary to the far greater Military Medical Organisation, and though the services of the few naval medical officers and sick berth staff were offered to the Army at this time, there was no doubt that the need for their presence in Singapore had ceased to exist. It seemed better that these personnel should be evacuated and utilised first in caring for sick and wounded evacuees at sea and later in building up a fresh Naval Medical Organisation elsewhere rather than that they should be wasted unnecessarily in useless captivity for the remainder of the war.

The British Forces in Singapore finally surrendered to the Japanese at 2030 hours on February 15, 1942. But already, on the morning of February 13, the Rear Admiral, Malaya, had decided to sail all the remaining ships and sea-going craft to Java during the night February 13–14 and to sail with them himself. There was accommodation in these small craft for about 3,000 persons in all, in addition to their crews. This was the last opportunity that could be foreseen for any organised parties to leave Singapore. The Rear Admiral, Malaya, called an Inter-Services Meeting at which passages were divided between the Services and the Civil Government.

The merits of personnel regarded as best entitled to these passages were carefully considered, and among others, it was decided that room should be found for all female members of the Military Nursing Services as well as trained staff officers and technicians no longer required in Singapore.

As planned, this flotilla of small ships left Singapore on the night of February 13–14. It was attacked by Japanese naval craft and aircraft. Many of its ships were sunk or disabled and there was considerable loss of life. Others were wounded and many were forced ashore and subsequently captured.*

---

* *London Gazette* No. 38215, Section LIV, para. 560. The flotilla included a patrol boat in which were the Rear Admiral, Malaya, and his party and the Air Officer Commanding, Far East. Both these officers lost their lives a few weeks later.

One Motor Launch (M.L.) became separated from the rest of this flotilla; in fact it would probably be untrue to claim that it ever joined the flotilla at all. Owing to early damage, the M.L. was delayed, and it finally left upon what proved to be virtually a solitary voyage.

On board the M.L. were 9 officers and 35 men. The majority belonged to the Royal Navy. Their experiences are here set down in some detail, for the reason, which at first seems paradoxical, that no medical personnel or nursing staff were actually involved. During the subsequent hardships which were endured, the impact of injuries and tropical disease was so severe that it is considered of the greatest importance to emphasise for the future, how vitally necessary it is that isolated parties should always contrive to include at least one member with medical experience and training. As will be seen, the inclusion on board this M.L. of even a junior sick berth rating with only the most elementary medical knowledge might yet have averted some of the tragic events which followed.*

The naval decision to leave Singapore was finally completed at 1400 hours on February 13, 1942, and a lieutenant, R.N. was instructed to make the necessary arrangements.

This lieutenant made his way to the docks with some difficulty, because Singapore itself was already showing an appearance verging on defeat. Heavy Japanese bombing had caused fires, the smoke of which mingled with that from burning oil installations on the Island. The town was covered with a black pall of smoke, water from burst mains flooded the streets and air attacks and gunfire were continuous.

The lieutenant arrived at the Telok Ayer Wharf which presented a busy scene, with the evacuation of civilians still proceeding and parties being ferried out to small ships in the harbour. The area was surrounded with anti-aircraft batteries the guns of which gave warning of the repeated Japanese air attacks on the docks. Each attack resulted in more casualties and wreckage on the dockside.†

By sunset, the arrangements made by this lieutenant were completed and the small craft began to approach the shore. By 1900 hours all the vessels were alongside the wharf, and a steady flow of personnel commenced embarking on this last organised sea evacuation.

At 2100 hours the embarkation was hastened following a strong rumour of a further Japanese advance, and all the craft were instructed to leave as soon as possible and to steer a course which would take them reasonably well clear of the area of probable air attack by the next morning.

---

* The medical aspects of this voyage have been based upon the factual account recorded by a lieutenant commander, R.N., who subsequently survived captivity in the hands of the Japanese.

† A naval observer makes special mention of a number of Australian nursing sisters who were among the hundreds waiting at the dockside. He states that after each air attack they attended to casualties and he pays tribute to 'the bearing and courage of these ladies'.

The last party to leave embarked in M.L.310, commanded by a lieutenant, R.N.Z.V.R.*

M.L.310 cast off at 2300 hours on Friday, February 13,† and slowly proceeded astern into the darkness of Singapore Harbour. She carried a crew of 2 officers and 14 ratings with a Chinese cook in addition.‡ Her passengers consisted of 4 Naval officers, 2 R.A.F. officers, 1 Army officer, 5 naval ratings, 6 Royal Marines, 8 Army and 2 R.A.F. other ranks.

Once clear of the jetty, the M.L. headed out through the breakwater,§ and then she increased speed down the swept channel.‖ Navigation was proving most difficult as navigational marks and buoys were shrouded in dense smoke from the burning oil installations. It was at this moment that M.L.310 suffered her first misfortune, for her steering gear suddenly broke down. By the time her engines had been stopped, the M.L. had been swept off her course. Within a few minutes, the auxiliary steering gear was working and the M.L. was once more under control. But she was now uncertain of her true position and, five minutes later, the M.L's. progress was checked by a series of jolts, and all on board realised that she was aground.

As the M.L. came to a stop she quickly took on an ever increasing list, and this list persisted in spite of throwing overboard a large amount of luggage and heavy equipment in order to 'lighten ship'. From the chart it seemed probable that the M.L. was aground on the edge of an island near the swept channel.¶ The tide was ebbing, so that there was obviously little chance to refloat the craft before daybreak when the tide would start to rise again.

The immediate anxiety of the M.L's. Commanding Officer was to ascertain whether the engines had been damaged by the grounding, and in particular, whether the propellers and their shafts had remained unscathed, so a lieutenant, R.N. tied a rope round his waist and went overboard in order to ascertain by touch the state of the craft. This officer found himself gripped by the strong tide, so the M.L's. small dinghy was now lowered to help him maintain his position. He was then

---

* The lieutenant R.N. responsible for the arrangements himself took passage in M.L.310. He has recorded that his last acts before embarking were to push his motor car off the jetty into the harbour, and to recover the White Ensign from the deserted, old ship H.M.S. *Laburnum*, headquarters of the Straits Settlement R.N.V.R.

† A lieutenant commander, R.N., later wrote: 'It was still Friday the 13th, and I afterwards wondered whether or not our luck would have been different had we stayed until the first minutes of the next day!'

‡ This Chinese cook has not been included in the official figure of the total personnel on board.

§ At this point M.L.310 was signalled by a minesweeper which had gone aground with a large number of troops on board. Unfortunately it was impossible for the M.L. to render assistance.

‖ Phillip's Channel.

¶ St. George's Island.

able to grope about beneath the M.L. and he found that she was undamaged and should have no difficulty in refloating on a rising tide.

The first medical incident now occurred. In trying to clamber back aboard the M.L., the lieutenant unfortunately slipped and crushed the fingers of one hand between the gunwale of the dinghy and the M.L. The bleeding was severe and he fainted on the tilting deck of the M.L. Rudimentary first aid was applied by those on board, but the officer's subsequent progress suggests that this first aid was not very effective.

At daybreak on February 14, the tide began to rise and the list of the M.L. gradually decreased. Singapore itself appeared quiet and no sound emerged from the haze of smoke overhanging the city.

At 0730 hours, in broad daylight, M.L.310 was able to refloat into the deeper water of the swept channel. Heading down the Channel at full speed, she altered course at 0800 hours into the Durian Straits in an attempt to overhaul the remainder of the flotilla of small ships. But a few minutes later an enemy reconnaissance aircraft appeared, which was likely to be the forerunner of heavy air attacks on the large number of small ships which was now passing south towards the Netherlands East Indies. In view of this probability, it was considered safer to steam the M.L. only by night and to seek shelter by day. At 1000 hours this decision was wisely put into practice, and the M.L. was steered into the cover of the Islands of the Bulang Archipelago.

The cover selected was a small bay, with a palm fringed shore occupied by a Chinese fishing village. The anchor was dropped close to the shore, and camouflage nets were at once hoisted over the M.L. Within a few minutes two large formations of enemy bombers flew overhead towards the south.*

The M.L. remained in shelter until the late afternoon, and during the day the hand of the injured officer was re-dressed with some difficulty. At 1700 hours it was judged a reasonable risk to continue passage again, so the M.L. once more steered south and made good speed during an uneventful night.

Daybreak on February 15 found M.L.310 in an open stretch of sea towards the northern end of the Banka Straits. Course was altered towards the Island of Katjangan where cover for the day was found in a tiny bay in which deep water ran close in to overhanging vegetation from the shore and which made camouflage nets almost unnecessary.

The forenoon passed uneventfully, but the damaged hand of the injured lieutenant now began to play its part in the misfortunes of the party.

By midday the officer's injured hand and arm had begun to swell, the pain was severe and he was becoming febrile. It was obvious to his

---

* These would appear to be the aircraft which carried out the attack described in *London Gazette* No. 38215, Section LIV, para. 560.

companions that somehow, skilled medical attention must be sought. With this in view therefore the senior officer decided that instead of remaining under cover for the rest of the day, the risk must be taken of making for the town of Muntok, in Banka, where there was sure to be a doctor and possibly a hospital in which the injured officer could be left if necessary.*

There was only some 30 miles of open water between the M.L's. present position and the island of Banka, so the journey was started and the M.L. left her safe cover at 1300 hours. As will be seen, this decision to seek medical assistance resulted in misfortune.

Within a few minutes of leaving cover, the M.L. was approached by a native sailing boat carrying two of the local islanders. One of these islanders had a letter which he delivered to the senior officer on board the M.L.† The M.L. resumed her course, and the lieutenant with the injured arm was put to bed below after being dosed with aspirin. But his fever continued to increase, and the pain of his hand and arm became so bad that he could not sleep, so he returned to the upper deck. He immediately sighted two Japanese cruisers on the horizon, and these were quickly joined by yet a third cruiser and two Japanese destroyers.‡

The lieutenant at once ordered an alteration of course away from the enemy. The M.L. was directed, at her maximum speed, back towards the shelter of the islands she had just left in the vain hope that she might have evaded detection.

But very quickly, a flash of gunfire was seen from the leading cruiser soon followed by a splash of falling shell some hundreds of yards astern of the M.L. Meanwhile, the second cruiser flew off an aircraft which quickly overtook the M.L.

The crew of M.L.310 stood to their guns and prepared to bring their craft to action. The aircraft was a single-engined float plane. As it approached, the M.L. 'zigzagged' violently and opened fire with all her armament. The aircraft dropped two bombs, which both exploded in the sea some 25 yards astern of the M.L. The aircraft turned back

---

* The injured officer has himself recorded: 'I was as keen as possible to see a doctor since I was conjuring up visions of losing my arm. But I was not so keen in being left behind in a part of the world I had not even heard about.'

† This letter purported to come from the Dutch Commandant of a military post on Tjebia Island, and gave the information that there were large numbers of Japanese warships in the vicinity.

‡ In the words of the sick lieutenant: 'After some minutes of tossing and turning in my high fever, I failed utterly to get to sleep and decided to come up to the wheelhouse and see how things were progressing. It was a perfect afternoon, blue sky with puffy cumulus clouds chasing one another across it, the deep blue sea flecked with "white horses", and every now and then a spray of cooling water would whip across the deck. On the port bow, the mountains of Banka Island stood up clearly, while on the starboard side a smudge of cloud betrayed the presence of the low lying coast of Sumatra. As I looked, I suddenly became aware of the masts and funnels of two ships standing up quite clearly. A second was sufficient to identify them as the unmistakable silhouettes of two Japanese cruisers.'

towards the cruisers, but the two destroyers were now seen to be steaming rapidly in the direction of the M.L.

M.L.310 had been severely shaken by the explosions of the two bombs. But she was still able to make a good speed, and with the destroyers approaching, she was able to round the promontory of the nearest island, thus placing the island between the enemy and the M.L. herself.* The M.L. was steered along the eastern side of the island which presented a long beach backed by coconut palms among which were the huts of a native village. At the far end of the beach was a small promontory, behind which the M.L. sought to take cover. A course was steered towards this promontory, but almost at once, M.L.310 ran aground firmly for what proved to be the last time.

There was now no time to be lost, and with the M.L. firmly wedged aground and already beginning to pound her hull on the coral sea bed, it was obvious that escape from the Japanese destroyers was probably unlikely.

A quick decision was made that the crew of the M.L. should remain on board her, while the passengers should be got ashore and should take cover in the jungle.†

All the passengers at once made for the island, wading breast high through the surf. On board the M.L. steps were taken to hide any evidence that the passengers had been in her.

The injured lieutenant was taken ashore in the dinghy. Feeling very unwell, he managed to make his way to some rocks behind which he hid. Almost at the same moment, a Japanese destroyer appeared round the point of the island. But, after inspecting the helpless M.L. from a distance, this destroyer circled round and steamed away.

After fifteen minutes ashore in the heat of the sun, the injured lieutenant felt so ill and his hand and arm were so painful that he decided that he had best return on board the M.L. Assisted by one of the R.A.F. officers, he attracted the attention of the crew of the M.L. The dinghy then came inshore and carried the two officers back to the M.L.‡

Meanwhile, examination of the M.L. had revealed extensive flooding in her engine room, with the deck plates almost submerged. Already the crew was attempting to effect emergency repairs with a view to refloating the M.L. so that further damage might be avoided through the constant pounding of the ship's hull against the coral.

---

* This was Tjebia Island from which the warning message had been received, as described earlier.

† This decision was in accordance with the instructions of G.H.Q., South-west Pacific. The policy adopted was that trained staff officers and technicians should be prevented from falling into the hands of the Japanese, as there was reason to suppose that attempts might be made to extract information from them—*London Gazette* No. 38215, Section LIV, para. 554 (b).

‡ The injured lieutenant has recorded: 'It was maddening to be in such a useless state physically just when almost every action required physical work'.

But the work had hardly begun, when another Japanese aircraft suddenly appeared and two bombs were dropped which narrowly missed the M.L. Within a few minutes a second Japanese destroyer appeared round the point of the island.

Those on board the M.L. discussed the possibility of a show of resistance, but decided against it. Instead, it was decided to continue to aim at securing the safety of the passengers who by now were hidden in the jungle ashore. Any remaining luggage of the passengers was quietly lowered into the sea, all confidential books and charts were burnt and the M.L's. wireless set was rendered useless. The injured lieutenant, the R.A.F. officer and the crew of the M.L. now settled down to await events.

The Japanese destroyer anchored a mile away, opened fire on the M.L. and, at the same time, sent off a motor boat containing an armed party. At once the Commanding Officer of the M.L. ordered all the ratings of his crew to wade ashore, which they did in safety. There now remained on board the M.L. only four officers, including the injured Lieutenant and the R.A.F. officer.

The motor boat from the Japanese destroyer took fifteen minutes to reach the M.L., and during this time shelling by the destroyer was maintained. The rate of fire was very slow and obviously intended merely to give cover to the motor boat. The majority of the shells passed overhead and exploded in the coral about a hundred yards beyond the M.L.*

The shallow draught of the Japanese motor boat allowed her to stop alongside the M.L., and immediately, the Japanese armed party boarded the M.L. and the four British officers found themselves being beaten about the face and shoulders until they were finally grouped around the stern of the M.L., covered by three sailors with light automatic rifles.

The armed boarding party was commanded by a Japanese midshipman who spoke a little English. He carried out an inspection and search of the M.L. He then addressed the British officers and expressed his regret that he could not take them aboard his destroyer which was too overcrowded. Thereupon, the four British officers were lined up with their backs against the guard rail faced by twelve Japanese whose weapons were loaded and aimed at them. The midshipman held his samurai sword and gave an order which indicated that the British officers were about to be shot.† Then, after a moment apparently lost in thought, the midshipman ordered the firing party to lower their arms. Hardly had the four British officers realised that their lives were to be spared, at least temporarily, when the midshipman ordered them to row

---

* The M.L. was actually hit once, but probably by accident, and the klaxon on the mast was blown away.

† One of the officers recorded: 'The midshipman was looking straight at us. Another Jap was looking away as if he did not wish to witness what was just about to happen.'

themselves ashore in the M.L's. dinghy. The four officers did as they were told, and even then they were convinced that the Japanese intended to shoot them in the dinghy rather than on board the M.L. Nevertheless, within a few minutes they had reached the shore and, quickly pulling the dinghy clear of the surf, they ran and took cover in the jungle at the edge of the beach. Peering back towards the sea, they watched the motor boat and boarding party return to the Japanese destroyer. As soon as the motor boat had been hoisted, the destroyer weighed anchor and steamed away until she was lost to sight over the horizon. Only then did these officers relax some of the tension and strain under which they had existed for the past hour.*

MAROONED

These survivors of M.L.310 were now cast ashore on the island of Tjebia, one of the Tuju or Seven Islands some 30 miles north of Banka Island. The island was owned by the Dutch, but the only inhabitants were a small number of islanders and a few Javanese troops whose duty was to man a small military observation post on a hilltop at the northern end of the island.

The islanders themselves had been alarmed by the gunfire of the Japanese destroyer, and had made up their minds to leave the island. In fact, some had already begun to do so by the evening of the same day, and before the next morning only the few Javanese troops and the survivors of the M.L. were left on Tjebia.

A short distance from the shore was a small clearing in the jungle, and here the passengers and crew from M.L.310 gathered about an hour after the Japanese destroyer had disappeared.

The officers held a quick conference to decide the best plan to adopt. The Japanese seemed to be in full command of the surrounding seas, and there was no knowing when they might not decide to return to Tjebia. It seemed necessary to get away from the island as soon as possible, and as a first step, some of the crew of the M.L. returned on board her to see if there was any chance of her being refloated and proving seaworthy.

Unfortunately, inspection of the M.L. showed that she could not be made seaworthy for at least several days. The fuel and circulating systems were smashed, and the engine room was half flooded through a leak as yet undiscovered. The wireless set was beyond repair.

Taking all these facts into consideration, it was decided to make preparations for the bulk of the party to remain on Tjebia for at least

---

* The injured lieutenant has described his thoughts while waiting to be shot, and his illness from his infected arm would seem to have made him relatively unconcerned about his immediate fate. 'A sort of mental and physical sickness stifled all thought, except that in the next second everything would be over. The feeling of utter helplessness was so great that there was no question of fear.'

a week. At the same time, it was decided that a small number should try to sail to Java in a native boat in the hope of being able to guide a rescue party back. For this latter purpose, a search was made in the local village for a suitable craft. But by now the last of the villagers had left the island and all that could be found was one small and leaky 'prau'.* This prau was obviously unfit to undertake a voyage to Java, 300 miles away. It was estimated that repairs to this craft would take some days.

Plans were now made to settle on Tjebia for several days. Food and essential stores were landed from the M.L., and the party took up residence in the deserted local village on the shore. Some rough latrines were dug and a freshwater spring was discovered. By 2300 hours on the night of their arrival on the Island of Tjebia these officers and men felt that they had done all that was possible for the time being, and they laid down to sleep on the floor boards of the village huts.

Viewed from the standpoint of preventive medicine, a subject about which the members of this party seem to have been singularly uninformed, it is probable that at this time the first step was taken which eventually led to tragic consequences. That night sleep proved impossible for most of these men. The floor boards upon which they lay were verminous and they were constantly attacked by mosquitoes. The officer with the injured arm rose towards dawn in order to re-dress his hand, and his record states that he was glad to do so in order to escape the discomforts of the night.†

At 0520 hours the prau was baled out and launched. Two officers and four men stored this small craft with provisions and managed to paddle it a short distance to another minute island nearby. Their object in doing this was to be able to repair the prau undisturbed should the Japanese decide to return to Tjebia. To paddle this prau a distance of three miles, and to keep her afloat by baling all the time, took nearly three hours.‡

The rest of the day this small party spent effecting repairs to the leaks in the prau, and by evening they had caulked and strengthened the hull and had patched the sails and renewed the rigging.

At 1800 hours they made their first attempt to sail this uncertain craft to Java. But after two hours against an adverse current and with little wind to assist them, the attempt was abandoned and they returned to the island.

---

* A wooden sailing boat.

† 'I longed for the dawn. The air was so thick with mosquitoes that it was hardly possible to breathe without getting them up your nose and into your mouth.'

‡ One of the persons on board the prau was the officer with the injured hand, and although he only performed the duty of steering the prau, it seems that his general condition had improved since the day before. But his condition got worse again later in the day.

They landed at about 2030 hours and settled down to spend the night in the open on the beach. From the standpoint of preventive medicine, it is probable that the second step towards subsequent ill-health had now been taken.*

The party rose at daybreak and made a breakfast off weak tea and biscuits.† The day was spent making the prau more seaworthy, but on two occasions the party had to take cover when Japanese aircraft appeared over Tjebia to bomb the M.L. again.

At 1700 hours a second attempt was made to sail the prau on the 300-mile voyage to Java. But this attempt also failed and at nightfall the prau was pulled back to the island where the party spent another night of discomfort.

The next morning a message was received from the senior officer ordering the prau to be paddled back to Tjebia. Later in the day the survivors were altogether again on the island of Tjebia, where certain developments had been taking place. The senior officer had been in consultation with the Commandant of the small group of Javanese troops who was now anxious to get his own men away. The senior officer had agreed that the repaired prau should be shared with the Commandant and one of his men, and this meant that two of the original naval party would withdraw. It was obvious that one of these should be the officer with the injured hand.‡

The whole of February 19 was spent re-storing and preparing the prau for the journey. That afternoon a fair breeze sprang up and at 1700 hours the prau set off on the third attempt to sail the 300 miles to Java. She made a good speed and by nightfall the party on the beach at Tjebia could barely sight her and her five occupants upon whom their hopes of rescue now rested. Unfortunately these hopes were not fulfilled.§

The assorted company of officers and men left on Tjebia Island now settled down to a novel existence of shipwrecked mariners. They took up permanent residence in the huts of the deserted village, and, after removing everything possible from the wrecked M.L., they devised a

---

* Describing this night, the injured lieutenant says: 'The place of bed bugs was taken by innumerable land crabs. The mosquitoes were no less vicious than they had been on Tjebia. My hand was useless and I knew I still had a fever, and these facts did nothing to help my frame of mind. Try as I might, I could not ward off the deepening sense of depression which came over me.'

† It seems probable that this meal represented yet a third step towards ill-health. One member of the party recorded: 'The biscuits tasted very odd. They were some we had brought from the Chinese village. They were all waterlogged, and were a mixture of salt, sugar, biscuit and sand.'

‡ The officer himself says: 'My hand was still useless but I felt better in myself. Once the suspense of the proposed journey to Java was off my mind I felt a lot easier and was able to eat and enjoy an evening meal.'

§ The prau was commanded by a lieutenant, R.N.Z.V.R. Two naval ratings acted as the crew, and the Javanese Commandant and one of his troops were passengers. Though too late to organise help for those left on Tjebia, this small group of men actually did sail the prau successfully to Java.

routine domestic life with a number of additional duties to pass the time away. One officer found another unseaworthy prau of considerable dimensions, and he commenced work on this with a view to its ultimate repair. Another officer organised the catering and cooking arrangements, while another supervised the collection of water,* firewood and fruit from the jungle.†

The whole party set out to scour and cleanse the huts of the village, but they were never able to diminish the swarms of bed bugs or the clouds of mosquitoes which appear to have attacked them by day and night.

They had ample tinned foods from the M.L., and to start with, a small number of chickens provided a very few eggs. Unfortunately, these chickens gradually disappeared and formed the subject of a minor international crisis between the British and the Javanese troops with whom contact had been maintained. Attempts to fish from the shore were made each day by various of the officers, but with a remarkable lack of success. Also, one officer narrowly escaped being attacked by a shark,‡ after which the others were less inclined to wade into the water of the lagoon.

During the next four weeks, three other castaways arrived on Tjebia. The first of these was a soldier, who had been drifting about for a number of days in a small boat.§ The second arrival was a naval stoker whose ship had been sunk, and who drifted up on to the beach on a piece of wreckage. The third was a civilian who had escaped from Singapore in a craft which had later been sunk by the Japanese. He had been drifting on wreckage from island to island, and had lived on coconuts.‖

From time to time, small numbers of the islanders returned for brief visits of a few hours. But it was impossible to invoke their assistance towards escape, because they reported great Japanese air activity in the neighbourhood, as well as the Japanese occupation of many of the islands. From time to time Japanese aircraft appeared and bombed the wrecked M.L. upon which work had long ceased. On one occasion a Japanese cruiser anchored off Tjebia and while the British party hid in

---

* There is no record that drinking water was ever boiled. It would seem always to have been drunk in its raw state.

† The main fruits available were bananas and papaya.

‡ The officer recorded: 'I was standing in some 2 feet of water at the time. Out of the corner of my eye I saw a swirl in the still water about ten yards away, and I instinctively flung myself headlong on to the beach. I was only just in time, because when I looked back, I saw the dorsal fin of a shark cut the surface. Had I been a little slower in my reactions I should have suffered severe injury, because the shark was at least 6 feet in length.'

§ This soldier was a private of the Gordon Highlanders who had survived after the ship had been sunk in which he had escaped from Singapore.

‖ This civilian was Australian by birth, and had been an employee in the Royal Naval Dockyard, Singapore.

the jungle, the Japanese boarded the M.L. and again inspected it, after which the cruiser sailed away.*

It was at the beginning of March 1942 that ill health began to manifest itself among these British officers and men on the island of Tjebia. Its advent was insidious, but once started its ravages gathered speed till a time came when even the strongest were struck down with dramatic suddenness.

The arm of the injured officer seems to have recovered within about three weeks because little mention is made of it thereafter. But a definite sick list was established on the island when the three extra survivors arrived. The soldier was obviously suffering from some form of dysentery when rescued, and his condition never really improved.† The civilian too was sick, and at the time of his arrival, was described as being 'covered in white sores from head to foot'.‡

The castaways on Tjebia Island had assumed that if the voyage of the prau proved successful, they themselves could expect to be rescued either by submarine or flying boat within about three weeks. As the first week of March drew to a close their hopes faded. From this time onwards there was a noticeable fall in morale, and a tendency towards listlessness on the part of everyone.§

The first to die was a naval officer who had been renovating another prau for some days. One morning he considered this old craft ready for launching, but, unfortunately, it capsized. This officer took no further part in the life of the island. He quickly became ill, and died on the morning of Sunday, March 7. He was buried on the same day.

The clinical details of this officer's illness were recorded as follows:

> 'For some days he had been delirious with a high fever, and had been getting worse rather than better. We were not at all certain what he died from, for he had only been sick for a few days and then only from what appeared to be a chill. This chill had developed into some kind of fever, and that was as much as our amateur diagnosis told us.'

This death seems to have had a most adverse effect on the remainder.‖

At that time there were some seven of the party ill from various causes, the most seriously affected being one of the Royal Air Force officers. This officer died on the afternoon of March 10, and was buried

---

* A peculiar incident is attached to this visit of a Japanese boarding party to the M.L. When the cruiser had departed, some of the British officers went on board the M.L. The only evidence they could find that the Japanese had visited her was a small piece of paper pinned to the engine room bulkhead and on which was written in English, 'How much bread?' The British party on Tjebia spent many hours trying to elicit the meaning of this strange message, if message it was, but without success!

† This soldier died on Tjebia Island.

‡ This civilian died on Tjebia Island.

§ One officer wrote: 'This drop in spirits, which up till then had been reasonably high, was added to by the knowledge that the sick had been increasing in number'.

‖ An officer recorded: 'From that time on the morale of all but a few sank never to be recovered'.

early on the following morning. The clinical description of his illness states:

> 'He too had caught a chill, probably from fishing in the evening, and he soon became delirious. In his delirium he constantly saw Japanese tanks coming through the jungle. At times during the night he would get up and wander away "to look for the elixir of life", and it took all our persuasive powers to get him back to bed. He was unconscious for a day before he died.'

The following week a second naval officer became ill, and he died towards the end of March. In this case the illness was more puzzling to the lay minds of his companions, and 'chill' is not mentioned as a clinical feature. One of his companions wrote:

> 'When he complained of feeling tired and said he would take it easy for a couple of days, nobody thought much about it. However, as the days passed into weeks and he showed no inclination to get up, we began to ask why. There did not appear to be anything much wrong with him, and it looked rather as if this lack of will-power to drive himself again to take his place in the life of the community was just laziness. However, he still remained where he was, in spite of every effort by us all either to persuade or bully him into making an effort. As the days passed, he began to take less and less care of himself, and finally he became so smelly and dirty that we had to put him in a hut by himself. It was a pitiful sight to see him, although at the time we had no sympathy. He died towards the end of March, a victim of sheer lack of will-power to fight against the depression and soul destroying lassitude which was becoming more marked among us each week.'

At first the numbers of sick were manageable, and devoted nursing duties were performed by a lieutenant, R.N. with the help of a naval stoker. These two tried to improvise treatment as best they could, but with little success. There were cases when a man would be struck down quickly and in a most frightening way. Such was the case of a naval petty officer.* One morning he complained of a sore throat which got worse during the day. He reported to an officer who stated:

> 'By midday he was unable to swallow anything, and I found that his throat had swollen up to the size of a football. He was put in the sick bay where he died that night.'

About the middle of March, the lieutenant who had recovered from the infected injury to his hand and arm again fell sick. His symptoms are best described in his own words:

> 'One morning I was having a good look round the horizon with my binoculars, just in case something should have turned up by some miracle. Suddenly, I could see nothing but a red haze. At first I thought that one of the colour filters had fallen, but as I removed the glasses from my eyes,

---

* This Petty Officer was a survivor from H.M.S. *Repulse*.

I found that it was my sight. After blinking and rubbing my eyes once or twice, it dawned on me that I could see nothing at all. After a few minutes, I found that I could just make out the blurred surroundings of the palms and village with my left eye.

'I staggered back to the village rather frightened, and wondering what had happened. No one could see anything wrong with my eyes, and it seemed as if there was no explanation. It was a couple of days before I could see well enough to move about, and two or three weeks before the sight returned to my left eye completely. My right eye took far longer, and it was almost four months before I could see sufficiently well to be able to read. Even then, I could only see the very top and bottom of letters and objects.'

By the end of March, about 25 per cent. of the party were sick. The hut used as a sick quarter was full, and all were suffering from what appeared to be some kind of fever and dysentery. The naval stoker who had been performing nursing duties now fell sick himself, and, before the end of the month, he is described as having died 'from what looked like a combination of everything'.

It is of interest to note that the outbreak of sickness was by no means confined to these European castaways on Tjebia Island. The Chinese cook attached to the party fell sick with fever, and reference has been made to the same form of illness among the few remaining Javanese troops.*

By this time food stocks were running low, and it was estimated that what the party had brought with them would be exhausted by the end of April, after which they would be forced to exist on the scanty supply of fruit provided by the island itself. The survivors now became obsessed with the fear that if they remained on the island indefinitely, they would all die of some form of sickness if not of starvation. Efforts were therefore concentrated upon devising some method of escape. Yet another disused prau was discovered on the edge of the jungle. Two of the naval ratings set to work on it, and this work was arranged on an organised basis in the days that followed, with the object of trying to render the craft seaworthy. Fortunately, the party included three sergeants of the Royal Engineers who had their tools with them and who were accustomed to working on wood.

The urgency of this work was not helped by the steady death rate from sickness which continued, and so many of the men had become so apathetic that the Senior Naval Officer instituted a strict and almost harsh working routine throughout the hours of daylight each day. Also, he was of the opinion that those who worked hard physically were less likely to succumb to the prevailing illness.

---

* 'The Javanese had gone really downhill as fast as our people. Their little hilltop post was dirty and unmanned, and they themselves were mostly to be found huddled in their blankets and shivering.'

The most unpopular duty now was that of helping to nurse the sick. These wretched men were usually in a poor state each morning, and are described as having been incontinent for the most part during the night.

One officer has described these nights most vividly:

'The day could always be passed doing hard work, which kept the mind away from the realities. But the nights were just an eternity of waiting, thinking and fighting off swarms of mosquitoes. Try as you might to ward it off, you were overwhelmed with loneliness, depression and frustration. This was bad enough for somebody who had the resistance to fight it off, but for those who had not, then the nights were just an agony of mind and spirit. Sleep was impossible. The heat made you drip with sweat if you pulled any form of covering over to protect yourself from mosquitoes. But otherwise, the mosquitoes bit you till you bled. At least once, and sometimes many times more, the unfamiliar fruit diet forced you to get up to relieve yourself.'

The fight against apathy was a formidable one, as is seen in the words of another officer:

'It was but a sign of our general lack of will-power that we were almost glad when the change in the monsoon brought the heavy storms and rain which swept across the island during April. These gave us just that excuse which we were ready to accept so easily, to put off facing the daily tasks.'

The monsoon added to their sufferings and appears to have brought with it even greater sickness of mind and spirit. For example:

'With the deluge would come the wind, rushing and tearing through the palms and leaving in its wake a chilling damp. This I enjoyed, because it took me, for a short space, away from the everlasting blue skies and blazing sunshine and reminded me of England. But this, as I realised, was sheer escapism, which as soon as I could, I strove to put aside and concentrate on the job in hand.'

Early in April the Island of Tjebia began to be visited by neighbouring islanders who, as the Japanese advance had extended southward, had now started to move about the seas again more freely. From one boatload of visitors the news was gleaned that the Lingaa group of islands to the north was still being administered by the Dutch. But the most important information was that there was a hospital functioning at Daboe, in Singkep Island, and that in it there was a number of wounded Europeans who were being cared for by nuns. It was decided to seek help from this hospital, and for the purpose the Chinese cook of the party was sent away in the boat of the islanders. He was told to get in touch with the Authorities and to charter a boat large enough to take all the survivors off Tjebia. Failing this, he was to make his way back by sea with medical supplies and a stock of food. For the purpose he was given 300 Straits dollars. Unfortunately he did not return.*

---

* Those who survived met this Chinese cook again some weeks later as a captive of the Japanese.

A few days later, Tjebia was visited by a boatload of islanders on passage to Banka. Relying on a rumour that Banka was still under Dutch control, two of the sergeants of the Royal Engineers volunteered to take passage with these islanders in order to try and obtain help. They set off the same evening, but they did not return.*

Throughout the whole month of March the sick list increased steadily, consistent with the reduced rations and the downward trend in morale which became evident as hope of rescue from outside diminished. A small number managed to carry on working and it is of interest to note that those who worked the hardest seemed to keep well. But the rest seemed to have no resistance to disease, and as they became unfit for work they merely lay about, some saying openly that they wished they could die. April was by far the worst month of sickness, and its last half saw the deaths of those who had sickened in the first half. At this late stage it had become almost impossible to nurse the sick in any degree worthy of the name.

In the last week of April the Senior Naval Officer died very suddenly and unexpectedly. The clinical details have been recorded as follows:

> 'We never knew what he died from, except that it was certainly not fever. For two days he had complained of indigestion and had even expressed a distaste for his scanty food. After lunch one day, he told us that he proposed to give himself an enema. He went away to do this. After some twenty minutes I found him unconscious and in what appeared to be a coma. We placed him on his bed and covered him up and he remained in much the same state until the evening. Just before the evening meal, I saw that he was dead.'

The death of the Senior Naval Officer was the sixteenth to occur since the party arrived on Tjebia Island. Its effect upon those who still lived may well be imagined. He was buried early the next morning.†

On the same day it was suddenly discovered that the few remaining Javanese troops had left with some of the visiting islanders.‡

If there had ever been any among the dwindling company who had doubts about the need of escaping from Tjebia Island as soon as possible, the question would seem to have been settled for them by this sudden death of the Senior Naval Officer. Every effort was now made to render the ancient prau seaworthy. The old, rotten hull had been surveyed and all the useless timbers removed, and new ones worked in to replace them.

---

* These two sergeants are not known to have reached their destination, and are still missing.

† A survivor wrote: 'As we stood round the grave I thought of how he had always read the Burial Service before, and now it was his turn to be lying wrapped in his blanket at the bottom of the shallow trench which was to be his last resting place. An air of unreality was with me, and it just did not seem possible that our lives should be as utterly changed as they had been in so short a time.'

‡ It is of medical interest that these Javanese left behind them almost as many graves as were left behind by the British party.

To make the craft more watertight, the hull was sheathed in a casing of metal contrived by beating out a number of 4-gallon fuel cans brought from the M.L. The timber for the new planking was obtained either by pulling down huts, or by choosing suitable palm trees and laboriously sawing them into planks. Nails and screws were obtained from the huts and from the M.L. Two naval ratings, one a survivor from the *Prince of Wales*, attended to the necessary rigging. Sails were cut and stitched by an Army corporal who was an upholsterer in civil life. The sails had been brought from Singapore in the M.L. They were of old canvas and mostly perished and rotten, but the corporal patched them with pieces of cloth from the clothing of the survivors.

By the beginning of May, the remaining food stocks were surveyed and mentally balanced against the progress of work on the prau. In consequence, a further reduction was made in rations and it was obvious that the boat must be ready to leave within 14 days.

At the same time, plans were made for the future after the boat had been rendered seaworthy. Of paramount importance was the need to remove living survivors from Tjebia Island as soon as possible. It was decided, therefore, first to seek some other island which would support life for a time while yet further plans were made. In the knowledge that the Japanese had advanced to the south and that a measure of Dutch control was believed still to exist in the islands to the north, it was planned to attempt to sail to the Island of Saaya, a distance of some 40 miles.

At the end of the first week in May the boat was considered to be seaworthy. The next problem was that of launching it, a task which was attended by difficulties. The prau itself lay some 50 yards from the edge of the sea and behind a line of palm trees. There were now only 10 men left in the party who were physically fit enough for manual work, but their strength was ebbing almost hourly and the task of lifting the prau by hand was already beyond them. An attempt was made to construct a complicated system of tackles, but without success owing to shortage of rope. The ten men next tried to dig a channel down to the sea, but this proved too heavy a task for their strength.

On May 10, just as these men had given up hope of getting the prau launched, a large party of islanders arrived at Tjebia by sea, and they at once agreed to undertake the launching of the prau. The arrival of these islanders at this particular moment was regarded as truly miraculous.*

Early on the morning of May 11, the islanders cut down large numbers of coconut fronds which they laid as skids under the keel of the prau. In the course of the day the prau was man-handled towards the sea

---

* One officer wrote, in reference to this event: 'By some miracle some islanders arrived and willingly agreed to assist us in getting the "Scriberganti" afloat. Such was her name, which I think means, in Malay, "By the grace of God".'

and finally launched. To the satisfaction of everyone the craft was found to be watertight and seaworthy.

The rest of the day was spent rigging the sails and storing the prau, after which a conference was held to decide who of the survivors should attempt to sail in her.

Desirable as it was for all the surviving members of the party to leave Tjebia Island as soon as possible, it was nevertheless obvious that such a policy would be both impossible and unwise. Should some of the sick sail in the prau, it was possible that some weakness of seamanship might arise in an emergency, resulting in disaster. It was well realised that to sail such a frail craft across the open sea under monsoon conditions would be hazardous in any event. Therefore, it was considered advisable that only those who were most fit physically should attempt the journey. It was finally agreed that the prau should be manned by a crew of six.* The remaining four survivors who were still capable of getting about, stayed behind on Tjebia to care for their sick colleagues. The object of the expedition which was to be given first priority was to effect the speedy rescue of those left behind on Tjebia Island.

It was decided to sail the prau for Saaya Island on the afternoon of May 15. Unfortunately, on the morning of the day of departure, the naval officer who was to navigate the prau amputated the top of his thumb while cutting open a coconut. He fainted, and was not particularly fit physically when the time came for the journey to begin.†

The crew of the prau had their last meal on Tjebia Island at noon on May 15, after which they set out on their voyage. Gathered on the shore to see them off were their companions in adversity whose instructions were, that unless help had been sent within one week, they were themselves to attempt to escape in the dinghy of the M.L. and also by means of constructing a raft for which purpose timber and fastenings were available.

Just before four o'clock, sail was hoisted and the prau passed very slowly out to sea before a gentle southerly breeze. Progress was little more than a drift, but the sea was calm. But two hours later, the sky began to darken and a breeze developed and quickly changed into a steady wind as part of a 'sumatra', one of the fierce and short-lived tropical storms of that area. In the first squall of wind and rain the prau was almost overpowered, while in a second phase of the storm the small craft was thrown about and sprang a leak. For some fifteen minutes vision was non-existent and the crew had no sense of direction at all.

---

* This crew consisted of 1 naval officer, 1 Army officer, 1 R.A.F. officer and 3 naval ratings. The naval officer was an experienced navigator. The R.A.F. officer spoke fluent Malay. The naval ratings were those who had had most experience of seamanship under sail.

† This was the same lieutenant who had previously suffered from an infected hand and arm.

The prau was driven, almost in a sinking condition towards a reef, but the strength of the breakers was such that it was carried clean over the rocks and escaped unharmed.

Within half an hour the storm had died away and the crew of the prau set about repairing the leak and managed to keep her still afloat. During the night, the wind was fitful and continued so during most of the following day.

On the evening of May 16, the prau started to make better headway and began to approach land towards midnight. Her crew, not being certain of the approaches to the shore, attempted to anchor for the night, but this proved impossible owing to the smooth nature of the sea bed. Eventually, a reef appeared through the darkness with heavy seas breaking over it, and despite all the efforts of her crew, the prau was driven ashore and wrecked upon this new hazard.

Fortunately, the six officers and men were able to clamber on to the reef itself carrying with them some of their precious stores from the prau. When the sun rose on May 17 they found themselves at the foot of a small rocky island less than 50 yards square. This island was separated from the main island of Saaya by a mere 50 yards of sea. But the current was so powerful through this narrow channel that the officers and men found it impossible to cross in their poor physical condition.

They might well have been marooned where they were indefinitely, had they not been able to attract the attention of a local fisherman who appeared in another small prau during the afternoon. The R.A.F. officer was able to converse with this fisherman, who eventually consented to rescue the party and sail them to Daboe, on Singkep Island, in return for the sum of 300 dollars each.

The prau of the fisherman was too small to carry six passengers, so it was arranged that the naval officer, 1 naval rating and the R.A.F. officer should take passage, the latter being essential to act as an interpreter. The Army officer and the 2 naval ratings remained on the rocks and the fisherman indicated that he would return and fetch them the following day.*

Just before noon the prau set off upon the 30 mile journey to Daboe, which was still believed to be under Dutch control. The voyage was uneventful and, towards midnight, the prau approached the shore and entered a small harbour, and finally came to rest alongside some steps up which the three British survivors climbed on to a small pier.

All three were completely exhausted, and the R.A.F. officer was in the throes of a fever attack. They lay down on the boards of the pier and fell asleep while the fisherman left to seek medical assistance. The

---

* This man kept his word. On the following day he returned and rescued these three men who by then were ill with fever. All three survived and were taken to Singapore where they became prisoners-of-war in the hands of the Japanese. The Army officer belonged to the Argyll and Sutherland Highlanders.

three men quickly awoke and found themselves surrounded by armed members of the local Javanese Gendarmerie, who had apparently been placed in charge of local civilian law and order by the Japanese. The three men were conducted to a motor lorry which conveyed them not to hospital, but to the local gaol where they were confined for the night in a small and badly ventilated cell. But, by the following morning, their physical condition was so poor that they were taken to a ward in the local Asiatic Hospital.

This ward consisted of a number of plain wooden beds mounted on iron trestles, with no mattresses. The ward had no other item of furnishing or equipment. The three men were placed in the care of a Chinese male nurse, while two of the gendarmes remained on guard in a corridor outside the ward. The R.A.F. officer was having frequent rigors and obviously needed urgent attention. After five minutes a Malayan 'doctor' arrived who, with a great deal of display, took a blood slide from each of the three patients. This 'doctor' then departed, but he soon returned and assured the three men that they were suffering from no kind of illness!*

During the next four days this Malayan 'doctor' frequently visited the three patients, but did little more than to talk to them and to adopt an attitude of great knowledge and superiority.† But the Chinese male nurse, who was an old man, proved a good friend to the three men. He was able to smuggle into the hospital extra food such as chicken and pork, albeit at an exorbitant cost.‡ But, in addition, his greatest asset to these men was to bring them up-to-date in the local news of the area. It seemed that the hospital at Daboe had become very busy soon after the fall of Singapore, and had received most of the survivors from the convoy of small ships which had left Singapore on February 13. The hospital had actually been full of casualties until a few days before, when some Japanese had arrived at Daboe and had transferred the casualties, Dutch doctors and nuns of a nursing order, to Sumatra. It seemed that the Japanese were expected to return again to Daboe within a few days, and that they would certainly do so now that they had been informed of the arrival there of these three British patients.

---

* One of the patients wrote: 'In a ridiculously short time he returned, and told us that we had not the slightest sign of any fever and were all perfectly healthy. This was in spite of the fact that one of us was shaking with ague at the time.'

† This Malayan ' doctor ' was, in fact, himself a male nurse. Originally, he had been the head dresser of the hospital when it belonged to the Dutch. After the Dutch surrender, the medical staff had been removed by the Japanese, who had left this dresser in control of the hospital. From then on he had conferred upon himself the title of 'doctor'.

‡ These three men did not give this Chinese nurse money merely for the purpose of providing extra food. They seemed to feel somehow that they were, as yet, unwilling to cease hostilities! One of them has recorded: 'We also gave him money with which to bribe some of the local hooligans to throw stones at the police station, as well as to make as much other trouble as possible!'

At the end of the second day, the three men were relieved to learn that the Army officer and two naval ratings left behind off the Island of Saaya had been rescued.

On the fifth morning a party of Japanese military police arrived at the hospital. The three men were closely interrogated, and then informed that they were now prisoners of the Imperial Japanese Army. During this interrogation their chief concern had been to make the Japanese Authorities aware of the presence of the remainder of the party on Tjebia Island, and of the urgent necessity to rescue them without delay.

Two days later, the men were removed from the hospital and were taken on board a small tugboat where, to their delight and relief, they found their companions from Tjebia who, although obviously extremely ill, were at least still alive.* Also on board the tug was the Chinese cook of the party. Other passengers in captivity were a Dutch planter with his wife, and a Russian civilian.

At 1400 hours on May 23, these survivors were landed at Clifford Pier in Singapore, approximately fourteen weeks after the original party had set off to escape.

As stated above, the total number on board the M.L. when she was wrecked on Tjebia Island was 45, including the Chinese cook. It will be remembered that 3 other survivors were washed ashore some time later, so that the total number cast ashore on Tjebia Island was 48, composed of 6 naval officers, 20 naval ratings, 6 Royal Marines, 1 Army officer, 9 Army other ranks, 2 R.A.F. officers, 2 R.A.F. other ranks, 1 naval dockyard civilian and 1 Chinese cook.

Of the 6 naval officers, 3, including the Senior Naval Officer, died on Tjebia Island; 1 naval officer eventually reached Java by sea. The other 2 naval officers survived as prisoners-of-war.

Of the 20 naval ratings, 10 died on Tjebia Island; 2 naval ratings reached Java by sea. The remaining 8 naval ratings became prisoners-of-war.

Of the 6 Royal Marines, 2 died on Tjebia Island, while the other 4 became prisoners-of-war.

The Army officer survived as a prisoner-of-war in company with 4 other ranks. Of the Army other ranks 2 died on Tjebia Island, 1 died at Singapore, shortly after being rescued from Tjebia, while 2 were missing after leaving Tjebia Island by sea.

The Senior R.A.F. officer died on Tjebia Island. The other R.A.F. officer and 2 other ranks survived as prisoners-of-war.

The naval dockyard civilian died on Tjebia Island.

The Chinese cook survived.

---

* One of these survivors, an Army corporal, died in the course of the following week.

The final figures for these men who were cast away on Tjebia Island therefore read as follows:

Died on Tjebia Island	19
Died shortly after leaving Tjebia Island	1
Missing at sea	2
Reached Java by sea	3
Survived as prisoners-of-war	23
Total	48

Apart from the two missing men, these figures represent a mortality rate from disease in this party of over 41 per cent. and in as short a period as fourteen weeks.

DISCUSSION OF HIGH MORTALITY ON TJEBIA ISLAND

As has already been indicated, even though no medical officer, sick berth rating or medical orderly was a member of this group of 48 men cast away on Tjebia Island, from the viewpoint of the Naval Medical History, many of the incidents which have been described in so great detail are considered to be of great importance. The story which has been told, though certainly enthralling, is not aimed merely at holding the attention of the reader. This story has been included by the Medical Branch of the Navy in the hope that its implications may be appreciated by all other Branches of the Service. It is also submitted that the implications may be appreciated by the non-medical Branches of the other Fighting Services, for it will be remembered that the men who suffered on this occasion belonged to the Navy, the Army and the Royal Air Force.

In order to justify this attitude, it is necessary to marshal the evidence which can be extracted from these events. Once elicited, this evidence may be supported by the views already expressed earlier in this History.*

To attempt to assess, in retrospect, the cause of death or of an epidemic illness is usually not only attended by difficulties, but is frequently unprofitable. Nevertheless, it is possible to effect a rough analysis of the events which have been described, which, though founded upon clinical details recorded by laymen, is yet illuminating to the qualified assessor.

The qualified medical assessor may best study the events described from the very beginning, pausing, from time to time, to consider incidents which tend to throw light sometimes on matters of pure preventive medicine and sometimes on matters of naval medical organisation which are little more than elementary.

---

* *See* Volume I, Chapter 12.

Taking the facts from the beginning, a party of 45 officers and men of the three Fighting Services left Singapore in a naval motor launch. They were later cast ashore on a tropical island, where their number was increased to 48 by the arrival of three independent survivors from elsewhere. Within fourteen weeks, approximately 41 per cent. had lost their lives from sickness, in addition to which other minor medical incidents occurred which tended to hamper the efficiency of these men. Two men are still missing, but probably lost their lives at sea, so the medical assessor need concern himself only with the remainder.

The original party which left Singapore included no doctor and no sick berth rating or medical orderly. The reason for this omission is not clear, but the general background of circumstances which existed at the time when this expedition was organised more than suggests the probability that the inclusion of some person with medical training was completely overlooked.

This omission proved to be very serious. To start with, an hour or so after the journey had begun, an officer had severely injured his hand. This injury quickly became infected, and exerted an adverse influence on the fortunes of the party from that very moment.

When this officer's hand was injured, first aid was given by some of his companions. There is no record of the particular nature of the first aid on this occasion, but that the infection which followed was both rapid and severe is certain.

Within 48 hours, the progress of this infection was such that plans had to be altered radically, and risks were taken in order to obtain medical assistance which led to discovery and pursuit by the Japanese, resulting in the final and disastrous arrival on the Island of Tjebia.

In relation to this, the injured officer himself recorded: 'My injured hand now played its part in our misfortunes.'

While such speculation may be idle, a medical reader cannot be blamed for concentrating on two facts at this point, the first of which is certain and the second less certain. The first fact is that the presence in the party of a person with medical training would have obviated the need to alter course to seek medical assistance elsewhere, in which case all the tragic events which followed might possibly have been avoided. The second fact is that the first aid applied was ineffective, which raises the proposition that among the whole party of 45, there would seem to have been nobody who had received first-aid instruction at the hands of his Service with a sufficiency to avoid a wound becoming infected. According to the patient himself, a 'first field dressing' was applied and held in place by a piece of fuse-wire.*

---

* When interrogated by the editor of this History, this officer agreed that the first aid was very elementary. He also volunteered the information that at the time of his injury, he himself knew very little first aid, having received but scanty instruction during his Service career.

On the other hand, such criticism is probably over severe, and the possibility must be admitted that this particular wound might have become severely infected even under the best and most skilled professional care.

Thus, this injury and infection could be regarded as inevitable. But the need for a doctor to treat it subsequently cannot be doubted, any more than it can be denied that had a trained medical man been present in the party at that time there is a remote possibility that the whole number might have survived and might even have evaded capture.

In considering the various medical incidents which occurred during the stay on Tjebia Island, it is necessary first to eliminate certain clinical features which were recorded, but were probably in no way due to the plight in which the party found themselves.

One such incident is that of the officer in whom there were sudden and prolonged disturbances of vision which began while he was using binoculars. It will be remembered that the first thing he noticed was a red haze, followed by a short period of complete blindness, followed by restricted vision which took some four months to recover completely.

This was the officer who had previously suffered from the infected injury to hand and arm. In the absence of any direct head or eye injury, and it being unlikely that any ophthalmic symptoms consistent with some deficiency disease could have arisen so soon after being cast away, it has been suggested that an indirect cause was some form of toxaemia from the old hand infection. However, the more acceptable diagnosis is that which has been offered by the Civil Consultant in Ophthalmology to the Royal Navy, who, in relation to the experiences of the particular officer, has given the following as his opinion:

> 'What he says fits in fairly well with the condition of erythryopsia which comes on as a result of exposure to bright light, . . . The colour is generally rather different having usually some purple in it, and the consequences are not so bad, complete recovery coming on fairly soon. I should think, however, that variations from the original course can be accounted for by the patient's general condition, and erythryopsia seems to me the most likely explanation.'*

Whether the presence of a medical officer in this party would have averted this ophthalmic incident is doubtful. But there is no doubt that his recognition of the state of affairs would have done much to allay the fears of the victim.

It is doubtful too, whether the presence of a doctor or skilled medical attendant would have made very much difference in the case of the death of the Senior Naval Officer. This officer was not a young man,

---

* This patient informed the editor of this History that while a prisoner-of-war, he was examined by an Ophthalmic Specialist who told him that his retinae had 'lifted' and that he must have had a blow on his head at some time or other. Any such history of injury was, however, strenuously denied by the officer.

and he had been subjected to considerable mental and physical strain and fatigue over a prolonged period. It seems probable that he died from some cerebrovascular catastrophe, sudden in onset and fatal within a few hours. It is submitted that the enema referred to played no part in what happened, although the theories of reflex syncope and air embolus have both been put forward by other clinical observers in retrospect.

The rapid death has been described of one naval rating following immense swelling of the throat 'to the size of a football'. There is no record that this man had anything wrong with him until about nine or ten hours before his death. The view of the layman is that the man noticed soreness of his throat during the forenoon, which was followed by swelling of his throat and neck to such an extent that he was unable to swallow. Apart from this swelling, there is no mention of any other physical signs up to his death.

One of his companions wrote: 'We all racked our brains to think what might have caused his death so suddenly. It was only long afterwards that his symptoms were thought to be similar to those caused by some form of sting.'

That this suggestion might not have been far wide of the mark is obvious, though it does not appear on record that the man himself had complained of any type of sting, either animal or vegetable. It is unfortunate that there is no past medical record of this man available, neither is it known whether there existed any former allergic susceptibility in himself or in his family.

However, whatever the cause, angio-neurotic oedema, followed by rapid and fatal dyspnoea, is a tempting diagnosis in retrospect. Should this have been truly the case, life-saving measures might have been adopted had a doctor been available. But the assistance of a skilled sick berth rating or medical orderly could only have been limited in this case, for it is doubtful whether he would have had either the courage or the ability to embark upon the tracheotomy which might have been the sole means of saving the life of this unfortunate man.

Mention has been made of the three extra survivors who arrived separately on the Island of Tjebia. One of these is described as having been covered in 'white sores from head to foot'. These were probably the 'salt water ulcers' which have frequently been described in persons wrecked at sea and immersed for long periods. Another of these three was obviously suffering from severe dysentery at the time of his rescue. This may well have been the cause of his death. But it seems likely that the other two men fell victims to the general 'fever' which is described as affecting all who took refuge on Tjebia Island.

It is with this 'fever' that the qualified assessor of what happened on Tjebia Island will be most concerned because, not only was it the cause of the high mortality, but it was also probably the one thing which might have yielded to correct therapy had a medical officer been present.

Also, the mind of the qualified assessor must of necessity consider the matter from the angle of preventive medicine, and he cannot fail to be puzzled by the fact that this large party of officers and men from the three Fighting Services seemed so incapable of either recognising the prevailing disease on the island or of taking more adequate measures to guard against it.

The whole of this question is best answered by recording the written words of one of the naval officers of the party:

'*The absence of any real medical knowledge among us was frightening.*'

These words themselves represent an admission which might well be regarded with dismay by the Medical Authorities of the three Fighting Services who have endeavoured for so long to implant into the minds of their lay colleagues the rudiments of medical precautions and self-help, particularly under tropical conditions.

Some of the officers on Tjebia Island were of very senior rank and were accompanied by members of their executive staffs. There was, in fact, present on Tjebia Island a section representing that Higher Administrative Authority which would have been responsible for appreciating and implementing the recommendations of its medical advisers in all matters of preventive medicine. From the moment they were cast away, the behaviour of these officers suggests that they could not have appreciated seriously all that their many medical advisers must have endeavoured to teach them in the past.

In this respect, it may be stated with confidence that much of what occurred on Tjebia Island, certainly as regards the Navy, is an outstanding example of the warning given by the Medical Director-General of the Navy himself.*

There is no doubt that the cause of death in these cases was malaria in one or more of its forms. That malaria was endemic on the island of Tjebia is true without question, as is the fact that this was something which was fully appreciated by the local inhabitants of the islands round about.

It would seem, in simple terms, that what actually happened subsequently was that in this small area in which malaria was already endemic,

---

* Reference should be made to Chapter 12, Preventive Medicine, in the Administration Volume of the Official Naval Medical History of the War. Surgeon Vice Admiral Sir Sheldon Dudley, F.R.S., in an address to the officers of the Royal Naval Staff College, issued a warning that the potential protection afforded by life at sea had itself insidiously become a dangerous doctrine in course of time, for the very reason that it was prone to be accepted as a matter of course. Hence, in successive generations of naval officers, an attitude of indifference had been fostered by their way of life afloat, and obviously complacency of this order had its dangers should the circumstances of Service suddenly transfer them from the comparative safety of the sea to the hygiene hazards of a shore environment. Sir Sheldon Dudley also stated at an Inter-Allied Conference on War Medicine convened by the Royal Society of Medicine, 'that executive and combatant officers must be taught that the enforcing of hygiene measures to preserve the health, morale and fighting efficiency of their troops is as important as any other military duty'.

the disease suddenly assumed epidemic proportions, a sequence which is all too common in malarious districts where no precautions are adopted. That the disease did become epidemic is supported by the fact that the Javanese troops on Tjebia were as severely infected as were the Europeans, and apparently with as formidable a mortality.

With all this in mind, it is difficult, at first, to understand why the officers of the party did not appreciate the dangers. Although warned that the island upon which they had landed was known as 'Fever Island',* and although they must have frequently been instructed by their medical advisers in the dangers of pitching camp too near to native villages in malarious areas,† this elementary precaution would seem to have been completely disregarded. In fact, these unfortunate men began life on the island by doing the worst thing possible. If any reservoir of malarial infection was likely to exist on Tjebia it would be in and around the small village near the shore. Yet, on the night of their arrival, the whole party took up residence in the huts of this village which had been abandoned by the local islanders a matter of a few hours before.

Nevertheless, Tjebia Island was shaped roughly like an hour glass with high land at either end. The whole island was $\frac{3}{4}$ mile long and up to $\frac{1}{2}$ mile wide except at the neck of the hour glass. The native village was situated on this narrowest part. The rest of the island, apart from an occasional track, was covered in dense and impenetrable jungle. Therefore, closer consideration reveals the fact that the village occupied the only habitable part of the island and there was nowhere else where these unfortunate men could have lived. Several attempts were, in fact, made to clear jungle and to erect alternative living quarters. But these attempts failed owing to the poor resources of the party as regards tools and materials.

Repeated and bitter complaints were made about the virulence of the mosquitoes which attacked the party without cessation. In the absence of adequate protection by way of mosquito nets or protective clothing, it might have been considered reasonable to search for the breeding places of these vectors and to take some steps to eliminate them. The party resided on Tjebia for several weeks and, certainly at one time, many hours each day were spent in performing manual work. But no mention is made of the filling in of pools and ditches, or of the burying of tins, etc., all of which must have provided breeding grounds. Also, large quantities of oil, in various forms, must have been available in the M.L., yet it does not seem that any

---

* One of the officers has recorded that the Commandant of the military post on Tjebia had informed the party, presumably at the time of their arrival, that the island was known locally as 'Fever Island'.

† One of the surviving officers has pleaded complete ignorance of this type of danger and has claimed that such knowledge was never imparted to him during his Service training.

attempt was ever made to employ any of it as a prophylactic measure against mosquitoes.*

But even more puzzling is the peculiar fact that when malaria obviously did begin to attack the community, the true nature of the disease would seem to have passed unrecognised. That it did pass unrecognised is obvious from some of the clinical descriptions which have been given in the case of those who died, e.g.:

(1) 'He had only been sick a few days, and then only from what appeared to be "a chill".'
(2) 'He too had caught "a chill" from fishing in the evening, and was now delirious.'†
(3) 'We noticed that in every case the man seemed to have caught "a chill" first.'
(4) 'In a number of instances "a chill" was undoubtedly brought on by men throwing off clothing during the night.'

Yet, although the epidemic of malaria, when it did occur, seems to have been unrecognised, an attempt was indeed made to enforce one line of preventive medicine by means of quinine prophylaxis. Quinine was available in good supply, and, from the beginning the whole party was instructed to swallow an unspecified number of tablets each day. But, as evidenced in the record,‡ this routine proved difficult to enforce and probably fell into abeyance in most cases.

It is a redeeming feature in this story to know that this attempt at prophylaxis was initiated by some of the more enlightened members of the party. That it failed is regrettable, but is not surprising in the light of that long experience of the difficulty of making combatant officers aware of their responsibilities in such matters, which experience eventually led, in 1942, to the realisation that preventive medical measures must be supported and enforced by disciplinary action where necessary.§

Unfortunately, there is no record whether this quinine was used in the treatment of those persons who developed the disease. But here, it

---

* Since this narrative was completed, the senior surviving officer has given further information on this point. While agreeing that very little was done towards eradicating the mosquitoes, he has pointed out the difficulties which would have had to be faced. There were only 50 gallons of lubricating oil available in the M.L., most of which was eventually utilised as additional fuel for cooking. There seems no doubt that the very nature of the island and its vegetation was such that the breeding grounds of mosquitoes could probably only have been eliminated by a major feat of engineering far beyond the capabilities of these men.

† This patient is known to have suffered badly from malaria, off and on, for many years. It is therefore surprising that, in this particular case, the symptoms were not recognised and promulgated by the patient himself.

‡ 'One item in the drug line of which we had a good supply was quinine, and in view of the Dutch Commandant's information that the island was known as "Fever Island", we endeavoured to make everyone take a daily dose. But this was only partially successful, the men going to extraordinary lengths to avoid taking it.'

§ Reference should be made to Volume I, Chapter 12.

is only fair to admit the possibility that the disease was manifesting itself in a cerebral form, in which case such administration by an unskilled person might well have been impossible.*

Apart from the very obvious malarial epidemic which must have afflicted those on Tjebia Island, other associated medical factors are suggested on reading the record. From time to time, reference has been made to dysentery, but it is not possible accurately to identify the particular type which prevailed. A supply of Asiatic food seems certainly to have been consumed, and this may well have been infected. It would seem likely that, apart from one of the extra survivors who arrived later and who was described as severely ill from dysentery, such cases of this type of disease which did occur were bacillary rather than amoebic. But it is not impossible that both types were present. Alternatively, it is not impossible that neither bacillary nor amoebic dysentery was present on Tjebia Island, but that the symptoms of enteritis to which reference has been made were due to varieties of food poisoning or to the unaccustomed diet in which tropical fruit would seem to have played a large part.

As regards diet, it is not possible, from the record, to assess the calorie value of what was consumed daily by each individual; but there is some evidence that what food was being taken was not adequate. There is no real evidence that any true symptoms or signs of deficiency diseases made their appearance, though reference was made to what was assumed to be pellagra. Naturally, in such a fever-ridden community the debility must have been severe. But a few of these men would seem somehow to have escaped infection by malaria, or to have been infected only lightly. Nevertheless, it has been emphasised that, towards the end, even those who were not on the sick list were almost too weak to work at the final task of preparing the prau for sea. It has also been emphasised that such small strength as they did possess was rapidly fading. It will be remembered too that of the six who left Tjebia Island by sea and were then wrecked on a small rocky island off Saaya, none had the strength to cross the 50-yard channel which separated them from the main island.

Rations were greatly restricted by the end of the stay on Tjebia, and all the evidence on record suggests that quite apart from obvious tropical disease, these men were suffering too from a slow but steady process of pure starvation.

The party arrived on Tjebia with a supply of tinned food which, it was estimated, would last for about two months if carefully conserved. These stocks were augmented under the direction of a naval officer who quickly organised a food store and cookhouse from which he managed

---

* This fact has since been confirmed. Attempts were made to administer tablets of quinine to those who were sick, but it proved impossible to get them to swallow the drug. A surviving officer has estimated that of the quinine which was actually given, probably not more than $\frac{1}{10}$ could actually have been ingested and absorbed.

to produce three meals a day which were described as 'excellent if unusual'.

After the first few days most of the party already complained of feeling perpetually hungry, but this hunger would seem chiefly to have been for normal European diet rather than due to lack of quantity of supplies of various commodities. For example, three large bags of rice were discovered in the local village, as well as some tapioca flour and two drums of coconut oil which could be used for cooking. At this time, the main meals were usually composed of rice with the addition of a tinned sausage, herring or sardine or on rare occasions a slice of bully beef. The few chickens mentioned gave a small supply of eggs, and the party learned how to collect turtles eggs from time to time.

It can be seen therefore that at the beginning the food situation might well have been worse. However, in the course of some four or five weeks the stocks of tinned food, rice and tapioca were almost exhausted, and the few chickens, which were shared with the Javanese troops, had begun to be progressively reduced in number as the days passed.

It was not long before the local vegetable produce of the island had become the main part of the diet to which it had previously been but a novel addition.

At this stage, sufficiency of diet became a paramount consideration, and Tjebia Island was soon being scoured for fruit and vegetables. A type of sweet potato was discovered, which eventually became the main article of diet. The art was acquired of removing the centre out of the coconut palm, and this 'coconut cabbage' was described as 'not unlike celery when eaten raw and cabbage when cooked'. Bananas* and papaya were abundant. Limes were plentiful, and there were pineapples available in small numbers.

Occasionally, a meal of fish was obtained, but this was rare and only possible when visiting islanders were able to supply part of their catch. For some reason unexplained, although members of the party constantly attempted to catch fish themselves, they never met with success.†

Therefore, after the first month, the basis of the diet was tropical fruit, with coconuts which were inexhaustible in supply. But a time came, during the last two or three weeks, when the consumption of fruit was constantly exceeding the supply. Also, the increasing weakness of

---

* One of the surviving officers stated: 'Towards the end of our stay I found I could comfortably eat up to forty bananas a day.'

† In the words of one officer: 'One of the extraordinary things about the whole of this period was our failure to catch the fish which would have been such a great help to our diet. We knew that the sea was swarming with many kinds of edible fish, which the local inhabitants of the islands seemed to have no trouble in catching. From the earliest days we tried with nets and with all kinds of lines, but with equally little success. The only success we did achieve was by stunning the fish by firing a rifle at the sea over the top of a shoal. The impact of the bullet striking the water sometimes stunned one or two fish, but they mostly recovered and got away before they could be picked up.'

the party restricted their ability to search for fruit in the jungle, with the result that coconuts, limes and bananas were the only things which they could obtain without great effort towards the end. To this shortage was added the increasing distaste which most of these survivors felt for the limited type of food which they could obtain. Hence the process of starvation which was gradually and insidiously overcoming them.

It must not be imagined that the officers of this party failed completely to initiate a number of measures of preventive medicine. Such a suggestion would not be true. These men did a great deal, and their mistakes of omission were in no way due to negligence. Rather were these mistakes due to ignorance coupled, perhaps, with many misguided traditions. Although the abandoned village was selected as the place in which to settle, a measure of cleanliness was achieved and strict 'Service Routine' established as regards such matters as working and cleaning parties. Nevertheless, it would seem that such hygienic precautions as were attempted were based upon many of the traditional customs and beliefs handed down through generations of sailors and soldiers on tropical service. For example, great stress was laid on the dangers of remaining uncovered in bed at night.

> 'To the very end we experienced the greatest difficulty in trying to get the majority to obey any orders or instructions in this respect.'

The dangers too were emphasised of eating unripe fruit, and in this respect, it was recorded, somewhat naïvely, that 'some men got the most unpleasant sores from unripe fruit such as pineapples'!

Thus it can be seen that there is a distinct possibility that outmoded custom and tradition held sway at the expense of more elementary and effective measures which were probably overlooked.

One of the features most open to criticism is the admission that it proved impossible to enforce such hygienic measures as were adopted. This difficulty of enforcement is something for which all due allowance must be made, however. To instil and enforce hygienic discipline is sometimes difficult enough in the case of troops who are physically and mentally fit. The men on Tjebia Island were neither. To maintain strict hygienic discipline is difficult enough even under peace-time conditions. But the men on Tjebia, some of whom were survivors from H.M.Ss. *Prince of Wales* and *Repulse*, recently sunk by the Japanese, had been involved in prolonged fighting in Singapore. They had escaped with great difficulty. Finally, they had been hunted by the Japanese up to the very moment of their arrival on Tjebia.

These men could be regarded as neither physically nor mentally normal, and it is to be wondered that their subsequent endurance was as high as it proved to be.

It is possible that hygienic discipline among them could have been better enforced had they themselves been in a better state of mental and physical health. But, from the beginning, physical health was something which they could not hope to preserve, living as they did. As sickness overwhelmed them, already mentally bruised as they were, so did their morale begin to suffer, resulting in that apathy and sense of despair which has been described above.

That this should have been the case bears out in full the claim made by Sir Sheldon Dudley, that:

> 'The enforcing of hygiene measures to preserve the health, morale and fighting efficiency of troops is as important as any other military duty.'

This statement is borne out by the experiences on Tjebia Island, where tropical sickness lowered the morale not only of the sick, but of those who managed to survive. Here again, mood was indeed the mirror of morale, and to those few on Tjebia Island who recognised this fact is due the greatest tribute. There was a small number of officers and men who managed somehow to make a stand against adversity. To these few, those who did survive undoubtedly owe their lives, and to no one more than the lieutenant commander, R.N., from whose personal records it has been possible to piece together this story.*

THE FALL OF HONG KONG

The garrison of Hong Kong was informed that the British Empire and Japan were at war, at 0645 hours on December 8, 1941, and the order for the cessation of all military resistance was given at 1515 hours on December 25, 1941.†

Various Naval and Royal Marine units took part in the strenuous defence of Hong Kong and, in spite of their recognised weakness, they carried out their duties, in very difficult circumstances, with the utmost gallantry.‡ Not the least of these units to fulfil the true traditions of the Senior Service was the Royal Naval Hospital, Hong Kong, and the events which led up to its final capture by the enemy when the Colony was forced to surrender on Christmas Day 1941, are worthy of being fully recorded.

By that time this hospital had contrived, for seventeen days, to perform its work of mercy with the battle raging around it. Casualties which consisted of Service and civilian patients, both European and Asiatic were received continually. The hospital is alleged to have been

---

* This officer, happily, is still serving afloat in the Royal Navy. After the war he was decorated for: 'Outstanding resource, bravery and initiative in action against the Japanese at Singapore in February 1942, and during the days which followed.'

† Supplement to the *London Gazette* No. 38190, page 704, para. 14 and page 724, para. 150.

‡ Supplement to the *London Gazette* No. 38190, page 700, para. 8, page 703, paras. 4 and 6, page 713, para. 63 (w) and page 720, para. 117.

hit approximately one hundred times by bombs* and shells, and to these dangers were added the hazards of machine-gun and rifle fire.

Supplies of gas, electricity and water soon failed, the operating theatres were wrecked during early enemy attacks, and other buildings were later demolished.

Towards the end, the pathetic predicament of this hospital can be appreciated by the fact that, for washing purposes, only one bowl of water was available between each twelve patients. Operations were carried out by candlelight in a passage between two wards. A patient in bed was struck by a shell fragment. The dead were buried under shell-fire in the grounds of the hospital.

Through all this the medical officers, nursing sisters and sick berth staff worked ceaselessly, and never failed to display that quiet and undemonstrative devotion to duty which is the essence of their vocation. Even during the last twenty-four hours when the battle had reached its peak and when the numbness of despair must have been looming largely, they did not fail. On Christmas Eve a Carol Service was held, and to the accompaniment of exploding shells and tumbling debris, a young naval sick berth attendant played a harmonium and led the singing. On Christmas Day, tradition was maintained in the face of a fate unknown, and the patients were given a Christmas dinner of roast beef and Christmas pudding procured somehow by the Chaplain, and even a tot of rum was not forgotten.

For the next twenty-one days after the capitulation, the hospital staff continued to attend to their patients and managed to restore some order out of the existing chaos. Then, with the knowledge that their work was well done, they marched away into captivity, there to undergo a further ordeal which they endured with equal fortitude.

It is considered that, as a lasting record, no better account of what was experienced in the Royal Naval Hospital, Hong Kong, can be set down than the following official reports by the Principal Medical Officer and Matron of the hospital.†

---

* This allegation is at variance with para. 11 (g) on page 701 of the Supplement to the *London Gazette* No. 38190, in which Japanese bombing is described as most accurate and confined to military objectives.

† The narrative of three nursing sisters in R.N. Hospital, Hong Kong, included in Chapter 5 of Volume I has treated the subject only from the more personal viewpoint of the Nursing Service.

This modified plan of the R.N. Hospital will help to make the ensuing text clear.

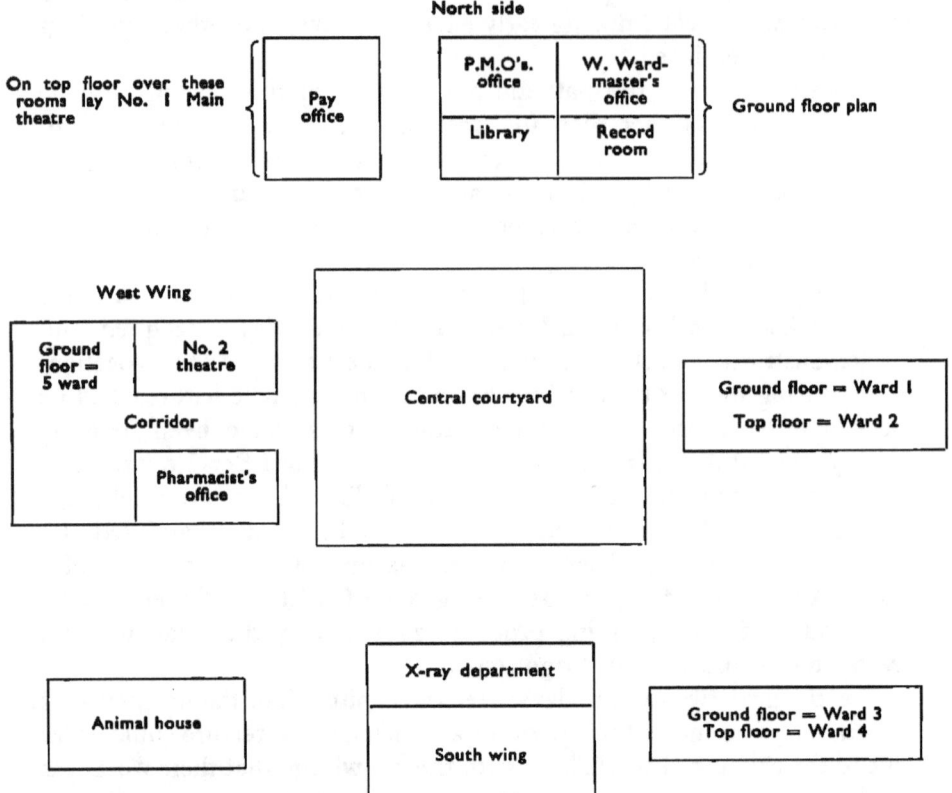

REPORT OF THE P.M.O. OF THE R.N. HOSPITAL, HONG KONG*

The 1st Day: December 8, 1941

On this day, all patients possible were discharged to duty. The remaining patients were transferred to No. 5 Ward on the ground floor. Gas masks were placed on bedside lockers, and each patient was given a wash-hand bowl as head protection and a mattress with which to cover himself during an air raid.

The prepared organisation for receiving and dealing with casualties was finally checked. All casualties were to be received in No. 1 Ward

---

* The Principal Medical Officer was a surgeon commander, R.N. He was later decorated, the citation reading: 'This officer worked untiringly in the interests of prisoners-of-war until his removal to Japan on April 20, 1944. He did at least a dozen urgent abdominal operations in the most primitive conditions. The Japanese refused to allow him to take his instruments into the prisoner-of-war camp, and he was never allowed the use of a properly equipped operating theatre. His only operating knife was a razor blade. He was a most trusted and sought after medical officer and, in spite of his own hardship, his services were always available to anyone needing them. His work is undoubtedly deserving of recognition.'

where they would receive first aid and resuscitation. They would then be transferred either to No. 2 Theatre and thence to No. 5 Ward, or to No. 3 Ward direct. The latter ward was reserved for minor surgical cases and for all medical cases.

The medical specialist* was in charge of No. 1 Ward and was assisted by 1 nursing sister, 1 L.S.B.A. and 2 A.N.S. nurses. A surgeon lieutenant commander, R.N., was in charge of No. 3 Ward, assisted by the same reception staff.

The Principal Medical Officer, who also performed the duties of surgical specialist, was in charge of No. 5 Ward and the operating theatres and also directed passive defence and the general administration of the establishment. He had an operating theatre staff of 1 nursing sister, 2 A.N.S. nurses and 1 sick berth rating. The Matron of the hospital was in charge of officer patients and the general nursing organisation of the hospital as well as its catering.

On this day 10 A.N.S. nurses were enrolled from the local voluntary organisation.†

A large supply of coal was ordered, as well as food and passive defence stores.

Passive defence arrangements were finally completed during this day, the Chinese employees of the hospital being divided into parties under the direction of sick berth staff. Other Chinese employees were also sent from the R.N. Dockyard, Hong Kong.

Blackout arrangements and lighting were in good working order, and continued to be so for some days.

The 18 sick berth staff of the hospital were augmented by 3 R.A.F. medical orderlies.

The 2nd Day: December 9, 1941

Continued air-raid alarms caused much time to be wasted, and it was decided that the hospital staff must carry on work, under cover, on the ground floor.

The hospital air-raid shelter was in the Pharmacist's Store. The walls were very thick, and the store was divided by two partitions with large shelves which were made into bunks and fitted with mattresses. At the beginning, these bunks were used as sleeping billets for the night duty staff, but later, all the staff slept in this shelter.

On this day the first trouble arose with the Chinese employees, who always ran down to the tunnels under the hospital when an air raid

---

* A surgeon lieutenant commander, R.N., who later died while a prisoner-of-war.

† This Auxiliary Nursing Service is believed to have been due to an order of the Hong Kong Government that any women remaining in the Colony after the evacuation of women and children in 1940, were to be prepared to carry out nursing duties, should hostilities occur, unless employed on other essential work. For some months before the outbreak of war with Japan, a number of these women had been undergoing practical nursing training each day at the Royal Naval Hospital, Hong Kong.

started. Here they would remain and refuse to emerge to perform their passive defence duties. It was necessary therefore to lock the entrance to the tunnels. Thereupon, the Chinese threatened to leave the hospital altogether. They only agreed to remain provided they were permitted to shelter in a baggage room attached to No. 1 Ward. But, with a few exceptions, these Chinese were petrified with fear during air attacks.*

The 3rd Day: December 10, 1941

Food rationing was instituted on this day.

The 4th Day: December 11, 1941

One chief petty officer was admitted in a very shocked condition with a wound of left foot and ankle joint.†

Four Chinese casualties were admitted, and after emergency operation were transferred to one of the civil hospitals during the night.

The Chinese employees lent by the dockyard for passive defence duties did not appear and were never again available for this duty.

The 5th Day: December 12, 1941

The first shell landed inside the hospital area. From this time onwards the hospital laundry was out of action, and all washing had to be done in one of the ward bathrooms.‡ The sterilising plant was also put out of action. Fortunately an ample supply of sterile drums and emergency dressings had been prepared. After this day all sterilising was carried out at the Bowen Road Military Hospital.

The 6th Day: December 13, 1941

Three surgical casualties were admitted on this day.

Arrangements were made for Army casualties to be admitted as necessary.

On this day the Chinese hospital coolies again threatened to leave, their grievance being that they were not permitted to join their families in the tunnels under the hospital during the night. Finally, in order to prevent them leaving, permission to join their families at night had to be conceded. As a number of these Chinese were employed as crew of the trailer pump, it was arranged that the hospital pharmacist and one member of the sick berth staff should learn to work this machine in case of an emergency. This foresight proved to be wise, as a time came when the Chinese crew of the trailer pump was no longer available.

---

* To retain these men, the Principal Medical Officer was forced to offer bonuses to the higher grade Chinese workmen and to double the pay of the ordinary coolies.

† This man's left leg was amputated, below the knee, the next day.

‡ Drying lines were also placed across the hospital tennis court and at other places in the grounds. But, in the words of the Principal Medical Officer: 'It was disappointing work. No sooner was the washing put out than shell fragments would land and either soil or destroy it.'

The 7th and 8th Days: December 14 and 15, 1941

These were fairly uneventful days except for a fair amount of shelling. During a lull the pharmacist and one sick berth attendant were leaning over a balcony behind the sick berth staff quarters when a shell burst immediately underneath the balcony supports. By good fortune, neither was hurt.

The 9th Day: December 16, 1941

A number of casualties was admitted at about 1500 hours. From then until 0500 hours the next day, the P.M.O. was operating continuously. The cases included one amputation through the left shoulder, one amputation through the left thigh and an officer with severe multiple gunshot wounds and a spinal paralysis.

The 10th Day: December 17, 1941

On this day the hospital's hot water system failed, and from then onwards all hot water had to be fetched from the galley and surgical instruments had to be boiled over a large four-jet primus stove.

The ward work had now become much heavier. Fortunately the hospital possessed a special spinal bed in which the wounded officer could be nursed. This patient was so heavy and had so many wounds that to move him in any other way would have been impossible.*

The 11th Day: December 18, 1941

There were only a few casualties on this day, but air raids and shelling became so heavy that ward work was greatly interfered with.

The beds were kept close up against the walls between the double windows of the wards. These windows were kept full open, but their 'typhoon shutters' were kept closed. This made the wards very dark but gave a modicum of protection against bomb and shell splinters.

On this day the zymotic wing of the hospital became a complete wreck as shells continually exploded in it.

In the evening two large bombs exploded in the road outside and interrupted communications with the Military Hospital.

In the evening news was received that the Japanese had landed, and later, in pouring rain, a small number of Army casualties was admitted.

The 12th Day: December 19, 1941

Many casualties were received from the strenuous fighting in the Wong Nei Chong Gap in which units of the Royal Navy took part. The Principal Medical Officer was again operating for several hours.

---

* This patient recovered.

On this day the electricity and water supplies failed. The hospital now had to rely on the underground water tanks in its grounds. The water was chlorinated and carried from these tanks in buckets.

The failure of electricity meant that the hospital X-ray apparatus could no longer be used, and this lack of X-rays naturally embarrassed the efficient treatment of casualties.

The 13th Day: December 20, 1941

This day started badly. A bomb* exploded outside No. 5 Ward, about 12 ft. from its wall. The blast shattered a number of the 'typhoon doors' and filled the ward with acrid smoke and dust. The main water and sewage pipes were fractured, which meant that the kitchens and lavatories of Nos. 5 and 6 Wards were out of action.

There were no casualties from this explosion.

During this day the hospital came under heavy and continuous shell fire from two directions, Kowloon Wharf and Leighton Hill, and the following were the main incidents of damage:

P.M.O's. residence. A shell burst in the drawing room.
The Sisters' Quarters.† Many direct hits, with the roof and top floor completely wrecked.
Sick Berth Staff Quarters.
Pharmacist's residence.
No. 2 Ward. Shell pierced the roof.
No. 4 Ward. Shells pierced the roof.
Main Operating Theatre. Shells pierced the roof.

The sick berth staff worked valiantly in repairing the damage of No. 5 Ward, and got it into reasonable working condition within a short time.

On this day a large sanitary pit was dug in the front lawn of the hospital in which soiled dressings and ward refuse could be placed. It was realised that this situation was not ideal, being too near to the water tanks. But steps were taken to chlorinate the refuse thoroughly, and in any case, it was necessary for the pit to be near the wards.‡

In the evening about 20 wounded sepoys were admitted to No. 1 Ward. These were also casualties from Wong Nei Chong Gap.

The 14th Day: December 21, 1941

Shelling continued over and around the hospital. By this time it had been noted that the enemy shelling usually commenced at about 1000

---

* According to the records, this would seem to be the only bomb which fell inside the hospital boundaries.

† It is to be regretted that some of the Chinese coolies took advantage of this confusion and looted the sisters' quarters at this time. They stole a considerable number of the personal belongings of the nursing sisters and then fled from the hospital.

‡ The Principal Medical Officer remarked that this fly-breeding nuisance caused much extra work after hostilities had ceased.

hours daily, after which time it was necessary to cover the patients up for protection. As a routine, therefore, all wound dressings were started very early in the morning, and were completed each day before 1000 hours. Needless to say, it was necessary to keep a large number of patients morphinised almost the whole time.

One Admiralty civilian employee was admitted with a severe wound of spine.*

The 15th Day: December 22, 1941

Shelling continued as usual.

In spite of the efforts of the staff, dirty linen had now accumulated, and there was a shortage of bed linen and clothing. Candles were also in great demand for lighting. The Naval Chaplain, who made many visits to the hospital, procured a large number of new sheets from the local Fleet Club which proved invaluable.

Graves had now to be dug in the gardens of the hospital, and this same Naval Chaplain conducted two funeral services.†

On this day the local Naval Passive Defence Officer‡ procured a quantity of candles and extra clothing for the hospital.

The 16th Day: December 23, 1941

Shelling continued, and by now, troops were in action on each side of the hospital, and machine-gun fire was very close outside the walls. Sniping also became a danger inside the hospital boundaries.§

On this day casualties included two Admiralty civilian employees.

The 17th Day: Christmas Eve 1941

Shelling continued and the hospital received a great deal of further damage. For example:

(1) A shell burst just outside the west end of No. 5 Ward.‖ A fragment of shrapnel pierced the 'typhoon shutter', and wounded one of the bed casualties.¶

---

* This patient recovered.

† These two burials were both of Royal Scots other ranks. One had been received dead on December 18, and the other, who was admitted with his left arm completely pulped, never rallied sufficiently to come to operation.

‡ A lieutenant, R.N.V.R., this officer made daily visits to the hospital and performed many useful tasks on its behalf. Each day he brought any stores which might be required and took away with him all weapons which had been removed from casualties. He also took the written record of daily admissions to the Office of the Commodore, R.N., so that the latter was aware of the presence in hospital of these casualties.

§ It is on record that the Matron went into a bedroom by candlelight, and was narrowly missed by a bullet which entered through the window.

‖ Owing to steeply sloping ground, it had proved impossible to build the usual hollow brick wall for protection at this point.

¶ This man was an Army corporal, who subsequently made a rapid recovery.

(2) A shell exploded outside the wall of the side-cabin of No. 5 Ward. A large fragment passed through the 'typhoon shutters' of the cabin, cut the electric light flex, traversed the substantial door of the cabin, passed across a corridor and came to rest buried in the door of the operating theatre. There were two bed patients in the cabin itself and people were standing on either side of the door of the theatre. Nevertheless, no person was hit!

On this day the Commodore, R.N., who himself had visited the hospital almost daily, brought H.E. The Governor of Hong Kong on a tour of inspection.

Later on this day, the Royal Naval Hospital, Hong Kong, found itself so much in the centre of the battle raging outside, that the P.M.O. frequently had to order off the premises groups of British soldiers who were attempting to take up strategic positions there. Also, having now been warned that the enemy might filter into the hospital at any time, the P.M.O. ordered all the valuables taken from patients for safe custody to be returned to them.*

The Last Day: Christmas Day 1941

Until the capitulation, fighting was severe on the Bowen Road, and all round the hospital in Wanchai, and up to the very end the hospital itself continued to be badly damaged.

(1) A mortar shell lodged behind the staircase of one of the hospital residences and failed to explode.

(2) Another hospital residence was struck by two shells, one of which passed through the wall and ended up, without exploding, on a landing outside a bedroom which was occupied by one of the nursing sisters at the time.

(3) A shell exploded at the entrance of one of the A.R.P. tunnels. Unfortunately, persons were standing nearby, and one of them had his left arm completely shattered. He was at once admitted to the hospital in a desperate condition and, as neither operating theatre was now usable, the Principal Medical Officer operated on this casualty and amputated his arm, by candlelight, in a corridor leading to No. 5 Ward.†

---

* In the words of the Principal Medical Officer: 'I disbursed all valuables to their owners to keep themselves, rather than that I should be forced to open my safe and surrender them'.

† This casualty was a Methodist Chaplain, R.N. He rallied well after operation, but unfortunately died the following day from delayed shock. He was buried in the garden of the Principal Medical Officer's residence. It is worthy of note that the Principal Medical Officer recorded: 'This was the only patient that I lost soon after operation, though three died subsequently from complications'.

In September 1943, all the bodies buried in the gardens of R.N. Hospital, Hong Kong, were re-interred in a common grave over which was placed a granite stone with a suitable inscription. A Service of Dedication was conducted by a Buddhist Priest and the ceremony was attended by a number of Japanese Naval Officers.

Eventually, on this day, the fighting outside died down, and news was then received of the capitulation.

At this point in his report, the P.M.O. placed on record his tribute to his medical and nursing staffs:

> 'It is difficult to make an appreciation of my medical staff, who could not have been more helpful nor remained more calm. I cannot adequately express my feelings of gratitude and affection for them.
>
> 'The three members of Queen Alexandra's Royal Naval Nursing Service were equally tireless and uncomplaining. They worked continuously. The Superintending Sister is especially deserving of praise.
>
> 'As regards the sick berth staff, I shall never forget their absolute tirelessness and cheerful willingness.'*

Also, at this point in his report, the P.M.O. makes reference to an apparent departure from the plans originally made for this hospital in the event of hostilities breaking out in Hong Kong. In his own words:

> 'We had originally planned to evacuate the hospital to Aberdeen† should the enemy arrive in Kowloon or should the hospital be rendered useless or untenable. But in the actual event, this seemed to me to be unnecessary, as Aberdeen would have been at least as dangerous and necessarily much less efficient.‡ On more than one occasion after December 20, the Commodore, R.N., asked me whether I advised evacuating the hospital. I knew that some of our worst casualties could not stand any journey, and I advised against transfer. I have no regrets on this point.'§

THE AFTERMATH

The period from December 26, 1941 to January 18, 1942

Immediately news of the capitulation was received, steps were taken to try to get the hospital into good working order. About a dozen of the Chinese staff returned, including three laundrymen, two cooks and some labouring coolies.

Many of the broken water pipes and punctured tanks were repaired, sanitary pits were dug and debris was cleared away. Large tarpaulins were placed over the holes in the roofs of Wards No. 2 and 4 and of the main operating theatre. Quantities of wood were cut into logs, and a store of coal was accumulated by hand.

---

* It is of interest that, owing to man-power difficulties and outside commitments, the sick berth staff of R.N. Hospital Hong Kong was nine short of the normal peace-time complement at this time.

† There was a small naval sick quarters in the district of Aberdeen, which was under the direction of a surgeon lieutenant, R.N.V.R., assisted by sick berth ratings of the Royal Naval Base, Hong Kong.

‡ This view is confirmed by the Supplement to the *London Gazette* No. 38190, page 706, para. 26 and page 710, para. 48 (c).

§ Needless to say, this attitude of the Principal Medical Officer was correct and was confirmed by his Higher Executive Authority.

One of the most important incidents of Boxing Day was the arrival at the hospital of a R.A.F. ambulance which had been preserved by an Admiralty and a R.A.F. employee, both English civilians. As the hospital had no transport of its own, this ambulance proved invaluable for the collection of provisions. On January 28 the Japanese provided the Principal Medical Officer and one of his medical staff each with a pass which permitted them to use this ambulance for the collection of food and the transfer of patients.

At the time of the capitulation there were 120 patients in the hospital. During the next fortnight 18 patients were received from the Queen Mary Hospital and 15 patients from the University Hospital. To make room for these extra patients, a number of Indian patients was transferred to the Tung Wah Hospital. The result was that, within a few days, food had to be provided for approximately 140 patients and a staff of 35. This food was obtained by a surgeon lieutenant commander, R.N., who visited the local Food Controller each day, and was very successful in obtaining supplies of flour, rice, beans and occasionally meat.*

Meanwhile the P.M.O. was operating almost continuously for some days and patients needing surgical attention continued to be received from other hospitals.

By the middle of January 1942, the work of the hospital was proceeding very smoothly and most of the patients were making a good recovery.

From the time of the capitulation, Japanese officials had been visiting the hospital almost daily. Finally, at 1000 hours on January 18, 1942, the P.M.O. was ordered by the Japanese to be prepared to evacuate the hospital by 1700 hours on the same day, and to transfer his patients and staff to St. Albert's Convent.

These orders entailed an enormous amount of work at short notice. Ten dangerously ill patients were transferred to Bowen Road Hospital, and called for very careful handling. Everything possible was done to transfer food and equipment at the same time.

In addition to organising this transfer, the P.M.O. was constantly harried by the Japanese Authorities. Finally, he had formally to conduct a Japanese officer over every room of the entire hospital, afterwards surrendering the keys to him. In the words of the P.M.O.:

> 'It is not surprising that, with these various duties on my hands, I had no time to attend to my personal belongings. I lost my attaché case with all my private papers, receipts, valuables and many of the hospital records. The Superintending Sister similarly lost her attaché case with many of her valuables and records. At first, the sisters and nurses were told that they would be permitted to take only one valise each, but, after representations, I managed to get permission for them to take much more. But even so, they lost a very considerable amount of their personal belongings.'

---

* As none of the hospital refrigerators was in working order, such meat as was obtained had to be brined.

One of the primary burdens, and one which weighed heavily on the shoulders of the P.M.O., was that he was responsible for the finances of the Royal Naval Hospital, Hong Kong, as well as the cash and valuables of his patients. He distributed equally among the members of his sick berth staff the proceeds of the staff canteen funds. Patients' cash and valuables had already been returned to them.* The remaining hospital funds he employed in the purchase of extra food, hire of coolies and the purchase of quantities of petrol at an inflated price.

St. Albert's Convent, January 18 to February 25, 1942

The convent of St. Albert, Hong Kong, had been previously converted into a hospital by the Royal Army Medical Corps. On January 18, 1942 this hospital was commanded by a lieutenant colonel, R.A.M.C. and it also accommodated the Commanding Officer and medical staff of the Tung Wah Hospital which had been evacuated a few days before.

On their arrival, the staff and patients from the Royal Naval Hospital, Hong Kong, were given a most cordial reception and everything possible was done to assist them. Part of the second and third floors of the hospital were set aside for their accommodation.

The Navy put its equipment and food supplies into the communal store and, in the words of the P.M.O.:

'During our stay at St. Albert's, we received far more from this store than we had ever put into it.'

From the day of their arrival at St. Albert's Convent, the naval medical officers and nursing staff from the Royal Naval Hospital, Hong Kong, were required by the Japanese to be constantly at twenty-four hours' notice to move elsewhere. This made their lives extremely uncertain, particularly as regards food for the future as, by this time, it was well realised that in the months or even years ahead food might mean ultimate survival. The Principal Medical Officer has stated:

'As always, securing food was one of our constant preoccupations for we never knew when we should be leaving or what we should be allowed to take with us. It was very difficult to plan our rations under such circumstances.'

During the period at St. Albert's Convent, the Principal Medical Officer himself showed some degree of reduced physical health which is hardly surprising considering the strain which he had undergone. He developed four separate whitlows, two on each hand, which finally had to be incised by one of his naval colleagues.

On February 24, 1942 the P.M.O. was informed that the naval staff from Hong Kong Hospital were to be ready to leave St. Albert's Convent

---

* In his report the Principal Medical Officer states: 'In my capacity as Accountant Officer to the R.N. Hospital, I made every effort to see that patients should not lose their valuables. No patient lost anything'

on the following day. This meant virtually the final splitting of the naval party as an individual unit.

On the morning of February 25, naval patients were transferred to Bowen Road Hospital with the exception of those who had almost recovered, who were sent to North Point Prisoner-of-War Camp. The P.M.O. and naval nursing sisters were transferred to Bowen Road Military Hospital. The remaining naval medical officers were sent to the Military Hospital in St. Theresa's Convent, Kowloon. The naval sick berth staff were sent as prisoners-of-war to North Point Camp.*

The P.M.O. remained at the Military Hospital, Bowen Road, until July, 1942, after which he was transferred to the prisoner-of-war camp at Argyle Street, Kowloon. He remained in this camp until May 1944.

In the prisoner-of-war camp at Argyle Street, conditions were very primitive and most unsuitable for the nursing of long-term cases. Nevertheless, it was only possible to transfer patients to one of the hospitals at very infrequent intervals. While at Argyle Street, the Principal Medical Officer operated on four cases of perforated duodenal ulcer and two of acute appendicitis.†

In May 1944, the P.M.O. of R.N. Hospital, Hong Kong, together with six other medical officers,‡ was moved to Sham Shui prisoner-of-war camp. He then embarked on a merchant ship which was carrying scrap metal from Hong Kong to Japan.

There were some 250 prisoners-of-war on board this ship, who were accommodated in one of the holds. The journey, broken by a short call at Formosa, was rendered more uncomfortable by the dysentery from which many of the prisoners-of-war were suffering.

---

* It would seem that the hospital at Bowen Road was intended to receive Royal Naval and Canadian sick from North Point Prisoner-of-War Camp. The hospital in St. Theresa's Convent was apparently intended for the treatment of sick British prisoners-of-war in captivity on the Kowloon side of Hong Kong. It is obvious from his report that the Principal Medical Officer was greatly concerned that his medical and nursing staffs should be split up at this time, for, naturally, he regarded their welfare as his personal responsibility.

Also obvious is his evident anxiety about the medical arrangements inside North Point Camp itself, and he made repeated representations to the Japanese Authorities on this matter as well as arranging the delivery of several consignments of drugs to the camp. The Army Medical Authorities also gave valuable assistance with drugs for this camp.

But the gravity of the difficulties with which this Principal Medical Officer had to contend are illustrated by the failure of his efforts to arrange for the continuity of the treatment of naval venereal patients in the camp to be maintained.

' I arranged for the genito-urinary specialist to be motored to the camp with a supply of novarsenobenzol and the records of all naval patients under treatment so that this treatment could be continued. The Japanese Authorities would not allow him to enter the camp!'

† In a letter to the Editor of this History, the Principal Medical Officer has written: 'These operations were performed under very primitive conditions indeed, which shows that the Japs would not play on the transport, or any other side'.

‡ 1 R.N.V.R., 1 I.M.S. and 4 R.A.M.C.

The journey ended at a port in Southern Japan where the Principal Medical Officer and a number of other Service doctors were landed and sent by train to Tokyo.

At Tokyo, three of these medical officers, including the P.M.O. of R.N. Hospital, Hong Kong, were employed at Shinagawa Prisoner-of-War Hospital. This hospital was the main reception centre for sick prisoners-of-war from all the camps in the Tokyo area. It was, however, most primitive, consisting of wooden huts with straw mats. There were no cots and there was no heating. The latrines were cisterns which had to be baled out once a week.

The P.M.O. remained at Shinagawa until released after the Japanese capitulation. Ostensibly, he performed surgical and administrative duties. But, in reality, and in his own words:

'We did what we were told, and did it "at the double". We did our medical work when we were not labouring in the fields or swimming for logs in the harbour. We had to collect the wood, saw and chop it, etc., for all our fuel which we needed for cooking, burning the dead, etc.'

When permitted to do so, the P.M.O. performed a number of surgical operations. As regards these operations, he has noted that no operation case ever developed pneumonia, despite the lack of heating in the hospital and the grim coldness of the Tokyo winter. He has attributed this fact largely to the splendid spinal anaesthetics which were given for him by one of his American colleagues.*

REPORT OF THE MATRON† OF THE R.N. HOSPITAL, HONG KONG‡

On December 8, 1941, when the Japanese assault on Hong Kong started, any patients who could be sent to duty immediately left the hospital. The remaining officers and men were accommodated in wards and cabins on the ground floor. The casualty ward was prepared for the resuscitation of wounded.

A sister was placed in charge of this casualty ward and of the adjacent ward for medical and minor surgical cases. A second sister took charge of the acute surgical ward and acted as theatre sister.

---

* A Captain of the United States Army Dental Corps.

† 'Matron' is here used for convenience. In point of fact, the correct designation, prior to 1943, would have been Superintending Sister. This latter rank was replaced by 'Matron' on April 1, 1943, following the recommendations of the Rushcliffe Committee. The reader is referred to the Chapter on Queen Alexandra's Royal Naval Nursing Service in Volume I.

‡ This person was appointed Matron-in-Chief of the Navy in July 1947. She held this appointment until August 12, 1950, when she retired from Queen Alexandra's Royal Naval Nursing Service. During this period she was appointed K.H.N.S.; she also was appointed Commander of the Most Excellent Order of the British Empire.

The Matron was responsible for officers and ratings in cabins; also the hospital catering, and she endeavoured to assist wherever help was required and also relieved the other two sisters from time to time.

At 0200 hours on December 11, shells started falling in Hong Kong. There was now a possibility of the hospital having to be evacuated to Aberdeen and, in view of this, supplies of linen, food, china and cutlery were prepared for transfer. However, before any transfer could be effected, Aberdeen itself was severely shelled.

On the following day, owing to the wrecking, by shellfire, of the sisters' mess, personal belongings and a certain amount of furniture were moved to one of the hospital residences. But it was still possible to use the sisters' mess for cooking and eating meals.*

The Chinese domestic staff soon ran away from the hospital. Unfortunately, they first ransacked the sisters' mess and stole quantities of money and articles of personal value.

Sisters and nurses were placed on a system of rationing on December 11. On December 14, the Matron obtained a quantity of food from the local Chinese contractor which included two sides of bacon, four boxes of cheese, cases of dried apples, apricots and prunes and various tinned foods.†

Gas and electricity supplies failed about December 19, and shortly after this the water main to the hospital became useless. The failure of electricity entailed work being carried on by candlelight not only at night, but also by day. This was because the wards were dark through the closing of the 'typhoon shutters' which was necessary to give protection from splinters and draughts.‡ No sterilisers, electric kettles or bed-cradles could be used, and the X-ray plant ceased to work. All drinking water had to be boiled and fetched from the main galley.

This cessation of water supply was really the most serious of the hospital's problems. For a time, use was made of the static water tanks from which it was possible to pump water into the main hospital tanks. But, after two days, the latter were rendered useless by shrapnel holes. One bowl of water had to be used for washing anything from six to twelve patients. For scrubbing up, one bowl of water had to be made to last a whole morning.

When off duty, sisters and nurses had little rest because, apart from the noise of shells and bombs, as the domestic staff had mostly deserted, they had to fetch and carry stores and water and prepare their own meals.

---

* 'We continued to have meals in our mess, until the kitchen stove was demolished!'

† The Matron could only obtain these supplies by paying for them with her personal cheque.

‡ The Matron's report is the only one which draws attention to the cold which prevailed in the hospital at this time. It was winter, the hospital lacked any form of heating and most of the glass in the windows had been shattered.

Nursing duties were very strenuous by day and by night. During air raids and heavy shelling, only one member of the sick berth staff could be spared for each ward as the remainder were required for fire parties and demolition squads as part of the hospital's 'passive defence' organisation. This often happened for long periods on end, so that the few sisters and nurses had all they could do to manage even the minimum requirements of nursing duties.

Casualties of all kinds and of all nationalities were received day after day. They included a number of Chinese men and women who were too severely injured to be moved elsewhere.* Wounded Indian soldiers and police were also received. The nursing staff soon became familiar with the management of casualties straight from the battle, even to the extent of taking possession of their weapons.†

On Christmas Eve, the Commodore, R.N., accompanied His Excellency the Governor round the hospital.

'This visit undoubtedly gave us all much comfort and encouragement.'‡

At this point in her report, the Matron pays tribute to the devotion which the local Royal Naval Chaplain displayed towards the welfare of patients and staff. In her words:

'On numerous occasions he came to the hospital and provided cigarettes and chocolate, the latter being particularly useful to hand round to the nursing staff at meal times when it was unsafe for them to go to their various messes. He also managed to obtain excellent beef, Christmas puddings, apples, oranges and sweets so that the patients were thus able to have a good Christmas dinner.§

'On the afternoon of Christmas Eve, the Chaplain held a Carol Service which all the off-duty staff and convalescent and less seriously wounded patients were able to attend. During this service shelling was severe and debris was falling outside the ward in which the service was held. I feel that I should like to record that a leading sick berth attendant remained at the harmonium for the whole service and played for us without faltering.'

After the capitulation on Christmas Day, the Matron was thankful that it was now possible to give more adequate attention to all patients.

---

* Several of these Chinese died of wounds.

† On removing the coat from one casualty, one of the sisters found herself holding a hand grenade with the pin out! Fortunately it did not explode, and was quickly disposed of by one of the male staff.

‡ The Matron's report states that during this visit, the Commodore's car was wrecked by a shell in the hospital grounds.

§ The Matron's report also makes mention of the kindness of the manager of one of the large British stores in Hong Kong, who sent a supply of Christmas puddings to the hospital as a gift.

It was also possible for the sisters and nurses to be given a definite period of rest in each twenty-four hours. This rest was badly needed as they were by now completely exhausted.

It was also possible to attend to the needs of the many Asiatics who now began to seek help at the hospital.*

After a few days the water supply was restored, though numerous holes in pipes projected water in all directions throughout the hospital. Some of the coolie staff were re-employed† and were kept at work for some days washing the vast accumulation of soiled linen.

Supervision of food supplies was one of the most difficult tasks of the Matron and her sisters and nurses. Tinned foods were augmented by occasional meat, fowls or deer. But these had usually been out of cold storage so long that they were on the point of putrefaction and had to be cooked immediately. In spite of the efforts which were made to maintain an adequate food supply, patients became very hungry and the strictest supervision was required over food distribution. Even drinking water, which could only be boiled on the one fire available, had to be kept under lock and key.

To add to these many difficulties, Japanese soldiers soon began to make their presence known, and they were quick to pilfer stocks of cigarettes and tinned food which had not been carefully hidden away.

To begin with, these strolling enemy soldiers caused the female nursing staff some apprehension but, in the words of the Matron:

'Apart from touching our wrists to indicate that it was watches they wanted, we suffered no harm. But had the hospital not been situated on a hill high above the main road, no doubt things would have been very different!'‡

As regards the conduct of the Japanese, the following incident, as related by the Matron, is worthy of a place in this History, recording as it does an act of quiet gallantry by the P.M.O. and the naval sick berth staff by which the thoughts of some enemy individuals were diverted from lust to loot:

'On December 30, at midnight, the hospital was invaded by some Japanese Army officers. They were interviewed by the P.M.O. who quickly ordered the two nurses on night duty to come to me with instructions that we were to lock ourselves in as best we could, while he delayed the men. When these Japanese demanded to be taken to the women's quarters, the P.M.O., at the point of a revolver, led them through the darkness to the sick berth staff mess, where they

---

* These included an Indian child who was brought in from an air-raid shelter nearby in a dying condition.

† These coolies were paid in rice.

‡ The reference here is to the sufferings of nurses in some of the other hospitals at the hands of the Japanese immediately after the capitulation.

occupied themselves in removing the watches, rings and fountain pens of the staff.'*

This incident was reported to the Japanese Authorities, who immediately placed a Japanese naval guard on the hospital and put a notice at the gate to forbid the entry of Japanese soldiers.

The presence of this Japanese naval guard, while giving some protection against such incidents as that of December 30, nevertheless was something of a mixed blessing. The sentries adopted a method of patrolling the hospital which was sinister and frightening until the staff became accustomed to it. For example:

'They usually wore black felt shoes and would appear, by day or night, in the Sisters' quarters without warning. We would not be aware of their presence until the candlelight flickered on a bayonet. The majority of the guard wore masks of white gauze.'

As an attempt to create some diversion, a concert was organised by patients and staff. But this and subsequent similar entertainments were subdued in character as the Japanese Authorities only permitted them to be held on the understanding that there was to be 'no music, no cheers, no clapping!'†

In her report, the Matron pays tribute to the conduct and bearing of her sisters and nurses. She also describes some of their truly miraculous escapes from injury before the capitulation. In her own words:

'My sisters at all times showed great presence of mind and coped sensibly with the unusual situations which they had to face.

'My casualty sister‡ adapted herself to conditions which became more and more difficult in an admirable manner and her resource and never-failing cheerfulness among staff and patients were of the utmost value.

'My theatre sister‡ carried on her work under most harassing conditions, without heating, with inadequate lighting, with makeshift sterilising and invariably during heavy shelling. Her nursing of the serious cases could not have been more ably carried out by anybody. Her personal attention to detail under these difficult circumstances was some of the finest nursing I have ever seen.

---

* It is in keeping with the reticence of the Principal Medical Officer that no mention has been made of this incident in his own official report. There is no doubt that his brave conduct and that of his sick berth staff saved his sisters and nurses from the terrifying experiences to which the nursing staff of another nearby hospital were subjected night after night at this time.

† In relation to this control of entertainment by the Japanese, an amusing story is on record.
On one occasion somebody was heard playing the British National Anthem on a piano. One of the hospital staff immediately ran to stop this playing, only to find that the offender was a Japanese sailor. This sailor then further displayed his prowess with a rendering of 'The Bluebells of Scotland', as an encore!

‡ In due course, both these nursing sisters were decorated 'for special devotion and competency in the performance of nursing duties in a Naval Hospital'.

T

'By their fearlessness and courage the sisters gave me the greatest confidence in them, and I feel that they fully lived up to the great traditions of our Service and our profession.'

Speaking of her Auxiliary Nursing Service nurses, the Matron says:

'These ladies, at all times during the hostilities, showed courage and keenness to do what their limited knowledge of nursing allowed. Their calmness and self-control during the heavy shelling did much to comfort our patients.'

On January 18, 1942, when the hospital patients and staff were transferred to St. Albert's Convent, the Matron and her staff made every effort to transfer food, bed linen and equipment at the same time. Mattress covers were filled with sheets, towels and pillow cases. Clothing and drugs were hidden under the blankets of stretcher cases as they were removed.

Unfortunately, when the staff had time to gather together their own belongings, they found that their quarters had been looted. Also, when the time came for them to leave the hospital, they were subjected to search, and all leather goods were removed from them, such as suit-cases, travelling bags and attaché cases. Certain articles of jewellery were also confiscated.

St. Albert's Auxiliary Military Hospital was a convent which had been considerably damaged during the fighting. There was accommodation for about 700 patients.

Most of the windows of the building had been shattered and many of the rooms were open to cold winds and mist. The water supply had been badly damaged and there was only one tap available on each floor. There was no electricity and lighting was by candles at first, and by lantern later.

There was some scarcity of food and the Matron has described the constant sensation of hunger which was soon felt. Nevertheless, she admits, in her own words:

'The food was excellent compared with what we were to have later on.'

On February 25, 1942, the naval nursing sisters were transferred to the Military Hospital, Bowen Road, where they reported for duty to the Matron, Queen Alexandra's Imperial Military Nursing Service. The naval sisters undertook duty in the wards set aside for tuberculous, dysentery and convalescent surgical patients.

The wards of which they had charge were very badly damaged, with windows and doors boarded up, laths hanging from the ceilings, walls shored up inside and outside and roofs leaking.

As would be expected, the accommodation for patients was the best which the hospital could offer. The accommodation for nursing staff was necessarily even more uncomfortable. However, there were certain advantages which were appreciated by the naval sisters. There was electric light, and fires could be lit as long as the fuel remained. Hot baths were also available.*

Food soon became scarce, and the daily supply of such items as bread, butter, powdered milk, cocoa and jelly was of such small quantity that it had to be locked away securely as a precaution against pilfering by hungry patients. The Matron has recorded:

> 'It was heart-breaking to watch so many cases having a retarded convalescence, entirely owing to lack of food and drugs.'

After doing much to augment the diet of their patients, the nursing staff themselves inevitably soon recognised the pangs of hunger. It was possible to purchase extra items of food in secret, with the assistance of local Chinese, but only at a very inflated price. Unfortunately the naval sisters had little money for such purchases. At the time of leaving St. Albert's Hospital, the Matron and each sister possessed but $10 and this was the sum total of their worldly wealth.† But, as in all other matters, the Army came to the assistance of the Navy and the Army Matron, for a time, was able to assist them with a little money for the purchase of vegetables from the town.‡

In May 1942 a canteen was opened in the hospital, and the P.M.O. managed to provide the Matron with Military yen 16 for the purchase of extra food.

As yet a further example of the splendid spirit which prevailed in this hospital, in June 1942 the officers of the Royal Army Medical Corps started a fund from which sisters and nurses were paid Military yen 7 per month. The naval sisters were included as beneficiaries from this fund.

In July 1942 the P.M.O. contrived to provide the naval sisters each with Military yen 10 per month from his own resources.§

Paying tribute again, the Matron of R.N. Hospital, Hong Kong, has described at length the strenuous efforts which were made by the Army Matron of Bowen Road Hospital to obtain the necessary recognition for all the nursing staff. At one time it seemed that she had succeeded in her aim, but, unfortunately, what was promised was not implemented.

---

* This was something which the naval sisters had not experienced since early in December 1941.

† This money had been given them by the P.M.O.

‡ The Matron has paid great tribute to the generosity of her Army colleague, e.g.:
'When we arrived at Bowen Road Hospital, I naturally offered the Army Matron such money as we had, towards our maintenance. But she refused to accept anything.'

§ Space has been given deliberately to this shortage of money on the part of female nursing staff in captivity. It would seem that, in spite of repeated representations, the Japanese Authorities refused to recognise nursing sisters of the Fighting Services as officer prisoners-of-war. Therefore, they were not eligible for any money allowance.

'We were led to expect it, but it did not materialise. It was indeed tantalising to suffer from lack of food, when money could have obtained adequate additions for us.'

In spite of this money provision, prices were so high and outside supplies so scarce that it soon became impossible to buy more than a little extra food. Once Army stores of food were exhausted, such bread as there was had usually to be eaten dry. The Japanese occasionally supplied sugar and salt, but the ration of meat which they provided was usually whale-meat or octopus. In due course, a further fund was inaugurated by the officers of the Royal Army Medical Corps for the provision of tinned meat, fish and tomato juice. These the sisters distributed among their patients and, though the amount was small, it was greatly appreciated.

On August 10, 1942, the female nursing staff of Bowen Road Hospital were transferred to the Civilian Internment Camp, Stanley, Hong Kong. The staff involved consisted of Queen Alexandra's Royal Naval and Imperial Military Nursing Services, together with sisters and nurses of the Hong Kong Volunteer Defence Corps Nursing Detachment.

The story of the actual transfer is best told in the words of the Matron herself:

'We were taken in buses to the waterfront in Hong Kong. We were paraded near the Law Courts. We were then addressed by Colonel Tggunaka* who told us, through an interpreter, that although he himself knew of the valuable work we had been doing for our sick and wounded, we were being sent to the civilian camp on orders from Tokyo. He told us that we should be sent back to our homes, but that we must be patient, as it would be "not very shortly". The Army Matron made a suitable reply.'

On their arrival at the Civilian Internment Camp, these sisters and nurses were searched by the Japanese. Later they were interviewed by H.B.M's. Representative in Hong Kong who was now acting as Commandant of the camp. Together, they now constituted a single nursing unit for work inside the camp. This unit consisted of 10 British Army, 2 Canadian Army and 3 Royal Naval Nursing Sisters. The unit was administered by the Army Matron.

Stanley Camp, until February 1944, was administered by the Japanese as a civilian internment camp, and the various blocks of buildings in which the internees lived were in charge of a number of Chinese superintendents. The camp guards were a mixture of Indians and Chinese.

---

* The Commandant of all the prisoner-of-war camps in the Hong Kong area.

After February 1944 the camp was taken over by the Japanese Military Authorities who administered it as a Military Internment Camp. Chinese now ceased to work in the camp and were replaced by Formosans.

The Naval Matron and sisters were accommodated in a building which had been considerably damaged during hostilities. There were 18 cubicles each of which was occupied by 3 persons. The Naval and Army Matrons shared a single cubicle. These cubicles were approximately 10 ft. × 14 ft. They were whitewashed and had frail wooden floors. All the cubicles were bug-ridden. The great majority of the windows were smashed and were stuffed with rags or roughly covered with wood and cardboard.

Sanitation was a difficulty. There was one European lavatory in this particular block, but it was broken and had to be flushed by hand. There were two Chinese lavatories. There were three shower baths in a large wash room. These facilities served some 70 women and children, and washing of persons, clothing and dishes had to be carried out in such a wash room. No warm baths or showers were ever available. Personal privacy seems to have been absent.

To start with, the naval sisters had to sleep on the floor, but later, following representations made to the Japanese by the Hong Kong Director of Medical Services, each sister was provided with a camp bed.

In the early days of its existence, the food at Stanley Camp consisted of two meals daily:

    10 a.m. Rice, soup, bread.

    5 p.m. Rice, soup, pastry or stew.

After January 1944, three meals a day were given:

    8 a.m. Rice congee with the addition of bran.

    11 a.m. Rice and vegetable soup.

    5 p.m. Rice, soup, hash or fishcake or fried fish, according to what was available.

From January 1944, there was no meat supply for a period of sixteen months. Fish was supplied about every third day, but in very small amounts, and the issue gradually became less frequent, e.g. during February 1945, the only fish received by naval sisters was one ration of tiny shell-fish which gave each person a teaspoonful when removed from the shells.

There was no bread ration after January 1944, and salt too was scarce so that vegetables were cooked in sea water.

Whenever meat bones were available they were ground into powder and given to the children for their calcium content. Also, such crisp rice as was left round the boilers in a thin layer after cooking, was given to the babies and children to chew.

Fish heads were a luxury and were given to internees in rotation so that they could cook them themselves.

Cooking of food was on a communal basis and was performed by men volunteers. Firewood was very inadequate, however, and eventually doors, banister rails and a proportion of the floor boards of the blocks had to be used as fuel. Most of the water-boiling had to be done on grass fires, the grass being cut by internees and dried. During the winter of 1944–45, fuel became so short that it was only possible to issue three-quarters of a pint of hot water to each person daily.*

As a means of augmenting the meagre food supplies in Stanley Camp, a canteen was organised from which small amounts of food and other articles could be purchased twice a month. But, as time went on, the items for sale became less while the prices steadily increased.

Here again, once they had arrived in Stanley Camp, the naval sisters soon found themselves short of money. When this camp had first been founded, the original internees had been permitted to make purchases in the town to the value of $75, which sum was paid by the Hong Kong Government Representative. Unfortunately, all the nursing sisters of the Services arrived in the camp too late to benefit from this arrangement. In fact, very soon they had no money at all, until the Camp Commandant was able to arrange for them to receive an *ex gratia* allowance of $10 in August 1942, $15 in September and $15 in October.

Meanwhile, the Army Matron had made a number of representations on this subject to the Swiss Representative of the International Red Cross Society. She pointed out that the Japanese had repeatedly refused to recognise Service nursing sisters as entitled to the prisoner-of-war officer allowance, and she appealed for some form of assistance from the Red Cross Organisation.

Such an allowance was very soon arranged, and money provided by the International Red Cross amounted to sums varying from Military yen 12·50 to 25·0 each month.†

The Naval Matron, in her report, has also expressed her appreciation and gratitude for gifts of money from Naval and Marine officers in the various prisoner-of-war camps.

To begin with, electric light was available in Stanley Camp, though the internees were expected to provide the bulbs themselves. It was

---

* It is worthy of note that all food shortages began to be righted by the Japanese as soon as the end of the war was in sight, e.g. in June 1945, a daily ration of meat was provided in Stanley Camp. In August, this ration was increased to an ample supply of meat twice daily.

† Soon after the occupation of Hong Kong by the Japanese, the rate of exchange of the Military yen was 4 to £1 sterling. By the end of 1944, the rate was 20 to £1. By the spring of 1945 the rate was 18 to the £1.

The purchasing power of this currency was very variable; e.g. in the Stanley Camp canteen, in February 1945, the price of ¼ lb. salt was Military yen 5·0. From outside sources, the same quantity of salt cost yen 25. In the camp canteen, the small quantities of sugar available were sold at the rate of yen 67 per lb. Outside the camp the price was yen 130 a lb. At this time, eggs could be obtained from outside sources at a cost of yen 40, equivalent to £2 sterling, each!

also possible to obtain primitive electric hot plates, constructed inside the camp, which allowed a certain amount of cooking to be carried out indoors. But gradually the electric power was curtailed, until the allowance was no more than one hour each day. In July 1944 all electricity was forbidden except for purposes of lighting, and by October of the same year it ceased altogether.

Naturally, with a large number of experienced and capable medical men among the internees, the health of Stanley Camp received constant attention.

A special Nutritional Clinic proved of great value owing to the number of ailments due to an insufficient and unbalanced diet. The remedies of this clinic depended upon its resources, but they included bran, yeast, shark-liver oil, nicotinic acid, peanut butter, multivit capsules,* soya-bean, milk, vitaminised caramels† and thyamine injections.

The naval nursing sisters found themselves in need of the assistance of the Nutritional Clinic from time to time, and their Matron has recorded her deep appreciation of what was done for them. That the Matron herself did not escape deficiency ailments, though not directly expressed in her report, is all too evident from a statement which she has recorded in another connexion and which reads:

'I used to help to make and repair clothing for the men until my sight forced me to give up sewing, in September 1944.'‡

Apart from their purely nursing duties, the Naval Matron and nursing sisters undertook many routine tasks inside Stanley Camp.

One naval sister supervised the cooking in a kitchen in the American Block of the Camp, which catered for 300 persons. To this kitchen was added a 'special diet' kitchen, which was placed under the supervision of the same naval sister. This 'diet' kitchen furnished meals for about 100 persons daily, for whom additional nourishment was provided through the Camp Welfare Fund.

In March 1943 nursing help was needed at Tweed Bay Hospital, and the naval sisters undertook this work for six hours each day.

In September 1943 the naval sisters assisted with a district nursing organisation which was arranged by the Naval and Army Matrons.

This organisation was initiated on behalf of sick persons in the camp who were not ill enough to be admitted to hospital. There were usually some 350 men, women and children to be visited twice daily. The sisters gave them treatment and advice, and made reports daily to the Camp Medical Officer, bringing to his notice any case who it was

---

* These were received from Canadian and American sources.

† These were received from the British Red Cross Society early in 1943.

‡ The reader is referred back to the statement of the Surgeon Commander of H.M.S. *Exeter*, earlier in this chapter:

'During the last two weeks at Pamalaa, I could not see the markings on playing cards.'

thought desirable to be visited by a doctor.* The Naval Matron has recorded, in great detail, her appreciation of the gifts which were received by the internees from a number of voluntary organisations.

The first British Red Cross parcels arrived in November 1942, and were distributed on a basis of 1¾ parcels to each person. Packages of men's clothing were divided and were easily utilised for women and children as well.† The bulk supplies of food were gradually distributed over a period covering six months and this enabled the majority of internees to have an adequate supply of food for the first time since the fall of Hong Kong. The medical supplies from the British Red Cross Society also fulfilled a much needed want, and the general improvement in the health of the community was soon obvious, most of the internees showing their first, slight increase in weight for several months.

In September 1944 each person received three Canadian Red Cross parcels. These arrived when food was extremely short, and the nourishment which they provided undoubtedly helped the community to face the cold winter months ahead. Here again, Canadian Red Cross medical supplies played a great part in improving conditions for the sick.

The Matron states in her report:

'The joy which Red Cross parcels gave, and the good they did, cannot be over emphasised.'

Stanley Camp received, from the Canadian Nurses' Association, 20 'comfort parcels'.‡ Each parcel was addressed to 'Nursing Sisters, British Army, taken prisoner in Hong Kong'.

The committee dealing with the distribution of parcels felt unable to decide for whom they were intended, particularly as the packing case containing them was marked 'Nurses Uniform'. Thereupon, the Naval and Army Matrons were invited to serve on a sub-committee of representatives of all the hospitals in Hong Kong, in order to decide to whom the parcels should be delivered. The parcels contained much needed toilet articles,§ and altogether about 100 nurses benefited.

In March 1945 each internee received one British Red Cross parcel.||

---

* In April 1945, the Naval Matron, on medical advice, was forced to relinquish this work. Her place was taken by an Army sister.

† As regards the acute shortage of clothing, toilet articles, etc., the Naval Matron made repeated official requests to the Japanese Authorities for permission for her sisters and nurses to obtain some of their belongings left behind in R.N. Hospital, Hong Kong. This permission was refused. In September 1943, the Matron was informed by a British electrician whom the Japanese had ordered to carry out regular electrical work at the hospital, that much of the belongings of the nursing staff was stowed away in the hospital store. This electrician himself represented to the Japanese that some of the articles should be delivered to their owners in Stanley Camp. He was informed that everything was 'captured property'. Later, he saw the linen and clothing of the nursing staff being packed for dispatch to Japan.

‡ Nine of these parcels were broken and incomplete.

§ One of the hardships suffered by women internees was lack of sanitary towels.

|| These parcels had been held back by the Japanese Authorities since 1942.

At the same time, some clothing for men, a few toilet articles, books and some medical supplies were received from the United States. Four American cigarettes were also given to each adult in the camp. But no food was distributed.*

The Naval Matron has recorded details of recreations and entertainments which were provided by the internees in the camp and which included variety concerts, classical music, plays, ballets and pantomimes. Lectures on many subjects could be attended and instruction was given in many educational subjects. Camp libraries were sufficient to provide all with reading material. During the summer months, a bathing beach was open for a certain time each day, but few internees had the strength to undertake the long walk involved.

Church services were held regularly on an inter-denominational basis, and religious plays were given at Easter and Christmas each year.

The naval internees of Stanley Camp received their first letters from the United Kingdom in February 1943. From then onwards, letters were delivered occasionally, but in haphazard fashion, being in no order of sequence whatsoever. In the same way, the few cards which the internees themselves were allowed to send were subjected to procedure and rules which were constantly changing, and the subject matter written was very limited.† Cards sent by naval sisters in June 1942 were not received in the United Kingdom until April 1945.

The Matron of the Royal Naval Hospital, Hong Kong, completed her report with a number of general remarks worthy of being recorded in this History.

'Though conditions were abnormal, we were able to lead a comparatively normal life within the camp community. With our work and the variety of outlets available, mental and physical, the majority of us had no difficulty in remaining happy and occupied.

'As our clothes wore out, we had no means of obtaining others. The problem of foot gear was partially solved by making rope-soled sandals, by clogs or by going barefoot as we frequently did.

'When we were first sent to Stanley Camp we were told that we were to be repatriated. In May 1943 the Japanese Authorities gave us to understand that women and children were to be repatriated that same summer. Our passports were brought up-to-date, but our expectations never materialised.

'No air-raid shelters were provided inside Stanley Camp, and it was not until bombs actually fell inside the camp that passive defence

---

* These stores are said to have been brought to Hong Kong by the relief ship *Awa Maru*.

† One naval sister wrote on a card the words, 'Hope to see you soon'. She was taken before the Japanese Authorities where she was required to explain the meaning of the word 'soon'.

precautions were taken.* International White Cross signs were laid out on the ground in various parts of the camp. First-aid parties, demolition squads and fire-fighting parties were organised among the internees themselves.

'I should like to record my deep appreciation and indebtedness to the Army Matron for her continual concern for our welfare in her dealings with the Japanese Authorities and with the Swiss International Red Cross Representative. Through the latter, in January and March 1945, she was able to send communications to the War Office regarding the safety of the Naval and Army Nursing Sisters in captivity.'

On August 30, 1945, Hong Kong was retaken by the Royal Navy. On the following day, the Naval Matron and her nursing sisters were taken on board H.M. Hospital Ship *Oxfordshire*. It was only then that the leader of this small unit of gallant women spoke those words which are typical of themselves, their Service and their profession.

'My Sisters have, at all times, remained cheerful and have made the best of everything. Among our memories of our time spent in a prison camp there will be many happy ones. Our one great disappointment was that we were unable to continue nursing our own sick men.'

The above narrative, extracted from the official reports of the P.M.O. and Matron of the Royal Naval Hospital, Hong Kong, is itself sufficient as it stands. The story is one of tenacity of purpose, gallantry and devotion to duty. It calls for no comment or criticism from the outside observer or historian.

Since the end of the Second World War, a new Royal Naval Hospital, Hong Kong, has come into being. This new hospital is modern and offers up-to-date surgical and medical facilities for the Fleet in Far Eastern Waters which are a great improvement on those which existed in pre-war days. Nevertheless, to the Royal Navy, the imposing, hillside building which represents the new hospital, will never fail to stand as a monument to the memory of that older Royal Naval Hospital, Hong Kong, which left behind a brief, but permanent record of gallantry in the pages of naval medical and nursing history.

---

* On January 16, 1945, Allied bombs fell inside Stanley Camp killing fourteen internees and injuring others.

CHAPTER 3

MEDICAL ASPECT OF THE CHIEF NAVAL EVENTS 1939-1941

The Year 1939

THE Second World War began on September 3, 1939. On the night of the same day, the S.S. *Athenia*, carrying refugees to Canada, was torpedoed and sunk by a U-boat. This disaster occurred in North Atlantic waters, and its impact was immediately felt by the Department of the Medical Director-General of the Navy to the extent of revealing that some changes in the medical organisation of small ships afloat might have to be effected in the very near future.

Survivors were rescued by H.M. destroyers *Escort* and *Electra*. Neither of these ships carried the medical officer of the Destroyer Flotilla, and the lesson learned was that such ships, acting independently, must be prepared to deal with many such emergencies in which medical care beyond the capabilities of a coxswain, trained in first aid, would be required. It was, however, some months before the evidence became sufficient to justify the appointment of a separate medical officer to each destroyer of the Fleet.*

Two weeks later, on September 17, 1939, the first serious naval loss occurred when the aircraft carrier, H.M.S. *Courageous*, was torpedoed and sunk in Home Waters. Survivors were picked up, within an hour, by destroyers and merchant ships. Unfortunately, all who abandoned ship did not survive owing to the cold and the absence of any means of support in the water. There seems to be no evidence that any float or raft was released when the ship sank.

One of the consequences was that very few wounded were picked up, and the only important casualty eventually to reach hospital was a man who had had a tourniquet applied to control the bleeding from a lacerated ankle. This tourniquet was still in position when the man was admitted to hospital 48 hours later, and the foot was then found to be gangrenous and infected with *B. Welchii*.

On the night of October 14, 1939, H.M.S. *Royal Oak* was torpedoed and sunk at her anchorage in Scapa Flow.

So unexpected and silent was the approach and attack of the U-boat on this occasion, that it was some time before other ships in the area became aware of the loss of the *Royal Oak*. In consequence, rescue work

---

* *See* Chapter 1 of this Volume.

was much restricted and the loss of life was heavy. Fortunately, the Hospital Ship *Aba* was at hand and received 40 severe cases of burns.

Some of these men had been in the water for three hours, and it was considered that their survival was due to oil fuel keeping out the cold. This was the only tribute paid to oil fuel at this stage in the war. It had already appeared in the Fleet as a 'bogey', and the sailor credited it with causing asphyxia, gastritis, conjunctivitis, sepsis and drowning. It was over two years before some of these opinions began to be discounted.*

Of far greater importance was the observation that a number of these cases of burns, which had been caused by 'flash', had been afforded a measure of protection by clothing, even thin underclothing. But the value of such protection had still to be fully appreciated and it was a long time before protective measures were instituted officially.*

On October 15, 1939, enemy aircraft attacked shipping in the Firth of Forth with both bombs and machine-gun fire. This was an event of some importance in naval medical history, for it announced a form of attack which was to be responsible for the greater part of the work of naval doctors for the rest of the war.

H.M.S. *Mohawk*, a destroyer, suffered 13 men killed and 32 wounded.

The casualties were admitted to R.N. Hospital, Port Edgar. They included eleven miscellaneous fractures due to men being thrown down by concussion and blast. All wounds were due to bomb splinters. It is again of interest that yet another case required amputation on account of gangrene following the prolonged retention of a tourniquet!

In this, the first bombing attack of the war to produce casualties afloat, no immediate conclusions were drawn from the fact that the track of the majority of the splinter wounds was from below upwards.†

In this Firth of Forth incident, H.M. cruisers *Edinburgh* and *Southampton* were also attacked, and it is of some interest that the senior medical officer of the latter ship reported that the present medical organisation for action was too inelastic and called for revision.

It was in November 1939 that the magnetic mine made its presence known. Throughout this month and, with a few notable exceptions, until the end of the year, the majority of casualties afloat were due to this particular weapon.

On November 13, 1939, H.M.S. *Adventure* was mined and suffered 30 casualties. These included fractures of the lower limbs and pelvis. Another feature reported by the Senior Medical Officer‡ of this ship was that personnel in the immediate vicinity of the explosion appeared apathetic and, though uninjured physically, made no effort to escape or help themselves.†

---

* *See* Chapter 1 of this Volume.

† *See* Chapter 1 of this Volume.

‡ This medical officer was decorated for his gallantry and devotion to duty on this occasion.

As the magnetic mine revealed its power, each report from damaged ships brought increasing evidence of the severe orthopaedic damage caused by this weapon. Fractures were reported, not only of the lower limbs, but also of the spine and jaw.

On November 21, 1939, H.M.S. *Belfast* was damaged by a magnetic mine. Over half her casualties were fractures and the remainder were chiefly suffering from sprains and contusions. Some men had been flung many feet off the deck into the air when the mine exploded. A number of these had struck obstacles overhead, and the casualties included 3 fractured skulls.

On December 4, 1939, H.M.S. *Nelson* was mined with a heavy list of casualties which included 25 fractures of lower limbs, 13 fractured skulls, 10 fractured spines, 6 fractures of upper limbs, 4 fractured jaws and 2 fractured pelves. The treatment of these casualties was complicated by the fact that none could be landed for five days.

During the last four months of 1939, 15 small craft were lost from enemy action, consisting of 11 trawlers, 1 tug, 2 minesweeping drifters and 1 boom defence vessel. Nine of these were sunk by magnetic mines. In only three was there more than one survivor, and the majority were lost with all hands. In such circumstances it did not appear possible to make any special medical provision in these small ships against the hazards of war.

Apart from the reports of the effects of air attack and magnetic mines, the Medical Department of the Navy, by this early stage in the war, had already had placed before it many experiences of rescue work at sea. Such work was still largely unorganised and had not, as yet, received that attention which it was to receive at a later date.

Another problem which was also starting to make its presence known was that of revising the existing medical organisation for action afloat. The view of the Senior Medical Officer of H.M.S. *Southampton*, following the Firth of Forth attack, was that the existing organisation was outmoded. This view was confirmed by the Senior Medical Officer of H.M.S. *Belfast*, when this ship was mined. The new conception was that the medical organisation for action afloat called for a greater mobility of medical personnel, with the dispersal of medical parties rather than their organisation in rigid teams, under cover. It was, in fact, already realised that the policy of sheltering medical parties below the waterline was unsuited to the circumstances of modern warfare at sea. This was a new idea which was to gain momentum after the Battle of the River Plate.

THE BATTLE OF THE RIVER PLATE

As regards medical experience for the future, this surface action, despite its international significance and its effect on the course of the war at sea, was of little importance, particularly when viewed later in its true perspective. The Battle of the River Plate was but a surface action between men-of-war. Such actions had been fought in former wars, and the medical incidents were much as would be expected. These incidents were the type which naval medical officers, during their peace-time training, had been led to expect. But their instructional value for the future was negligible when compared with the effects of enemy air attacks and damage by magnetic mines which had occurred in the weeks before. Indeed, in view of what was to come in the few months ahead, in naval operations associated with Norway and Denmark, the medical incidents of the Battle of the Plate tend to fade into insignificance.

The details of this battle are well known. The cruisers *Exeter*, *Achilles* and *Ajax* brought the *Graf Spee* to action soon after dawn on December 13, 1939. Heavily damaged, the *Graf Spee* withdrew into Montevideo, shortly after midnight. The *Graf Spee* blew herself up at 1540 hours on December 17, in shallow water six miles south-west of Montevideo.

The medical organisation for action in H.M.Ss. *Exeter*, *Achilles* and *Ajax* was based on peace-time complement and existing regulations,* with the ship's sick bay and wardroom as dressing stations, first-aid haversacks distributed to various persons and stretcher parties operating from medical centres. H.M.S. *Exeter* had been in commission for three years. This ship had had the experience of riots in Trinidad and of the earthquake at Concepçion, in Chile, so medically she was as fully prepared for action as experience up to that time indicated was necessary.

H.M.S. EXETER

The action opened at 0618 hours, with little warning. Within three minutes of the medical parties having been fallen in for duty, the *Exeter* was straddled by the third salvo fired by the *Graf Spee*. A near miss killed most of the crew of the starboard torpedo tubes and casualties began to arrive in the dressing stations almost at once. As recorded by one of her medical officers:

'The S.B.P.O. and the wardroom mess man were erecting the operating table. As I was taking the instruments, drugs and dressings from a cupboard, there was a loud crash and a sudden blast of air. Large holes appeared in the side of the cabin opposite, and pieces of metal hurtled inboard.'

The ship's Master-at-Arms, who was assisting in the preparation of this dressing station, was at once among the wounded.

Six minutes after the first shot was fired, H.M.S. *Exeter* received a direct hit which killed or wounded nearly all the personnel on the bridge and half the gun's crew of the Marines' turret.

---

* *See* Chapter 1 of this Volume.

Shortly afterwards, the ship was hit by two 11 in. shells which caused a fierce fire amidships, and flooded a magazine.

The sick bay was wrecked by a shell passing through it and bursting a water main. This caused a flood 12 in. deep, and further water poured in through many holes on the upper deck. Wounded had to be removed to adjacent compartments and, in view of their concentration in the sick bay, it was fortunate that the medical staff survived.

By 0650 hours, H.M.S. *Exeter* had a list of 7 degrees but, though forced to fall out of the action, she continued to fire with one gun until 0730 hours.

The work of clearing up then began. The dead were prepared for burial, and 5 officers and 55 ratings were committed to the deep during the afternoon.

Within half an hour of the commencement of the action, *Exeter* had 5 officers and 50 ratings killed, 2 missing and 82 wounded. Five of the wounded died soon after the action. Five or six died later, after being disembarked.*

Of the wounded, 63 per cent. had lacerations due to fragments of metal. While most of these injuries involved only superficial skin and muscle, nine of them included compound fractures. Seven of these compound fractures were of lower limbs and two of upper limbs. There were also three simple fracture cases. One patient had an ulnar nerve severed at the elbow.

There were eighteen cases of burns, all of which were above the waist and involved only the exposed parts of the body.†

There were three cases of eye injury. In two of these, small particles of metal and debris were embedded in the cornea. In the third, a fragment of metal had penetrated more deeply and the eye had to be enucleated.

It is of the greatest interest that among a large number of casualties, there was no instance of blast injury. The absence of this feature, in the case of shell fire, was very different from the injuries caused by blast, during bombing attacks, later in the war.

Owing to her extensive damage and the very frequent calls made upon her medical personnel in so short a time, immediate first aid was, of necessity, rudimentary in H.M.S. *Exeter*. Even when this had been completed, the task of rendering effective surgical aid was hampered

---

* Of these latter five, three died of multiple injuries and burns, on the day they were landed at the Falkland Islands. One died a month later, during an operation on the stump of what had previously been a traumatic amputation of an arm. The fifth case died nearly four months after the action, from a penetrating wound of the skull.

† During this action, the ship's company wore tropical shorts and shirts. No anti-flash gear was worn. Had the attack been made with bombs, which were later found to cause more severe burns by 'flash' than those caused by shell explosions, there would certainly have been a greater number of men suffering from severe burns. (The reader is referred to Chapter 1 of this Volume and Chapter 12 of Volume I.)

by the conditions on board this damaged ship. Not only had a large quantity of medical stores been destroyed, but lighting and water supplies had failed. Sterilisation was impossible and antisepsis, rather than asepsis, was practised.

During the day of the action, the principal efforts were directed towards immobilising fractures and dressing burns with a tannic acid spray. All wounds were dressed with acriflavine in oil, but many of them subsequently became septic with particularly adverse results in the case of compound fractures.*

It was three days before H.M.S. *Exeter* could reach harbour, and the demands of nursing on her medical staff were very great. The ship arrived at Port Stanley, in the Falkland Islands, and landed all her casualties at 1015 hours on December 16.

H.M.S. ACHILLES

The two medical officers of H.M.S. *Achilles*† had less work to do than the doctors in H.M.S. *Exeter*. The few casualties in *Achilles* all occurred in the forward part of the ship. There were no direct hits, but four men were killed and ten wounded as a result of shell fragments coming inboard from near misses. The wounded were all lacerations and splinter wounds, with one compound fracture of a lower limb.

H.M.S. AJAX

H.M.S. *Ajax* was straddled by shells from the *Graf Spee* three times, at 0720 hours. Five minutes later, she received a direct hit which killed four and wounded six of the crew of a gun turret. Subsequent near misses caused a small number of other casualties. Altogether, casualties in H.M.S. *Ajax* amounted to seven killed and fifteen wounded. There were only four serious cases, three being multiple lacerations and the other a compound fracture of upper limb.

THE AFTERMATH

Owing to operational requirements the casualties in *Ajax* and *Achilles* were detained on board for nearly eight days, so it was fortunate

---

* It cannot be over-emphasised that where casualties are to be treated in a damaged ship, during or following an action at sea, a large number of the peace-time standards of surgery have to be abandoned. This proved to be the case time and time again in the course of the war at sea. Circumstances and conditions vary from ship to ship, and from action to action. It is as impossible to dictate which surgical principles shall be observed as it is to lay down hard and fast rules of clinical procedure. (Editor's Note.)

† H.M.S. *Achilles* was a unit of the Royal New Zealand Navy. It is of interest that the junior of the two medical officers, an ophthalmic specialist, had only left his consulting practice in Auckland on August 28, 1939, at an hour's notice. He had joined H.M.S. *Achilles* as she was on the point of sailing. Having no uniform, he wore plain clothes. After the action, his specialist experience was of great value to the ophthalmic casualties of H.M.S. *Exeter*.

that their numbers were small and that the sick bays of these ships remained intact. No undue difficulties arose and all the necessary treatment was given during this long period.

On the day of the action, mere first aid was all that was possible. On the next day, a large number of wounds were X-rayed on board.* Subsequently, under anaesthesia,† wounds were cleaned and excised and foreign bodies removed. All wounds remained clean and healing was rapid.

The Battle of the River Plate took place in waters far remote from any British Naval Base, and there was no hospital ship in the vicinity. Casualties could not be landed at Montevideo or Buenos Aires because of the danger of internment. They were, therefore, conveyed to the Falkland Islands. The King Edward VII Memorial Hospital at Port Stanley had been designed for seventeen patients. As this hospital could not possibly deal with nearly a hundred wounded, many had to be accommodated in the private houses of the local residents.

Unfortunately, there was no ambulance in which to transport cases from the jetty, and the journey along very rough roads, in improvised transport, was difficult for some of the wounded to bear.

The population of Port Stanley included two medical officers of the Colonial Medical Service, a matron and a small number of probationer nurses. This small staff was supplemented by an ex-matron who returned from retirement, and by the sick berth staff and bandsmen of H.M.S. *Exeter*.

The nearest source of British naval medical supplies was in South Africa, so that the overall strain on local resources at Port Stanley was very considerable and it was soon obvious that outside assistance was necessary.‡

It was not long before the condition of a number of these casualties ashore in the Falkland Islands gave cause for anxiety. In particular,

---

* This was impossible in the case of H.M.S. *Exeter*, owing to the failure of electric power.

† Evipan sodium was employed in H.M.S. *Ajax*. Fortunately, a large supply of this anaesthetic had been purchased ashore. Otherwise, in both *Ajax* and *Achilles*, medical stores proved more than adequate, though it was suggested that more plaster bandages and hypodermic syringes could have been used.

‡ Offers of such assistance were at once forthcoming but, unfortunately, could not be fully accepted owing to their possible impact on diplomatic matters outside the sphere of knowledge of doctors and nurses whose main concern must always be the welfare of their patients.

H.M.Ss. *Ajax* and *Achilles* arrived in the Falkland Islands on December 22. H.M.S. *Exeter* had arrived on December 16. It was with relief that the medical officers of these ships received news from Buenos Aires that a surgeon, radiologist, radiographer and some twelve nursing sisters had volunteered to travel to the Falkland Islands to render assistance. Also, the British community in Buenos Aires had fully equipped the Falkland Island vessel *Lafonia* with medical stores and equipment.

For some reason, however, the surgeon turned back at Montevideo. The *Lafonia* did reach Port Stanley, but all except two of the nursing sisters remained on board. Nevertheless, the X-ray facilities of the *Lafonia* were made good use of.

some of the orthopaedic cases needed specialised treatment and, in due course, an orthopaedic surgeon was sent out from England by air.

Meanwhile, three dangerously ill men were transferred to Buenos Aires. One of these died there, and another was taken on board H.M.S. *Dorsetshire* on February 9, 1940, to prevent his being interned.

Eventually, on March 10, 1940, the remaining cases were taken on board H.M.S. *Dorsetshire* and transferred from the Falkland Islands to the Royal Naval Hospital at Simonstown, South Africa. Many of these had to remain in South Africa until the end of 1940 before they were fit enough to return to the United Kingdom.

Numerous official reports of the Battle of the River Plate have paid tribute to the outstanding conduct and devotion to duty of the medical officers* and sick berth staffs in the three British cruisers. The final analysis of casualties was as follows:

H.M.S. *Exeter* (complement 602)

Killed	55
Died of wounds on board	5
Died of wounds at Port Stanley	4
Died of wounds in Buenos Aires	1
Wounded who recovered	71
Total	136

H.M.S. *Ajax* (complement 644)

Killed	7
Wounded	15
Total	22

H.M.S. *Achilles* (complement 572)

Killed	4
Wounded	10
Total	14

Total casualties of this action were 172, of whom 76 did not survive.

The Year 1940

THE NORWEGIAN OPERATIONS

The part played by the Royal Navy in these operations was chiefly the transporting of troops and stores to Norway, and later back to the

---

* The Senior Medical Officer of H.M.S. *Achilles* and the Junior Medical Officer of H.M.S. *Exeter* were both decorated with the Distinguished Service Cross for their part in this action. The Senior Medical Officers of H.M.Ss. *Exeter* and *Ajax* were both Mentioned in Dispatches.

United Kingdom, with some service in support of the advance on Narvik. Action was also joined during minelaying operations, and skirmishes took place between units of the Home Fleet and German men-of-war. Enemy air activity was severe and its effects upon naval medical organisation afloat were now fully realised.

As a precursor of future events in Norway, south of Bergen, on the night of February 16, 1940, the German store ship *Altmark* was attacked and boarded by a naval party from H.M.S. *Cossack*, commanded by Captain Philip Vian.*

A number of British prisoners-of-war was freed from the *Altmark*. Seven of their German guards were killed, but there was only one British casualty, a wounded officer.

On April 8 H.M.S. *Glowworm* was minelaying in Norwegian Waters. A member of her ship's company fell overboard and *Glowworm* stopped to search for him. As a result of this delay, the ship was sighted by superior German forces. With great gallantry, *Glowworm's* Commanding Officer joined action with the enemy.† H.M.S. *Glowworm* was lost with her entire ship's company of 112 missing.

On the following day, H.M.S. *Gurkha* was sunk by bombs from enemy aircraft. Sixteen of her crew were killed, but 190 men, including 7 wounded, were rescued by H.M.S. *Aurora*.

On the same day H.M.S. *Glasgow* was damaged by bombs and suffered a few casualties.

THE FIRST BATTLE OF NARVIK

On the morning of April 9, nine British destroyers, under the command of Captain Warburton-Lee, were directed to patrol the entrance to Vest Fjord. At 1600 hours on the same day, it was learned that six modern enemy destroyers were inside the fjord at Narvik. At dawn on April 10, Captain Warburton-Lee in H.M.S. *Hardy*, led H.M.Ss. *Hotspur*, *Havock*, *Hunter* and *Hostile* to attack the enemy.

The medical officers of these destroyers had been warned to expect a heavy engagement with many casualties.‡ These medical officers did their best to prepare for all contingencies, but their facilities were limited. These destroyers had minute sick bays which were inadequate for treating more than one or two patients at a time. The forward messdecks were therefore cleared and converted into medical stations. Mess tables were scrubbed and blankets and pillows were prepared. Hot water, stimulants, sterile dressings, tourniquets and splints were collected and surgical instruments were placed in bowls of spirit and

---

* Now Admiral of the Fleet Sir Philip Vian, K.C.B., K.B.E., D.S.O.

† The Commanding Officer of H.M.S. *Glowworm* was awarded the Victoria Cross posthumously.

‡ Each of the destroyers carried one medical officer. Four of the five medical officers were R.N.V.R. with little previous experience of life at sea and none of action afloat.

firmly lashed under clean blankets. These preparations on the forward messdecks had to be carefully arranged so that they did not interfere with the passage of ammunition through that part of the ship from the forward magazine. The remaining medical stores and equipment were dispersed throughout the ship. First-aid equipment was supplied to the bridge, engine rooms, guns' and torpedo tubes' crews. In each ship the medical officer stationed himself on the forward messdeck, and stationed his sick berth attendant in the ship's wardroom, aft.

The British destroyers made three attacks on the enemy ships. Three enemy destroyers were sunk or seriously damaged and six merchant ships were sunk.

As the British Flotilla turned away after the second attack, fresh enemy destroyers were sighted and engaged. These latter sank H.M.S. *Hunter* and disabled H.M.S. *Hotspur*. H.M.S. *Hardy* was also disabled but was beached. The remaining British destroyers retired under the cover of gunfire from four other destroyers and the cruiser *Penelope*.

In H.M.S. *Hotspur* a heavy concentration of fire inflicted severe damage and many casualties. Both medical centres were quickly put out of action and the ship took on a heavy list. At first, all that could be done was to give the wounded morphia and to remove them to the limited shelter available. As the action died down, it was possible to begin the cleaning, dressing and splinting of wounds. But the lights soon failed and the Medical Officer was warned that the ship was in a sinking condition. With all the ship's boats holed the survival of the wounded presented a problem. Fortunately, H.M.S. *Greyhound* was able to come alongside and the Medical Officer of *Hotspur* contrived to transfer not only his wounded, but a large quantity of his undamaged medical stores.

Treatment of the wounded was resumed in H.M.S. *Greyhound* until later in the same day, when the casualties were transferred yet again, this time to H.M.S. *Penelope*.

The adventures of these unfortunate casualties were not yet over because at 1430 hours on the following day, while steaming at high speed, H.M.S. *Penelope* hit a rock. Her Medical Officer was told that there was a grave possibility of the ship foundering and that his patients must be evacuated as soon as possible. All were transferred by boat to H.M.S. *Kimberley* and were carried to Gravdal, where they were discharged to the civil hospital ashore on April 12.

When H.M.S. *Hardy* was beached, Captain Warburton-Lee was already mortally wounded on the bridge of his ship. He was placed in a Neil-Robertson stretcher to which cork lifebelts were attached. The stretcher was lowered into the water, and the surviving officers swam ashore with this improvised float in tow.* Many other casualties were

---

* Captain Warburton-Lee was awarded the Victoria Cross posthumously.

landed in the same way by the ship's Medical Officer who was later to become a prisoner-of-war at Calais.

H.M.S. *Hostile* had only one minor casualty during the action. This was fortunate because her Medical Officer had fractured a femur in rough weather on the day before the battle. However, he too took on board a number of the casualties of H.M.S. *Hotspur* and these he attended to, while using a broom handle as a crutch. These casualties were also landed at Gravdal.

THE SECOND BATTLE OF NARVIK

In the interval between the first and second Battles of Narvik, a small number of British destroyers patrolled Vest Fjord and awaited reinforcements.

On April 12, aircraft from H.M.S. *Furious* bombed enemy shipping at Narvik, and in the early morning of April 13, H.M.S. *Warspite*, in company with nine destroyers, proceeded to attack the enemy.

As before the previous action, medical officers were warned of impending events. The morale of the ships' companies was superb and they are reported to have faced the action in a spirit of pleased expectancy.

In H.M.S. *Punjabi*, although, as part of the preparation for action, the ship's company was given the time-honoured injunction to bath and don clean underwear, the dispersal system for action was adopted, which was to be favoured later in the war.

The second Battle of Narvik began at 1243 hours on April 13, and at 1400 hours H.M.S. *Punjabi* was in close action with the enemy for some fifteen minutes. This ship sustained much damage and was on fire in three separate places when she retired from the action. The value of the dispersal system with alternative dressing stations was well illustrated, as one became untenable owing to fumes from calcium flares in a flooded compartment nearby.

In H.M.S. *Cossack* there were heavy casualties. This ship was struck by eight shells and most of her casualties occurred through explosions around the guns and in the boiler rooms.

H.M.S. *Eskimo*, having avoided seven enemy torpedoes, was struck by an eighth. The explosion carried away the bows of the ship and the forward medical station disappeared with its staff. The ship remained afloat, and turned in uncontrolled circles while her Medical Officer crawled about in water and oil fuel to attend to casualties trapped in wreckage.

The casualties from H.M.S. *Eskimo* were taken on board H.M.S. *Forester* which already had a small number of casualties of her own.*

---

* H.M.S. *Eskimo* was towed to the Lofotens by H.M.S. *Punjabi*. Later she was towed to safety by H.M.S. *Vindictive*. It was not until June 5, at Barrow-in-Furness, that it was possible to remove many of the dead from her wreckage.

Other destroyers taking part in this action were H.M.Ss. *Foxhound, Icarus, Bedouin, Hero* and *Kimberley*. All these escaped with a comparatively light list of casualties, which is accounted for, to some extent, by the fact that the action was fought at very close range, so that many shells passed clean through a number of destroyers without exploding. In H.M.S. *Foxhound* there were a few casualties from rifle bullets fired from the shore by German snipers.

H.M.S. *Warspite* had no casualties, but she took on board casualties from H.M.Ss. *Eskimo, Cossack, Punjabi, Foxhound* and *Forester*. *Warspite's* sick bay had been damaged, so the forward medical flat was converted into an operating theatre in which 59 major surgical casualties were treated. In due course, the walking casualties from H.M.S. *Warspite* were transferred to the S.S. *Franconia*. Cot cases were kept on board for twelve days and were then transferred to H.M.H.S. *Isle of Jersey*, on April 26. In due course, these casualties arrived at the Royal Naval Auxiliary Hospital, Kingseat, Aberdeenshire.

It will be noted that in this action H.M.S. *Warspite* virtually performed the duties of a hospital ship for a time, which meant that the numerous casualties were subjected to far less handling and hardship than those of the first Battle of Narvik.

OPERATION 'RUPERT'

After the second Battle of Narvik there was little local interference by the German Navy. But men landing for such purposes as the investigation of damage in beached destroyers, were still exposed to snipers and enemy air attack which increased daily.

With a view to the capture of Narvik itself, British troops arrived, on board H.M.S. *Southampton*, on April 14, and on April 15 in three transports escorted by H.M.S. *Valiant* and some destroyers. These Army units were based in the Harstad area.

The enemy held Narvik in considerable strength and direct assault was impossible pending harassing action by a number of naval units.

On April 20, H.M.S. *Enterprise* bombarded enemy shore establishments in the Narvik vicinity. On May 4, *Enterprise* was continuing her bombardment in company with the Polish destroyer *Grom*. Enemy air attacks were heavy, and the *Grom* was hit and sank in three minutes. Fortunately the sea was calm and H.M.S. *Enterprise* was able to rescue 30 survivors, 4 of whom were severely wounded. At the time of this rescue, the survivors were drenched with oil fuel and the comment was made that although the temperature of the water was 34° F., the survivors noticed relatively little discomfort during their immersion lasting half an hour.*

---

* Destroyers also took part in this rescue work, and out of a complement of 220, 165 survivors of the *Grom* were finally transferred to H.M.S. *Resolution*.

By May 5, H.M.S. *Enterprise* was the only British ship operating in the Fjord. Intense enemy air attacks were directed against this ship, and near misses caused a number of casualties on board.

During the rest of the month of May, H.M. ships were active in assisting the Army advance which finally led to the capture of the port of Narvik on May 27. Among the ships taking part in bombardment and covering operations, were H.M.Ss. *Resolution, Effingham, Aurora, Cairo, Coventry* and *Southampton*, and the Polish destroyer *Blyskawica*.

These ships were constantly under intense enemy air attacks, and casualties were numerous.

The larger units engaged not only operated against the enemy on their own account, but also acted as clearing ships for the casualties from the smaller units. They also received casualties from the heavy fighting ashore.

H.M.S. *Aurora* received a number of Army casualties, and her Senior Medical Officer reported:

'By May 1, Allied patrols had advanced close to Narvik on the harbour side, and a platoon of the South Wales Borderers was in position along a road running parallel to the shore. There were many casualties among these troops and stretcher-bearers had to run a gauntlet of fire to get to them. On one occasion, wounded had to be left out overnight, and when the stretcher-bearers reached them the following morning, they found that these wounded had not survived the night in the snow. Also, there were four casualties among the stretcher-bearers. These latter were brought on board *Aurora*.'

On May 7, H.M.S. *Aurora* received a direct hit by a bomb which killed seven of her crew and wounded seven others.

H.M.S. *Resolution* received a steady stream of wounded over a period of fourteen days. Among these were men from the trawlers *Northern Spray, Northern Gem, Northern Dawn* and *Northern Wave*, from H.M.S. *Vansittart*, and from the *Blyskawica*. Nine German casualties were also received.

On May 17, 160 bombs were dropped around H.M.S. *Resolution*, and the ship was hit. She now returned to Scotland where 98 casualties were transferred to H.M.H.S. *Amarapoora*.

By May 25, a naval base staff, with its medical officer, had been established at Harstad, 33 miles north-west of Narvik. Work proceeded under great difficulty owing to continuous enemy air attacks. Among other losses were H.M.S. *Curlew** and the S.S. *Mashobra*, the latter carrying a large quantity of medical stores.

The withdrawal of forces from the Harstad area began on June 3 and was completed on June 5, 1940.

---

* H.M.S. *Curlew* was the last British ship to be lost in a Norwegian fjord. She was bombed in Lavengs Fjord on May 26, 1940. The death roll in this ship was remarkably small and only five casualties required admission to hospital.

OPERATIONS AROUND NAMSOS

On April 14, about 350 seamen and marines from H.M.S. *Sheffield* were landed at Namsos. A similar number from H.M.S. *Glasgow* was landed at Bangsund.*

The object of these landings was to hold the anchorage of Namsos until the arrival of the Army. There was a good medical liaison with the local authorities ashore and a medical organisation was set up with a view to a stay ashore of some permanency. However, no action took place and the landing parties were re-embarked in a destroyer on April 17, and transferred to a cruiser at sea.

This evacuation was quickly followed by that of the Army, and during the next two weeks a number of H.M. ships saw a great deal of action.

On the night of May 2–3, H.M.S. *Afridi* went alongside at Namsos and evacuated troops from 2200 to 0400 hours. At 1100 hours on May 3, *Afridi* rescued survivors from the French destroyer *Bison*. Unfortunately, *Afridi* herself was bombed and sunk at 1400 hours on the same day and her survivors were picked up by H.M.Ss. *Griffin* and *Imperial*.

H.M.S. *Griffin* went alongside the *Afridi*. There was a swell which made the passage of wounded from one ship to another very difficult and two survivors of the *Bison* fell between the ships and sustained crush injuries from which they later died. Altogether *Griffin* took on board 3 officers and 129 survivors of the *Afridi*, 3 officers and 44 survivors of the *Bison*, and 5 Army officers and 17 other ranks. Within half an hour of performing this work of rescue, H.M.S. *Griffin* was herself subjected to severe air attacks. Her Medical Officer found himself with more than 50 dangerously wounded casualties in addition to those which this overcrowded ship already had on board.†

The Medical Officer of H.M.S. *Janus* was also busily occupied during the last days at Namsos. On April 30, the trawler *St. Goran* had signalled from Namsen Fjord asking for medical assistance for three casualties caused by a dive bombing attack. Almost simultaneously, H.M.S. *Bittern* was hit by a bomb which blew off her stern and killed 15 of her crew outright. As H.M.S. *Bittern* was sinking, H.M.S. *Janus* came alongside and took off her survivors, including 30 wounded. Seven of these wounded died in H.M.S. *Janus*. The remainder were treated

---

* H.M.S. *Glasgow* had been heavily attacked from the air only five days previously, and had sustained 57 casualties.

† H.M.S. *Griffin* already had wounded on board, following the bombing and sinking, on May 2, of the trawlers *Gaul*, *Arab* and *Aston Villa* two miles from the entrance of Namsen Fjord. *Griffin's* Medical Officer was sent ashore in a dinghy to deal with the casualties. He found 50 survivors sheltering in a snow covered rocky bay. One of the trawlers was burning 70 yards away, and presently blew up. Some of these survivors had been living in the snow, under constant bombing, for three days. They were taken on board H.M.S. *Griffin* where some 50 per cent. of the survivors were found to have been wounded by bomb splinters.

on board until, during the brief hours of darkness,* it was possible to transfer them to the cruiser H.M.S. *Carlisle*, where two more died.

The Medical Officer of H.M.S. *Bittern* had himself done a great deal in caring for the casualties on board H.M.S. *Janus*, although he was wounded and suffering from shock.

Having transferred these casualties to H.M.S. *Carlisle*, H.M.S. *Janus* was immediately called upon to give passage to 100 Chasseurs Alpins. By this time, the ship was getting so short of food supplies that the stock of medical comforts had to be expended in victualling these passengers.

In addition to casualties from H.M.Ss. *Bittern* and the *St. Goran*, H.M.S. *Carlisle* had on board wounded from the Lincolnshire and King's Own Yorkshire Light Infantry Regiments. With these casualties on board, *Carlisle* had to fight her way to safety under almost continuous bombardment from the air.

H.M.S. *Maori* also performed good service evacuating Army casualties from Namsos to Scapa Flow. She herself suffered casualties from air attack, and 1 man was killed while 20 were wounded of whom 4 died later.

It must be recorded at this point that, during the brief period of operations around the Namsos area, H.M. ships had more experience of dealing with casualties afloat than at any time up to this stage in the Second World War.

OPERATIONS 'SICKLE' AND 'PRIMROSE'

On April 13, 1940 it was decided to land a force of 300 naval ratings and 400 marines, which was to establish Allied control of Romsdal Fjord by occupying Aandalsnes, the railhead to Dombaas. This force was drawn from H.M.Ss. *Hood*, *Barham* and *Nelson* as well as from the A.A. Detachment, Royal Marines. The force embarked at Rosyth on April 14 in the sloops *Auckland*, *Bittern*, *Black Swan* and *Flamingo*.

There was no enemy opposition on passage, though these ships were shadowed from the air.

Disembarkation took place at 0400 hours on April 17. Seamen and Royal Marines from H.M.S. *Barham* were sent to Aalesund, those from H.M.S. *Hood* to Setnesmoen while the unit from H.M.S. *Nelson* remained at Aandalsnes.

From April 20 onwards, enemy bombing attacks on the Aandalsnes neighbourhood were of an unprecedented intensity† and by the night of

---

* As recorded later in this Volume, the work of medical officers was frequently embarrassed by the short hours of darkness in Arctic Waters during the spring and summer months.

† At this time the Norwegian gold reserve is believed to have been in railway trucks at Aandalsnes. Some members of the Norwegian Government were also present in the area. These factors may have played some part in the intensity of the enemy air attacks.

April 29, few buildings remained intact, and British forces began to withdraw.

The evacuation of Naval, Royal Marine and Army units from this region presented great difficulties. On the night of April 29–30, 1,200 men were to have been embarked but, owing to transport limitations and heavy bombing and incendiary raids, only about 350 could be got away. The wounded were subjected to severe strain and exposure and had to spend many hours at the water's edge without any shelter from the machine-gun attacks of low flying aircraft. H.M.S. *Fleetwood* took off as many casualties as she could embark. The following night 230 casualties were taken off by H.M. Ships *Wanderer* and *Sikh*.

The evacuation of the Aandalsnes area was completed by 0400 hours on the morning of May 1. Ships taking part were H.M.Ss. *Walker*, *Westcott*, *Somali*, *Birmingham*, *Arethusa* and *Auckland*. The medical officers of all these ships were busily employed treating the wounded on the way back to Scotland and they received great assistance from the personnel of evacuated Army Field Ambulance Units.*

MOLDE

H.M.S. *Curacoa* carried 100 officers and men of the 5th Leicestershire Regiment from Rosyth to Molde, where a safe landing was effected. During April 21, 22 and 23, *Curacoa* was bombed continuously. Nevertheless, she managed to receive and care for a number of casualties from stricken trawlers. On April 24 *Curacoa* received two direct hits, her sick bay was destroyed and there was a large number of casualties.†

Meanwhile, H.M.S. *Pelican* was bombed and hit off Molde on April 22. The stern 40 ft. of the quarterdeck disappeared leaving what was recorded as:

'A shambles of wreckage in which some 25 bodies were strewn about. Further forward the messdecks were in complete darkness and the remains of the ship were shrouded in silence save for the groans of her wounded.'

H.M.S. *Pelican* was carrying the Molde Naval Base Staff of whom 16 were killed and 9 wounded. Of *Pelican's* own ship's company which numbered 186, 39 were killed and 29 wounded.‡ Her Medical Officer and sick berth rating had managed to treat 30 of the wounded by the

---

* It is noted in the records of H.M.S. *Arethusa* that, of four British regimental medical officers whom she carried to Norway, only one returned.

† H.M.S. *Curacoa* managed to reach Scapa Flow under escort on April 26. This ship was refitted and subsequently performed valuable service on the Atlantic Convoy Route.
H.M.S. *Curacoa* was sunk in collision with the liner *Queen Mary* on October 2, 1942. Her Senior Medical Officer did not survive.

‡ This total of 93 killed and wounded is the highest incidence recorded during the war in a small ship which was not sunk.

time that outside assistance arrived and all casualties were transferred to H.M.Ss. *Fleetwood** and *Jackal*.

STAVANGER

During operations in the area around Stavanger, H.M.S. *Suffolk* was hit by a bomb on April 17, 1940. One officer and 26 ratings were killed, and 40 were wounded of whom 5 died later. H.M.S. *Suffolk* was fortunate in that she was able to discharge her casualties to H.M.H.S. *Amarapoora* at Scapa Flow twenty-four hours later. She did not have to suffer the anxiety, experienced in so many other ships, of retaining casualties on board for prolonged periods during further enemy air attacks.†

MEDICAL ORGANISATION ASHORE

Aandalsnes Area. The medical personnel attached to the naval force landed in this area consisted of 4 medical officers, 1 sick berth petty officer and 6 sick berth attendants. Sick bays were established ashore and the policy was to act as a casualty receiving centre and to evacuate to H.M. ships during the hours of darkness.

On April 18, the Senior Medical Officer established a temporary hospital in which, in spite of its limited accommodation and equipment, many major surgical cases were dealt with. On April 25 the building received a direct hit and had to be abandoned.

The hospital was transferred to cellars underneath some houses but these too became untenable as a result of incendiary bombs.

The hospital was next accommodated in a house some five miles away from the main target area and here the Senior Medical Officer worked in conjunction with the 158th Field Ambulance Unit.

On April 22, the naval medical personnel ashore was increased by 1 medical officer and 1 sick berth rating. Further inland, another naval medical officer, with 3 sick berth ratings, established a sick quarters inside what had formerly been a hospital attached to the Norwegian Military Camp at Setnesmoen. Here adequate medical stores and a staff of Norwegian nurses permitted everything possible to be done for casualties.

Namsos Area. The medical party ashore in this area consisted of a medical officer and 2 sick berth ratings as well as a number of Royal Marines as stretcher-bearers. Nothing was known in advance of the existing medical facilities ashore. It was assumed that a regimental aid

---

* H.M.S. *Fleetwood* performed a remarkable feat of endurance by being constantly in action in Norwegian Waters for a period of six weeks. During this time she carried on board not only her own wounded, but large numbers of casualties from other ships and from the Army. Her Medical Officer received great assistance on board from a Major of the R.A.M.C. The ship was described as appearing 'more a hospital ship than a sloop'.

† This was a problem which medical officers frequently had to face on Arctic convoys later in the war.

post would have to be set up in some building or other and the necessary equipment was landed for this purpose. This arrangement proved unnecessary as 60 beds of the local civil hospital were handed over to the use of the naval medical party, which meant that excellent facilities became available unexpectedly for the care of casualties.

Narvik Area. A medical officer and 2 sick berth ratings established a sick bay ashore in Harstad. In practice this sick bay functioned solely as a transport centre. It had been intended to establish a small sick quarters, but lack of accommodation and loss of equipment made this impossible. But in any case, the 22nd General Hospital at Harstad already provided ample local facilities, in addition to which the Hospital Ship *Atlantis* was available.

For local inland waters the Army adapted two 350-ton pleasure steamers each capable of carrying 70 stretcher cases and these were available for naval wounded.

MEDICAL STORES AND EQUIPMENT

Medical stores and equipment to accompany the British Expedition to Norway were sent from the Royal Naval Hospital, Haslar, at short notice, and were assembled at Rosyth. The Senior Medical Officer also gathered everything which he could from local stores in the Firth of Forth area and in particular, from the Royal Naval Hospital, Port Edgar.

Unfortunately, the speed of events was so great that the distribution of all these stores and equipment was not as well organised as it might have been. Loading into ships had to be done in the dark at the same time as troops were embarking and while general stores and ammunition were being placed on board. For some reason no written or printed list of medical stores seems to have been available, so that it was necessary to rely entirely on the outward appearance of packing cases when arranging distribution of the whole between various ships. Once loaded on board the ships, medical stores were placed wherever there happened to be a vacant space and this meant that they became widely scattered. An attempt was made to identify medical packing cases during the voyage, and to paint red crosses on them. But, unfortunately, a number remained unmarked.

The impact of these original defects of organisation was felt when stores and equipment were unloaded and put into use at the various points of disembarkation in Norway. For example, unloading was effected mainly in the dark and medical stores were not collected into separate dumps. The result was that, wherever packing cases had not been adequately marked, it proved impossible to identify medical as opposed to other kinds of cases. Then again, the speed of events had been such that there had been no opportunity to open and check the contents of packing cases before they were loaded at Rosyth. One unfortunate result of this omission was that a number of packing cases were found to contain nothing but several dozens of empty medicine bottles! Not only did this error mean a waste of stowage space, but one such packing case proved to be the only emergency medical store supply which was available to an isolated landing party. Fortunately in this instance, one of H.M. ships was at hand and was able to supply dressings and drugs in lieu of the useless contents of the packing case.

Further difficulty arose because little was known of the state of the medical facilities ashore, and this meant that there was frequently some doubt regarding the quantity of stores which should be landed in a particular area. Naturally, in view of what they could see going on in front of their eyes, some medical officers well realised, even before their stores were landed, that they would probably have to be re-embarked very soon even if they could be salved at all.

In point of fact, enemy action gave rise to a shortage of drugs and equipment in only one area. This was when the *Mashobra* was damaged at Narvik with the loss of the bulk of her medical supplies.

Naturally, the local Norwegian hospitals placed their medical supplies at the disposal of the British. But, in some areas, it was not long before medical stores became gravely diminished and it was realised that, if further fighting was to continue, more medical equipment would have to be sent from the United Kingdom. This shortage was particularly obvious in some of the smaller Norwegian hospitals, especially at Gravdal where many Service casualties were treated. In such cases urgent local needs were satisfied by supplies from H.M. ships and by handing over such medical stores as could be salvaged from the many damaged and beached vessels. Also, all H.M. ships returning to their bases in the United Kingdom left behind them in Norway all the medical supplies which they could spare to supplement the stocks of medical stores ashore.

In spite of the defects of organisation which have been outlined, by dint of a high degree of co-operation between the Services and the Civilian Medical Authorities ashore, most contingencies were covered and not only did medical supplies prove adequate in the end, but large quantities were also safely re-embarked at the time of the evacuation.

From the point of view of this History it is important to emphasise that the experience of supplying the medical stores and equipment for the campaign in Norway proved of the greatest value when future operations were being planned later in the war. Not the least of the lessons learned was the importance of the logistics and loading priorities of medical stores and equipment.

MEDICAL TRANSPORT

The nature of the operations in and around Norway necessitated the transport of casualties from scenes of action by a number of methods both ashore and afloat. Casualties were received by sick bays, temporary hospitals, hospital ships and combatant units of the Fleet. These various and dispersed reception centres dealt with the casualties nearest to them so that, as a rule, transport over long distances was minimised.

Short journeys were made by a variety of vehicles and vessels. Ashore, in some cases horse-drawn sledges were used on which casualties were placed in wicker baskets and amply covered with blankets.*

Cars and motor lorries were frequently available ashore but their use was limited owing to the bad state of the roads and also lack of fuel.

From the quays, wounded were often embarked in destroyers which were able to come alongside. In deeper waters, they were then transferred from the destroyers to larger men-of-war. Whenever weather conditions permitted, this direct method was used and casualties suffered a minimum of disturbance by being kept on Army type stretchers the whole time. But in rough weather, the direct method could not be used and a great variety of small craft was employed to transfer casualties from quay to ship and from ship to ship. Norwegian 'puffers' or fishing boats were mostly used, supplemented by every variety of ship's boat. When small craft were used, the Neil-Robertson stretcher had to be employed not only for safer transference afloat, but also because there was insufficient deck space to carry Army type stretchers.

ASSESSMENT OF CASUALTIES

FIRST BATTLE OF NARVIK

This naval encounter was exceptional in that it was a destroyer engagement with no capital ship in company, and it occurred in a place where casualties could not be landed. Thus, medical officers in small ships were required to deal with casualties on board on a large scale.

About 800 officers and men were in the five destroyers engaged, and of these 146 were killed, 35 were wounded and 8 died of wounds.

During the course of the action, the removal of wounded to relative shelter between decks, first aid and rough treatment for shock were all that could be attempted. Once the action was over, it became possible to assess the state of the casualties and roughly to place them in some order of priority for surgical attention. The actual injuries were nearly all the result of direct hits by enemy shells, and 75 per cent. of the wounded had lacerated wounds in which shell fragments and metal splinters from ships' hulls were embedded in the soft tissues. There were very few compound fractures and only one peripheral nerve injury was recorded.

---

* Sledge transport was chiefly used to carry casualties from the quayside to the hospital at Gravdal.

It was one or two days before these casualties reached hospitals ashore, which meant that a large amount of major surgery had to be performed in small ships under fairly primitive conditions. The operations performed included the repair of ruptured bowel, limb amputations, and one case of a shattered mandible with much loss of tissue and the evisceration of an eye. Local and general anaesthetics were used and prophylactic chemotherapy was instituted in many cases. It is of interest that the subsequent progress of these casualties showed nothing more than a very mild degree of wound sepsis, and no case developed tetanus or gas gangrene.

SECOND BATTLE OF NARVIK

The type, treatment and disposal of casualties in this action were very different from that above. Although some injuries were caused by shellfire, torpedo hits were responsible for many more. The latter included a high proportion of fractures. For example, H.M.Ss. *Punjabi* and *Eskimo* had fractures in 35 per cent. of their casualties, while in those ships damaged only by shellfire fractures amounted to less than 10 per cent.

The presence of H.M.S. *Warspite* in this action meant that a large number of casualties could be transferred to her from the destroyers, and better surgical treatment and subsequent nursing were possible on *Warspite's* large messdecks which were cleared to form a satisfactory hospital. However, it is of interest to note that though conditions in *Warspite* were less primitive than in the destroyers which treated casualties at the first Battle of Narvik, chemotherapy was not employed, and more than 50 per cent. of all wounds became infected.

EFFECTS OF BOMBING ATTACKS

Nearly half of the 60 cruisers, destroyers and sloops which took part in the Norwegian Campaign were damaged by direct bomb hits or near misses. In the individual ships so damaged the percentage of casualties in each ship's company varied from 15 per cent. to 50 per cent. This very high percentage of personnel disabled in those ships which eventually reached harbour was unusual in the history of naval medicine. But it is also worthy of record that such casualties would never have reached shore at all but for the advanced degree of damage control achieved in many ships and which led to many wounded being saved who, prior to the modern system of damage control, would undoubtedly have been lost with the foundering of their ships.

As a result of bombing attacks, a total of 540 casualties was suffered in the Norwegian Campaign; 236 were killed and 304 wounded. The majority of these casualties were sustained in H.M.Ss. *Suffolk, Pelican, Curacoa, Cairo, Bittern, Afridi* and *Curlew.*

In ships which suffered direct bomb hits as opposed to near misses, the ratio of dead to wounded was approximately 1 to 1. The ratio as a result of near misses was approximately 1 to 3.*

Forty-six per cent. of these casualties suffered lacerations, a figure very much less than the 75 per cent. which the Navy had come to expect from shellfire in sea actions in former wars.

Twenty-three per cent. were cases of burns which was in striking contrast to the negligible numbers caused by shellfire.

In addition, there were about 10 per cent. of casualties suffering from multiple contusions due to violence of explosions and about 10 per cent. from fractures, mainly of the lower limbs. There was a small number of penetrating wounds of chest and abdomen.

Owing to the fact that vessels damaged were usually in company with other ships, direct transfer of casualties from ship to ship was possible. In this way, the added trauma of immersion was seldom seen in those already wounded.

Small auxiliary craft taking part in these operations were subject to bombing on a very heavy scale and the official record shows that 18 trawlers were sunk. Survivors were either picked up by other ships or were able to swim to the shore. The point here to be made is that, had medical officers been carried in these trawlers, they obviously would have been wasted because sinking was so rapid and widespread among these small craft that no medical officer would have been able to give any assistance to casualties.

MACHINE-GUN ATTACKS AND SNIPING

Naval personnel were only occasionally exposed to the risk of bullet wounds, the occasions being confined to sniping from the shore and machine-gun fire from low flying aircraft. The latter form of attack produced negligible casualties in H.M. ships and was only really successful against survivors swimming in the water.

The bullet wounds inflicted presented characteristic features. They were mostly clean, through and through perforations, though the bullet was still *in situ* in some cases. Both tracer and dum-dum bullets would seem to have been used by the enemy.

MORALE

Although the operations in Norway produced few circumstances comparable with the later evacuation of the Army from Dunkirk and Crete, yet the very fact that they were prolonged and frequently carried out in the face of overwhelming enemy air attack, introduced an equally potent element of mental strain.

---

* This ratio was subsequently shown to be consistent in later bombing attacks at sea throughout the whole war period.

Added to the mental strain of operating in strange waters difficult to navigate, and in the unfamiliar settings of deep fjords, was the lack of repose which is always felt by those unaccustomed to the long Arctic twilight. Ships' companies were frequently required to be at their action stations, at first degree of readiness, for 24 hours each day. The cumulative lack of sleep and the monotony of this existence required as much fortitude for its endurance as did some of the more spectacular actions afloat.

Under such conditions it is encouraging to read in the Journal of a Senior Medical Officer that:

'The display of fortitude, devotion to duty and consideration for others was most remarkable, especially in the case of the younger inexperienced members of the ship's company.'

Loss of emotional control was indeed very rare, even among those wounded at Narvik who later had to abandon ship three times after the action. Psychomotor retardation was sometimes seen and a medical officer reported, after continuous bombing attacks:

'Many men were affected with an intense lethargy, loss of appetite and vomiting.'

Very naturally, mental and emotional shock was greatest in ships which were hit in their first experience of a bombing attack, and then had to face further attacks with reduced defences and loss of personnel. But it has been recorded that in most cases the wounded stood up remarkably well to the strain of further air attacks and everlasting gunfire.

In relation to the whole question of morale in the course of these operations, it is indeed worthy of record that officers in command of H.M. ships contrived, whenever possible, to give their ships' companies some traditional contrast to compensate for their long periods of mental strain. In the case of many ships every use was made of a few hours' respite in remote anchorages, and the mind of the sailor was quickly diverted into such absorbing ship activities as boat-pulling regattas, deck hockey, boxing contests,* tugs o' war and concert parties.

NAVAL AIR ARM

Apart from H.M.S. *Glorious*, the losses among naval airmen during the Norwegian Campaign were small. Those in H.M.S. *Ark Royal* in her raids on Trondheim, Stavanger, Bergen, Molde and Narvik were very light in comparison with those of the enemy, while H.M.S. *Furious* had only 2 killed and 1 wounded.

---

* One Commanding Officer, who later rose to Flag-rank, considered that it was essential for his sailors to be given the chance 'to hit something' whenever they had been subjected to heavy enemy air attack. He found that boxing was the best means of permitting men 'to let off steam'!

THE MEDICAL LESSONS OF THE NORWEGIAN CAMPAIGN

The resolution with which medical officers, particularly in small ships, refused to accept the medical limitations imposed upon them was largely responsible for the outstanding work which they did, frequently amid scenes of great destruction.* Also, the meticulous records and reports furnished by some medical officers were of the greatest assistance to the Department of the Medical Director-General of the Navy in assessing the need for certain changes in medical organisation afloat which had far reaching effects later in the course of the war.

At the time of this campaign medical action organisation afloat remained, in general, that of the First World War. Two dressing stations were employed, one of which, in cruisers, was the sick bay. The early destruction of both these dressing stations in H.M.Ss. *Cairo* and *Curacoa* confirmed the need for a wider dispersal of medical stores and personnel in action.

The campaign revealed that circumstances could arise in which a capital ship would be required to act for lengthy periods of air bombardment as a parent ship for smaller vessels. It became apparent that in such a capital ship major surgery must be carried out on board and that for this purpose it was desirable to have allocated to the medical department of the ship a suitable space as an operating theatre, which would be remote from the noise of battle and reasonably protected.†

The campaign revealed the need for anti-flash gear in the case of personnel exposed to bomb explosions and, though this type of protection had already been provided for, it was not taken seriously afloat until the effects of neglecting its use were observed during the numerous actions in Norwegian waters.

On the whole, medical stores and equipment in H.M. ships were found to be adequate with two exceptions. These were the allowance of Neil-Robertson stretchers per ship and the supply of morphia which some ships found fell short of their actual requirements.

In the less familiar environment of landing parties and shore-based operations, the Navy found that its medical preparation was far from adequate. The whole speed of events had been so rapid in the first place,

---

* Among decorations for gallantry and devotion to duty in these operations were the awards of the Distinguished Service Cross to the Medical Officers of H.M.Ss. *Hotspur, Eskimo, Afridi* and *Cossack*. The Senior Medical Officer of Operation 'Primrose' was similarly decorated, as was the Base Medical Officer at Narvik. The Medical Officers of H.M.Ss. *Aurora, Afridi, Cairo, Resolution, Curacoa* and *Griffin* were mentioned in dispatches.

† When put into practice, this provision did not usually fulfil the requirements which had been considered desirable. For example, the noises of exploding bombs, the rattle of splinters against the ship's side and the blast of the ship's own guns could never be conducive to efficient surgical technique. Later in the war, as in the case of the convoy battles on the routes to Malta and North Russia, depth charge explosions proved to be an added impediment as did the movement and frequent alterations of course of the ship itself.

CASUALTIES IN H.M. SHIPS, NORWEGIAN OPERATIONS, 1940

H.M. Ships Lost: L Damaged: D		Date	Cause of casualties	Total casualties* Dead	Total casualties* Wounded	Types of injuries † see footnote. 1	2	3	4	5	6	7	8	9	10	11	12	13	14	15	16	N/S
Glowworm	L	April 8, 1940	Shellfire	112	5	4																
Glasgow	D	April 9, 1940	Bombing	2	5		2															7
Gurkha	L	April 9, 1940	Bombing	16	7	7																
Hardy	L	April 10, 1940	Shellfire, Torpedo	21	12	7	2	2	1			1										1
Havock	D	April 10, 1940	Shellfire		3	3																
Hotspur	D	April 10, 1940	Shellfire	18	16	14	3		1				1					1				
Hunter	L	April 10, 1940	Shellfire	115	4				1													
Cossack	D	April 13, 1940	Shellfire	11	19	13			3			1	2							5		
Eskimo	D	April 13, 1940	Torpedo	19	16	6	5		1			1										
Punjabi	D	April 13, 1940	Torpedo	7	15	6				1 rib												
Forester	D	April 13, 1940	Shellfire	1	2	1				1 rib												
Foxhound	D	April 13, 1940	Shellfire, Machine gun		2	2						1	1									
Kimberley	D	April 14, 1940	Shellfire, Machine gun	5	6	5							1									
Suffolk	D	April 17, 1940	Bombing	32	40	2	2								1							4
Furious	D	April 18, 1940	Bombing	2	1	1																
Carlisle	D	April 20, 1940	Bombing	1	6	4	1					1	3		1							
Pelican	D	April 22, 1940	Bombing	41	27	16	1	3	3	3 rib	1	1							1	36		
Curacoa	D	April 24, 1940	Bombing	41	42	18			1		2					2				5 8		
Black Swan	D	April 28, 1940	Bombing		3	2	1																
Fleetwood	D	April 29, 1940	Bombing	2	3	3														3		
Bittern	L	April 30, 1940	Bombing	22	12	8	1					1	1		1							
Maori	D	May 2, 1940	Bombing	5	19	16													1	16		
Afridi	L	May 3, 1940	Bombing	53	30	4	5		4													
Enterprise	D	May 5, 1940	Bombing	1	7	7						1	1									
Aurora	D	May 7, 1940	Bombing	7	29	5	11	11												2		
Vansittart	D	May 8, 1940	Bombing	2	4	4	1																
Penelope	D	May 10, 1940	Bombing	5	15	14							1										
Warwick	D	May 15, 1940	Bombing		1	1																	
Somali	D	May 15, 1940	Bombing		3	2	1																
Resolution	D	May 14, 1940	Bombing	1	28	5	12		2			1			1					11		
Resolution	D	May 17, 1940	Bombing		3	2									3					1		
Firedrake	D	May 23, 1940	Bombing, Machine gun																			
Cairo	D	May 25, 1940	Bombing	12	16	8							4									
Southampton	D	May 25, 1940	Bombing		10	7																	
Curlew	L	May 26, 1940	Bombing	9	4																	
Acasta	L	June 8, 1940	Shellfire	158	1																	4
Ardent	L	June 8, 1940	Shellfire	154																		1
Glorious	L	June 8, 1940	Shellfire	1,204	34																	34

* Includes 'Killed in action', 'Died of wounds' and 'Missing, presumed killed'.
† Numbers 1–16 Classification of wounds. N/S = Not Stated

1. Lacerations
2. Contusions
3. Simple Fractures. Upper limb
4.   "   Lower limb
5. Simple Fractures. Spine
6.   "   Skull
7. Compound Fractures. Upper limb
8.   "   Lower limb
9. Penetrating Wounds. Skull
10.   "   Chest
11.   "   Abdomen
12.   "   Spine
13. Wounds of Blood vessels
14. Wounds of Peripheral Nerves
15. Burns
16. Blast injuries

that the choice of a Senior Medical Officer to supervise the medical organisation ashore in any area was fortuitous. In consequence, he had no previous knowledge of the medical officers who would be co-operating with him in his particular area nor the opportunity to discuss with them the details of any proposed medical organisation. The inevitable result was that it was not possible for any individual to inform himself of local conditions beforehand. This failure in organisation of personnel led directly to the failure to make the best use of local medical facilities ashore. There is no doubt that, certainly as regards the Navy, little was known about the distribution of Norwegian hospitals ashore. Medical officers frequently were landed at destinations well prepared to set up a medical organisation and sick quarters ashore, only to find themselves redundant in a civilised town of considerable size which already offered excellent hospital facilities.

One outstanding example of wastage and inconvenience which the Navy suffered from this lack of knowledge was the incident of organisation which required the Navy to send casualties ashore to the Military Hospital at Harstad. From the naval medical point of view there would have been overwhelming reasons for selecting the local civil hospital at Gravdal instead. The latter would have offered deep water facilities and easy access to ships of all classes. There was a good jetty and an excellent fleet of local transport. The climate was equable and food plentiful and not the least of the advantages were the absence of any large town or concentration of ships or troops to attract enemy bombers. Though used to some extent, Gravdal would have made an ideal medical centre for all ships operating in Norwegian waters and one in which the central naval medical organisation ashore might well have been set up with advantage had the Naval Medical Authorities been better informed of local conditions.

EVACUATION OF THE BRITISH EXPEDITIONARY FORCES FROM THE CONTINENT, MAY–JUNE 1940

PRELIMINARY EVENTS

On May 10, 1940 Germany invaded the Low Countries and a number of H.M. ships concentrated in the Dover area was immediately involved.

H.M.S. *Whitshed* proceeded, at top speed, to Ijmuiden with a party of 200 men whose task was to demolish industrial plant and canal machinery at Ijmuiden and Amsterdam.

Whitshed was joined by H.M.Ss. *Versatile* and *Wivern*, and in the face of heavy enemy opposition from the air, local evacuation of troops was begun by these and other ships at a number of points on the Dutch and Belgian coasts.

H.M.S. *Versatile** had casualties from a direct bomb hit received on

---

* The medical officer of H.M.S. *Versatile* was mentioned in dispatches for his devotion to duty on this occasion.

May 13 and from two near misses on the jetty at Ijmuiden. She received other casualties by machine-gun and cannon-fire from aircraft which attacked her while she was embarking the Welsh and Irish Guards and Royal Army Service Corps at the Hook.

On May 15, off the Dutch coast, the Fourth and Fifth Minesweeping Flotillas were attacked by German aircraft. A salvo of twelve bombs straddled H.M.S. *Hussar*, killing 3 and wounding 10 of her ship's company.

Meanwhile, H.M.S. *Wivern* had been bombed and machine-gunned off the Dutch coast. She returned to Dover with 24 of her ship's company killed and carrying 41 wounded including a number of soldiers.*

On May 17, H.M.S. *Whitshed* and the S.S. *Mona's Queen* evacuated 1,500 British refugees from Ostend. *Whitshed's* Medical officer recorded:

'There was nothing of medical interest during this evacuation except for one woman who threatened to go into labour unless she was given passage in a destroyer!'†

On May 19, H.M.S. *Whitley* was sunk off Nieuport and her survivors were rescued by H.M.S. *Vimiera*.

OPERATION 'DYNAMO'

The main evacuation from Dunkirk and the beaches stretching ten miles eastward began at 1857 hours on Sunday, May 26. Approximately 1,300 men of the British Expeditionary Force had been safely carried to Dover that same night. In planning this operation, an orderly procession of 'personnel vessels' had been visualised as coming alongside the jetty at Dunkirk every four hours. Other vessels were to lie off the beaches further east and to these men would be transported in a variety of small craft selected for work close inshore. Hospital ships were made available for the reception of casualties.

However, these preparations were quickly compromised by the loss of Calais, and the enemy, manning the guns of Les Hemmes, Fort Grande Philippe and other heavy coastal batteries extending to Gravelines, were able to open fire on ships in the western approaches to Dunkirk. On May 27, no less than five transports and the Hospital Ship *Isle of Thanet* were shelled by these guns and forced to return to England without fulfilling the purpose of their journey. As a consequence this route could only be used under cover of darkness, and by day ships could only approach Dunkirk by the Zuydecotte Pass, a long swept channel to the east which added 92 miles to the round journey from

---

* The sick berth attendant of H.M.S. *Wivern* was decorated with the Distinguished Service Medal on this occasion.

† Naval medical records show a remarkable absence of obstetrical practice during the evacuation of civilians from the Continent.

England. On this same day, five other transports completed this round trip and lifted some 4,000 soldiers from the Jettée de l'Est at Dunkirk. One of these, the S.S. *Mona's Isle*, was machine-gunned by enemy aircraft; 7 soldiers were killed and 100 wounded in addition to 7 of her ship's company. Medical aid was given by H.M.S. *Windsor*.

By May 28, in view of the damage inflicted by shellfire and air attack, which had now resulted in the loss of the S.S. *Queen of the Channel*, it was decided that evacuation during the hours of daylight must be confined to destroyers and other small craft. Moreover, it appeared at this stage that the evacuation might well be strictly limited owing to the time available for the operation. Any system of organised reliefs was abandoned, and as many destroyers and small craft as possible were employed together and some 14,000 troops were evacuated from the beaches on this day, despite a moderate surf which reduced the rate of embarkation and tended to exhaust boats' crews. Some 10,000 of these troops were given passage in 17 destroyers, while the remainder were brought home in minesweepers, trawlers and a miscellaneous assortment of small power boats only 4 of which were damaged or sunk by enemy action. At 1100 hours on May 28, the destroyer *Windsor* was bombed and had 2 of her crew killed and 25 wounded. Nevertheless, *Windsor* made six journeys altogether on this and subsequent days, carrying from 600 to 1,000 troops each time.*

At 1830 hours on the same day, news was received that by midnight the 3rd Corps of the B.E.F. would be concentrated on beaches near La Panne. The rescue of this force was begun during the night by H.M.Ss. *Calcutta*, *Gallant*, *Wakeful*, *Verity* and *Grafton* and a number of small craft. During the early hours of May 29, some of these ships suffered heavy casualties. H.M.S. *Wakeful*, while proceeding to Dover, was hit amidships by a torpedo and broke in two. The two portions sank in 15 seconds, and only those troops on her upper deck and a small number of her crew managed to get clear†

Among the ships which attempted to pick up the few survivors from *Wakeful* was H.M.S. *Grafton* which was immediately herself torpedoed.‡ *Grafton's* bridge was also hit by shellfire and her Captain was killed. An additional 15 of her ship's company were killed and 11 wounded. In the same action, the minesweeper *Lydd* rammed and sunk the motor drifter *Comfort*. The Medical Officer of H.M.S. *Grafton*§ recorded:

---

* The Medical Officer of H.M.S. *Windsor* was mentioned in dispatches for his devotion to duty.

† Approximately 500 soldiers and 80 per cent. of the crew of H.M.S. *Wakeful* were lost, including her Medical Officer.

‡ These torpedo attacks were carried out by a German motor torpedo boat which was engaged and destroyed by H.M.S. *Grafton* after the latter had been hit.

§ This Medical Officer had only joined *Grafton* the day before, having volunteered to take the place of the previous medical officer who had fallen sick. He was decorated with the Distinguished Service Cross for his gallantry on this occasion.

'At 0300 hours on May 28, 40 miles N.W. of La Panne, we were carrying about 1,000 men of the B.E.F. Literally every space on board seemed to be taken up with soldiers. Many of them were casualties with fractured legs and gunshot wounds of all kinds some of which were infected with gas gangrene. I was below, fully clothed and wearing gum boots. The next thing I knew was a crash and I found myself in water, in complete darkness and with no boots on. Water was pouring down from somewhere overhead and I could see faint daylight through a gap in the ship's side. Having gradually grasped the situation, I did a breast stroke and broke my way through some smashed bulkheads and got up a twisted ladder to the upper deck. I was very wet and shivering. I found a man in great pain and I could feel a fractured tibia but not haemorrhage. I gave him some morphia and used his sound leg as a splint.'

The dawn revealed a scene of great destruction and heavy mortality. H.M.S. *Grafton* was abandoned and her survivors were transferred to H.M.S. *Ivanhoe** The latter ship was on her way to Dunkirk so that the unfortunate survivors from H.M.S. *Grafton* had to endure further hours of ordeal before they eventually reached Dover.

May 29 was a day of heavy action. In the forenoon, H.M.Ss. *Jaguar*, *Gallant* and *Grenade* were heavily attacked by enemy dive-bombers while approaching Dunkirk, and H.M.S. *Gallant* was damaged and one of her crew killed. H.M.S. *Saladin* was also damaged and had to return to Dover being no longer seaworthy. On her way back to England, loaded with troops, *Jaguar* was again attacked by enemy aircraft and a large number of casualties was caused by bomb splinters from near misses. Fortunately, her Medical Officer received great assistance from a R.A.M.C. officer on board. Nevertheless, it became necessary to transfer some of the wounded to H.M.S. *Express* and so many were involved that the available stretchers proved insufficient and casualties had to be passed from ship to ship in blankets.

It was on May 29 that enemy air attack seemed to reach its peak, and one naval medical officer recorded:

'For each ship there was this constant menace from the air which was capable of reducing her to a mass of mangled metal. Distributed along the upper decks and through the messdecks were soldiers who showed exemplary fortitude. Happily extreme exhaustion acted somewhat as an anaesthetic. Some had marched long distances and all, including wounded, had waited for long periods on the shelving beaches. Many had had no food for 48 hours and had been on half rations since May 23.'

Throughout the whole of this day transports operated through the northern route. They began to enter the harbour of Dunkirk at daybreak and their return journey proceeded smoothly for a few hours. But at 1600 hours shipping alongside the mole was very heavily bombed for

---

* Unfortunately, during this transfer, a number of soldiers fell and were crushed between the sides of the two ships.

two hours. As this attack developed, the S.S. *Canterbury* and H.M.S. *Jaguar** managed to leave harbour, but both were hit and damaged by bombs. The S.S. *Fenella* was sunk alongside, and H.M.S. *Grenade*, on fire and sinking, had to be abandoned after being towed clear of the fairway. H.M.S. *Verity* was continually bombed for 35 minutes, but managed to escape at 1800 hours. By that time evacuation from the harbour had completely stopped temporarily, and later ships arriving could only report absence of life and the presence of burning and stricken ships.

Meanwhile, a steady embarkation of troops continued from the beaches. Here too, enemy air attacks were heavy, and the paddle-minesweepers *Gracie Fields*, *Waverley*, *Devonia* and *Brighton Belle* were lost. The S.S. *Crested Eagle* was set on fire and had to be beached, with the loss of about half of the 600 soldiers she was carrying.

In the evening H.M.S. *Bideford* was dive-bombed while embarking 400 troops from Bray-Dunes. Bombs hit her quarterdeck and destroyed the after part of the ship, and she was raked by machine-gun fire. Four of her officers and 24 ratings were killed, while the soldiers who died on her crowded upper deck or in the small boats alongside her could not be calculated. In her after dressing station all the first-aid party were either killed or wounded as were all those on her quarterdeck. As darkness fell movement was difficult and casualties had to be treated where they had fallen. Her Medical Officer† recorded:

'Besides the dead there were about 60 casualties varying in severity. The more severely injured had mainly multiple compound fractures from splinters. Immediate impromptu stretcher parties used anything they could improvise as stretchers including the door of the sick bay which had been blown off. I rapidly examined them and dealt with them in accordance with their severity and urgency as best I could. I was greatly assisted by a Corporal of the R.A.M.C. who was thoroughly competent, tireless, willing and self-sacrificing. When, some time later, he had the chance of being transferred to another ship, he refused to leave and insisted on staying with me.'

During the hours of darkness the surviving troops who could be moved were transferred from *Bideford* to the minesweeper *Kellett*. At dawn on May 30 H.M.S. *Bideford* was taken in tow by H.M.S. *Locust* and she eventually reached Dover after a passage lasting 30 hours.

In all, some 38,000 troops were carried in H.M. ships on May 29, but losses were heavy, and other ships lost were the S.Ss. *Normania*, *Lorinin* and *Mona's Queen*, while H.M.Ss. *Intrepid* and *Greyhound* were damaged.

---

* The Medical Officer of H.M.S. *Jaguar* was mentioned in dispatches for his devotion to duty on this occasion.

† The Medical Officer of H.M.S. *Bideford*, a surgeon lieutenant, R.N., was awarded the Distinguished Service Order for his gallantry on this occasion.

During May 30, approximately 48,000 troops were carried and there were many less casualties to ships and personnel. This must be attributed mainly to the fact that a mist hung low over the beaches and, combined with the heavy cloud of smoke flowing from Dunkirk, prevented accurate enemy attacks from the air.

Once again it was possible to send transports into the harbour of Dunkirk, and these fared much better than on the day before. The *Princess Maud* was damaged by gunfire from the shore batteries at Gravelines, and the *King Orry* was severely damaged by near misses of bombs inside the harbour and finally foundered when towed away.

A grave incident on this day was the deliberate attack made by enemy aircraft on the Hospital Ship *St. Julien*. The *Isle of Thanet* had already been shelled on May 27, and the attack on the *St. Julien* was the second made against a hospital ship with apparently complete disregard for the sanctity of the Red Cross.

Evacuation from the beaches continued on this day when increasing numbers of small power boats did much to increase the rate of embarkation. H.M.Ss. *Sabre* and *Anthony* were damaged by enemy aircraft but neither suffered casualties.

During the night of May 30–31, shelling of the evacuation areas was heavy and at 0530 hours on May 31, air attacks on the harbour of Dunkirk and the beaches developed more strength and continued throughout the day. In spite of this, embarkation of troops continued at all points. At La Panne piers of pontoons and lorries had been built which greatly speeded the process of evacuation which was attended by the loss of the H.M.S. *Devonia* and damage to H.M.Ss. *Hebe* and *Express*. All the troops in this area were embarked by midnight and La Panne was in the hands of the enemy by the following day.

Approximately 58,000 troops were evacuated on this day.

On June 1, two hospital carriers returned to England, only one of which had succeeded in entering the harbour of Dunkirk. The other had been forced to return after enduring heavy shellfire for some 4 hours. A number of light transports managed to enter the harbour despite repeated air attacks. The *Mona's Isle* was damaged by fire from shore batteries and the *Prague* was also damaged, taken in tow back to England and finally beached opposite Sandown Castle.

More hospital carriers were repeatedly demanded, but the momentum of evacuation had now increased to such a degree that all the available large ship berths in the harbour of Dunkirk were reserved for transports and destroyers. On shore therefore, no attempt was made any longer to segregate casualties in anticipation of them being given passage in vessels specially designed for them. They were merely embarked in whatever ship was the next to arrive with the result that every ship of every kind had its quota of casualties to be catered for by its harassed medical officer.

With the loss of La Panne evacuation from beaches had to be effected from those nearer Dunkirk. This meant that a concentration of shipping presented a tempting target which the enemy was not slow to attack. Soon after dawn heavy bombing and machine-gunning developed over the whole area and by 0900 hours nearly every ship had faced an attack of some kind. While embarking troops, H.M.S. *Basilisk* was put out of action by a direct hit aft which killed 8 and wounded 4 of her crew. She tried to struggle back to England but sank on the way.

H.M.Ss. *Keith*, *Salamander* and *Skipjack* were heavily bombed. *Keith* had to be abandoned with the loss of 35 of her crew and 16 wounded. *Skipjack* received several direct hits while she was carrying some 800 troops. She turned turtle and sank taking down with her most of the soldiers who were below decks. Those who survived the sinking were machine-gunned in the water and 29 of her crew were killed and 30 wounded. H.M.S. *Salamander* returned safely to England.

The destroyer *Havant* was sunk by bombs as was the gunboat *Mosquito*. H.M.Ss. *Ivanhoe* and *Vivacious* were damaged while crowded with troops. H.M.S. *Worcester*, with 1,000 troops on board, was dive-bombed and machine-gunned by 30 aircraft for nearly an hour. In such an overcrowded ship casualties were inevitable even in the absence of a direct hit and, although only 6 of her crew were killed and 33 wounded, casualties among soldiers on board amounted to 60 killed and over 200 wounded by bomb splinters and bullets. The ship's sick bay was severely damaged and most of the medical supplies were destroyed. The sick berth attendant was wounded and *Worcester's* Medical Officer did his best alone.*

In addition to losses by air attack, H.M.S. *Sandown* was damaged by shellfire, the *Grive* was blown up by a mine and the trawlers *Argyllshire* and *Stella Dorado* were sunk by torpedoes.

In spite of these losses 60,000 troops were carried back to England on this day by ships which executed a succession of round voyages interrupted only by time for necessary refuelling. At this stage of the evacuation some 226,000 troops had been landed in the United Kingdom; 95,000 had been lifted from the beaches and the remainder from Dunkirk Harbour. Of the latter, 49,000 were carried in transports and hospital ships and 82,000 by H.M. ships. By now the majority of the surviving vessels had been operating ceaselessly for some five days and officers and men were approaching a state of complete exhaustion.

Partly under cover of darkness, embarkation continued between 0200 and 0900 hours on June 2 and during this period some 31,000 troops were evacuated. It was then intended to suspend further concentrations of shipping around Dunkirk during the daylight hours, and to concentrate all efforts towards a mass evacuation the following night.

---

* This Medical Officer was mentioned in dispatches for his gallantry.

However, at 1039 hours an urgent signal was made from Dunkirk which read:

> 'Wounded situation acute and hospital ships should enter the harbour during the day. Geneva Convention, it is felt, will be honourably observed.'

It was felt that this signal had probably been made without the full knowledge of the attacks already made on hospital ships in the area. However, two hospital carriers were despatched from Dover.

The first to sail was the *Worthing*, which sailed alone at 1300 hours. At 1400 hours she was attacked by a formation of twelve German aircraft and, although not seriously damaged, she was forced to return to harbour.

The *Paris* followed the *Worthing* later in the day, but she too was deliberately attacked from the air at 1915 hours. She was badly damaged and her engines were rendered useless. Tugs were sent to her assistance, but she eventually sank.*

At 1700 hours on June 2, a large armada of ships left England for Dunkirk. This consisted of 13 transports, 11 destroyers, 14 minesweepers and several hundreds of small craft. There were also some French destroyers and about 120 fishing boats. These ships were filled with troops and returned to England without enemy interference.

During June 3, the same fleet of ships was made ready for yet another journey during the coming night. This fortunately proved to be the last journey, as there was no doubt that naval officers and men who had been involved in this evacuation had almost reached the full limit of human endurance. The embarkation was begun at 2330 hours on June 3 and by 0340 hours on June 4 the evacuation was completed as an organised evolution, H.M.Ss. *Express* and *Shikari* being the last to leave; 27,000 troops, mostly French, were lifted during the night.

Operation 'Dynamo' was now considered to be complete, although occasionally stragglers continued to be picked up at sea and were even rescued from the beaches until as late as June 12.

Much has been written elsewhere about the evacuation from Dunkirk, and it is not the duty of this History to add anything more than medical comment. The number of wounded embarked from Dunkirk itself and from the beaches was invariably a matter of chance and varied greatly. Some destroyers carried as many as 80 cot cases on one voyage. Some of these would be recent casualties who had been wounded while waiting for embarkation, while others had wounds which had occurred some

---

* This was the last attempt made to rescue wounded in and around Dunkirk by means of hospital ships. It was now realised that many wounded could never hope to be evacuated and, as is now known, Army chaplains, doctors and medical orderlies drew lots to decide who should remain with them.

days before and were gravely infected. At first it was regarded as a record when 600 soldiers, including 50 wounded, were carried by a destroyer in a single passage. But after a few days this became an average number and all considerations of overcrowding were waived. On May 31, H.M.S. *Whitehall* made two journeys and embarked 2,250 troops. H.M.S. *Sabre* made nine journeys in all as did H.M.S. *Vanquisher*, carrying between them almost 10,000 troops. H.M.S. *Basilisk* was the only destroyer to make as many as three journeys in one day during which she carried approximately 1,500 troops. These figures have been given as an illustration of the overcrowded conditions under which the medical officers of these ships had to perform their duties, and also as an indication of the mental and physical strain to which the crews of these ships were subjected.

BOULOGNE

At dawn on May 22, H.M.S. *Whitshed* escorted units of the Welsh and Irish Guards to Boulogne.

At dawn on May 23, two medical officers were sent from the Royal Naval Barracks, Chatham, to Dover. One of these doctors was attached to a party of 80 Royal Marines in H.M.S. *Vimy*, whose task was to assist in holding the approaches to Boulogne. The other was attached to a party of seamen from H.M.S. *Wild Swan* whose task was that of demolishing harbour and dock installations at Boulogne. By noon these medical officers found themselves attending to casualties amid the ruins of the station of Boulogne Docks. Each was accompanied by a sick berth attendant and six stretcher-bearers, and each contrived to form a Regimental Aid Post as best he could. Under continuous attack from the air and by gunfire from the surrounding hills, these small medical parties amalgamated with some personnel of the R.A.M.C. and formed a casualty reception centre in a corridor of the station. Here first aid was given, and wounded were transported to a number of destroyers. The wounded included a large number from two hospital trains.

As evening approached enemy air attack was intensified and German artillery and tanks were engaged by destroyers at point blank range. Meanwhile, H.M.Ss. *Keith*, *Wild Swan*, *Vimy*, *Venetia*, *Whitshed*, *Venomous* and *Vimiera* made repeated journeys across the Channel removing troops and wounded. *Keith*, *Wild Swan*, *Vimy* and *Venetia* were damaged by bombs. As many as 500 troops and 80 stretcher cases were carried at one time. With messdecks crowded to capacity, room was gradually made for the living by the removal of the dead, and ships' medical officers did their best in the face of heavy bombing attacks until the safety of Dover was reached.

By nightfall Boulogne Docks were surrounded and the small naval medical party was ordered to embark in H.M.S. *Venomous*. Here casualties continued to be treated in the ship's galley which was improvised into a sick bay, and these casualties included a number of the crew of *Venomous* herself.*

CALAIS

At noon on May 23, H.M.S. *Whitshed* escorted the last troop convoy into Calais.

On May 24, H.M.S. *Wessex* was bombed and sunk in the harbour of Calais. Her survivors were picked up by H.M.S. *Vimiera*. *Vimiera* herself was now heavily attacked from the air and there was no lighting on her messdecks so that treatment of the *Wessex's* casualties had to be carried out by the light of hand torches. In addition to their wounds these men were suffering from shock due to prolonged immersion.

H.M.S. *Greyhound* was bombed outside the harbour of Calais on May 26 and sustained casualties on her bridge.

On that day news was received in Dover that although the evacuation of Calais had been considered as completed as regards the Navy, there was a number of wounded left behind in a tunnel running east from the Gare Maritime, near the railway pier. In the afternoon it was arranged that the motor yachts *Gulzar* and *Grey Mist* should attempt to rescue these men. A medical officer and one sick berth attendant took passage in the *Gulzar*, and one sick berth attendant in the *Grey Mist*. These ships arrived at Calais at 0130 hours on May 27. The moon had risen but its light was virtually outshone by the glare of blazing buildings along the waterfront. In the words of the Medical Officer:

'We crept into a deserted harbour with no sign of life, and only the sound of the crackle of flames and the occasional fall of a roof or building.'

A landing was effected, but challenges and machine-gun nests discouraged prolonged reconnaissance. It was with some dismay that the medical officer saw a steady file of dim figures trooping on board the *Gulzar*, but they proved to be a party of 3 officers and 48 men of the Rifle Brigade, Royal Corps of Signals and Royal Marines. It was now learned that these men had taken shelter on one of the wooden piers where they had decided to fight to the last. Their rescue was effected and the medical officer was informed that the wounded who he had been sent to seek had already been taken off in some French boats. He also searched for but could not find a naval medical officer who had been sent to Calais with a party of Royal Marines.†

ST. VALERY-EN-CAUX

On June 9, a medical officer was lent from R.N. Barracks, Portsmouth,

---

* Both the medical officers ashore in Boulogne were mentioned in dispatches.

† This Medical Officer had survived the loss of H.M.S. *Hardy* at Narvik. At Calais he was made a prisoner-of-war. The Medical Officer of the *Gulzar* was mentioned in dispatches.

to H.M.S. *Hampton* for special service. He was provided with medical stores and two sick berth attendants. H.M.S. *Hampton* was a former train ferry which had been converted for minelaying. She was not well equipped for medical activities. She arrived off the harbour of St. Valéry at 0430 hours on June 11. Her task was to evacuate British troops who left the shore in boats towed by a motor boat. The *Hampton*, which also saw service off Le Havre, came under shellfire from the shore and was heavily attacked from the air, being near missed by sixteen bombs.

Other ships operating off St. Valéry were H.M.Ss. *Broke*, *Codrington*, *Saladin* and *Harvester*. All evacuated British troops, including casualties who were discharged to R.N. Hospital, Haslar, within a few hours. All came under enemy attack and *Harvester* was fortunate to escape with only three members of her crew wounded.

ST. NAZAIRE

On June 17, H.M.S. *Highlander* began the evacuation of men of the B.E.F. from St. Nazaire. During embarkation the S.S. *Lancastria* was bombed and sunk with great loss of life. The *Lancastria* had sunk very quickly and her survivors could remember little except the explosions, the collapse of their surroundings and the surge of water in which they found themselves clinging to wreckage. H.M.S. *Havelock* rescued approximately 500 survivors including some 250 cases of wounds and burns who were treated by *Havelock's* Medical Officer and sick berth attendant during the next 36 hours. A small number of survivors was also rescued by H.M.S. *Highlander* including wounded who were later transferred to the S.S. *Oronsay*.

A number of British Army casualties and 300 Polish troops were evacuated from St. Nazaire by H.M.S. *Punjabi*. The rescue of these Army patients was effected chiefly by the zeal of *Punjabi's* Medical Officer.*

---

* This Medical Officer, a Surgeon Lieutenant, R.N., was awarded the Distinguished Service Cross for his outstanding initiative and determination during the evacuation of these troops from St. Nazaire. The official citation reads:

'At 0824 hours on June 20, 1940, H.M.S. *Punjabi* was berthed at the entrance to Penhouet Basin, St. Nazaire, for the purpose of evacuating Polish troops. The main German forces had reached Nantes, 30 miles away. An advance party had already entered St. Nazaire the evening before to make arrangements for taking over the town. The town had been bombed earlier in the morning, the main objective being apparently the hospital, and German land forces were expected to enter at any moment.

'When embarkation was nearly completed it was reported, at 0940 hours, that a number of British wounded soldiers, mostly survivors from S.S. *Lancastria*, was ashore in the local Army Hospital. The Surgeon Lieutenant commandeered a motor lorry which he found on the wharf nearby. Driving the vehicle himself, and syphoning petrol from the tanks of other abandoned motor vehicles on the roadside, he made three journeys to and from the hospital some three miles distant. He cleared the hospital of all the British wounded, of whom 12 were cot cases. The work was completed most expeditiously so that H.M.S. *Punjabi* was just able to leave before the dangerous time of low water.

'The Surgeon Lieutenant showed the most commendable initiative and determination in carrying out this valuable work.'

MEDICAL ORGANISATION FOR THE EVACUATION OF THE B.E.F.

In general the medical organisation of the evacuation was of necessity improvised to meet requirements as they arose. Also, it was greatly dependent on the personal initiative and resourcefulness of medical officers in destroyers and other small ships.

But many ships did not carry a medical officer so that, early in the evacuation, it was found necessary to appoint a special medical unit for duty with the Vice Admiral, Dover. This unit was provided by the Royal Naval Barracks, Chatham, and served from May 29 until June 4.

The unit consisted of 6 medical officers and 26 sick berth ratings. On arriving at Dover, they were distributed between the *St. Helier*, *Tynwald*, *Manxman* and *Lady of Man*, while 2 medical officers and 8 sick berth ratings were detailed for duty with the Senior Naval Officer, Dunkirk.

When the latter party arrived at Dunkirk, on May 30, the jetty was under heavy fire and the concentration of troops rendered progress ashore impossible. Eventually the party collected some 15 wounded which they brought back to England in the *St. Helier*. On reaching Folkestone, these 2 medical officers were returned to Chatham as their services were no longer necessary.

The remaining medical officers sent from the Royal Naval Barracks, Chatham, performed valuable services in a number of ships. These medical officers were completely unfamiliar with the various ships to which they were attached. They did not remain in any one ship for long, but were moved from one to another.

RECEPTION AND DISPOSAL OF CASUALTIES IN ENGLAND

Soon after the invasion of the Low Countries on May 10, 1940, the harbours on the south-east and south coasts of England, from Harwich to Plymouth, began to receive troops and refugees many of whom were casualties.

At Dover, in H.M.S. *Lynx*, prior to the commencement of the Dunkirk evacuation on May 26, the medical staff consisted of 5 medical officers and 19 sick berth ratings distributed as follows:

H.M.S. *Sandhurst* . .	2 medical officers, 7 sick berth ratings
R.N. Sick Quarters .	2 medical officers, 9 sick berth ratings
Dover Patrol Sick Bay .	1 medical officer, 3 sick berth ratings

In addition, two stretcher parties, each consisting of 1 petty officer and 8 ratings, had been trained and were available at the Base. The plan was that all information concerning casualties should be transmitted from the Naval Staff Office to the local Senior Medical Officer at the R.N. Sick Quarters, who would be responsible for making the necessary arrangements. His task, having been acquainted with the expected numbers, nature, place and time of arrival of casualties, was to muster the necessary transport and reception staff at the various landing stages. These landing stages were:

Admiralty Pier	Suitable for large vessels.
Prince of Wales' Pier	Suitable for trawlers and drifters.
West Jetty	Suitable for vessels up to Destroyer Class.
Eastern Arm	Suitable for large vessels.
Grenville Dock Steps	Suitable for motor boats and small yachts.
H.M.S. *Sandhurst*	A destroyer depot ship, suitable for berthing destroyers.

On the reception of casualties, after confirming that all necessary first aid had been rendered, minor cases were sent either to H.M.S. *Sandhurst* or to the local Royal Naval Sick Quarters. Serious cases were sent directly to a base hospital. An agreement had been made with the local Military and Civil Authorities to pool resources in an emergency, but, at this time, this was only a superficial scheme of co-operation which applied principally to the pooling of transport facilities.

Some extension of this naval medical organisation in Dover became necessary on May 11 and 14, when casualties were received from H.M.Ss. *Whitshed* and *Wivern*. Of the casualties, 13 were sent to the E.M.S. Hospital, Dover, 16 to the Military Hospital, Shorncliffe, and 8 to the Royal Marine Infirmary, Deal.

From May 20 onwards, wounded were being landed in Dover almost continuously. On May 25, it was necessary to obtain additional naval medical staff. On the same date an emergency routine was developed to deal with the very large numbers of casualties which it was anticipated would be received between May 26 and June 3.

Within these few days 180,982 troops were landed in Dover of whom 6,880 were casualties requiring hospital treatment. In addition, there were approximately 600 naval casualties, including 54 dead. The 'peak day' was May 31, when 34,484 troops were landed from 129 different ships, and included 1,200 wounded.

Casualties arrived in Dover in every sort of ship. Each ship which came alongside was met by an ambulance with a medical officer and 2 sick berth ratings. Should the ship carry her own medical officer, the information regarding requirements was quickly available. But where no medical officer was carried, the shore doctor had to board the vessel and ascertain the number of casualties and estimate their seriousness, etc. Casualties were classified as follows:

Urgent stretcher cases, to be sent to nearby base hospitals.
Non-urgent stretcher cases, to be sent further afield.*
Walking cases, some to be sent to local sick bays and others to the more remote hospitals.

---

* These were mostly sent by hospital train to E.M.S. Hospitals.

Each ambulance which met a vessel carried first-aid equipment and a Neil-Robertson stretcher in addition to the four fitted stretchers of the ambulance itself.

In most of the destroyers and larger vessels very efficient first aid had been rendered to casualties on passage, either by the ship's own medical officer or by R.A.M.C. passengers, and frequently by both. But in the case of trawlers and smaller craft, of which there was a very great number, it was usually necessary for a considerable amount of first aid to be rendered before casualties could be moved from ship to ambulance.

Once the organisation at Dover had been fully developed there was excellent co-operation, pooling of resources and distribution of labour between the local Naval, Army and Civilian Services. To start with the Navy had endeavoured to deal with all Service casualties as ships arrived. But once every landing stage was being used at the same time this became impossible and the R.A.M.C. dealt with casualties from ships which berthed at Admiralty Pier. This pier received about 60 per cent. of ships arriving at Dover, all of whose casualties were dealt with by the R.A.M.C. At this particular landing stage ambulances could be parked right alongside the ships, and wounded could be transferred into them in the shortest possible time. Also, 200 yards away was a railway station in which were hospital trains into which casualties from the ships could be quickly transported.

The Navy now became concerned with the more remote landing stages, and at these conditions did not always favour the reception of large numbers of casualties. Steep gangways and slippery steps had to be negotiated, and patients had either to be man-handled or conveyed to the quayside in Neil-Robertson stretchers. Unfortunately, once the casualty had been transported to the point where ambulances were waiting, the patients had to be transferred to an Army pattern or A.R.P. stretcher so that the Neil-Robertson stretcher could be used again.

The nearest available base hospitals for the reception of these casualties were:

E.M.S. Casualty Hospital, Dover*	1½ miles distant. 100 beds. 2 surgical teams.
Royal Marine Infirmary, Deal	9 miles distant. 150 beds. 2 surgical teams.
Military Hospital, Shorncliffe	11 miles distant. 200 beds. 3 surgical teams.
Royal Naval Hospital, Chatham	43 miles distant. Full general hospital facilities.

---

* *See* E.M.S. Volume I, Chapter 4; 354 casualties were admitted to this hospital.

As numbers increased great care had to be taken to avoid swamping these hospitals of which the capacity was limited by the strength of surgical teams rather than by beds. Large numbers of casualties were sent to hospitals inland and to E.M.S. Hospitals throughout the South of England. Where possible, naval wounded were segregated and sent to Service hospitals.

Although there is no doubt that casualties arriving at Dover were dealt with expeditiously, a number of difficulties existed which militated against that smooth reception and disposal of wounded which would have been desirable. The chief adverse factors were:

Much of the work had to be done at night, and often during air-raid alarms.

The unsuitability of a number of the landing stages, with crowding which meant that ships frequently had to be berthed alongside each other.

An 18 ft. rise and fall of tide sometimes caused the gangways to be almost vertical.

The transport of wounded from ships was often hampered by troop movements, refugees and stray dogs.

That these difficulties were overcome must be attributed not merely to medical personnel, but also to the crews of the ships involved who, though invariably fatigued, were always ready cheerfully to assist in disembarking wounded.

At Ramsgate the local naval base was used as a clearing station. Once troops had been landed, there was very little delay in clearing the wounded from ships as they berthed. At the height of the evacuation two additional naval medical officers were sent from Portsmouth, and these were employed to proceed to sea and make contact with ships carrying casualties, which had broken down and found difficulty in entering the harbour.

A Naval and an Army Medical Officer were always available at the pierhead at high tide, the only time at which many of the larger vessels could enter harbour. A pierhead rallying point was established for medical personnel, and here large stocks of dressings, medical equipment and stretchers were held in readiness.

At Ramsgate large numbers of Army casualties were received and transferred by military ambulances to hospitals at Tunbridge Wells, Farnborough, Maidstone, Dartford and Canterbury.

Other casualties were landed at Sheerness, Southampton, Portsmouth and Plymouth.

CLINICAL ASSESSMENT OF CASUALTIES

The destroyers and the large number of miscellaneous ships engaged in the evacuation of the B.E.F. from the Continent were subjected to almost continuous attacks by enemy aircraft. As a result of bomb explosions, most casualties were caused by metal splinters from bombs and from parts of the ships themselves. Burns were caused through cordite charges becoming ignited. Other burns were the result of oil fuel blazing on the surface of the sea around men struggling in the water. Scalds were caused by bombs exploding close to ships and lifting some of the plates and fracturing connexions in engine and boiler rooms. Persons immersed in the sea were exposed to blast injuries from exploding mines, depth charges and bombs.

Some ships were attacked by enemy motor torpedo boats, but the damage which they inflicted was negligible compared with the attacks of enemy aircraft.

In H.M. Destroyers there were approximately 220 naval officers and ratings killed, 100 missing and 420 wounded. These figures cover the whole period of operations along the Dutch, Belgian and French coasts, from May 10 to June 18. The figures represent not more than 10 per cent. casualties among the ships' companies of all the destroyers involved. The majority of these casualties occurred during Operation 'Dynamo' between May 26 and June 3. During this short period 40 destroyers were engaged. Of these, 5 were sunk and 18 damaged. In the 5 sunk naval casualties were 175 killed, missing or died of wounds, and 81 wounded. In the 18 damaged, 15 were killed and 163 wounded. In all a total of 478 casualties occurred in a number of destroyers whose total complement was approximately 5,500.

In the auxiliary ships such as H.M. minesweepers, trawlers, drifters, tugs and gunboats, during the same short period, naval losses were 60 killed, 50 missing and 160 wounded. Thirty-five auxiliary ships were sunk and these figures represent approximately the same percentage of casualties as in the case of the destroyers.

Naval casualties therefore, in both destroyers and auxiliary ships, were less than 800 during the course of Operation 'Dynamo'. This, it is submitted, was an unbelievably light cost in relation to the magnitude of the evacuation and the valuable results achieved.

TYPES OF WOUNDS

The numerous reports of medical officers show that wounds of most descriptions were encountered; 60 per cent. of wounds were caused by flying fragments of metal, with wounds due to machine-gun bullets the next highest in frequency.

The lacerations caused by metal splinters varied from slight superficial flesh wounds with tiny particles under the skin to large wounds with great destruction of tissue and internal damage. Compound fractures, traumatic amputations and penetrating wounds of the skull chest and abdomen were all seen. Some of the metal splinters were as large as an orange, with sharp ragged edges, and caused tearing rather than penetrating wounds, with extensive tissue destruction and wide gaping of wound edges. In many cases men were lying face down during bombing attacks, and this undoubtedly reduced the number of fractures and penetrating wounds of abdomen and chest wall. This practice of lying down is thought also to have played some part in the low incidence of damage to the larger blood vessels and of all nerve injuries. Among 300 lacerated wounds recorded only two cases of nerve injury occurred. In one case, typical of the more serious type of laceration, a naval rating who had thrown himself on his face had the whole of one buttock severed down to the ileum, but the large vessels and nerves were undamaged.

As regards injuries caused by the direct blast of bomb explosions, numerous widespread contusions and ruptured tympanic membranes were observed, but direct blast injuries to chest and abdomen were very uncommon. Of the latter there is only one case reported by a destroyer's Medical Officer, who states:

'I came across my first case of chest compression from blast. I recognised a man's voice and removed him from under two dead bodies. He complained of a pain in his chest. He was dyspnoeic and there were signs of froth and blood on his lips. There was absolutely no sign of external injury, but it seemed obvious that he had some form of internal chest lesion involving his lungs.'

Almost all the reports of medical officers remark the fact that after a bombing attack, personnel were not fully conscious or rational for some minutes and frequently seemed unable to give or to obey orders.

Another possible hazard of bombing appears in the report of one Medical Officer of a destroyer which states:

'A stick of bombs exploded alongside and the whole of one gun's crew disappeared overboard. Whether they were blown into the sea by blast, or whether they were thrown overboard by the ship suddenly altering course, or whether they merely jumped will never be known.'

Machine-gun bullets fired from aircraft and rifle bullets fired by snipers ashore caused a relatively high mortality among exposed personnel. Factors which played a part were the absence of sufficient steel helmets and the difficulty of finding cover on the ships' crowded decks. Penetrating wounds of skull and chest were more frequently caused by bullets than by bombs and usually resulted in instant death.

The wounds caused by bullets were characteristic and in many cases the missile remained deeply embedded in the tissues. The wounds caused by cannon shells from aircraft were different in that the missile exploded on contact and broke up into innumerable small particles of metal. In a typical case some hundreds of tiny fragments would be distributed through the tissues at various levels.

TREATMENT ON BOARD DESTROYERS

The reports of medical officers show how the customary medical organisation was adapted for the treatment of large numbers of casualties in all parts of a ship, during constant and prolonged action, and amid overcrowding the like of which had never been visualised.

In most ships the Captain's cabin was transformed into a dressing station, while officers' cabins, chart room, etc., were reserved for serious cases. Apart from these positions, wounded were placed in every possible position between decks. In one ship as many as 72 wounded, on Army type stretchers, were arranged in layers on the forward messdeck, the top layer being supported by kit lockers, the middle layer on mess tables and the bottom layer on the deck itself. In some destroyers stretcher supports were constructed of three equidistant loops in a rope hung from hammock hooks. The Army stretcher handles could then be fitted into these loops and the stretchers accommodated in tiers of three.

Fortunately, the majority of Army wounded had been well dressed by the R.A.M.C. before embarkation. The chief task which medical officers of destroyers had to perform was concerned with efficient attention to shock and exhaustion, with a minimum of surgical intervention. The treatment during passage to England usually consisted of giving morphia and anti-tetanic serum as necessary, allowing the men on board to empty their bladders, providing hot drinks and distributing clothing where it was needed.

Although the general policy was to interfere with these Army casualties as little as possible, there were occasional cases where there had not been time for a casualty to be dealt with fully before embarkation. In some cases adequate splinting of fractures and the re-dressing of wounds required general anaesthesia. Occasional bleeding points had to be ligatured and 'sucking' chest wounds were sutured.

But the situation described became more exacting, and almost overwhelming conditions arose when the loaded ships were strongly attacked on passage to England. Then medical personnel, already fully occupied, found themselves burdened with additional casualties, often in large numbers. The Medical Officer of one destroyer has recorded:

> 'While transporting 1,000 soldiers we were attacked by enemy aircraft. There were 20 casualties among the ship's company, including 3 killed, and 70 casualties among our passengers, 10 of which were fatal. All these occurred within the space of a few minutes. At the time of the attack I was busy treating soldiers who had been injured before embarkation. I was overwhelmed by ambulant casualties, but I found other more serious cases in almost every section of the ship, who had to be treated where they lay.'

Another destroyer which was attacked while carrying 1,000 troops had 240 casualties of which 40 were fatal. Her Medical Officer recorded:

'The wardroom was plastered with pieces of viscera and limbs, but I did find some living entangled in the twisted wreckage.'

Under these extraordinary conditions it was almost impossible to find space for the segregation and treatment of casualties in these small ships.* The detailed examination of wounds newly inflicted on board was impracticable, and the medical staff was never adequate to deal efficiently with everyone.†

This virtual impossibility of adequately coping with casualties in such overcrowded conditions meant that such routines as the intermittent loosening and tightening of tourniquets were not always possible. Consequently there are a few reports of limbs being lost owing to gangrene where a tourniquet was left *in situ* for too long. Nevertheless some medical officers have claimed in their records that there was one small advantage which was brought about by overcrowding. This was that the impossibility of moving casualties about in such great congestion did at least have the merit of avoiding any further increase of shock by man-handling.

As regards severe burns, tannic acid sprays and 'Tannafax' jelly were used, but for first and second degree burns flavine emulsions were found quicker and more easy to handle.

Anti-tetanic serum was administered to the wounded military and also to any naval personnel who had been wounded on the beaches or in a ship alongside. But the demand for this serum much exceeded normal naval requirements and discretion had to be shown in its use. In many cases, because of the lack of supplies and also because of lack of opportunity it was not given at all. Likewise, the small supplies of anti-gas gangrene serum which were carried in destroyers were quickly exhausted. A number of gas gangrene cases was reported among soldiers wounded before embarkation. But no cases were reported among naval wounded, despite the proximity of the grossly infected to those with wounds newly inflicted on board.

The great number of casualties to be treated in destroyers involved the expenditure of very large quantities of medical stores of all kinds. Dressings and bandages carried according to service afloat scale were generally found to be adequate for dealing with anything up to 50 cases. After that ships' emergency chests had to be opened and used in most cases. These were found to contain too much lint and not enough gauze, and field dressings were required far in excess of the number carried. In some ships R.A.M.C. stores were brought on board, and the Army shell dressings were found most valuable on account of their larger size. The unexpectedly small numbers of fractures did not overtax the

---

* Some medical officers contrived to move badly shocked casualties to the approaches to the engine room, for greater warmth.

† This was particularly so when the medical staff had themselves become casualties.

normal supply of splints. But some medical officers felt the need for an 'aeroplane' type of splint or some form of material from which this could have been constructed.

The value of the small number of Neil-Robertson stretchers in H.M. Destroyers was found to be inestimable. They allowed some of the more seriously wounded to be stowed away in places which otherwise would have been quite inaccessible to them.

The 'Novox' apparatus proved its value on several occasions when men were rescued from the sea. But some ships reported that resuscitation and the treatment of shock were gravely hampered by the lack of sufficient blankets for the many men who had to remain in exposed positions.*

PSYCHOLOGICAL EFFECTS

The naval casualties received from the Hook of Holland and during the latter part of May were all very cheerful and made light of their experiences. But the legacy of psychological trauma which was left by Operation 'Dynamo' was probably limited only by the number of men who were present.

From the actual cases recorded, it is apparent that the psychological effects were most manifest and most prolonged in seamen over the age of 45, in pensioners and reservists. On the other hand, younger men with no previous experience of action seemed to be less prone to anxiety.

In many instances soldiers arrived on board H.M. ships in a condition of advanced nervous exhaustion and in no state to face further enemy attacks. Occasional cases were so hysterical that morphia was necessary. One Medical Officer records that men 'had to be strapped in Neil-Robertson stretchers and given morphia, both to prevent suicide, and to prevent their anxiety spreading to others not so badly affected.'

As regards mental strain, ships' companies were more fortunate than their military passengers on board. The vigil of the latter was uninterrupted by any form of occupation. Also, naval personnel were employed in corporate units and had that sense of mutual support which is present in the closely knit comradeship of a ship's crew. But the Army units on board had inevitably become extensively disorganised in some cases.

One of the most severe tests of morale was that imposed upon the destroyer *Bideford* when she lay disabled. Her Medical Officer recorded:

> 'During hours of suspense and uncertainty we were all watching the clock and anxiously wondering whether 0400 hours would bring with it rescue or hostile aircraft.'

The hope of help to this ship was very dim, and the prospect of air attack was a conviction among men who had had no sleep for sixty hours. When dawn brought a relief ship and an attempt was made to

---

* Some survivors reached England wrapped only in tablecloths.

tow *Bideford* off the mud, her Medical Officer has recorded the dramatic moments when 'We moved, ever so slightly, but we moved. The suspense was terrific as we watched the stern yaw.' Nevertheless, in this ship there was no sign of breakdown, only that of the most intense alertness.

Coupled with the usual background of the incidents of battle, continued loss of sleep was the factor which contributed most toward psychological disturbances. It seems probable that, had sleep not been denied to the crews of so many ships through force of circumstances, there would have been hardly any hospital admissions for psychiatric reasons as a result of this operation. In actual fact, there were probably many more hospital admissions than were warranted by the number of genuine cases because, under the conditions existing at Dover, admission to hospital was often the only means of securing sleep, rest and regular meals for some men who were obviously badly in need of relief. There came a time when some seamen had been on almost continuous watch for six days. The type of case in which exhaustion and not lack of courage was the factor involved is illustrated by one seaman who showed a marked generalised tremor and was unable to walk. This man had been on watch for some six days and nights and had also dived overboard to rescue a drowning soldier.

Individual hysterical manifestations were rare and very few are recorded. H.M.S. *Whitshed* reported one case of hysterical aphonia and amblyopia. The need for isolating such few cases as did occur, in order to avoid others becoming infected by such symptoms, is shown by events in H.M.S. *Hebe*. On Saturday June 1, *Hebe* was damaged by bombs during the evacuation of Dunkirk. No one in her had slept for five days and nights. One young officer suddenly had an attack of hysterical epilepsy on the bridge. Some 30 members of the ship's company now became similarly affected with generalised clonic movements and incoherent mumbling. The Medical Officer who had to deal with these cases himself finally succumbed to this mass suggestion. It is in point that these psychological manifestations did not appear until the ship's crew ceased to be actively engaged and found themselves safely in harbour after a long period of physical and mental fatigue had culminated in the last severe air attack. It is also on record that in H.M.S. *Hussar*, men became hyper-emotional and broke down and wept when given an order.*

The measures adopted for controlling threatened psychological breakdown in these ships varied, but always called for the combined efforts of Doctor and Commanding Officer working hand in hand. Reassurance by a Medical Officer frequently proved successful when

---

* The reader is referred to the description of Arctic Convoys given in Chapter 4 of this Volume.

CASUALTIES IN H.M. DESTROYERS
May 10–June 10, 1940

H.M. Destroyers Lost/Damaged	L/D	Date	Cause of casualties	K	M	W	D/W	1	2	3	4	5	6	7	8	9	10	11	12	13	14	15	16	N/S
Whitshed	D	May 10, 1940	Bombs	7	0	9	0	2	0		1											1			
Versatile	D	May 13, 1940	Bombs and cannon fire	7	0	26	3	24	1	2								1					1		2
Wivern	D	May 14, 1940	Bombs and machine gun	24	2	29	7	17	1				1	1	1								8		
Valentine	D	May 15, 1940	Bombs	0	1	2	0	2	1																
Whitley	L	May 19, 1940	Bombs	4	0	3	0	1																	
Malcolm	D	May 20, 1940	Bombs	2	0	25	3	14	3		1			2					1			1	4		1
Keith	D	May 23, 1940	Bombs	2	0	5	0	3			1														1
Whitshed	D	May 23, 1940	Bombs	1	0	1	0	11						1											
Wild Swan	D	May 23, 1940	Bombs	3	0	13	0	6	1				1												4
Venetia	D	May 23, 1940	Bombs and bullets	7	0	13	0	2						1	1			1							
Vimy	D	May 23, 1940	Bombs	2	0	2	0																		
Wessex	L	May 24, 1940	Bombs	0	14	6	1		2						1								2		2
Greyhound	—	May 26, 1940	Bombs	2	0	3	0	2				1 rib													1
Wolsey	—	May 27, 1940	Bombs	0	0	2	0																		1
Vivacious	D	May 28, 1940	Bombs	0	0	3	0	2																	1
Gallant	D	May 28, 1940	Bombs	1	0	25	0	22	1		2	1 rib			1			1							1
Windsor	D	May 28, 1940	Bombs	2	0	11	0	9	3																
Grafton	L	May 29, 1940	Torpedo	16	16	56	0	5															36		9
Grenade	L	May 29, 1940	Bombs	0	0		0																		
Greyhound	D	May 29, 1940	Bombs	6	0	31	2	24															1		6
Jaguar	D	May 29, 1940	Bombs and bullets	3	0	17	1	16	1									1					1		
Intrepid	D	May 29, 1940	Bombs and bullets	2	0	22	0	19		1				1									1		2
Saladin	D	May 29, 1940	Bombs	0	0	3	0	3																	
Bideford	D	May 29, 1940	Bombs and machine gun	13	2	21	0	16	3																	
Wakeful	L	May 29, 1940	Torpedo, bombs	86	13	5	0	3																	
Shikari	—	May 29, 1940	Torpedo, bombs	1	0	3	0	1																	
Basilisk	L	June 1, 1940	Torpedo, bombs	8	0	4	0	3																	2
Ivanhoe	D	June 1, 1940	Torpedo, bombs	18	0	12	1	10															2		
Icarus	—	June 1, 1940	Torpedo, bombs	0	0	3	1	3																	
Worcester	D	June 1, 1940	Bombs and machine gun	6	0	33	0	31	2		1					2							1		3
Scimitar	D	June 2, 1940	Machine gun	1	0	9	0	9																	
Sabre	D	June 5, 1940	Bombs	0	0	1	0	1																	
Boadicea	D	June 10, 1940	Bombs	2	5	1	2	1					1												
Keith	L	June 1, 1940	Bombs	3	32	15	1	5	2		1		1												

* K = Killed, M = Missing, W = Wounded, D/W = Died of wounds. Classification of wounds. N/S = Not stated.
† Numbers 1–16,

1. Lacerations
2. Contusions
3. Simple Fractures.
4. " "
5. Simple Fractures. Spine
6. " " Skull
7. Compound fractures. Upper limb
8. " " Lower limb

9. Penetrating wounds. Skull
10. " " Chest
11. " " Abdomen
12. " " Spine

13. Wounds of Blood vessels
14. Wounds of Peripheral nerves
15. Burns
16. Blast injuries

CASUALTIES IN H.M. SHIPS

H.M. Ships	Date	Casualties			Types of injuries															
		Dead	D/W	Wounds	1	2	3	4	5	6	7	8	9	10	11	12	13	14	15	16	N/S
Gloucester	July 8, 1940	14	4	9	7					1											
Hereward	July 9, 1940		1	1		1															
Vampire	July 11, 1940				1																
Liverpool	July 12, 1940	3		3	1						2								1		

Notes: All these casualties were caused by bombs. Seven of the *Gloucester's* including the four who died had burns in addition to other wounds. Except in the case of H.M.S. *Gloucester*, H.M. Ships were undamaged.

Numbers 1–16, Classification of wounds. *See* p. 307. N/S = Not stated.

THE CHIEF NAVAL EVENTS, 1939-1941

combined with the natural leadership of the professional naval officer and senior rating. In fact, in many ships it called for skilful judgement and resolution to decide how far it was possible or wise to drive a ship's company suffering from prolonged strain.

ACTION OFF CALABRIA, JULY 1940

In common with other operations in the Mediterranean before the arrival there of units of the Luftwaffe, this action lacked any great medical significance, and therefore merits only brief reference in this History.

The Mediterranean Fleet left Alexandria on the night of July 7/8, 1940, its object being to cover the passage of a convoy of merchantmen from Malta to Alexandria.

On the morning of July 8 the Italian Fleet was reported to be at sea, but the first hostile action came in the form of heavy air attacks which continued throughout the day. H.M.S. *Gloucester* was hit by a bomb which exploded on her compass platform; 14 persons were killed instantaneously and 4 others soon died of wounds. A further 9 wounded survived. Among those killed were the Captain, Commander, Navigating and Torpedo Officers. *Gloucester's* dead were buried at sea immediately and her wounded were treated under conditions of difficulty as the ship continued in company with the main Battle Fleet and remained at first degree of readiness for action in spite of her damaged state.

Contact was established with the enemy fleet at 1500 hours on July 9 and surface action and air attacks continued until about 1925 hours on the same day. Although H.M.S. *Neptune* was damaged by bomb splinters, the only British casualty recorded was in H.M.S. *Hereward*.

The Fleet was repeatedly bombed during the return passage to Alexandria. On July 11 an officer of H.M.A.S. *Vampire* was wounded by multiple bomb splinters, and died after being transferred to H.M.S. *Mohawk*.

On the following day 3 men were killed in H.M.S. *Liverpool* in the course of two bombing attacks, while her Commander and 2 ratings were wounded. All these injuries were caused by bomb splinters in personnel in exposed positions on the upper deck, and all were wounded in the upper parts of the body.

ACTION OFF CAPE SPADA, CRETE, JULY 1940

At dawn on July 19, 1940, H.M. Destroyers *Hyperion*, *Ilex*, *Hero* and *Hasty* sighted the Italian cruisers *Giovanni Delle Bande Nere* and *Bartolomeo Colleoni*. This sighting was reported to H.M.A.S. *Sydney* which, with H.M.S. *Havock*, was in position off Cape Spada. At 0726 hours, the enemy engaged H.M.Ss. *Hyperion* and *Ilex* soon after which the *Sydney* joined action.

At 0921 hours H.M.A.S. *Sydney* received her only hit and suffered one minor casualty. Two minutes later the *Colleoni* was seen to be stopped and on fire. She was then torpedoed and lost the last hundred feet of her bows. The *Colleoni* had many casualties including her Captain and though little attempt was made to lower boats or rafts, it proved possible to rescue a remarkable number of survivors. The *Colleoni* sank at 0959 hours, and 545 survivors were rescued by the British ships concerned. These survivors included 58 wounded of whom 3 died.* A great number of these survivors was rescued by H.M.S. *Havock* and this ship reported that her work of mercy was interrupted by enemy bombing attacks in the course of which *Havock* herself suffered 2 casualties in her boiler room as the result of a near miss. This incident is of some importance in that it led the Commander-in-Chief, Mediterranean, to issue a Memorandum to the Fleet, on July 22, 1940, which reads:

'Rescue of Survivors from Enemy Ships

While the instincts of the British race and the traditions of the sea produce in us all a powerful urge to rescue the survivors of sinking ships, it must be remembered that there are other considerations to be weighed against this humane work. We are waging a relentless war against odds, and here in the Mediterranean not only are we competing against numerically superior naval forces, but we have also against us very considerable air forces which our own Air Force is not yet in a position to attack, except in Eastern Libya. It follows that no favourable opportunity must be lost of destroying enemy forces, and the rescue of survivors must never be allowed to interfere with the relentless pursuit of enemy ships. It must also be borne in mind that practically the whole of the area of our operations is subject to enemy bombing. Therefore ships cannot usually afford to hang about picking up survivors, for not only do they thus expose themselves to bomb attack under very disadvantageous conditions, but also subsequent operations are liable to be delayed. Moreover a destroyer with a large number of persons on board is bound to be considerably reduced in fighting efficiency. Difficult and distasteful as it is to leave survivors to their fate, Commanding Officers must be prepared to harden their hearts for, after all, the operations in hand and the security of their ships and ships' companies must take precedence in war.'

OPERATIONS OFF DAKAR, SEPTEMBER 1940

In these operations on September 23 and 25, 1940 unexpected resistance by French forces was encountered.

The old battleships *Barham* and *Resolution* were engaged on this occasion and it is of some medical interest that conditions on board them resulted in a number of cases of heat exhaustion. In H.M.S. *Barham* the dry bulb temperature on the messdecks was between 100°

---

* The Captain of the *Bartolomeo Colleoni* subsequently died on board the Hospital Ship *Maine*.

and 110° F., while in the forward dressing station it reached 140° F. In the presence of a high relative humidity it is surprising that only 9 cases of heat exhaustion reported sick. Unfortunately the numbers in H.M.S. *Resolution* were greater and she had 64 cases of heat exhaustion altogether, of whom 1 died. Included in these were 12 per cent. of the engine room complement who had been exposed to temperatures in the boiler and dynamo rooms which varied between 126° F., and 136° F.

Certain of H.M. cruisers and destroyers were damaged in the Dakar operations. H.M.S. *Dragon* had 10 wounded, all due to shell splinters and including two cases with comminuted fractures of the upper limbs.

H.M.S. *Cumberland* was hit amidships by a shell which exploded 6 ft. inside the ship. A fire started in the affected compartment and a number of steam pipes was broken. Seven men were killed instantly and two wounded were removed each suffering from severe burns of the upper half of the body. Only one of these latter survived.

H.M.S. *Foresight* had 9 casualties 4 of which were fatal. One shell passed through the ship's forecastle without exploding but it passed 20 ft. away from a rating who suffered from spinal concussion with motor and sensory paralysis below the waist for the next twelve hours. One of the 4 dead was also the victim of a shell which passed through the ship without exploding. This man was in the direct path of the shell and was completely disintegrated. The remaining 3 fatal cases were all members of a gun's crew and received compound fractures of the skull.

H.M.S. *Inglefield* received a direct hit by a shell which exploded in the vicinity of her wardroom and she was fortunate to escape with as few as 6 casualties, all suffering from lacerated splinter wounds and minor burns.

ACTIONS INVOLVING ARMED MERCHANT CRUISERS

H.M.S. *Rawalpindi* was sunk by the *Deutschland* and another enemy raider while on patrol in Arctic waters on November 23, 1939.* The *Rawalpindi* sank about twenty minutes after the action commenced. Twenty-six of her crew were rescued by the enemy and made prisoners-of-war. Eleven other survivors were rescued by H.M.S. *Chitral*. These latter had spent 18 hours on improvised rafts exposed to a sea temperature of 46° F., and an air temperature of 31° F. One man was found frozen across the keel of an upturned ship's boat. He recovered and stated that three other men who started with him had died and been washed away. All the survivors were semi-conscious when rescued and were suffering from frozen and swollen extremities. Some subsequently developed pulmonary congestion, but all recovered.

---

* This incident has been included in this section for reasons of convenience, although it occurred in 1939.

H.M.S. *Alcantara* fought an action for ninety minutes against a German raider in the South Atlantic on July 28, 1940. Two of her crew were killed by large shell fragments which caused very destructive wounds; 30 men were wounded and suffered lacerations by splinters. But it is of some interest to record that no less than 9 of the casualties were accidental, and due to members of guns' crews dropping projectiles on themselves in the heat of action.

The gallant action of H.M.S. *Jervis Bay* against a German warship in the Atlantic took place on November 5, 1940. After being repeatedly hit, the *Jervis Bay* was abandoned under conditions most unfavourable to her wounded, who had to face semi-darkness and a bitterly cold rough sea; 65 survivors reached Halifax, Nova Scotia, a week later. Only 1 officer and 6 men had survived among the casualties. These 7 wounded all had splinter lacerations and 1 had extensive burns in addition. All wounds were infected, but all recovered. The survivors were able to report that it had been impossible for the most severe casualties to abandon ship.*

Of the *Jervis Bay* survivors who were not casualties, a number suffered from sprains and bruises through being buffeted in rough sea while awaiting rescue. It is considered of interest that 6 of these men had lost their dentures while vomiting into the sea.†

H.M.S. *Carnarvon Castle* was in action in the South Atlantic on December 5, 1940 with an enemy armed merchant cruiser. The action commenced at 0757 hours and was broken off at 0911 hours. The *Carnarvon Castle* carried 2 medical officers and 2 sick berth staff. There was plenty of room to deal with casualties, and as these occurred at steady intervals there was no really heavy concentration of medical work.

The type of shell used by the enemy had a high power of fragmentation, and on bursting sprayed the decks with small splinters of high velocity. These splinters were ragged, sharp and varied from the size of a split pea to fragments 3 in. long and 1 in. broad and thick. The type of wound tended to be superficial, though some extensive lacerations of surface tissue were seen. These wounds are recorded as having been relatively painless and caused little shock. There was a minority of deep wounds with splinters embedded in the muscles. The majority of wounds were in the lower half of the body particularly the feet and legs.

---

* The Medical Officer of H.M.S. *Jervis Bay* was last seen attending to wounded on her forecastle. He was lost with the ship.

† The loss of dentures during bouts of seasickness was not confined to men adrift in open boats. Many Medical Officers have recorded it as a fairly common occurrence among seasick ratings in all classes of men-of-war. In some cases a problem was created by the unscrupulous naval rating afloat who would deliberately lose his dentures overboard and would then plead that he had lost them while seasick, in the hope that he would avoid sea service until such time as his dentures could be replaced. Such an event called for careful and tactful assessment by the Medical Officer, and in some cases ended in disciplinary measures being taken against the malingerer.

The *Carnarvon Castle* lost 6 men killed and there were 22 wounded. There were 5 cases of burns of which 1 was numbered among the 6 killed.

As regards the burns cases it was observed that the need for having cordite charges close to the guns and on the open wooden decks of this class of ship meant accepting a risk of ignition and of consequent severe burns among guns' crews. Such burns occurred at very high temperatures, but the flash was of short duration so that unless the clothing happened to catch fire, they were of first or second degree with the maximum effect on the exposed skin and especially on the moist flexures. Though the epidermis was blackened and charred in some cases it pulled off easily leaving only slightly damaged tissue underneath. All these cases of burns showed profound shock, however.

OBSERVATIONS ON THE EFFECTS OF PARTICULAR WEAPONS

By the end of 1940, it was possible for the Medical Department, Admiralty, to make an overall assessment of the effects of the various types of weapons to which naval personnel had so far been exposed, ashore and afloat, up to this stage of the war.

SHELLFIRE

In addition to the experience of shellfire in the case of the armed merchant cruisers described above, a number of other men-of-war were involved with this type of weapon. The ships involved were the battleship *Barham*, the battle cruisers *Hood* and *Renown*, the cruisers *Ajax*, *Berwick*, *Dragon*, *Australia* and *Cumberland*, and a number of destroyers.

H.M.S. *Ajax* engaged units of the Italian Fleet during the early hours of October 12, 1940. The ship was in a high state of preparedness and medical personnel and first-aid parties were sleeping at their action stations in accordance with the usual night routine at sea. The value of this latter routine was shown by the speed with which subsequent events occurred. The first warning of action which was received by the Senior Medical Officer, was the firing of the ship's main armament, and within a few moments casualties began to occur. The final casualty list was 13 killed and 22 wounded, all being due to shell splinters. There were no cases of fracture and only one was complicated by burns. The ship's after dressing station received only 3 casualties while the remainder were all taken to the sick bay in the forward part of the ship. The consequence was that the latter dressing station was quickly overcrowded and the position was aggravated by smoke and water which entered from damaged adjoining compartments. This was yet another example to add to the growing list of illustrations of the need for a wider and more even distribution of medical first-aid facilities throughout H.M. ships.

This need for a revised medical organisation for action afloat was demonstrated even more forcibly in the case of H.M.S. *Berwick*, in an

EFFECTS OF WEAPONS 1940—SHELLFIRE

H.M. Ships	Date	Casualties			Types of injuries															
Lost : L Damaged : D		Dead	D/W	Wounds	1	2	3	4	5	6	7	8	9	10	11	12	13	14	15	16	N/S
Inglefield D	September 23, 1940	7	1	6	2		1												3		
Cumberland D	September 23, 1940			1															1		
Foresight D	September 24, 1940	4		5	3				1 rib										1		
Australia D	September 25, 1940	3		10	These 3, ftr. lt. and crew missing presumed killed.
Dragon D	September 23, 1940			1	7	1															
Barham D	September 24, 1940			2	(1 eye injury, not serious.)																
Hood D	July 3, 1940				2							2									
Rawalpindi L	November 23, 1939	242		12	12 sequelae exposure. (Means of rescue not stated.)
Alcantara L	July 28, 1940	2		30	19	8					1			1					1		1
Jervis Bay L	November 5, 1940	184	10	17	5	1					1								1		9
Carnarvon Castle D	December 5, 1940	6		22	10	1	(1 sequelae immersion.)				1			3					4		3
Renown D	April 9, 1940			1	1																
Kimberley D	October 21, 1940			1	1																
Ajax D	October 12, 1940	13		22	21			1			1	1		1					1		
Berwick D	November 27, 1940	7		9	2																
Westminster D	December 23, 1940			5	5																3

Note: 1-16, Classification of wounds. *See* p. 307. N/S = Not stated.

action with units of the Italian Fleet in the Western Mediterranean on November 27, 1940. The *Berwick* had 7 men killed and 9 wounded. Of the wounded, 6 sustained splinter lacerations, one involving lung tissue. Three had fractures, but it is of interest to record that these were not directly due to shell splinters themselves, but were caused by the normal hazards of action, such as jamming fingers in scuttles and, in one case, being hit by a door which was blown open by blast.

In this action, the first casualty occurred in the after part of the ship, and he at once was carried to the forward dressing station. The way having been paved, so to speak, all subsequent casualties from the after part of the ship were also carried to the forward dressing station. Under the conditions existing, this journey was a hazardous one but was necessary as the Medical Officer and medical personnel of the after station had already been killed and all their dressings and equipment destroyed.* Nevertheless, the journey could have been avoided had intermediate first-aid posts existed between the two stations.

A month later, on Christmas Day, 1940, H.M.S. *Berwick* was again involved in a surface action.† Two men were killed instantly and two died soon after being wounded. One of the wounded had a compound fracture of the skull.‡

This action illustrated the tendency for a doctor to be unnecessarily summoned in an emergency. A medical officer was called urgently to a gun deck where he found only one dead man and another requiring morphia and removal to a first-aid post, which could easily have been effected by a first-aid party in the vicinity.

TORPEDOES

The assessment of the types of wounds likely to result from this weapon was most difficult, because the majority of men-of-war attacked by torpedoes during 1940 were sunk, while those that did survive had relatively minor damage and very few casualties.

In the case of larger ships it was found that casualties varied according to the compartment hit and the number of men in the vicinity. In H.M.S. *Andania*, torpedoed on June 15, 1940, the torpedo hit the ship aft and the only two casualties of note were men who were working at the very site of the explosion. One of these was flung 40 ft. and both had fractured skulls. When H.M.S. *Resolution* was damaged by a torpedo on September 25, 1940 there were no casualties at all.§

---

* This fact was not realised for a considerable time by the medical personnel of the forward dressing station as telephone communication between the stations had been interrupted.

† The figures for this action have not been included in the following table.

‡ This man died three months later having developed a cerebral abscess.

§ An even more outstanding incident was the case of H.M.S. *Ark Royal*, sunk later in the war. *Ark Royal* was lost without a single casualty directly attributable to the torpedo which hit her.

Another ship with no casualties was H.M.S. *Calypso*, torpedoed and sunk on June 11, 1940.

Already, by this stage of the war there was enough evidence to suggest that, provided a ship survived, the limited number of casualties caused by the actual torpedo explosion was recorded too frequently to be accepted as merely fortuitous.

Among the casualties which were directly caused by torpedo attack certain features were revealed which allowed a number of very general conclusions to be formed. Fractures predominated, and appear to be caused by men being thrown down.* There was a conspicuous absence of such severe disabilities as dislocated knees or fractured spines, etc. It seemed too that there was no definite ratio of 1 to 1 between killed and wounded as had come to be expected in the case of men in the neighbourhood of mine or bomb explosions. Torpedo casualties showed few lacerations, neither was there a high incidence of burns.

This statement regarding burns might seem to be refuted in the case of H.M.S. *Liverpool*, torpedoed between Crete and Alexandria on October 14, 1940. But close investigation shows that her large number of casualties, which included many cases of burns, was not directly due to the torpedo explosion. Some casualties did occur immediately, but the great majority resulted from the explosion of the ship's petrol tank which occurred twelve minutes after the torpedo itself exploded. There was a total of 64 casualties of whom 14 were killed and 18 died within two days. Only 4 orthopaedic injuries and 1 laceration were recorded. Burns from the second explosion comprised the bulk of these casualties.

The information available showed that although, in general, there was relatively little clinical information to be obtained after torpedo damage, yet such attacks were not without their effect on medical organisation in the larger ships. Various attacks showed the need for medical centres and stores to be situated above the water-line. When H.M.S. *Kent* was torpedoed in the Mediterranean on September 17, 1940, 4 of the medical party were lost when part of the ship was flooded below the water-line.

In particular, the disaster in H.M.S. *Liverpool* stressed the need for dispersed medical centres. In this ship the sick bay was the only forward medical centre, in accordance with the current practice at that time. Fire and damage caused the sick bay to be abandoned, but casualties continued to go there in search of aid and then, though severely burned, continued to walk and crawl about the ship uncertain of an alternative place where such aid could be found. The *Liverpool* casualty list also brought home the need for more protection against burns than that afforded by simple tropical clothing at sea.†

---

* This differed from the force exerted by a mine explosion, where the common effect was an upward thrust transmitted through the skeleton.

† The majority of the fatal burns cases had been wearing shorts only.

MINES

In 1940 the effects of mining in producing fractures became established. Indeed, some observers went so far as to state that the casualty lists from ships damaged by mines were so characteristic that the cause of the disaster could be deduced merely by glancing at the diagnoses. In general, the casualties differed little from ship to ship, provided that the ship was not sunk outright as was frequently so in the case of smaller vessels.

Where a ship was struck, in some cases the effects were remarkably local. For example, in the case of one destroyer with a broken back, which quickly had to be abandoned, her Medical Officer recorded:

'I was in my cabin reading a book. At 0450 hours I felt the thud of an explosion, but I did not regard it seriously. However, realising that I had not heard anything similar before, and hearing a trickle of water in the compartment next door, I got up to see what was wrong.'

Meanwhile, observers only a few yards further forward in the same ship recorded that they 'saw the bows bend rather slowly towards them first upwards and then downwards, much as one bends a thin piece of metal to break it in two.'

When the Medical Officer of this ship made his way to the scene of the explosion, his report states:

'A sight of indescribable horror met me. Men were cut in two, scalped, internal viscera strewn about and intestines wrapped around the mast which was visible when I looked up through a large hole in the upper deck. I had three seamen with me when we suddenly noticed a messdeck hatch covered with debris. We worked with frantic haste to uncover the hatch and managed to open it to be greeted by a voice from below. By the aid of a hammock rope I got down with a torch. I landed knee deep in a mixture of oil and water on an insecure deck which had been torn away from the rest of the ship. I found 7 injured stokers and we got them up through the hatch. I then found an eighth. This was a man who had slept with his lifebelt inflated and had been concussed by the explosion, but otherwise unhurt. His life was probably saved by his head being kept above water and oil by his lifebelt. We got him out. By this time I was up to my hips in the rising oil and water and the ship was lurching. I found the darkness and the silence, broken only by an occasional splash, uncanny and terrifying. I hurriedly looked round for the last time and could only see here and there signs of quivering protoplasm as the only evidences of life in its last throes. I left as quickly as possible and secured the hatch.'*

---

* This Medical Officer, a surgeon lieutenant, R.N.V.R., was decorated with the Distinguished Service Cross, having shown 'great devotion to duty in attending to wounded with complete disregard for his own safety'.

In another case in which mine damage was even more severe, one of the ship's medical officers was unaware of the situation as long as half an hour later when he emerged from his cabin.

In most ships damaged by mines casualties were confined to the immediate neighbourhood of the explosion, and the ratio of those killed to those wounded was found to be roughly equal.*

At this stage of the war most damage was caused by the German delayed action 'Y' type of mine. The 'Y' type mine invariably exploded about 15 ft. aft of the ship's bows, which meant that casualties were generally confined to the messdecks normally situated in that part of the ship. The numbers of casualties therefore depended upon the time of day or night and the ship's routine, according to whether or not messdecks were occupied at the time.

The casualties which survived were the kind which would be expected in a patient who had fallen from a height. The injuries were more commonly in the lower extremities and simple fractures of leg or thigh, occasional dislocations and torn lateral ligaments of knee and ankle joints were all recorded. More rarely the pelvis was fractured. As might be expected from the transmission of the force, compression fracture of the lower dorsal vertebrae was reported as fairly common in some ships, and there were also cases of fractured base of skull and maxillae. Burns and scalds were relatively rare and there are few references to the effects of blast.

DEPTH CHARGES

By the end of 1940 depth charges exploding in the vicinity of survivors in the sea had proved an unexpected menace. The first report of their effects came from the Medical Officer of H.M.S. *Penzance*, himself a victim when she was torpedoed on August 24, 1940. He describes his immediate sensation as of a violent blow in the back which knocked the wind out of him and transient loss of power in the limbs which might have caused drowning. Later, some men from this ship suffered from paralytic ileus, and perforation of the bowel and internal haemorrhage were suspected. These observations all received confirmation by research later in the war and are described elsewhere in this History.

AIR ATTACK

During 1940 approximately 260 of H.M. ships of various kinds suffered damage and casualties as a result of bombing attacks.

The surprise of this form of attack and its frequently long and sustained nature were qualities peculiar to it in the history of naval

---

* e.g. in the ship whose Medical Officer's report is quoted above, 18 were wounded and 19 killed.

warfare. The torpedo was usually unexpected, but the attack was brief. Surface actions between men-of-war had their lulls. But the instances of continuous attacks by waves of bombers over many hours presented a special problem in the maintenance of both nervous and physical endurance.

The physical effects of a bombing attack differed according to whether the cause was a near miss or a direct hit. In the case of the near miss men were thrown into the air and suffered fractured limbs, spines or skulls. But the majority of casualties caused by near misses suffered from wounds by bomb splinters. These splinters tended to strike a ship about 20 ft. above the water-line. The danger to personnel exposed in the open is obvious, but splinters were also capable of passing through steel plates of a ship's side $\frac{7}{8}$ in. thick. In this latter respect it was found that splinters which penetrated the sides of a ship did so in an upward direction.

The wounds caused by splinters corresponded to the characteristics of flight of the missile so that the vast majority of men were wounded in the upper half of the body and the tracks of wounds were usually from below upwards. One ship reported 70 casualties all of whom were wounded above the waist, while another reported that nine-tenths of her casualties were in the upper part of the body.

These observations did much to encourage the custom of ordering unoccupied personnel to lie down during bombing attacks, and there seems no doubt that this practice of lying down with the head inboard did much to reduce the casualties caused by bomb splinters.

As regards direct hits by bombs, the total mortality tended to be 50 per cent. of those in the immediate vicinity or in the immediate path of the blast from the explosion. In these cases practically every survivor, whatever his other injuries, was burned according to the amount of exposed skin. Those who suffered most from burns were personnel scantily clad, and they showed an 80 per cent. mortality, hence the introduction of various Admiralty Fleet Orders on the subject of the wearing of anti-flash protective clothing. Cases of burns were frequently complicated by the effects of acrid fumes and hot gases which damaged the upper respiratory tract and led to broncho-pneumonia. This was also the case whenever bomb splinters ignited cordite, quite apart from the intense heat generated.

Gas gangrene was an extremely rare complication of wounds in men-of-war, but the few cases which were recorded during 1940 occurred in men wounded by bomb splinters. The infection was seen in wounds of the thighs and usually resulted from splinters from near misses which had not touched anything before striking the man. Clothing or skin must therefore have been responsible, and undoubtedly justified the old sea-going maxim of going into action with a clean body and clean clothes.

MACHINE-GUN AND CANNON-FIRE AT SEA

Bullets and cannon shells fired from enemy aircraft were weapons unfamiliar to naval personnel and in consequence there was a tendency in the early stages of the war to neglect the use of steel helmets and not to take cover.

However, these weapons only caused appreciable damage when employed against ships whose upper decks were grossly overcrowded, as in Operation 'Dynamo', and the total casualties from machine-gun fire in a series of thirteen ships attacked in other operations during 1940 was only 24, of whom 2 were killed immediately. These latter were small ships lacking upper deck cover or appreciable armament.

In connexion with this form of attack, it was quickly found that tracer bullet wounds sometimes showed a considerable destruction of tissue and delayed healing due to phosphorus.

BOMBING OF NAVAL SHORE ESTABLISHMENTS

Air raids on shore establishments in the Navy caused relatively few casualties during 1940.

During the second quarter of the year an air raid on H.M. Dockyard, Chatham, resulted in only 1 man wounded. There were three further raids on this dockyard in the third quarter of the year, with casualties totalling 3 dead and 27 wounded. In the last quarter of 1940, however, the casualty figures were 7 killed and 62 wounded.

In five air raids on H.M. Dockyard, Portland, only 6 persons were killed and 9 wounded.

In a heavily concentrated attack on the Royal Naval Air Station, Lee-on-Solent, on August 16, 1940, casualties were very moderate with only 6 killed and 20 injured. At the same establishment in November 1940 a direct hit on the W.R.N.S. Hostel resulted in 10 dead and 13 wounded.*

Overseas, aircraft attacked Gibraltar on seven occasions, but only 16 naval casualties were caused including 1 dead.

---

* Though originally believed to be due to a direct hit by an enemy bomb, these casualties were caused by an A.A. shell. They were taken to the Royal Naval Hospital, Haslar, within a very short time and it is of some interest that resuscitation measures were greatly handicapped by the difficulty which surgeons experienced in performing blood transfusions by the intravenous route in the case of young adolescent women in their late 'teens. This difficulty was well expressed in the words of the Surgical Specialist, who described the surface veins as being 'collapsed and buried in "puppy fat" '.

This difficulty was again referred to at a Conference of Naval Surgeons held at the Royal Naval Hospital, Chatham, in 1941, when it was observed that in such cases intra-arterial transfusion might have to be resorted to, and measures evolved for intravenous transfusion to be effected under pressure greater than that customary under the normal practice at the time.

RESCUES AT SEA 1940

By the end of the year 1940, the Medical Department, Admiralty, had been able to study numerous valuable reports concerning rescues at sea.

Picking up survivors of torpedoed merchantmen was a common experience on the convoy routes, and in many cases provided naval medical officers with their first experience of wounds received in action. The medical care of Merchant Navy survivors commonly became the task of the escorting naval vessels, many of them no larger than destroyers and corvettes. This task frequently placed a heavy strain on the restricted accommodation and limited medical facilities and supplies of these small ships.*

On occasions, following surface actions, survivors from sunken enemy men-of-war were rescued by H.M. ships. But, as has been mentioned, experience in the Mediterranean showed that such rescue work was highly imprudent. In some cases the risk was taken of informing the enemy by wireless signal in plain language of the position of their survivors and to suggest that a hospital ship be sent to the locality.

In addition to survivors from ships at sea, survivors from aircraft were also rescued on many occasions by H.M. ships. These included enemy airmen as well as Allied. Regarding the rescue of enemy airmen, the following account is of some interest:

'On July 1, 1940 H.M.S. *Black Swan* sighted a German aircraft in a sinking condition and four of her crew in a rubber dinghy nearby. The enemy aircraft, a Heinkel 115, was painted white with red crosses on the wings and body. Her crew all wore red cross brassards. One of the four claimed to be a medical student, but he had not attempted to render first aid to one of his wounded colleagues, neither was any medical equipment carried by the aircraft.'

The treatment and care of survivors following rescues at sea was not particularly dramatic. There were many times when artificial respiration was employed even where there was no evidence to show how long a man had been apparently drowned but records show that instances of the successful use of Schafer's method were almost completely lacking, even when employed on persons whose chances of survival might have been regarded as relatively good. In H.M.S. *Javelin*, 2 survivors of the S.S. *Cedarbank* were resuscitated by this method after $3\frac{1}{2}$ hours, though 5 others could not be revived. Most of His Majesty's ships kept a number of teams trained and available for the performance of artificial respiration on a large scale should it prove necessary.

As regards survivors suffering from the effects of exposure, the first observations on 'immersion foot' were by the Medical Officer of H.M.S.

---

* At this time the system of Rescue Ships in convoy had not been built up, as it was later in the war.

Versatile. In February 1940, this ship rescued 13 survivors from H.M.S. *Cape Howe* who had been adrift for six days on a raft in the Atlantic. It was noted that those who had foot covering, even if the feet were wet, suffered from less oedema than did those who had no covering.

Further information on the subject of 'immersion foot' was forthcoming after the loss of H.M.S. *Glorious*. The *Glorious*, in company with the destroyers *Ardent* and *Acasta*, was in action with the *Scharnhorst* and a German cruiser on June 8, 1940, inside the Arctic circle. Within an hour the aircraft carrier had received twelve direct hits and was listing heavily. Within two hours the final order to abandon ship could no longer be delayed. Some Carley floats and ship's boats were launched and a considerable number of men managed to reach them in spite of the long breaking seas and extreme cold. The majority of these men died within an hour, by which time H.M.S. *Glorious* and the two escorting destroyers had all been sunk. The floats and boats soon became separated and deaths were rapid and numerous. On one float only 4 survived of the 80 men who clung to it. It was estimated that after 24 hours some 1,500 men had perished.* After 64 hours six floats were found by a Norwegian trawler,† and 36 men were saved. Of these 35 survived, the number being composed of 34 from the *Glorious* and 1 as the sole survivor from the crews of the two destroyers.

The detailed accounts of these survivors did much to stimulate research into the survival of life among shipwrecked personnel, which subsequently threw much light upon such problems of exposure as thirst, hunger, cold and exhaustion. A further feature mentioned in the accounts of these survivors was that of 'mass hallucinations' as a phenomenon experienced among shipwrecked persons in company.

Further views on exposure were also given following the loss of H.M.S. *Grenville* which was mined on January 19, 1940. Her survivors were immersed from 20 to 55 minutes in a sea temperature of 38° F. It was noted that a number were unconscious when rescued and of these only 3 survived. As regards these unconscious survivors it was observed by the Medical Officer of H.M.S. *Grenade* that they had all been immersed in the sea for a minimum of 40 minutes and all were thinly or sparsely built.

CLINICAL PRACTICE IN CONVOY

By the end of the year 1940, the convoy system for merchantmen had become well established and some indication has been given of the part

---

* This number included the medical personnel of the three ships, none of whom survived. It is known that the Senior Medical Officer and Dental Officer of H.M.S. *Glorious* managed to reach a submerged motor boat, but they died of exposure within two hours.

† The attention of the Norwegian trawler was drawn to the floats by a boiler suit being waved on the end of a paddle.

played by the medical personnel of escorting H.M. ships in caring for Merchant Navy survivors whose ships had been sunk. But the medical officers of men-of-war escorting merchant ships in convoy soon came to realise that their duties were not merely concerned with the care of casualties. When a large number of ships was proceeding in convoy naval medical officers would find themselves confronted with the needs of a busy medical and surgical practice afloat, for few merchantmen carried medical staff of their own. A large convoy would contain many hundreds of merchant seamen in some dozens of scattered ships, and among these a variety of medical or surgical conditions might arise necessitating the attention of the nearest naval medical officer either by direct or indirect methods. The direct attendance of a medical officer from a man-of-war could frequently only be effected with great difficulty because it involved either a boat being lowered or, more usually, the medical officer would be required to be hoisted across to the merchantman or even 'to jump for it'. Visits of this nature obviously involved delicate ship-handling and a high degree of seamanship. In bad weather the personal attendance of a medical officer would clearly be impossible. More commonly the medical officer would have to treat and nurse his Merchant Navy patient indirectly at a distance, by means of a series of signals. Examples of indirect treatment are given below:

H.M.S. AUSONIA

For a period of a week *Ausonia's* Medical Officer had instructed, by signal, the Master of a merchantman how to treat one of his crew who appeared to be suffering from an ischio-rectal abscess, but progress was not satisfactory as is indicated by the following signals between the ships:

'*Merchantman to Ausonia*, 1015, 31.3.40.
"Patient's temperature 0600 101, pulse 100. Heavy discharge of pus and blood during night. Very restless. Having trouble in breathing. Mouth broken out in sores."'

'*Ausonia to Merchantman*, 1045, 31.3.40.
"Keep patient well propped up with pillows. To wear vest and nightshirt. Have scuttles open and heat on. Give excess of fluids and sugar. Brandy one tablespoon every four hours. Cough medicine three times daily. Do not bath. Hot bottles. Mouth Wash. How old is patient?"'

'*Merchantman to Ausonia*, 1135, 31.3.40.
"Patient 39. Believed to have had blackwater fever in December."'

'*Merchantman to Ausonia*, 0815, 1.4.40.
"Temperature 100. Pulse nil. Body very cold. Breathing difficult. Semiconscious."'

'*Ausonia to Merchantman*, 1005, 1.4.40.
"Condition obviously seems grave. Patient probably has infective pneumonia with blood poisoning and constitution weak following blackwater. Continue treatment as yesterday. Make further report at 1400."'

'*Merchantman to Ausonia*, 1230, 1.4.40.
  "Regret patient passed away at 1300 G.M.T."'
'*Ausonia to Merchantman*, 1300, 1.4.40.
  "We are exceedingly sorry to get your signal especially after your untiring efforts in a most difficult case. Both the doctor and myself feel that even if it had been possible to transfer the patient to this ship we could probably have done no more under the circumstances than has already been done."'

H.M.S. DUNVEGAN CASTLE

In July 1940 the Medical Officer recorded:

'Recently one personal visit was made on the high seas to the S.S. *Corinaldo*, whose Master was suffering from a hypostatic lung oedema associated with a failing myocardium. Thereafter daily reports of progress were made to us by signal and further treatment of the case advised. I am pleased to report that when our ships parted company he was convalescent.'

H.M.S. ABERDEEN

The Medical Officer recorded on October 14, 1940:

'Another of our escort reported by signal that one of the crew had gone sick the previous day with a temperature of 103 and pain in the chest. He had been given aspirin and had slept for ten hours, but on waking the pain was still present. Both our ships were on the same side of the convoy, but our Captain did not feel justified in stopping us both so that I might go across and examine the patient. Following a succession of signals I decided to treat the man as a case of pneumonia. A supply of sulphapyridine, with full instructions as to dosage, etc., was fired across by Coston gun.'

H.M.S. AUSONIA

On July 27, 1940, a supply of drugs was passed to the S.S. *Thala* for the treatment of a sick merchant seaman. On this occasion, in spite of bad weather, the drugs and instructions were sealed in a tin, made fast to a lifebuoy and floated across the bows of the merchantman which picked the tin up with a grapnel.

H.M.S. WESTON

The following account of the Medical Officer of H.M.S. *Weston* is an example of long distance treatment of a casualty in a merchantman following a bombing attack on a convoy:

'On September 25, 1940, while in convoy in the Atlantic, we were bombed. Following the attack we were closed by one of the ships in convoy, the S.S. *Natia*. Her Master announced by megaphone that his second engineer had been wounded in the stomach by a bomb splinter. U-boats were known to be in the vicinity and our Commanding Officer did not propose to stop for the transference of the patient or myself. Some verbal first aid was given and later the following signals were flashed by light:

'*Natia* to H.M.S. *Weston*, 26.9.40.

" Patient has jagged wound on left side of abdomen 1 in. long by ¾ in. wide at surface. Dull pain around wound. Red strip of flesh showing in wound 1 in. long by ⅛ in. wide." '

'*Weston* to *Natia*, 26.9.40.

"Do you think it is intestine sticking through the wound?" '

'*Natia* to *Weston*.

"No." '

'*Weston* to *Natia*.

"Put clean piece of gauze over wound and strap edges together. Wind binder firmly round abdomen. Keep flat on back. Give sips oxo, cocoa, soup. Keep hourly record of pulse. If steady it is a good sign. If it increases he may be bleeding internally. Report if blood is passed in water or motions." '

'*Natia* to *Weston* 27.9.40.

"Comfortable. Temperature 98. Pulse 72." '

'*Weston* to *Natia*.

"A good sign." '

'Unfortunately our ships parted company on this day, and I have no more information about the progress of this patient.'

These and many other reports were made during the year 1940 and it is worthy of being recorded that Naval Medical Officers were unstinting in their admiration for the skill displayed by Merchant Navy Masters and Officers in the care and nursing of sick members of their crews.

The Year 1941

OPERATION 'EXCESS'

The object of Operation 'Excess', in January 1941, was to convoy a number of troopships from Gibraltar to Greece. This convoy was protected by naval units comprising Force 'H' based on Gibraltar, and by the main Mediterranean Fleet based on Alexandria. The convoy was escorted on part of its journey by Force 'H' alone, and the Mediterranean Fleet joined this force in the Sicilian Narrows.

On January 10, when the convoy was approaching Malta,* the escort sighted and engaged two Italian destroyers. One of these, the *Vega*, was sunk and the other forced to retire.

Fifteen miles west of the Island of Pantellaria, Force 'H' was attacked from the air by eight Italian S.79s. The formation of these aircraft was broken by A.A. fire from the escort, and two of them were shot down by fighters from H.M.S. *Ark Royal*. The remaining aircraft dropped

---

* A subsidiary commitment of this operation was to fly five Swordfish aircraft from an aircraft carrier to be landed at Malta. This commitment was fulfilled successfully.

their bombs ineffectively and there were no casualties in any ships although H.M.Ss. *Malaya* and *Gloucester* suffered near misses.

Meanwhile the main Mediterranean Fleet was approaching Pantellaria from the east, and H.M.S. *Gallant* was mined and had her bows blown off. She lost 55 men killed or missing, and 27 were wounded out of a total complement of 160. But H.M.S. *Gallant* did not sink. Her casualties were taken off by H.M.S. *Griffin,* and she was towed to Malta by H.M.S. *Mohawk* protected by H.M.S. *Bonaventure.*

These brief encounters with the enemy on January 10, 1941 occurred early in the day, and they were but a prelude to attacks by enemy aircraft which were delivered on a scale hitherto never experienced by any fleet in time of war.

The main air attack developed shortly after midday when dive bombers, high level bombers and torpedo bombers were used against the merchant ships and their naval escort. These enemy aircraft included a proportion of German Ju.87s. which, in contrast to the Italian machines, were handled with great skill, and their pilots pressed home their attacks with great determination.

The aircraft carrier *Illustrious* was singled out by these German dive bombers for special attention and she was hit by 7,000 lb. of bombs, and in addition she suffered a large number of near misses. The bombs exploded at different levels inside the ship and caused extensive damage, fire and flooding; 125 officers and men were killed and a greater number wounded. The majority of these casualties occurred in the aircraft hangar and there were few survivors among the Naval Air Arm personnel on board. In spite of this damage, H.M.S. *Illustrious* continued to fight back against her attackers. Her Fulmar fighters shot down six enemy aircraft, and the ship made her way into Malta under her own steam.

H.M.S. *Illustrious* had withstood the main enemy onslaught, and attacks against other ships of the Fleet were almost negligible on this day. A near miss on H.M.S. *Valiant* resulted in four casualties, one of which was fatal, and one man was wounded during a machine-gun attack against the bridge of H.M.S. *Warspite.*

The convoy continued on its journey but now was without air protection. On the afternoon of January 11, further air attacks developed. H.M.Ss. *Gloucester* and *Southampton* were both hit. In *Gloucester,* 7 men were killed and 25 wounded, though her damage was merely superficial. But in *Southampton* the damage was severe, and 75 men were killed and 90 wounded. A severe fire broke out which involved the after engine room and magazine, and the ship had to be abandoned and sunk by our own forces. Survivors and casualties were taken off by H.M.S. *Diamond* and most of them later transferred to H.M.S. *Gloucester.*

Operation 'Excess' was concluded when the majority of the troopships reached Piraeus at noon on January 12, 1941. Meanwhile, H.M.S.

Illustrious was still at Malta where she was undergoing emergency repairs in the face of almost continuous dive bombing attacks by German aircraft. She received two more direct hits and numerous near misses caused further damage. During this period in Malta she suffered another 40 casualties. Nevertheless, on January 23, H.M.S. *Illustrious* left Malta under her own steam and arrived at Alexandria without further damage on January 25. (*See* Plate XII).

Naturally it is with the events in H.M.S. *Illustrious* that this account is mainly concerned. At the time of Operation 'Excess', the whole question of the medical organisation for action afloat was under review in Admiralty and was soon to be recast with a view to the dispersal of medical personnel and stores and the provision of first-aid posts distributed throughout all men-of-war.* The damage to H.M.S. *Illustrious*, and the sequence of events when about 25 per cent. of her large complement became casualties within a few minutes provided an added impetus towards the initiation of the new policy for medical action organisation afloat.

The Senior Medical Officer of H.M.S. *Illustrious* was a surgeon commander, R.N.† who was assisted by two junior medical officers. From the official reports of these medical officers it has been possible to piece together a most graphic description of the various medical incidents in *Illustrious* from the time of the first attack on January 10.

The following account describes what happened in the two Medical Distributing Stations:

'In the forward M.D.S., within a short space of time, 50 casualties were brought to the main bathroom flat. None of them had received first aid,‡ and in the overcrowded conditions which resulted only morphia could be given. The flat was then gradually cleared to a messdeck above where the long work of cutting off clothing, dressing and splinting was begun. All these casualties were stretcher cases, but other minor cases continued to report for attention all day. The accommodation of these large numbers necessitated the use of a number of messdecks.

'The after M.D.S. received its first minor casualties within a few minutes of the ship being hit. While these were being treated in the ship's laundry, a direct hit occurred in the neighbouring wardroom flat and the blast wrecked the Operating Theatre which was in the Dental Surgery. Lighting and water supplies failed, the M.D.S. filled with smoke and fumes, and the situation was aggravated by heat from the burning hangar and by the noise of exploding aircraft ammunition. Lighting was quickly

---

* *See* Chapter 1 of this Volume.

† The Senior Medical Officer was awarded the Distinguished Service Order for his gallantry on this occasion. He subsequently became the first Editor of the Naval Medical History of the War.

‡ One of the chief principles to be emphasised in the re-formed medical organisation for action afloat was that *first aid should be carried out on the spot or at the nearest first-aid post*.

restored and casualties continued to be dressed in the laundry and were then passed on into the ship's chapel and to neighbouring bathrooms. The serious casualties treated in this after M.D.S. were less than those treated in the forward M.D.S. This was because the majority of casualties in the wardroom flat were killed outright, while those further aft were isolated by fire and were removed to the ship's quarterdeck.'*

At about 1500 hours, one of the junior medical officers was sent to the quarterdeck in order to confirm deaths and to dispose of bodies. He gave morphia to 18 severely wounded men and he disposed of 4 dead bodies by committing them to the deep. Immediately afterwards severe fire underneath the quarterdeck made its evacuation essential and, as there were no stretchers, the wounded were placed on camp beds and man-handled up a broken ladder to the Admiral's quarters. This was a long and painful procedure.

Meanwhile, between decks, groups of wounded had by now been collected together in ten different places throughout the ship. Delay in attending to all these men was inevitable, as little assistance could be rendered by the ship's company who were all fully occupied fighting fires and working the ship. This meant that the task of coping with these isolated groups of casualties devolved on the three medical officers† and their small sick berth staff.

One of the places in which a group of wounded had assembled was the ship's sick bay, and the official report of one of the medical officers states:

'The lights were still burning in the main ward, wounded lay on all the twelve cots and stretchers filled the gangways. The first stretcher contained a dead man, the second a marine suffering from multiple lacerated wounds from which he quickly died, and in the third stretcher was another marine profoundly shocked and with a compound fracture of femur. Someone had already applied a splint before transporting him to the sick bay. The next two stretchers contained severe cases of burns to whom Tannafax was rapidly applied. In the next was a man with a fractured tibia. The floor of the sick bay was covered with slowly widening pools of blood which was dripping from the wounded on the cots overhead.

'I was short of Tannafax so I made my way to one of the two treatment rooms to get some more, but I found the room wrecked and in darkness. Beyond was the Operating Theatre in complete darkness and with some 4 in. of water swilling about the tiled deck. In the centre of the theatre I found a stretcher in the water, and on it a casualty who was still alive and appeared to have a tourniquet around his left thigh. But at this point I had

---

* At this time an attempt was made to reach a number of casualties isolated by fire in this part of the ship, but the volunteer stretcher party of 6 ratings was killed outright by a further direct hit.

† The war complement of H.M.S. *Illustrious* allowed for 4 medical officers, but only 3 were on board at this time. No reason for this reduction by 1 medical officer is given in Admiralty records. However, there was a dental officer on board who rendered valuable assistance to the Medical Department of the ship.

to suspend my investigations as the A.A. guns above the theatre opened fire with a tremendous concussion and noise as the ship was attacked by torpedo bombers. I had some difficulty in reassuring the man on the stretcher, as the darkness, the noise and the water had convinced him that the ship was sinking. I now approached the second treatment room and found the door jammed, but I was able to get inside by breaking and climbing through the upper door panel. Inside I dropped into a foot of water and my torch revealed some tins of drugs and drums of dressings among the wreckage. These I removed and found that the contents of the drums were still usable.'

The futility of bringing wounded men to such a place is obvious and there is no doubt that individual action should have been assumed throughout the ship with first aid being rendered on the spot instead of being left to the Medical Department alone. This was in fact the plan, and the failure of the existing medical organisation to cope with the medical incidents of modern naval warfare is revealed in the official report of the Senior Medical Officer:

'The arrangements in existence on board were in accordance with the design of the ship and with the experience passed on from the last war, exercised through the intervening years, and still in force in the majority of H.M. ships.

'In each M.D.S. there was organised a major surgical centre for one case at a time, a minor centre for numbers visualised as up to ten at a time and a ward for bed patients.

'In addition there were 46 first-aid bulkhead boxes fully stocked round the ship. There were 4 emergency surgical dressing chests in different positions. A selected number of men, trained in first aid, was distributed through the ship. Forty-four Neil-Robertson stretchers were secured to bulkheads throughout the upper deck ; 240 doses of morphia, gr. $\frac{1}{4}$, were distributed among 10 officers. All officers and flying personnel had received first-aid instruction.

'In frequent lectures the importance of local action had been stressed, and in view of this extensive and apparently comprehensive peripheral first-aid organisation the central medical parties were in teams with surgical, dressing, nursing and recording units.

' In a naval action of long duration, when ships are firing at each other and the chances are in favour of only one or two hits with an interval between, this organisation may be appropriate provided that the periphery co-operates fully. But when the attack is from the air the actual engagement may be over in a few seconds, and if the attack is accurate the ship may be hit in several places at once. This is what actually happened in H.M.S. *Illustrious* at 1230 hours on January 10, 1941. The existence of extensive damage, fire, flood and darkness, and the fact that the first-aid men themselves had other duties to carry out is a partial explanation of why so little first aid was performed on the spot. But the unfortunate fact remains that as soon as casualties occurred in large numbers the wounded were man-handled from every part of the ship and concentrated in the two Medical Distributing Stations. Had the wounded been left where they were after the first attack, and had they been attended to on the spot, no matter how perfunctorily, by the men who devoted time and energy to their removal much would have been gained. Neither the organisation nor the situation of the central medical parties were suited to this great influx of untreated and severely wounded men. Also the Medical Distributing Stations were lacking the stores which had been placed in first-aid boxes around the ship.

'A dispassionate consideration of this complete breakdown of the existing first-aid organisation in this ship has suggested that it is unsuited to modern conditions of war at sea. Where many severe casualties occur over a wide area simultaneously, the unit concept and Medical Distributing Station organisation is no longer appropriate. In a ship the size of *Illustrious*, distances up to one furlong have to be covered in order to reach the nearest M.D.S. from certain positions. The M.D.Ss. themselves become grossly overcrowded, and personnel become too concentrated in one spot which may be struck in a subsequent attack. It is a waste of technical knowledge and surgical equipment for medical officers to be employed in cutting off clothing and applying bandages, and it is an equal waste for them to be summoned away from their stations in order to give morphia or certify death.

'The situation resulting from the breakdown in first aid was that at first there was no room to move among the wounded forward, and later all treatment had to be carried out by 3 medical officers, 1 dental officer and 6 sick berth ratings who were unable to perform any surgery of a life saving degree or even to give special treatment for shock.

'It is strongly recommended that the medical officers, sick berth staff and men attached to medical parties should be divided into multiple units of one skilled and one unskilled person, and distributed as widely as possible in established first-aid posts throughout the ship. These first-aid posts should be so selected as to be near positions where casualties might be expected to occur. They should be reasonably sheltered and each should be capable of receiving up to 15 casualties at a time. They should be near a water supply and telephone, and they should not obstruct the main thoroughfares of the ship. They should be conspicuously marked with a red cross and the importance of this conspicuous marking is considerable in a ship of this size and complexity, whose personnel work in widely separated sections and many of whom are frequently out of the ship in shore establishments such as Air Stations for long periods and are thus not fully acquainted with the internal geography of the ship itself. The units attached to these posts should not leave them, and each post should have a large cupboard containing blankets, hot water bottles and other nursing equipment in addition to the normal first-aid gear. Each post should thus be self-contained.

'This system would avoid undue overcrowding, difficulties in the transport of wounded, or the sudden annihilation of the entire medical party or destruction of large quantities of essential medical stores. Its chief advantage would be to dispense with the unreliable features of the present peripheral system.

'The present siting of Medical Distributing Stations in new construction appears to aim at protection from attack by high explosive shells and the non-magnetic mines of the last war by placing them behind armour and far below the waterline. In this war such positions are very vulnerable to underwater attack, in addition to which access is so difficult that in practice they are hard to use. In the case of H.M.S. *Illustrious* only the bathrooms on the deck above the forward M.D.S. could be used. Even had it been possible, further descent to the M.D.S. itself would have been most difficult, would have led to impossible overcrowding and would certainly have been purposeless. Also, in due course the forward M.D.S. was so damaged by an underwater explosion that anyone stationed there would have been seriously injured. A further disadvantage of this low position below the waterline is that it is impossible to dispose of waste water except by carrying it to the deck above. A further small point, but one which is of some importance as regards morale, is that an M.D.S. shut away below a watertight hatch which must always be clamped down, and above two oil fuel tanks and a room in which bombs are stowed, is not calculated to give even the most sanguine a feeling of elation during the course of a long action at sea!'

It is of interest to mention that this report also brought to light a number of relatively minor points of detail of medical action organisation. For example, attention was drawn to the need for more water ready for use and better emergency lighting, for increased quantities of splints and dressings, and, in particular, it was stressed that rubber-capped morphia bottles and Wildey's syringes should be provided in great numbers. The point was made that men allocated to medical parties should never be the type who, owing to physical or mental drawbacks, had proved themselves unsuitable to perform any combatant function. It was emphasised that such men for medical work should be volunteers who would be more capable of real assistance.* It was also recommended that a member of the Regulating Branch† should be attached to groups of medical parties in order to avoid delay in rendering returns of dead and wounded. The early removal and disposal of the dead while the exaltation and 'mental anaesthesia' of action was still operating were also considered to be of importance.

These reports and their recommendations did much to assist the Medical Department of the Admiralty in evolving the new medical organisation for action in H.M. ships afloat which was promulgated by Admiralty Fleet Order in March 1942. In particular, the site and construction of the sick bay of H.M.S. *Illustrious*, and other ships of her

---

* This submission by the Senior Medical Officer in his report, while desirable and understandable, would be impossible to implement in practice. In any man-of-war, the general action organisation comprises so many essential duties of a combatant character that few men are likely to be left over for allocation to medical parties. To nominate these few only on a volunteer basis would clearly be a most impossible task for the ship's Executive to attempt in practice.—Editor.

† Broadly speaking, the Regulating Branch may best be described as the 'Ship's Police', the senior member of which would be the Master-at-Arms.

In the case of H.M.S. *Illustrious* identification of the dead was rendered most difficult by the fact that few men had bothered to wear their identity discs.

class, were reviewed and the policy of greater dispersal of personnel and stores was approved.

As has been described, H.M.S. *Illustrious* managed to make her own way to Malta where the arrangements made for the reception of her wounded included the provision of 6 Naval medical officers, 2 Army medical officers, 6 sick berth ratings and a chaplain, all of whom met the ship on her arrival. Twenty ambulances and large quantities of medical stores and equipment were available on the quayside. With the exception of 22 minor cases, all the casualties of H.M.S. *Illustrious* were landed by 0200 hours on January 11, and were admitted to the Military Hospital, Imtarfa, 13 miles away.*

The fact that these casualties were at once transported over rough roads for a distance of 13 miles to the military hospital was made the subject of some comment by the Senior Medical Officer of H.M.S. *Illustrious* in his official report:

> 'In view of the gravity of the cases, the fact that their removal occurred at a time when vitality was at a low ebb, that a long cross country journey to the military hospital lay before them, and that 11 ratings and 1 officer died soon after arrival, it is advanced for consideration whether arrangements should not in future be made at Malta for the treatment of certain dangerous cases to be carried out in the dockyard surgery and ward in the tunnel† for 24 hours so that they might recover more completely from shock before being subjected to the strain of long transport.'‡

The landing of the wounded from H.M.S. *Illustrious* was by no means the only commitment of the local medical organisation ashore in Malta. Casualties from H.M.Ss. *Gallant* and *Bonaventure* were landed at the same time as those from *Illustrious*, and the resources of the shore medical organisation were taxed to the full.§

Dead bodies from H.M.Ss. *Illustrious*, *Gallant* and *Bonaventure* numbered 95, and they were removed forthwith to the naval hospital. Here they were prepared for burial at sea by the hospital sick berth staff, and the funerals took place on January 13.

---

* The Royal Naval Hospital, Malta, had been badly damaged by enemy action and was functioning solely as an Out-Patient Department at this time. (*See* Chapter 15 of Volume I—Administration.)

† The 'tunnel' referred to was part of the elaborate underground system of shelters which had been constructed in the dockyard area at Malta.

‡ These views of the Senior Medical Officer cannot fail to be the object of comment by other medical authorities, and in any case they should not be regarded as reflecting adversely on the steps taken to get these casualties under the care of an up-to-date hospital in the shortest possible time. It must also be remembered that where a local medical organisation exists, such organisation must be permitted to accept responsibility and to exercise its own discretion when casualties from a ship are landed and promptly come under the local jurisdiction.—Editor.

§ A temporary relative shortage of staff in the Military Hospital at Imtarfa was slightly eased by the transfer of the Medical Officer of H.M.S. *Gallant* who worked in the hospital for a period of three days.

At first, 22 minor casualties and the remainder of the crew of H.M.S. *Illustrious* remained on board while the ship underwent emergency repairs. But in subsequent days air attacks against the ship became so severe that by January 19, she had to be evacuated except for damage control parties. At this time all her medical stores and records were removed to the shelter of the tunnel ashore. Two parties each of 300 officers and men were accommodated in the country at Rest Camps at St. Andrews and Ghain Tuffieha. Each party was accompanied by a medical officer and 2 sick berth ratings, while 1 medical officer and 2 sick berth ratings remained with the ship and conducted their medical duties in a sick bay which was set up in the shelter of the dockyard tunnel.

As stated on page 349 H.M.S. *Illustrious* sailed from Malta to Alexandria on January 23.

CLINICAL ASSESSMENT OF CASUALTIES IN OPERATION 'EXCESS'

Analysis of the casualties in H.M. ships damaged or sunk during Operation 'Excess' provided further convincing evidence of the effects of modern weapons in sea warfare which had already been remarked during 1940. In H.M.Ss. *Illustrious* and *Southampton*, 50 per cent. of the casualties were burns which had by now become regarded as characteristic of bomb flash. In H.M.S. *Warspite* the only casualty due to a machine-gun attack was a rating on the bridge. In H.M.Ss. *Valiant* and *Bonaventure* near misses by bombs produced splinter wounds. In H.M.S. *Gallant*, following an underwater explosion of undefined origin, the characteristic fractures were lacking, but in any case it was the forward part of the ship which had borne the brunt of the explosion and which was blown off and sank at once still carrying the killed and wounded. The fact that the surviving casualties of H.M.S. *Gallant* were cases of burns bears no relation to the underwater weapon which damaged this ship, because these burns were due to fire and the ignition of cordite on board the after two-thirds of the ship which remained afloat. Although H.M.S. *Gloucester* was hit by a bomb she had no casualties due to burns, and it would seem that men in the immediate vicinity were all killed, while the other injuries were due to bomb splinters.

As regards the burns due to bomb flash in Operation 'Excess', the majority were second and third degree. They ranged in severity from superficial burns of a single limb to extensive lesions involving half the body surface.*

An analysis of the burns in H.M.S. *Illustrious* shows the parts of the

---

* There seems to be no doubt that the failure to use anti-flash gear and other clothing to cover the body was responsible for a large number of these cases of burns.

body affected and also the extent to which burns were complications of other injuries, and *vice versa:*

Burns Alone

Burns of face and neck	4
Burns of face, neck and hands	8
Burns of face, neck, hands and forearms	6
Burns of face, neck, hands, forearms and arms	6
Burns of face, neck, hands, forearms, arms and legs	4
Total	28

Burns Plus Multiple Injuries

Burns, lacerations and simple fractures	5
Burns and compound fractures of the upper limb	2
Burns and compound fractures of the lower limb	2
Burns and lacerations	6
Burns and blast	1
Total	16

A single case of blast injury is shown above, and it is surprising that this was the only casualty who was suffering from such effects. However, it must be assumed that the majority of the dead were killed by blast.

In all the ships concerned in Operation 'Excess' the simple fractures caused as a result of direct bomb hits were approximately equal to the number of compound fractures. The compound fractures were all due to bomb splinters and mainly affected the lower limbs. The simple fractures mainly affected the upper limbs and were due to men being knocked down by blast. In most of the compound fractures there was much destruction of the soft tissues and extensive splintering of the bones beneath.

The multiplicity of wounds due to bomb explosions was very striking and most cases of compound fracture had other injuries as well. Complications of small splinter wounds were very common, with damage to tendons, major nerves and blood vessels. One casualty developed a large traumatic aneurysm of the *profunda femoris* artery which was later successfully treated by operation.

Only three eye injuries were recorded. Two were due to foreign bodies, one of which called for enucleation later. The third was a subconjunctival haemorrhage and iritis due to blast.

All casualties received first-aid treatment on board their respective ships. H.M.S. *Gloucester* carried her own casualties as well as those from H.M.S. *Southampton,* and in some cases more advanced treatment was carried out including the amputation of an arm, the ligating of major bleeding vessels and the X-ray location of metallic foreign bodies. The casualties from these two ships were landed at Alexandria and transferred to the 64th General Hospital.

In the case of casualties landed at Malta, between 12 and 16 hours had elapsed between the time of the action to the time of admission to the Military Hospital, Imtarfa, and secondary wound shock was very common. The burns cases were treated by cleansing all the burnt areas under nitrous oxide and ether anaesthesia, followed by the application of tannic acid and acriflavine compresses to trunk and limbs. Tannafax was used for facial burns and gave good results. In general, these cases of burns did very well and no instances of scarring or deformities are on record as having developed subsequently.

Fractures and splinter wounds were treated on the standard lines in vogue at the time. It is recorded, however, that where fractures were complicated by burns, secondary shock proved fatal in a small number of cases.

Five cases of severe abdominal wounds were admitted to Imtarfa. Three of these were moribund on admission. The other two underwent laparotomy with repair of damaged viscera. Both these cases died.

It is of interest that the official report on these casualties from the Military Hospital, Imtarfa, stated that:

> 'Six cases developed gas gangrene (5 per cent. of those suffering from open wounds). These wounds were all caused by large pieces of shrapnel and from 24 to 30 hours had elapsed before the cases were actively treated. The development of gas gangrene was diagnosed clinically, as the wounds presented a typical appearance and odour and the presence of gas in the tissues was felt and confirmed by X-ray. But laboratory reports on smears taken in three cases were inconclusive.'

This report was viewed with some concern in the Medical Department of the Admiralty owing to the fact that gas gangrene had always been considered as an unlikely complication of battle casualties in war at sea. In the absence of bacteriological confirmation, it was argued that the presence of gas as felt and shown by X-ray might well have been air forced into the tissues by the missiles themselves, and it was felt that the appearance and odour of wounds might be insufficient evidence of gas gangrene. Nevertheless, if these cases were true examples of gas gangrene, the distribution of the wounds which involved buttock, thighs and popliteal fossa does suggest the possibility of autogenous infection. The final view of the Naval Medical Authorities was to regard the presence of gas gangrene in these six cases with some doubt. This view was supported by the progress of the cases themselves. In two of the cases amputation of the lower limbs was undertaken. One recovered while the other died, but the latter case was moribund on admission and in any case was suffering from secondary shock with a compound widely comminuted fracture of femur. The other four cases all recovered following wide excision, incision and drainage in three cases, and excision and plaster-of-paris in the fourth.

CASUALTIES—OPERATION 'EXCESS', JANUARY 1941

H.M. Ships	L/D	Date	Cause of casualties	Total casualties*				Types of injuries†														
				K	M	D/W	W	1	2	3	4	5	6	7	8	9	10	11	12	13	14	15	16	N/S
Gallant	D	January 10, 1941	Mine	3		4	23	3														17		
Illustrious	D	January 10, 1941	Bombs	125	52	26	128	44	2	3		1	3	8	12		3	7		3		43	1	3
		January 11–23, 1941	Bombs				40	(14 anxiety states, 1 iritis, 5 ruptured T.M.'s, 20 minor wounded.)																
Warspite	D	January 10, 1941	Machine gun bullet				1	1						1										
Valiant	D	January 10, 1941	Bombs	1			3	2																
Bonaventure	D	January 10, 1941	Bombs	1			4	4																
Southampton	L	January 11, 1941	Bombs	20	55	7	83	12	8		4	2		2	3	1						42		7
								(Also 1 F.B. in cornea, and 1 intraocular F.B. enucleated.)																
Gloucester	D	January 11, 1941	Bombs	7		4	21	11			1				2									
								(Many of '1' had F.B.s *in situ*.)																
S.S. *Essex*	D	January 16, 1941	Bombs	14			3								1							2		7

* K = Killed, M = Missing, D/W = Died of wounds, W = wounded.
† Numbers 1–16, Classification of wounds. See p. 307. N/S = Not stated.

Also of interest is the following extract from the report of the Military Hospital, Imtarfa:

'On the whole the casualties admitted did not seem to be as badly shaken up as might have been expected, and no true psychoneurotic state was produced. In a few instances, mostly among younger ratings, a mild anxiety state was noticed, evidenced by agitation on hearing air-raid warnings and inability to sleep. These cases reacted well to sedatives and rest.

'Ten cases of a true anxiety neurosis were admitted who had suffered no physical injury during the dive-bombing attacks while at sea and also during the period spent in Malta.'

The ordeal suffered by H.M.S. *Illustrious* in Operation 'Excess' and the magnificent manner in which this ship was fought, handled and eventually sailed safely to Alexandria brought glory to her name, and no small part of the tribute paid to her officers and ship's company was directed towards her small group of medical officers and sick berth staff.*

With regard to the figures given above, where 40 casualties from H.M.S. *Illustrious* are shown as having occurred at Malta between January 11 and 23, only 2 of these can be directly attributed to attacks from the air during the period spent at Malta. These 2 were cases of wounds by bomb splinters. The remaining 38 included 14 persons who developed anxiety states as a result of the total series of attacks, and the rest were either those originally wounded at sea on January 10, but who reported late, or whom it was first possible to treat on board. This negligible casualty incidence at Malta must be ascribed to the policy, also adopted by H.M.S. *Penelope* at a later date, of evacuating all non-essential personnel from the ship while emergency repairs were being carried out.

THE SINKING OF THE BISMARCK

The *Bismarck* and *Prinz Eugen*, raiding in the North Atlantic, were sighted at 2032 hours on May 23, 1941, 75 miles west of Iceland and were shadowed by H.M.Ss. *Norfolk* and *Suffolk* during the night. Early the following morning the enemy ships were intercepted off Greenland and brought to action by H.M.Ss. *Hood* and *Prince of Wales*. At 0600 hours H.M.S. *Hood* received a direct hit and blew up with the loss of 1,421 lives, including both her medical officers.† Only 3 survivors

---

* In addition to the award of the Distinguished Service Order to the Senior Medical Officer of H.M.S. *Illustrious*, one of her junior medical officers was mentioned in dispatches. The sick berth chief petty officer was also decorated with the Distinguished Service Medal, the official citation reading:
'For exemplary conduct during the actions on January 10, 1941, when for 13 hours he worked with speed, initiative and cheerfulness under exacting conditions. He continued to work on board during the subsequent air attacks at Malta.'

† A surgeon commander, R.N., and a surgeon lieutenant, R.N.

were picked up by H.M.S. *Electra*, all suffering from shock and exposure.

Meanwhile H.M.S. *Prince of Wales* was damaged and had a small number of casualties.

During the remainder of the day both enemy ships escaped further contact with our forces although still pursued by H.M.Ss. *Norfolk* and *Suffolk*. Just after midnight naval aircraft flown from H.M.S. *Victorious* scored one torpedo hit on the *Bismarck*.

It was now some forty hours before contact with the enemy was re-established. Then, the *Bismarck*, now separated from the *Prinz Eugen*, was located by a shore based Catalina flying boat. At 1930 hours on May 26, Swordfish aircraft from H.M.S. *Ark Royal* scored two torpedo hits which reduced the speed of the *Bismarck*. The only damage inflicted by the *Bismarck* in retaliation was by the bursting of one of her 15 in. shells fifty yards from H.M.S. *Sheffield* resulting in 10 casualties, 3 of them fatal.

During the following night the *Bismarck* was attacked in bad weather by the destroyers *Cossack*, *Maori*, *Sikh* and *Zulu* and further torpedo hits reduced her speed. H.M.S. *Zulu* alone suffered casualties, 3 men being badly injured. At daybreak on May 27, these same destroyers and H.M.S. *Norfolk* were engaged by the *Bismarck* until, at 0848 hours, H.M.Ss. *King George V* and *Rodney* drew her fire. During the ensuing exchange of heavy shells no casualties were suffered in the British ships. Within little more than an hour the *Bismarck* had been silenced by repeated hits, and she finally sank at 1101 hours after a torpedo attack delivered by H.M.S. *Dorsetshire*.

An eyewitness account of the last hours of the *Bismarck* is provided by the journal of the Medical Officer of H.M.S. *Mashona* which was escorting H.M.S. *Rodney*:

> 'At 0830 hours we first contacted the *Bismarck*. *King George V* and *Rodney* opened fire. *Tartar* and *Mashona* left the battleships and cruised about hopefully, waiting to be told to attack with torpedoes. But this was not to be. Instead we watched the battle from our seats in the grandstand. As we were to windward of the big ships we could hear little noise but we saw the smoke, flashes and explosions and a rapid kaleidoscope of motion. In the distance I could make out a dull shape on the horizon from which came smoke, flame and fire. We could follow the course of all the British shells from gun to target.'

The rescue of about 100 survivors of the *Bismarck* was carried out by H.M.Ss. *Dorsetshire* and *Maori* in very unfavourable circumstances as the day was overcast, with rain squalls and a wind of nearly gale force which broke the sea into a heavy spray. Most of the survivors were hauled from the sea by means of lines with the ships rolling so deeply that the work of assisting these men on board was far from easy.

On May 28, the British ships were subjected to enemy air attacks. H.M.S. *Mashona* was straddled by a stick of bombs and soon had to be abandoned. Her Medical Officer recorded:

> 'There was a rush of casualties, many being seriously injured. I found it impossible to keep my hands clean and I had to work by torchlight. The ship was heeling over with the decks awash, and I somehow had to hold on to casualties and contrive to stop myself sliding about at the same time. Evacuation of the casualties was difficult to organise as all our boats had been pierced by splinters and none of them was serviceable. All I could do was to lower the wounded into the water where other people helped them. Eventually I myself had to leave and swim away from the ship. After half an hour in the water I got aboard a Carley float and managed to pull some other fellows in with me.'*

The survivors of H.M.S. *Mashona* were picked up by H.M.Ss. *Sherwood* and *Tartar*. One rating had been killed in the *Mashona*; 21 of her wounded were picked up, but 6 wounded were never rescued; 18 other men were missing, making the total missing up to 24. In addition, 11 men picked up died from shock and exposure on board the ships which rescued them.

CLINICAL ASSESSMENT OF CASUALTIES AND OBSERVATIONS ON ACTION MEDICAL ORGANISATION

Apart from the great loss of life in H.M.S. *Hood*, the casualties suffered in British ships involved in the *Bismarck* action were very few. They were all due to the bursting of heavy shells, and no features were revealed which have not already been dealt with. Neither did their treatment present any outstanding clinical or medical administrative problem.

However, an item of interest revealed by study of the action reports of the battleships engaged in this action is the suggestion that, had there been a large number of casualties, the wrecking of the sick bays in this class of ship, due to blast from their own guns, might have had an adverse effect on the ship's medical organisation. The Senior Medical Officer of H.M.S. *King George V* reported:

> 'A great deal of destruction was caused in the sick bay by blast from our own guns when they were fired at low elevation. The most notable damage was the complete dislocation of every tile in the Operating Theatre and bathroom. The bath itself was overturned. The theatre lights collapsed and were shattered. Several of the cots were rendered useless by their main supports being fractured off the deckhead fittings. The ventilation trunks collapsed, bottles were broken and most of the bedding was damaged by the amount of water which found its way in.'

---

* The Medical Officer of H.M.S. *Mashona* was decorated with the Distinguished Service Cross for his gallantry on this occasion.

A very similar report came from H.M.S. *Rodney* whose sick bay also became untenable pending extensive repairs.*

The officers and men who took part in the four day chase of the *Bismarck* were at action stations for very nearly the whole of this time, and in those ships which were subjected to the subsequent bombing attacks the crews maintained action stations for yet a further thirty-six hours. At this stage of the war this period at action stations was remarkable for its long duration and it imposed a heavy strain, both mental and physical, particularly in view of the attendant lack of sleep. In H.M.S. *Norfolk* the lack of sleep necessitated by the maintenance of the constant vigil over the movements of the *Bismarck* was countered by the use of benzedrine. The medical officer recorded:

> 'I had a private stock of benzedrine, held for just such an occasion, and it certainly came in very useful. During five days and nights there was only a single period of some thirty minutes which was available for sleep. I administered benzedrine to the Admiral, the captain, the flag lieutenant, the gunnery officer and the warrant telegraphist all of whom found it most valuable in helping them stay awake.'†

As regards morale, in all H.M. ships there was a feeling of dejection following the loss of H.M.S. *Hood*. But spirits rose when it became known that the chase was still in progress, and this heightening of morale continued with the ultimate pride of victory.

The behaviour of the survivors of H.M.S. *Mashona*, to whom the added ordeals of abandoning ship and immersion came at the end of a severe period of stress, was generally good, apart from a small number of cases of incipient hysteria. Her Medical Officer recorded:

> 'One stoker would not help to dry himself, but began to shiver and shake all over. He was stopped by a hearty slap on the back and an

---

* Commenting on these remarks, the Director of Naval Construction has since pointed out that it was, nevertheless, decided not to seek new positions for sick bays in these ships. The existing positions held many advantages in matters of accessibility, daylight and ventilation. Also, it was thought that the peculiar circumstances of the *Bismarck* action had led to a scale of damage which would probably not be repeated in subsequent actions. It was accepted that in major actions it might be necessary to abandon the sick bay and proceed to an emergency position.

The lesson was however fully applied with the building of H.M.S. *Vanguard* at a later date. In this ship two sick bays were provided, one in the usual position and one behind armour and away from blast.

† The opinions of naval medical officers varied considerably regarding the use of benzedrine in circumstances of prolonged action at sea. Records suggest that on the whole, it was not employed as a routine. Moreover, some experienced medical officers observed that, where benzedrine was administered, it could exert an adverse effect by virtue of the insomnia which was likely to be induced during the period of reaction when the battle was over. This period of reaction following some days of strain was studied by many medical officers not only in their messmates, but also in themselves. It was noted that the reactionary period always tended to translate great physical exhaustion into an aftermath of mental excitability and disorientation. It was suggested that this excitability and disorientation were aggravated in those persons who had taken benzedrine during the course of the action.—Editor.

SINKING OF BISMARCK
May 24–28, 1941
Casualties in H.M. Ships and Bismarck Prisoners

H.M. Ships Lost (L) / Damaged (D)	Date	Cause of casualties	Total casualties* K	M	D/W	W	1	2	3	4	5	6	7	8	9	10	11	12	13	14	15	16	N/S
													Wounded (excluding Died of wounds) Types of injury†										
Hood — L	May 24, 1941	Shells		1,421		3	(Shock and exposure only.)																	
Prince of Wales — D	May 24, 1941	Shells	11		3	12	9	2		1														
Sheffield — D	May 26, 1941	Shells			3	7	5	1							1									
Zulu — D	May 27, 1941	Shells				3				1	1	1												
Mashona — L	May 28, 1941	Bombs	1	24	11	21	7	3	2					1		(Shock only 4)					2			2
Bismarck Prisoners in																								
Dorsetshire	May 27, 1941	Shells				80	1	1				2	{'In addition to those shown, there were many minor injuries from flying splinters, contusions, sprains and slight burns'.											
Maori	May 27, 1941	Shells				24							{'None seriously injured. Most had cuts and abrasions and only one had a metal splinter embedded (in thigh). All more or less shocked from immersion'.									1		

* K = Killed, M = Missing, D/W = Died of wounds, W = Wounded.
† Numbers 1–16, Classification of wounds. *See* p. 307. N/S = Not stated.

admonition to dry his ——— self and get on with it! Another survivor was a rating who had already been rescued from the sea on three previous occasions. He presented a picture which might easily have been mistaken for acute alcoholism. He was incoherent, tremulous, emotionally labile, weeping and unable to do anything for himself. Firm words and encouragement quickly restored him, and within half-an-hour he was behaving normally.'

As regard the German survivors from the *Bismarck*, all were greatly affected by exposure and shock and artificial respiration was applied in a number of cases, and not always with success. Many had swallowed considerable quantities of sea water and oil fuel, the majority had minor wounds and abrasions, but no serious casualties were rescued. Some who recovered obviously appreciated the medical assistance which was accorded them and were grateful for their rescue. But others remained distrustful and uncommunicative, and it was with the greatest difficulty that these could be persuaded to part with their life-jackets in order to accept the warm dry clothing which was offered them by their rescuers.

GREEK AND CRETAN OPERATIONS

The end of Greek neutrality and the operations of the R.A.F. in this new theatre of war in 1940 had little effect upon naval medical organisation for some months. To start with Greek harbours were not used by the Mediterranean Fleet and no patients were landed there. The only small naval medical commitment was at Suda Bay in Crete, which was a shelter for oiling ships and where a signal station was manned by naval personnel.

At the end of October 1940, the Suda Bay base was augmented by a further 130 naval officers and ratings,* and a week later by a detachment of Royal Marines including a junior medical officer.

This initial naval landing party was accommodated around Calami Prison, 75 per cent. being in dugouts while the remainder were in barracks or billets. A naval sick bay was established in the prison until February 1941, after which it was moved to the former Greek Army Sick Quarters at Suda Naval Base. In spite of the difficulty in maintaining hygienic standards the health of these men was greatly improved by living ashore and by the fresh food obtainable. No case of waterborne infection or of malaria occurred among them.

The 189th Field Ambulance set up four small hospitals over an area up to eight miles from Suda. These dealt with 9 casualties from H.M.S. *Glasgow* which was torpedoed in Suda Bay on December 3, 1940. But

---

* These were survivors of H.M.S. *Liverpool*, torpedoed on October 14, 1940. The naval medical stores and equipment salved from H.M.S. *Liverpool* were also transported to Suda Bay.

apart from this incident there was little medical activity locally during the first five months which followed the establishment of this base at Crete.

This period of tranquillity ended with the torpedoing of H.M.S. *York* at Suda Bay on March 26, 1941. The *York* was rendered uninhabitable and her ship's company lived ashore while repairs were attempted locally. But during further bombing attacks this ship became a total loss. Meanwhile the medical staff of H.M.S. *York* set up a sick bay ashore accommodated in two tents.

Further naval medical provision in Crete was made by the arrival of the First Naval Tented Hospital unit on the Island on May 9.*

NAVAL OPERATIONS—GREECE

The events which led up to the German invasion of Greece and Yugoslavia on April 6, 1941 are well known. The next day there was a heavy air raid on Piraeus when the explosion of an ammunition ship caused casualties in H.M.Ss. *Ajax* and *Hyacinth* which were at that port. By April 12, minesweepers of the Mediterranean Fleet were operating off Piraeus.

On April 23, the Greek Government moved to Crete and on the following day the planned evacuation of Allied Forces from Greece was begun.†

As in the case of Norway and Denmark this evacuation had to be carried out mainly from places with inadequate port facilities, so that ships usually had to lie off while troops were ferried out to them in small craft.‡ Ships taking part were H.M.Ss. *Glengyle, Calcutta, Phoebe, Stuart, Voyager* and *Glenearn.*

On the first night embarkation took place from Navplion and from beaches east of Athens, and 10,750 troops were successfully removed. Numerous wounded were among those evacuated, and H.M.S. *Voyager* carried 160 Army nursing sisters. This first night of the evacuation passed most successfully without losses to personnel, and with scarcely any interference by the Luftwaffe over the evacuation beaches.

On the night of April 25, 5,700 troops were evacuated from the beaches at Magara, some 20 miles from Athens. This number included 100 nursing sisters and 1,000 wounded. They were embarked in the transport *Thurland Castle*, in H.M.A.S. *Waterhen* and in H.M.Ss. *Coventry, Havock, Decoy* and *Vendetta.*

---

* The activities of this tented hospital have already been described in Chapter 2 of this Volume.

† Operation 'Demon'. 1,300 troops and some vehicles had already been evacuated from Piraeus by this date.

‡ Berthing facilities would actually have been available at the port of Navplion save for the early foundering of H.M.S. *Ulster Prince* in a position which blocked the fairway.

On April 26, a large force of ships approached the coast to evacuate troops from Navplion and Drepanon. These were the transports *Slamat* and *Khedive Ismail* with H.M.Ss. *Calcutta, Isis, Hotspur, Diamond, Havock* and *Glenearn*. These ships were attacked by dive bombers at 1800 hours. H.M.S. *Glenearn* was hit in her engine room and had to be towed to Crete, and there were casualties and damage to the two transports. The depleted force reached Navplion and Drepanon just before 2200 hours. Information received showed that enemy air attacks could be expected in force around daybreak, and the instructions of the evacuating ships were that they should cease embarking troops by 0300 hours, in order that they might be within the range of fighter protection from Crete by dawn. During the five hours available 4,450 troops were embarked. Unfortunately the enthusiasm of the masters of some of the small merchant craft engaged in the task was such that they continued to embark troops long after the appointed hour. This kindness of heart meant a delay until 0400 hours on April 27, which meant that tragedy lay ahead. At 0700 hours the convoy was attacked from the air. Within ten minutes the *Slamat* had again been hit and was soon a mass of flame. H.M.S. *Diamond* went alongside her and transferred survivors, and H.M.S. *Wryneck* now appeared on the scene and rescued others from the sea. In all, these two destroyers rescued about 500 troops, but by now they were alone and at 1300 hours they were attacked by dive bombers. H.M.S. *Diamond* was hit twice and sank immediately, and her survivors were machine-gunned in the water. H.M.S. *Wryneck* was hit by a bomb on the forecastle which killed or wounded every member of a gun's crew. Other bombs exploded on the bridge and in the ship's sick bay. Though still moving at 18 knots the ship took on a list to port which gradually became steeper until she rolled over and disappeared. During the following night a small number of survivors was picked up by H.M.S. *Griffin* and one boat from H.M.S. *Wryneck* made its way to a cove 60 miles north of Suda Bay. But, in the end, only 1 officer, 43 ratings and 8 soldiers were rescued from these three ships.

Meanwhile, a successful evacuation of troops had taken place from the beaches at Raphthis and Raphena by H.M.Ss. *Carlisle, Kandahar, Kingston, Glengyle*, and the transport *Salween*. Some 6,300 men were taken off.

At much about the same time another evacuation took place from Kalamata by H.M.Ss. *Phoebe, Defender, Hero, Hereward* and *Flamingo*, and the troopships *Dilwara, Costa Rica* and *City of London*. Between them these ships carried 8,000 troops. The convoy was attacked at 1440 hours on April 27 and the *Costa Rica* was damaged and eventually sank. Some 3,000 troops were rescued from her by the *Hereward, Hero* and *Defender*. The only man lost from the *Costa Rica* was a rating who dived overboard and fractured his skull by hitting a raft.

THE CHIEF NAVAL EVENTS, 1939–1941

Similar evacuations of troops were effected on April 28, 29, 30, and on May 1, and the total number of troops withdrawn was approximately 47,500.

During all these evacuations, which included numerous casualties on each occasion, the involvement of the medical departments of H.M. ships was much as has been described already in the case of Norway and Dunkirk, with first-aid measures predominating and overcrowding making anything in the way of detailed examination or treatment an impossibility.

NAVAL OPERATIONS—CRETE

Some account has already been given of the naval operations in and around Crete,* and it is not the purpose of this History to give the complete story of the multifarious activities of H.M. ships at this time.

Broadly speaking, units of the Mediterranean Fleet were in action around Crete for a period of one month from May 1, 1941. By the second week in May it was known that the invasion of Crete was imminent and the commitment of the Fleet was to thwart any attempt of the enemy to land on the Island. A short period of waiting followed, the only incidents of importance being two dive bombing attacks on the Army Hospital Ship *Aba* on May 17 and 18. The second of these attacks was driven off by a naval force which included H.M.S. *Coventry* and this ship suffered 9 casualties, 2 of them fatal.† On the same day there was intensive dive bombing at Suda Bay. H.M.S. *York* was again damaged and H.M.S. *Salvia* suffered casualties.

On the forenoon of May 20 the invasion proper of Crete began and a generalised sea battle ensued between H.M. ships, attacking aircraft and invading troops. The first record of this period is that of the Medical Officer of H.M.S. *Juno*:

> 'When the Germans began their invasion the *Juno* was patrolling off Crete in company with H.M.Ss. *Naiad* and *Perth*, both cruisers, and the destroyers *Kandahar*, *Kingston* and *Nubian*. At dusk on May 20 we slipped through the Kaso Straits where we successfully beat off torpedo bombers and E-Boats, sinking two of the latter and damaging two more.
>
> 'At dawn on May 21, we were soon spotted and dive bombers gave us no peace. During an attack at midday I was in the sick bay, and I was astonished to see a cupboard crash down, spraying me with the contents of several broken bottles. Suddenly there was a blinding flash, the lights went out and I could just sense redness. I have no recollection of any noise or great concussion. I and my small first-aid party climbed up a ladder and quickly followed others who were jumping overboard. Looking up from

---

* *See* the account of the first naval tented hospital and the sinking of H.M.S. *Gloucester* in Chapter 2 of this Volume.

† One petty officer displayed extreme gallantry after being mortally wounded by a machine-gun bullet. He was awarded the Victoria Cross posthumously.

the water I could see the bows sliding under as the ship sank with no suction and hardly a ripple.

'In the water things were not too unpleasant, though there was nothing floating to hang on to, it was a bit cold, and there was a thick layer of oil fuel which rather hampered one's style. However, the company was cheerful and there was much jocularity. I found it possible to float on my back and blow up my Admiralty pattern lifebelt. Near me was a leading seaman with a small flask of rum, and he soon collected many friends around him in the water.

'We had sunk in under a minute and soon, through a pall of smoke, we could see the *Kingston* and *Kandahar* returning to pick up survivors. They lowered boats which were soon filled, but I carried on swimming for about twenty minutes and managed to get alongside *Kandahar* with some difficulty. It was only when I tried to climb up a rope which they threw me that I realised how cold and weak I felt. I just could not grip it at all, but managed to tie it under my arms and was so hauled aboard.'*

The total survivors from H.M.S. *Juno* were 6 officers and 91 ratings.

On the night of May 21–22, the cruisers *Dido*, *Orion* and *Ajax* and the destroyers *Janus*, *Kimberley*, *Hasty* and *Hereward* engaged a convoy of some 30 troop-carrying schooners escorted by Italian torpedo boats. After sinking the bulk of these enemy ships the British force was attacked at daybreak on May 22 by enemy aircraft and was forced to fall back on the supporting Battle Fleet. Meanwhile, the cruisers *Naiad*, *Perth* and *Carlisle* and the destroyers *Kandahar*, *Kingston* and *Nubian* had also attacked a troop-carrying convoy off Milos. This force, too, was heavily attacked from the air and retired towards the Battle Fleet. H.M.Ss. *Naiad* and *Kingston* sustained casualties.

Shortly after conjunction of the Battle Fleet with these two smaller naval forces, H.M.S. *Warspite* was hit by a bomb and sustained 112 casualties.

H.M.S. *Greyhound* was detached to sink a small schooner in the Kythera Strait, but was herself sunk by air attack soon afterwards. H.M.Ss. *Kandahar* and *Kingston* attempted to pick up survivors but with little success owing to continuous bombing and the merciless machine-gunning of survivors in the water.

Limited rescue work was later effected under the cover of fire provided

---

* This description of the Medical Officer of H.M.S. *Juno* is very typical and came to be well recognised in the course of the war. Wherever survivors were suffering from immersion and exposure, the actual moment of their rescue was a crucial one in many cases. The extent of the weakness and exhaustion of survivors was sometimes not fully appreciated by either the rescuers or the rescued, and the result was that a survivor's strength might suddenly fail altogether at the moment of being picked up so that he would fall back into the sea and disappear. This sequence of events was very likely to happen when oil fuel made it difficult for rescuers to take firm hold of a survivor. It was also occasionally recorded that a survivor whose strength was ebbing, though alive and conscious at the moment of being taken from the water, would be dead on the deck of the rescuing ship a matter of some seconds later.—Editor.

by the cruisers *Gloucester* and *Fiji*, both of these cruisers themselves being sunk by enemy aircraft within the next few hours.*

Heavy air attacks on the Fleet continued on May 23 and resulted in the loss of H.M.Ss. *Kashmir* and *Kelly*.

The Navy's task of evacuating the Army from Crete began on May 27, by which time further damage to units of the Fleet had resulted from heavy enemy air attacks. H.M.S. *Barham* sustained a direct hit on a gun turret, the aircraft carrier *Formidable* was hit twice by heavy bombs, and H.M.S. *Nubian* had her stern blown off with 15 men killed and 4 seriously wounded.

The evacuation from Crete took place from two points of embarkation, Heraklion and Sfakia.

A force consisting of the cruisers *Dido* and *Orion* and the destroyers *Decoy, Jackal, Imperial, Hereward, Hotspur* and *Kimberley* arrived at Heraklion at 2330 hours on May 28. The cruiser *Ajax* should have been in company but had been forced to return to Alexandria following bomb damage and casualties at 1935 hours. The destroyers embarked troops from the jetties and ferried them to the cruisers, and by 0245 hours on May 29 the whole of the Heraklion garrison, amounting to 3,641 soldiers, had been withdrawn.

Unfortunately all these men did not finally reach safety. At 0330 hours the steering gear of H.M.S. *Imperial* failed and after her passengers and ship's company had been transferred to H.M.S. *Hotspur*,† she was abandoned and sunk by our own forces.

At 0625 hours, H.M.S. *Hereward* was bombed and hit and was last seen making her way slowly towards Crete. Her surviving personnel, including her medical officer, were later made prisoners-of-war.

At 0645 hours, H.M.S. *Decoy* was damaged by a near miss which resulted in casualties and she sustained other casualties due to machine-gunning from the air.

H.M.S. *Dido* was also hit by a bomb and severely damaged, and she suffered 82 casualties on her crowded messdecks.

At 0730 hours, H.M.S. *Orion* was heavily attacked by enemy aircraft. Her commanding officer was mortally wounded by an explosive bullet and the ship also received a direct bomb hit on a gun turret. The *Orion* was attacked again at 1045 hours when a bomb pierced her bridge, passed through the ship's superstructure and exploded in the sick bay flat. At this time this ship was carrying 1,090 troops, and her passengers embarked from Heraklion included 13 cot cases and 4 women. She continued to be attacked from the air until 1500 hours, by which time she was so damaged as to make her abandonment a probability. Nevertheless, H.M.S. *Orion* reached Alexandria by 2000 hours, having had 262 sailors and soldiers killed and over 300 wounded.

---

* See Chapter 2 of this Volume.
† The *Hotspur* now had a total of 900 persons on board.

Altogether 800 soldiers were killed, wounded or captured following this evacuation from Heraklion.

The evacuation of troops from Sfakia was complicated by the fact that the village lay at the bottom of an escarpment 500 ft. high which had to be descended by a precipitous track. There were no jetties, and troops had to be embarked in small boats and ferried to destroyers lying close inshore. Among these soldiers were many wounded, classified as walking cases merely because of their personal endurance. Others were sick from evacuated hospitals. These sick and wounded were factors which contributed to the reduction of the number which could be evacuated each night, particularly as the rescuing ships were required to leave by 0230 hours in order to preserve the protection of darkness against air attack for as long as possible.

On the night of May 28–29, 654 men were embarked in the destroyers *Napier*, *Nizam*, *Kelvin* and *Kandahar*. On the return voyage this force was attacked from the air and the *Kelvin* suffered a small number of casualties from machine-gun bullets.

On the night of May 29–30, 6,000 men were embarked by the cruisers *Phoebe*, *Perth*, *Calcutta* and *Coventry*, the destroyers *Jervis*, *Janus* and *Hasty*, and H.M.S. *Glengyle*, the latter carrying landing craft which were of great value. On passage to Alexandria H.M.A.S. *Perth* received a direct hit, but the other ships escaped unscathed from enemy air attacks. The final party to be evacuated from Sfakia was taken off just before dawn on June 1 by H.M.Ss. *Phoebe*, *Abdiel*, *Kimberley*, *Hotspur* and *Jackal*. This force had an uneventful passage to Alexandria, which was fortunate in view of the fact that H.M.S. *Phoebe* was carrying 1,400 troops, including 3 officers and 50 other ranks wounded.

By June 1, 1941, a total of 16,500 troops had been evacuated from the Island of Crete. Unfortunately on the last day H.M.S. *Calcutta* was sunk by air attack, 23 officers and 232 ratings being rescued by H.M.S. *Coventry*.

It is worthy of record that of the 2,000 Royal Marines who fought out a rear-guard action in Crete at this time, 1,400 became casualties or prisoners-of-war.

ASSESSMENT OF CASUALTIES

The casualties in H.M. ships operating in the Eastern Mediterranean and the Aegean Sea between April 7 and June 1, 1941, were caused almost entirely by bombs. Enemy aircraft also inflicted casualties by machine-gun and cannon fire, more particularly against survivors in the water. There were no casualties as a result of a small number of engagements between H.M. ships and enemy destroyers and E-boats.

Naval personnel in H.M. ships suffered 246 killed and 1,430 missing; 44 men died of wounds and 479 were wounded. The total number of 2,199 represents approximately 15 per cent. of the total complement of all British men-of-war engaged. The figures do not include numerous casualties among naval personnel who were manning transports and auxiliary ships of the Merchant Navy.

Of the men missing 1,397 belonged to three cruisers and eight destroyers which were sunk. The small remainder missing were in ships which did not sink but which were badly damaged. The bodies of these men were never recovered from the wreckage and they must be presumed either to have been blown overboard or else to have been disintegrated by the force of explosion.

As regards particular types of wounds, there is little to be added to what has already been described previously in this volume. But it is of interest that most reports of medical officers remarked on the large number of burns which was seen among casualties, and that these burns, almost without exception, involved the exposed surface areas of the bodies of men who were seeking comfort rather than protection during action by wearing neither anti-flash gear nor sufficient clothing. That these factors considerably influenced the degrees of burns which occurred is certain, and it is scarcely surprising that extensive burns were the most frequent cause of death among those men who died after reaching hospitals.

In relation to the problem of protective clothing against burns the Senior Medical Officer of H.M.S. *Warspite* stated in his report:

'Anti-flash gear is not the answer for personnel between decks in this climate. The temperature in the fore medical flat ranges up to 95° F. at sea, and if heavy anti-flash gear is worn symptoms of heat exhaustion with impairment of efficiency are bound to result. But between anti-flash gear and comparative nudity there is a happy mean, which is the covering of the whole body with a light overall so that only the head and hands are exposed. Valuable protection may also be afforded by wearing anti-gas eye shields. The risk of burns on the skin which remains exposed would have to be accepted, but should they occur, the total area involved would be small and the fatalities infinitesimal.'

This Medical Officer did, however, consider that anti-flash gear was an essential on the upper deck in the open.

A report from H.M.S. *Dido* illustrates the efficiency of anti-flash gear as a protection against burns by flash from bomb explosions:

'All the men in "B" turret which had received a direct hit were killed by blast, burns and gross crushing injuries. But all their ordinary clothing, except boots, had been burnt off while their anti-flash gear was still intact. It was very noticeable that this gear had protected the skin of the areas which it covered.'

As regards Army casualties carried in H.M. ships, several cases of gas gangrene in wounds were recorded, and other wounds were found to contain maggots. Prolapse of abdominal contents through broken down infected wounds was also seen, and faecal fistulae had to be treated. Needless to say most of these casualties were at least seven days old when they were received on board.

In addition, many soldiers were suffering from blistered feet and jagged laceration of the hands as a result of scrambling over cliffs. Some were also suffering from dysentery, enteritis and malaria which required attention while on passage.

The treatment of Army casualties during passage in H.M. ships was of necessity limited. But H.M.S. *Janus* reported that a soldier with gas gangrene was isolated and given sulphapyridine and 100,000 units of A.G.G. serum of which 40,000 were administered intravenously. The man's wounds and infection were of the arm, and he was discharged to hospital ashore with his condition greatly improved.* By contrast however, the Medical Officer of H.M.S. *Griffin* amputated an upper limb of a soldier for gas gangrene.

In most of H.M. ships which were carrying wounded troops, the situation was complicated by further action and frequent damage during the sea passage. Examples of these difficulties are given in the official reports of the Medical Officers of H.M.Ss. *Orion* and *Dido*.

In H.M.S. *Orion*:

'Bombing attacks began early in the day and casualties soon began to arrive, mostly with splinter and machine-gun wounds. First aid was rendered and morphia administered in ½ grain doses. From 0730 hours onwards the stream of wounded was constant and included many of the soldiers on board.

'At 0906 hours "A" turret received a direct hit which wiped out the gun's crew.

'At 1045 hours, a large bomb hit the bridge, passed through the superstructure and sick bay bathroom, and burst below the stokers' messdeck. The deck of the sick bay immediately buckled, bulkheads were stove in, the lighting failed, all the cots and fixtures and fittings were destroyed as well as our medical stores. The occupants of the sick bay were blown in various directions. I had difficulty in getting out owing to debris and smoke as did the junior medical officer and 3 ratings with us. The S.B.P.O. suffered severe concussion.

'The casualties among our ship's company were 107 killed and 84 wounded. But I found it impossible accurately to check the numbers killed or wounded among the troops on board owing to confusion among the units which we carried and the general chaos at the time.'†

As regards H.M.S. *Dido*:

'At 0815 hours, the ship sustained eight near misses in quick succession. A ninth bomb hit "B" turret. The blast of its explosion travelled downwards and wrecked the marines' messdeck which was crowded with troops at the

---

* This soldier recovered and amputation was not necessary.
† The figure is believed to be 155 soldiers killed and 216 wounded.

time. The explosion was followed by a serious fire; 27 of our ship's company were killed and 19 soldiers; 10 naval ratings were wounded and 28 of our Army passengers.

'My medical parties worked well and got the wounded out quickly, but with the ship so overcrowded and littered with wreckage and water, it was difficult to find anywhere convenient for the treatment of casualties. Also, most approaches were blocked by fire hoses and damage control parties. The Army dead together with our own were buried at sea.'

DISPOSAL OF WOUNDED IN EGYPT

Following the withdrawal from the Greek mainland, naval and military wounded were nearly all taken direct to Egypt where the majority of the naval cases were admitted to the 64th General Hospital, the remaining few being dealt with in H.M.H.S. *Maine*. A small number of naval casualties which occurred about this time, particularly in ships at Suda Bay, was admitted to the 7th General Hospital in Crete.

During the sea battle off Crete H.M. ships operating from Alexandria landed their casualties at this base where the 64th General Hospital continued to deal with most of them, although rather more now went to H.M.H.S. *Maine*. A small number of casualties was also admitted to the 8th, 11th, and 19th General Hospitals in Egypt.

Disembarkation of casualties at Alexandria was carried out most efficiently by the Australian Royal Army Medical Corps with the help of medical personnel of the 'harbour' based H.M.Ss. *Resource*, *Woolwich* and *Medway* in accordance with the local Fleet organisation for the reception of casualties arriving at Alexandria by sea.

The hospitals and hospital ship already mentioned continued to receive casualties until the completion of the Greek and Cretan campaigns. The following report by the Senior Medical Officer of the Naval Wing of the 64th General Hospital mentions some of the difficulties experienced by this large influx of patients:

'In the month of May no less than 1,200 sailors were admitted, the majority following the evacuation of Crete. These patients, together with a large number of Army casualties from Greece and Crete, placed a considerable strain on our hospital resources. It was only by the continual transference of patients by hospital train and ambulance convoy that it was possible to cope with each successive wave of casualties which arrived. During the peak period of congestion 400 naval patients were transferred to Cairo. At one time the number of patients exceeded the number of beds available in the establishment, so that casualties had to be accommodated in the Dining Hall on mattresses placed on the floor. Although the nominal bed strength of the hospital was 1,200, by crowding it was possible to receive 1,306 patients; but on this occasion 1,340 patients were accommodated.

GREEK AND CRETAN OPERATIONS
April 7–June 1, 1941
Casualties in H.M. Ships

H.M. Ships Lost L / Damaged D	Date	Cause of casualties	Total casualties* K	M	D/W	W	1	2	3	4	5	6	7	8	9	10	11	12	13	14	15	16	N/S
Ajax D	April 7, 1941	Explosions of nearby ammunition ship which was bombed	1			2	1		1															
Hyacinth D	April 7, 1941	Bombs																						
Glenearn D	April 25, 1941	"	1		1	4	4																	1
Orion D	April 26, 1941	Bombs		5		1	1																	1
Diamond L	April 27, 1941	Bombs		155		5	5																	6
Wryneck L	April 27, 1941	Bombs		108		19	19																	21
Ajax D	April 28, 1941	Bombs	5			7	5																	
Coventry D	May 17, 1941	Bullets and bombs	1		1	5	5															2		
Salvia D	May 17, 1941	Bombs	2	116		8	1																	
Juno L	May 21, 1941	Bombs	8		4	21	25						1											26
Naiad D	May 22, 1941	Bombs	6		1	31				3			2	1	1							1 (D/W)		
Carlisle D	May 22, 1941	Bombs	13		1	25	28	9		3	1			3	1							35		19
Warspite D	May 22, 1941	Bombs	8	24	11	69	3																	
Greyhound L	May 22, 1941	Bullets and bombs	1	83		23	2																	
Kingston D	May 22, 1941	Bombs	1			2																		
Gloucester L	May 22, 1941	Bombs		182		4	2			1														4
Fiji L	May 22, 1941	Bombs	5	271	2	24	8			3				1								6		20
Kelly L	May 23, 1941	Bombs	3	127		17	9			3														
Kashmir L	May 23, 1941	Bombs		82		14																			
Kipling D	May 23, 1941	Bombs	1	4		10	1				1						1							1
Havock D	May 23, 1941	Bombs	15			1																			9
Griffin D	May 24, 1941	Bombs				1																			1
Perth D	May 24, 1951	Bombs	4			3	1																		3
Glenroy D	May 26, 1941	Bombs				2	1								1										
Jaguar D	May 26, 1941	Bombs			3	10	2																3		6
Formidable D	May 26, 1941	Bombs	9		1	3	3			4													3		
Nubian D	May 26, 1941	Bombs	14		2	6	2																		9
Barham D	May 26, 1941	Bombs	5			6	10																		1
Ajax D	May 28, 1941	Bombs	6			19		2																	3
Imperial L	May 29, 1941	Bombs				1																			
Hereward L	May 29, 1941	Bombs	5			3																	3		
Decoy D	May 29, 1941	Bullets and bombs	1	165		8	2			1															
Orion D	May 29, 1941	Bombs	107		8	76	4									2							1		76
Dido D	May 29, 1941	Bombs	27			10	1	2	1	1															2
Kelvin D	May 29, 1941	Bullets and cannon shell			1	4	4																		
Perth D	May 29, 1941	Bombs		108		4	4																		
Jervis D	May 30, 1941	Bombs				4																			
Calcutta L	June 1, 1941	Bombs	1		8	40	4	4		1	3												27		5

* K=Killed, M=Missing, D/W=Died of wounds, W=Wounded.
† Numbers 1–16, Classification of wounds. See p. 307. N/S=Not stated.

'As regards the Army casualties received, the majority were walking cases. Their most urgent need was food, sleep and re-dressing before being transferred on to hospitals in the Nile Delta, Palestine and elsewhere in the Middle East.'

OPERATIONS IN THE RED SEA, EAST AFRICA AND THE PERSIAN GULF

The chief medical historical interest attached to operations in and around the Red Sea, East Africa and the Persian Gulf is centred around the general health of personnel in H.M. ships involved. These areas are well noted for discomfort afloat even under the most ideal conditions of peace-time cruising. But under war-time conditions, in overcrowded ships, not designed or equipped for tropical service, it was to be expected that the effects of heat would be reflected in daily sick lists.

During July and August 1941, the upper deck shade temperature in H.M.S. *Sea Belle* averaged 93° F. in the Persian Gulf. During the period this ship recorded six cases of heat exhaustion.

In H.M.S. *Ceres*, off the East African coast, the average messdeck temperature during April 1941 was 101° F. at sea, and 94° F. in harbour.

In H.M.S. *Shoreham*, in the Red Sea, the engine room temperature reached 150° F. in January 1941. Most ships in this area reported one or more cases of collapse in the engine room each quarter.

During April 1941, H.M.S. *Hermes* recorded 27 cases of heat exhaustion in the Indian Ocean out of a ship's company totalling 719; 22 of these cases belonged to the engine room department.

Another aspect of hot weather conditions afloat was revealed by the skin diseases which produced large attendances at ships' sick bays. 'Prickly heat' and mycotic conditions made up the bulk of these skin diseases which were aggravated by the constant watch-keeping which reduced the leisure available for bathing and laundry, in addition to which the fresh water supply in the older men-of-war was often restricted.

In these tropical and sub-tropical areas the shore hospital facilities were anything but ideal at some of the smaller ports, and many naval medical officers were of the opinion that the visits of their ships to certain ports of call were more likely to add cases to their sick lists in the form of malaria, rather than to relieve them of their burdens on board.

In the third quarter of 1941 H.M.S. *Eagle* had 21 cases of benign tertian malaria after a visit to Aden, while H.M.S. *Ceres* recorded 12 cases. Malaria was also seen in H.M. ships operating in the Shatt-el-Arab. H.M.S. *Sea Belle*, whose ship's company numbered 220, including personnel of the naval base at Basra, had 71 cases of malaria during the second quarter of 1941. The benign tertian type predominated, and the outbreak occurred principally during May, when the Shatt-el-Arab was at its highest level and had inundated the low lying country around.

In spite of the hardships suffered in the older ships operating in these areas, it is of some interest that on the only occasion on which disease is known actually to have interfered with naval operations, the disease concerned could not be described as one peculiar to the Tropics. The occasion was when H.M.S. *Shropshire* developed 148 cases of streptococcal tonsilitis and was out of action for ten days, between January 25 and February 4, 1941. These cases represented 20 per cent. of the ship's total complement. A further 60 similar cases were also recorded in the following quarter of 1941, but without interference with the ship's operational routine. This outbreak did not spread to any other ship in the same area.

NORTH AFRICAN COASTAL OPERATIONS
1940 *and* 1941

With the entry of Italy into the war and the commencement of the first military campaign in North Africa, units of the Navy were required to afford both combatant and domestic support to the Army ashore in a number of ways.

On December 7, 1940, the Army began an advance which, as is well known, was to reach a climax a month later with the fall of Benghazi. During the night of December 8, H.M.Ss. *Terror*, *Ladybird* and *Aphis* left Alexandria and bombarded the Italian encampment at Maktila. On subsequent nights similar operations were carried out against Sidi Barrani and Sollum. These ships experienced little more than formal opposition by coastal batteries, and there were no casualties at this stage.

On December 16, 1940, Sollum fell to the Army, and the Navy took on the task of delivering water and supplies to this port as well as that of removing prisoners-of-war from it. H.M.Ss. *Terror*, *Ladybird* and *Aphis* now operated freely from Sollum, and the shallow draught of the old monitor and two river gunboats made them well suited to carry out attacks close in to the gently shelving sands of the coast.

On January 20, Tobruk fell to Australian Forces and the Navy was able to ferry supplies to this port.

These later sea operations were not unopposed and it became necessary for H.M. ships to combat attacks from the air by dive and torpedo bombers. By now casualties afloat were becoming commonplace, and ships maintaining the ferry services between the newly won North African ports and Alexandria found themselves faced with the additional task of carrying wounded troops from ashore. For example, at noon on December 24, 1940, a bomb exploded on the jetty at Sollum and inflicted heavy casualties among troops. The wounded were attended to by the Medical Officers of H.M.Ss. *Terror* and *Chakla*, and these ships embarked Army casualties from this air raid to full capacity.

H.M.S. *Chakla* took 81 casualties on board, and assistance was given by the loan of 5 R.A.M.C. orderlies. Before this ship could leave

Sollum, she was heavily attacked at 1600 hours on Christmas Day. Thirty bombs fell in her immediate vicinity, and conditions became so adverse that it was necessary to land the wounded who had been taken on board and they were sent to Sidi Barrani Casualty Clearing Station some sixty miles away. Meanwhile, H.M.S. *Terror* had left Sollum, but was ordered to return and she too was forced by circumstances to land her wounded and send them away by road.

H.M.S. *Terror* was eventually sunk by a mine off Derna on February 24, 1941. For the next three months H.M. ships continued to maintain sea communications along the coast. At 1615 hours on May 12, H.M.S. *Ladybird* was attacked and sunk by enemy aircraft while at anchor in the harbour of Tobruk. Her Medical Officer recorded:

'I was standing on deck when we were first hit by a large calibre bomb. I went to the sick bay to fetch some surplus dressings as the ship was now on fire. As I entered, another bomb struck the ship and passed through the sick bay. The blast threw me down and I hit my head on the splintered plating. But although I was knocked out, my tin hat saved me from more serious injury. I recovered after a few seconds, and realised that it was impossible to go aft because of the fire, so I went forward. I at once dealt with several casualties including some with amputated legs. While I was dressing one casualty he was struck by some splinters and I myself was hit in both elbows. The casualties were taken off in shore boats and I made sure there was nobody left behind. I then had to abandon ship owing to fire in the magazine.'*

Three ratings of H.M.S. *Ladybird* were killed and 1 later died of wounds. The ship suffered 25 other casualties.

A heavy commitment of the Royal Navy at this time was the transport of prisoners-of-war by sea. Enemy prisoners ashore numbered approximately 100,000 and this capture of so great a proportion of the Italian Army required much improvisation in the matter of their transport away from the battle area. At first they were evacuated in every available ship which plied between Egypt and the Libyan ports, but on December 12, 1940, H.M.S. *Knight of Malta* was commissioned as a prisoner transport.

The *Knight of Malta* was, in peace-time, a mail steamer running between Malta and Syracuse. Equivalent to a small cross-channel steamer, she not only lacked accommodation for any considerable number of passengers, but her water supply and sanitary provisions were grossly inadequate. She carried only 31 tons of fresh water. This quantity had been adequate enough for the ship's peace-time routine, but the journeys from Tobruk to Alexandria took almost four times as long,

---

* This Medical Officer, a surgeon lieutenant, R.N., was decorated with the Distinguished Service Cross for his gallantry on this occasion. The citation states:
  'He showed no thought of his own safety and continued his efforts in the vicinity of a fierce oil fuel fire until given the order to abandon ship.'

and on her first mission she carried 1,000 prisoners-of-war. Fortunately there were no casualties among them, though most were suffering from varying degrees of exhaustion and semi-starvation. The lack of relation between the accommodation of these men and their numbers provided the ship's medical officer with an insoluble problem. They were accommodated in the holds and on all the available deck space. The lack of sanitary facilities did not seem to bother the prisoners themselves unduly. Demoralised and accustomed to the absence of such provision in the Desert, they disregarded it. But for the medical officer, the failure of these prisoners to make use of the petrol tins and sanitary bins provided for their natural functions meant that by the time the ship arrived at Alexandria, she could hardly be regarded as habitable.

These men were inoculated and vaccinated on board. The ship's water supply soon became contaminated with B. coli, and eventually had to be boiled. After each trip the decks and holds were in a disgraceful state of contamination and usually could not be properly cleansed and fumigated before putting to sea again. In addition, each fresh batch of prisoners introduced a new quota of lice and fleas. Altogether the *Knight of Malta* transported 11,500 Italian prisoners-of-war.

The only other ship to carry considerable numbers of prisoners-of-war was H.M.S. *Fiona*. She carried a total of 5,000 Italians between Mersa Matruh and Alexandria. Among these were some with bullet wounds, but these were not infected. It was recorded that although a small number of these men suffered from thirst and exposure, in general, their physical condition was very good and they were free from desert sores.

At this time medical organisation ashore was uncertain owing to the vast areas of conquered territory and the difficulties of communication. At Benghazi the brunt of the work fell at first on the overworked Italian Civilian Hospital. Fortunately at most of the ports there were vast quantities of medical stores of which good use could be made. A stabilised system of medical centres ashore was beginning to be evolved satisfactorily when, on April 3, 1941, Benghazi was evacuated and, during the rest of the month, the retreat took place across Cyrenaica to Tobruk. The following two months saw the loss of H.M.Ss. *Ladybird*, *Grimsby* and *Auckland* and H.M.A.S. *Waterhen*. A number of small vessels was lost in the harbour of Tobruk, including H.M.S. *Chakla* which had to be beached, and H.M.Ss. *Gnat*, *Greyhound*, *Flamingo*, *Cricket*, *Decoy*, *Vendetta* and *Phoebe* were damaged.

During the siege of Tobruk there were few naval personnel actually ashore in the town apart from Royal Marines who were manning A.A. defences, and among whom there were a few casualties from dive bombing attacks.

The Army made extensive medical provision in Tobruk, and the Navy had a sick bay ashore at Admiralty House. At first the requirements of this sick bay were met by medical officers from H.M.S. *Terror*. But in general, full medical facilities on land in Tobruk were provided by the Army in the 62nd General Hospital, the Beach Hospital, and at the 21st Casualty Clearing Station. In addition there was the fully equipped 4th General Hospital, and the R.A.F. maintained No. 21 Medical Receiving Station eight miles east of El Adem.

The Navy appointed a medical officer for duty in the Desert with the Fighter Squadrons from H.M.S. *Grebe*, and he had the assistance of the No. 22 R.A.F. Medical Receiving Station at Fuka. The facilities of this latter station included an Air Blood Transfusion Service which could be made available at very short notice.

The small naval sick bay in Admiralty House, Tobruk, had a number of cots and was in the charge of a surgeon lieutenant, R.N. Following extensive damage by air attack, this sick bay eventually had to be moved into air-raid shelters some 60 ft. below ground. These shelters had the advantage of being bomb-proof, but they lacked sanitation and water supply, though a primitive water supply was improvised later. Even so, water had to be limited to half a gallon per man per day for all purposes and much of this was brackish and unpleasant to drink. The washing of personnel and clothing became difficult, and scarcity of paraffin restricted the boiling of water even for surgical purposes. This scarcity of water was a considerable handicap as the wounds of most casualties were very dirty, and their clothes, skin and hair were completely covered with thick layers of dust.

Flies increased as the weather grew warmer and the disposal of refuse and waste water became a problem which, fortunately, was overcome with the aid of the Field Hygiene Section of the R.A.M.C. Bed bugs presented a further problem which was never satisfactorily overcome.

However, the general health of the Navy during the siege of Tobruk remained good. There were few cases of serious illness. Odd cases of sand-fly fever occurred and skin diseases were seen with epidermophytosis predominating. The absence of fresh meat and the scarcity of fresh vegetables combined with the poor quality of drinking water led to several minor digestive disturbances. At this time the general diet consisted of bully beef and tinned stewed meat and vegetables. Eggs, ham, sausages and fruit were occasionally sent from Alexandria. As a precaution, all naval personnel were issued with marmite and anti-scorbutic tablets from Army supplies.

One of the major naval medical incidents during the siege of Tobruk was the bombing of the Hospital Ship *Vita* which has already been described in Chapter 8 of the Navy's Administration Volume of this History.

In consequence of the attack on H.M.H.S. *Vita* it became necessary to evacuate casualties by warship during the remainder of the siege of Tobruk. Between April and November 1941, this 'ferry service' ran regularly from Alexandria to Tobruk with stores and supplies, and returned carrying wounded. Wounded were first carried by Australian 'V' Class destroyers operating in pairs, and later supplemented by a small number of British 'D' Class destroyers. The pairing arrangement allowed the ships to have alternate nights at sea and in harbour. To begin with, these ships had little protection against air attack during the daytime, and none at all during the hours of darkness. Within the first few weeks two destroyers had been lost and one damaged, all three with large numbers of troops on board.

During the second half of the siege all the Fleet destroyers operated the ferry service in turn and were augmented by fast minelayers. The dangers were further relieved by increasing fighter protection against air attack. The destroyers engaged on this task each averaged fourteen voyages to and from Tobruk before its relief.

The journeys made by these ships were usually begun by leaving Alexandria at 0800 hours carrying from 40 to 60 tons of stores. Apart from U-boats, there was little enemy interference until west of Mersa Matruh. There were usually high level bombing attacks between Mersa Matruh and Sidi Barrani, which was usually passed at about 1600 hours. West of Sidi Barrani the ships increased speed to 28 knots and usually had fighter protection until dusk. Enemy torpedo carrying aircraft usually had to be contended with at sunset. After this, allowing for further U-boats and mines, the rest of the journey would be peaceful if the night was dark, but would be otherwise interrupted by aerial torpedo and bombing attacks by moonlight.

Having surmounted all these dangers, these ships would proceed to Tobruk in the gathering night. The difficulty of finding the harbour entrance in the low coast was often decreased by an air raid being in progress which thus marked the way. Having felt their way among the wrecks and mines these ships would go alongside either a jetty, a wreck or a lighter. Gang planks would now be run out and the whole ship's company would deal with wounded, frozen meat, mail, ammunition, etc.

The average number of wounded to be embarked was 30 stretcher cases and 150 walking cases. If the ship happened to be alongside, the embarkation of stretcher cases was simple. But they were usually brought off in lighters and had to be lifted about 6 ft. on to the ship's upper deck. They were received on board by organised stretcher parties from the ship's company, but the number of personnel available for this task of taking in wounded on one side of the ship depended upon the number engaged in disembarking and unloading stores from the ship's other side. The essence of this unloading and loading was speed, the object being that ships should be away from Tobruk and well clear of enemy dive bombers by daybreak. Also, the harbour of Tobruk was well within range of enemy artillery fire. A competitive spirit was observed between the ships involved, and it was the constant attempt of everyone to unload and load faster than his neighbour. Everybody was expected, and was usually willing, to work to this end, irrespective of rank or quality. In this respect a medical officer recorded in his journal that:

'During one of these races with time the man-power of my ship was severely taxed. I saw an Australian standing by idly so I damned his eyes for doing nothing. I ordered him to take one end of a stretcher and, thus admonished, he promptly did so. It was only later that I discovered that he was a full Colonel who was in charge of the embarkation! However, he bore no resentment.'

There came a time when most ships kept to a definite schedule which read:

'Leave Alexandria with stores and personnel at 0800 hours.
Arrive Tobruk 2330 hours.
Unload stores, disembark personnel, embark wounded.
Sail 0100 hours.'

This meant that the average time spent in Tobruk before setting out on the return journey to Alexandria was a mere one-and-a-half hours.

These conditions of the ships of the ferry service were obviously strenuous and attended by great risk, and the losses of ships and personnel were by no means light. The general impression of medical officers employed on the task is reflected in the journal of one of them, who recorded:

'Taking it by and large, the Tobruk period was pretty grim, not only because of the dangers involved, but also because the ship was constantly cluttered up with all sorts of people and things. By night it used to take about twenty minutes to get from the bridge to the wardroom. One was likely to step on the faces of soldiers lying on the decks and the presence of groaning wounded between the hot messdecks resembled an inferno.'

On the night of October 25 the fast minelayer *Latona* was attacked by aircraft and hit by a bomb in the after engine room at 2008 hours. Fire immediately broke out among inflammable material. The after medical dressing station was soon put out of action by the spread of flames and 20 naval ratings and 14 soldiers were killed. There were 4 serious casualties and 13 minor ones. The first casualties were transferred to H.M.S. *Encounter* which came alongside, and the others, with the *Latona's* Medical Officer, to H.M.S. *Hero*.

Among the ships lost were H.M.Ss. *Huntley*, *Stoke* and *Svana*. On November 27, H.M.A.S. *Parramatta* was torpedoed off Tobruk and only 19 survivors were rescued by H.M.S. *Avon Vale*, who lost one of her own men when one of the rescuing boats capsized in heavy seas.

Before the end of December 1941 the siege of Tobruk was raised and, as soon as circumstances permitted, naval medical centres ashore were expanded.

The morale of naval personnel at Tobruk had remained good. There were occasional cases of anxiety state, and it is on record that some men

NORTH AFRICAN COASTAL OPERATIONS 1940-1941

Analysis of Casualties

H.M. Ships	Lost/Damaged	Date	Cause of casualties	Total casualties			Types of wounds† (excluding wounds of men who died as a result of them)														
				K	M	D/W	W	1	2	3	4	5	6	7	8	9	10	11	12	13	14	15	16	N/S
Decoy	D	November 13, 1940	Bombs	8			1	1					M.O. among killed.										
Ladybird	D	January 1, 1941	Shellfire			3	2																1
Aphis	D	January 1, 1941	Shellfire	3	5	1	31	2	11	2	2	1										7		2
Huntley	L	January 31, 1941	Bombs	12	3	1	1	6	(Sequelae of exposure.)															3
Southern Flow	L	February 11, 1941	Mine				1																
Ouse	L	February 20, 1941	Bombs				4								1										2
Terror	L	February 24, 1941	Bombs	13		3	2	6		1	1			M.O. among killed.											1
Dainty	L	February 24, 1941	Bombs	13			17			1														
Hasty	D	February 24, 1941	Bombs	2			2																	
Rosaura	L	March 18, 1941	Mine				1						1											
Skudd II	D	April 12, 1941	Bombs				5	4																
Draco	L	April 11, 1941	Bombs			1	3	2		(1 hysteria.)														
Vita	D	April 14, 1941	Bombs		51																			
Gnat	D	April 15, 1941	Shellfire			1																		
Fiona	L	April 18, 1941	Bombs				3	1																
Greyhound	D	April 21, 1941	Bombs				1	1	2	1														
Chakla	L	April 29, 1941	Bombs	8			18	7	6	1		(3 fr. femora.)								1					
Abingdon	D	May 1, 1941	Bombs																					
Stoke	L	May 7, 1941	Bombs					6	4																1
Svana	L	May 7, 1941	Bombs					7	3					1											10
Urania	D	May 9, 1941	Bombs				25								2		(includes 1 eye injury)							11		3
Ladybird	L	May 11, 1941	Bombs	11	3	1	10			1															
Grimsby	L	May 25, 1941	Bombs	1			13																		
Sindonis	D	May 29, 1941	Bombs					5	1			1													
Decoy	D	June 1, 1941	Bombs	1			5	9			(1 hysteria.)							1					2	2	
Falk	L	June 3, 1941	Bombs	9	25																				
Southern Maid	D	June 24, 1941	Bombs					2	4	1															
Auckland	L	June 29, 1941	Bombs				7																		
Waterhen	L	June 30, 1941	Bombs		1																				
Flamingo	D	June 30, 1941	Bombs																						
Cricket	D	July 9, 1941	Bombs																						
Decoy	D	July 15, 1941	Bombs																						
Vendetta	D	July 15, 1941	Bombs																						
A.10	L	August 3, 1941	Mine																						
Sotra	L	August 12, 1941	Bombs	8			3	1		1			(1 oil immersion)	1			1								
A.14	L	August 19, 1941	Bombs				6	3																	
Thorbryn	L	August 27, 1941	Aircraft-torpedo			1	17																		
Phoebe	D	August 27, 1941	Bombs	3	2	1	19	2	(17 effects of immersion)						(includes 1 eye injury)							3		5
Skudd III	L	October 25, 1941	Aircraft-torpedo		20										(includes 1 fr. mandible)									8
Parramatta	L	November 27, 1941	Torpedo		152		1		(1 eye injury)																
May	L	December 7, 1941	Bombs				1					1 rib													
A.2	L	December 15, 1941	Bombs																						
Salvia	L	December 26, 1941	Bombs		60		1	1																	

* K = Killed, M = Missing, D/W = Died of wounds, W = Wounded.
† Numbers 1-16, Classification of wounds. See p. 307. N/S = Not stated.

were anxious not so much about themselves as about the safety of their families in air raids on their homes in the United Kingdom. This type of anxiety was naturally aggravated by the loss and delay of mails from home which had to travel by the long sea route *via* the Cape at this time.

In the ships operating along the Libyan coast the morale was excellent. This was especially so in the case of H.M.Ss. *Terror*, *Aphis* and *Ladybird*. Quite apart from skilful and successful leadership, there is no doubt that the incongruous appearance of these three peculiarly constructed ships when compared to the rest of the Fleet went some way towards engendering a community sense of responsibility and pride. In these three ships, under conditions of enormous fatigue and stress, there was never the slightest indication of any breakdown from mental or physical causes other than direct wounding. This is the more remarkable in that on two occasions, when these ships had exhausted their ammunition, the Commander-in-Chief specifically ordered that ammunitioning parties should be supplied by other ships so that the ships' companies of H.M.Ss. *Terror*, *Aphis* and *Ladybird* might gain a few hours of needed sleep.

THE LOSS OF H.M.Ss. *PRINCE OF WALES* AND *REPULSE*

Singapore had its first Japanese air raid in the early hours of December 8, 1941, following which H.M.Ss. *Prince of Wales* and *Repulse* prepared to put to sea. In the late afternoon both ships sailed to investigate a reported Japanese landing at Kota Bharu on the east coast of Malaya. On December 9, towards evening, the ships were sighted by a Japanese reconnaissance aircraft.

At 0400 hours on December 10, the ships' companies had breakfast and then went to action stations, anticipating a probable dawn attack by the enemy. However, the first enemy air attack was delayed until about 1115 hours, in the face of a tremendous anti-aircraft barrage from the *Prince of Wales*.

At about 1145 hours, H.M.S. *Prince of Wales* was struck on her port side aft by an aerial torpedo and her port engines were disabled. The ship immediately listed to port, the lighting in the after medical distributing station was extinguished, and telephonic communication with other parts of the ship was interrupted. Secondary lighting was immediately employed, but within a short time cordite fumes sucked in through the punkah louvre ventilation trunks were so overpowering that the station had to be evacuated. It was decided to utilise the ship's chapel overhead as the main medical station and the many wounded, the majority suffering from severe scalds from fractured steam pipes, were diverted there. The chapel had no lighting, neither was there any fresh air supply, but the wounded were given morphia, dressed and placed on stretchers by torchlight. Some 40 casualties were so dealt with in the ship's chapel.

A passage way outside the chapel was also used as a dressing station, but this soon became useless as water was being forced into it from above and below through fractured ventilation shafts. It was then decided to use the Admiral's and Captain's quarters as dressing stations, but before this could be done there were three or four more torpedo hits on the starboard side of the ship, the last one of which was very close to the chapel and disabled the starboard engines.

At this point it was decided to keep the wounded below owing to a warning of impending high level bombing attacks. It was some time before a bomb hit the ship amidships. The explosion was tremendous and a medical officer took some stretcher parties forward and returned with a considerable number of casualties. At the same time the ship was rocked by a number of near misses.

Shortly afterwards a call came from the quarterdeck for medical assistance, and a medical officer recorded:

'I went on deck to find the port side of the quarterdeck awash. I found a few casualties underneath "Y" turret, one of whom was actually rolling across the deck towards the port side. I attended to these men on the deck and when I had finished I saw the Captain come aft. He called for volunteers among the ship's company to assist in getting the wounded up from below and a number was so transferred up to the quarterdeck. The destroyer *Express* came alongside the starboard side of the *Prince of Wales* and a gang plank was placed in position for a short while. Stretchers were passed by hand between the two ships and those wounded able to walk across did so.'

While the *Express* was alongside the order to abandon ship was given. By this time the *Prince of Wales* was listing heavily and smoke was billowing up from between her decks. Then, at 1320 hours, the ship slowly rolled over and turned turtle. There were hundreds of men in the oily water trying to swim towards rescuing destroyers. Others were picked up from floats, rafts and boats.

About 900 survivors from H.M.S. *Prince of Wales* were transferred to H.M.S. *Express* just before the *Prince of Wales* sank. Among these survivors were about 45 casualties, two-thirds of whom had extensive third degree burns of the hands, face and chest. Treatment of these was confined merely to the administration of morphia and the application of Tannafax. Owing to the congestion on board *Express* it was impossible to do more for these men pending their arrival in Singapore eight hours later.

As regards these burns cases, it was observed that, owing to the heat, few of the men had been wearing any anti-flash protection. It is also of interest that the landing of these cases from the *Express* at Singapore presented a problem as it was found that the standard Neil-Robertson stretcher was a painful method of lifting burns cases from the confined spaces of a small man-of-war. It was found best to sit these men in a

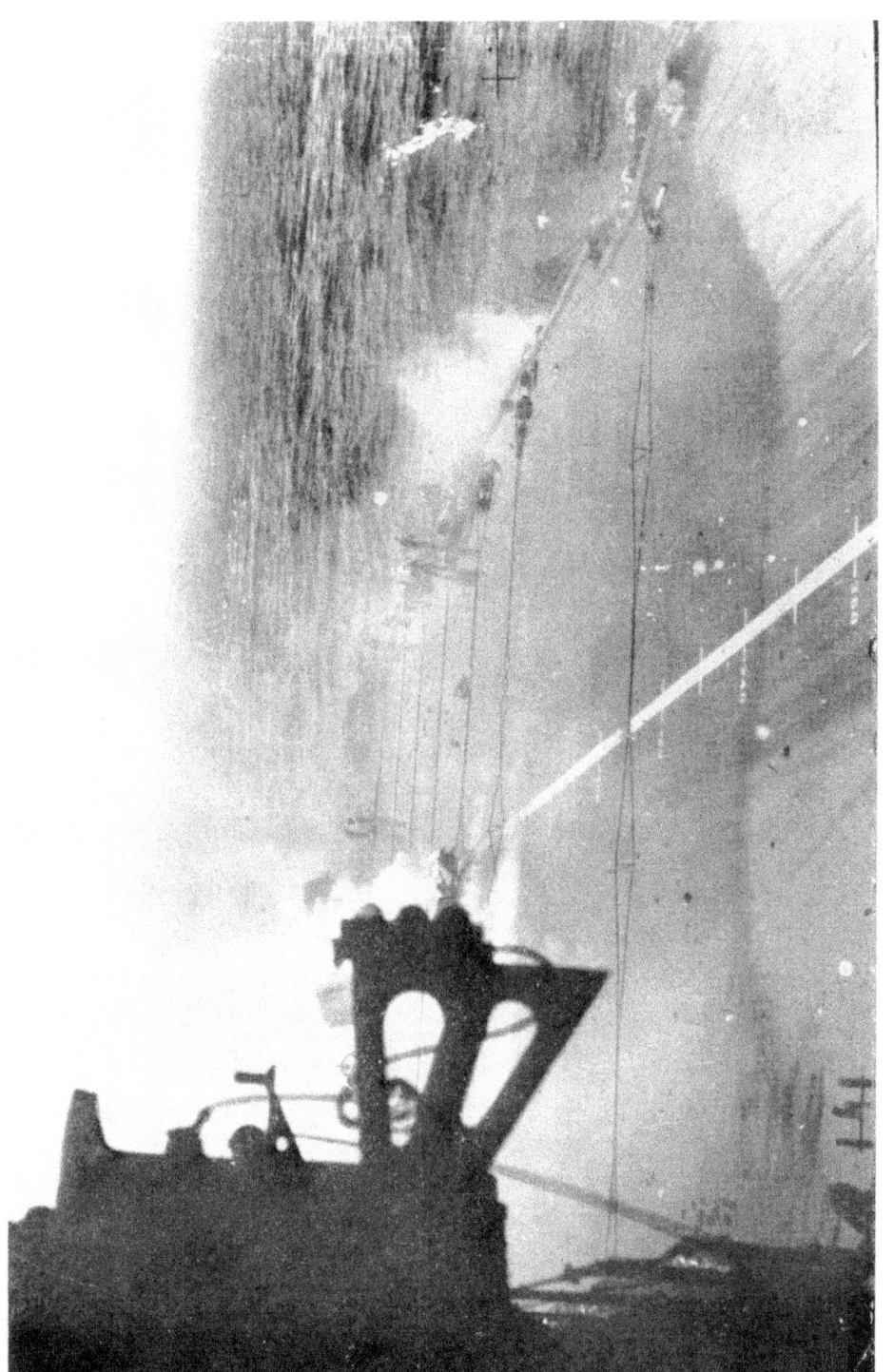

Plate XII. Damage to H.M.S. *Illustrious*.

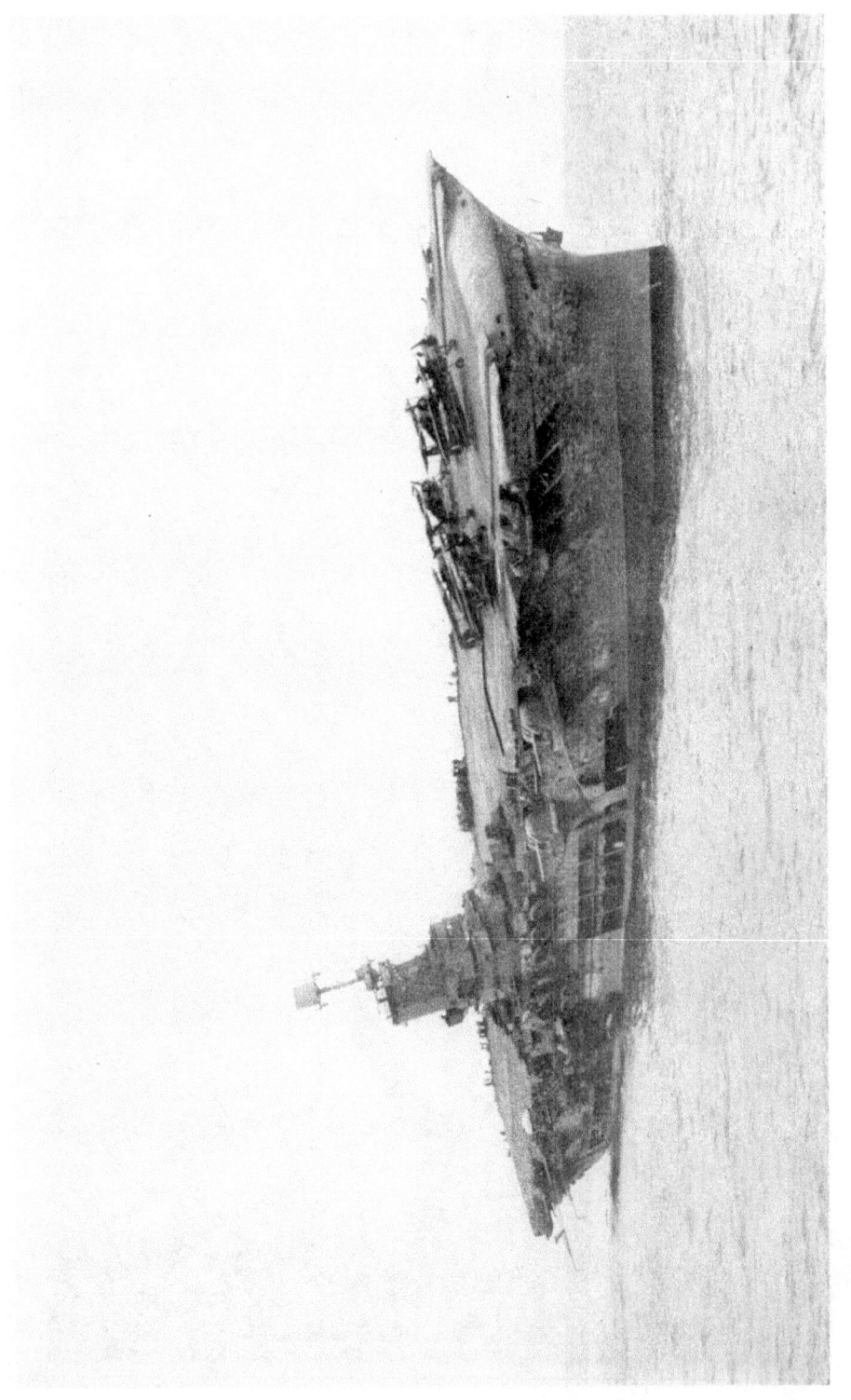

Plate XIII. Sinking of H.M.S. *Ark Royal*.

'Bosun's Chair' and so to lift them out by the ship's ammunition hoists.*

Meanwhile, in H.M.S. *Repulse*, events had developed on almost parallel lines to those in the *Prince of Wales*. Action with Japanese aircraft was begun soon after 1100 hours, and a medical officer who survived recorded:

'Very soon a loud explosion was heard. We were in the after medical station and smoke began to enter the space from the deck above. I thereupon ordered the armoured hatch to be closed. Loudspeakers then announced that a bomb had pierced the marines' messdeck and had exploded, causing a fire to break out. We heard tapping on the armoured hatch and opened it to receive five casualties. The first man was dead from severe head injuries. Two were severe cases of burns. One of the others had a lacerated wound of his forearm and one was a boy with a large haematoma of his buttock caused by being thrown to the deck by the bomb explosion.

'One of the telephones in direct communication with "Y" turret asked for help and the surgeon lieutenant (D) made his way there and found a seaman with a compound fracture of his humerus due to a machine-gun bullet. The dental officer rendered him first aid and gave him morphia.†

'While this was happening I was informed that several casualties had been collected in the Captain's lobby, so I made my way there *via* the quarterdeck. I found about a dozen men, mostly cases of burns and scalds, and one had a fractured femur. I gave them morphia and what first aid I could. But I had no time to label these cases then, and I meant to return and do so later, but I was never able to. I saw that the wardroom lobby just below me was full of smoke and steam.

'I arrived back in my station to find more messages reporting casualties in other parts of the ship. At that moment there was a loud explosion so I ordered the armoured hatch to be closed again, thinking that bombs were falling. Actually this explosion was a torpedo hit somewhere amidships.

'A few minutes later there was another torpedo hit and the lights went out momentarily.

'About two minutes later there was a very heavy explosion of a torpedo quite close to us. At once the ship began to list, so I decided to investigate and ordered the armoured hatch to be opened once more. As soon as the hatch began to open water started to pour into the station, so I ordered the hatch to be opened at full speed and told everybody to get out. Fortunately, the two men whose duty it was to turn the winch did not lose their heads, and they continued to open the hatch until there was space enough for men to scramble through. It was only just possible to climb the vertical ladder against the fall of water through the hatch, and unfortunately it was out of the question to move the two badly burnt casualties.

---

* It is of interest that this view was confirmed yet again while this volume was in the course of preparation. Following an explosion of petrol vapour on board H.M.S. *Indomitable* on February 3, 1953, it was recorded that the Neil-Robertson type stretcher was unsuitable for patients with burns.—Editor.

† This casualty survived and made a full recovery.

'We made our way to the quarterdeck which was listing heavily to port to such an extent that it was difficult to climb up to the starboard rails. I saw that many men had already jumped into the sea.*

'I should think the ship sank within about seven minutes. We blew up our lifebelts, though this was not very easy to do in a hurry. Many men jumped from the starboard side of the ship and injured themselves by landing further down the ship's side.† As the ship was still moving forward, those who jumped were soon left clear in the sea, but there must have been some danger from the propellers which were still revolving.

'Destroyers soon started to pick up survivors, and I myself was fortunate enough to be rescued by H.M.S. *Electra*. I was then able to help her medical officer organise resuscitation parties, and afterwards to sort, treat and label patients till we arrived in Singapore some ten hours later.

'Most of the casualties rescued were burns, cuts and fractures. Everybody was suffering from the effects of swallowing and inhaling oil fuel. Two cases of severe burns died before reaching Singapore. Fractures of *os calcis* seemed frequent.

'There were some 800 survivors on board the destroyer, but in the crowded ship we made the casualties as comfortable as possible though, apart from morphia, first aid and supplies of hot sweet tea, there was very little we could do. Many of the casualties were all but naked, but it seems probable that shock was lessened by the warmth of the climate.'‡

Unfortunately, owing to the confusion which soon existed in Singapore itself and owing to the later loss of ships involved in the rescue work, detailed medical records of the casualties from the *Prince of Wales* and *Repulse* are scanty. It is on record however, that the only cases of bad burns of the trunk were seen in casualties from the *Prince of Wales*, while in the *Repulse* the burns were confined to hands and face and were mainly seen in engine room personnel. It is perhaps significant that in H.M.S. *Repulse* all men working on deck had received anti-flash gear and had been instructed to wear shirts with long sleeves, and long trousers tucked into their socks. A number wore boiler suits which gave good protection against burns on the body.

---

* An armoured hatch of the type described on the previous page is opened by a winch mechanism, hand operated by two persons detailed for the purpose.

† It was later recorded in Singapore that among some 250 casualties from H.M.Ss. *Prince of Wales* and *Repulse*, there were numerous Pott's fractures and fractures of *os calcis* due to men jumping from the deck and landing on the ship's bilge keel.

‡ This medical officer was mentioned in dispatches for 'outstanding devotion to duty in tending the wounded in action in H.M.S. *Repulse*'. A sick berth attendant of H.M.S. *Repulse* was also mentioned in dispatches, his citation reading: 'He remained below in the fore medical station after everyone had been ordered on deck, in order to try to help a wounded man to escape. Although he failed in this, he only abandoned the attempt when the ship began to turn over and was about to sink.'

LOSS OF H.M. SHIPS PRINCE OF WALES AND REPULSE
DECEMBER 10, 1941

Casualties

H.M. Ships Lost L	Approximate no. of ship's company	Cause of casualties	Total casualties				Types of injury	Disposal of wounded
			K	M	D/W	W		
Prince of L *Wales*	1,400	Bombs and torpedo	4	328	3	10	2 burns, 1 multiple injury and 1 fractured clavicle are recorded. (Remainder not known)	No. 1 Malayan G.H. and M.H. Alexandria, Singapore, on December 11, 1941
								H.M.S. *Express* landed these and approximately 900 other survivors.
Repulse L	1,300	Bombs and torpedo	4	400	1	5	2 penetrating wounds of abdomen are recorded. (Remainder not known)	M.H. Alexandria, Singapore, December 11, 1941
								H.M.S. *Electra* landed these and approximately 900 other survivors.

This statistical list is in accordance with the Casualty Register, Admiralty, in April 1943. It is incomplete in detail because:

(1) M.Os., H.M. ships *Express* and *Electra* could not keep lists of those treated on board, while so many were present during only a short emergency passage. In any case, H.M.S. *Electra* was herself lost soon afterwards.

(2) Singapore Hospital records were not available following the capitulation.

AIR RAIDS AFFECTING NAVAL ESTABLISHMENTS ASHORE AND SHIPS IN HARBOUR*

During 1941, air raids were so frequent and so widely distributed that a detailed survey is impossible. The following examples have been selected with a view to illustrating some of the main effects on naval establishments, etc.

UNITED KINGDOM

Portsmouth Area. On January 10, 1941, the biggest raid occurred. The local power station was damaged resulting in the failure of current in many naval establishments, few of which escaped some degree of damage by fire.

---

* Some account has already been given in Volume I, Chapters 14 and 15.

The next date on which the raids were severe was the night of March 10–11, when damage was widespread and many small ships in the harbour were involved and sustained casualties among seamen manning their lightly protected guns. The bombs were mainly of small calibre as illustrated by one which exploded in the boiler room of H.M.S. *Witherington*. The stoker on duty in the boiler room received only a small cut as he 'swam up the ladder' out of the flooding compartment.

In this raid damage was done to the Training Establishment at Fareham, H.M.S. *Collingwood*, and also at the Naval Air Station at Lee-on-Solent. Other establishments damaged were H.M.S. *Excellent*, the Naval Gunnery School, H.M.S. *Dolphin*, a submarine base, and the Royal Dockyard. But casualties were relatively light and were generally incidental to fire fighting.

The relative lightness of casualties is shown in the following examples extracted from records for the first two quarters of 1941:

(1) In H.M.S. *St. Vincent*, a shore establishment at Gosport, during the first quarter there were 5 casualties among 1,080 personnel, and 3 of these were due to explosive incendiary bombs.

(2) In H.M.S. *Vernon*, a shore establishment on the edge of Portsmouth Harbour where damage was extremely severe, there were 66 wounded and 31 killed out of 2,135 personnel during the first quarter of the year. In the second quarter the figures fell to 7 wounded and 2 killed out of a complement of 1,474.

(3) In the Royal Naval Barracks, Portsmouth, with personnel of 9,276, there were 23 wounded and 2 killed during January 1941. In the next two months there were 48 wounded. On one occasion a bomb pierced a shelter and killed 7 naval ratings, and another bomb badly damaged a dressing station injuring 2 medical officers and a sick berth attendant. Fortunately these dressing stations were numerous and widely dispersed and most of them continued to function though various other parts of the barracks were burned out.

The Royal Naval Barracks was even more badly damaged on the night of April 17, when a landmine fell on a block of buildings which contained the Dental Department.* On this occasion there were 33 killed and 71 wounded.

On April 27, the barracks was again damaged and there were 4 dead and 41 wounded. Once again the damage was caused by a landmine.

(4) A landmine also caused extensive damage at the Royal Marine Barracks, Eastney, when two wards in the Royal Marine Infirmary and the Dental Department were completely wrecked.

Plymouth Area. On the night of April 20–21, a block of the Royal Naval Barracks, Devonport, was hit by two large high explosive bombs together with a large number of incendiary bombs. The bombs

---

* *See* Volume I, Chapter 16.

penetrated to the basement which was used as a refuge for barracks' personnel. Fire was extensive and the roof and walls of the building collapsed burying a large number of men. 105 men were killed and 99 injured, and it was a number of days before all the dead could be dug out.

In the same raid other blocks of buildings in Devonport Barracks were damaged, including part of the sick quarters. This latter damage, concurrently with damage to the Royal Naval Hospital, Plymouth, made it necessary for 100 emergency beds to be set aside for use by the Navy in King's Tamerton School, St. Budeaux.

Damage and minor injuries were appreciable at the Royal Naval Engineering College, Keyham, but the mortality was fortunately low.

Air raids were frequent and prolonged in April and early May, and the Royal Naval Hospital, Plymouth, was severely damaged, as has already been described in Chapter 14 of the Administration Volume of this History.

During all these raids ships in the harbour escaped with relatively little damage, only the minesweeper *Assama* being sunk on March 21, with the loss of 1 officer and 5 ratings.

Barrow-in-Furness Area. The first heavy air raid occurred at 2300 hours on May 3, when a naval ambulance and first-aid party were involved as is described in the following record:

> 'A heavy bomb fell 150 yards away. The blast broke the windows of the ambulance and loosened the panels. We dismounted and took shelter on the ground behind the far side of the ambulance. Before we could rise a landmine fell about eighty yards away. We got up and went to the craters and found one person slightly injured and two elderly persons dead. The next landmine fell a quarter of a mile away and we went there and found several people dead and rendered first aid to a large number of injured.'

On May 8, at 0025 hours, bombs were dropped in Vickers-Armstrong's yard in the vicinity of a number of naval ships. One naval rating was killed by two machine-gun bullets which had perforated his steel helmet.

On the next night a naval Mobile Medical Unit went on board a damaged merchant ship and extinguished burning wreckage and removed a number of casualties some of whom were dead.

Liverpool Area. Considering the presence of many men-of-war in the dock area the damage and casualties were comparatively small. Damage in local naval establishments on shore was widespread, and it is remarkable that only one naval rating is recorded as having sustained injuries which were of a very minor nature.

Swansea Area. Here there was a great deal of enemy air activity, particularly during February. Damage to naval establishments included the naval sick quarters but only 6 casualties occurred among naval personnel.

Bristol Area. The only air raids causing naval casualties occurred on January 3 and March 16–17, and these were very minor in degree and small in numbers.

Skegness Area. The Training Establishment, H.M.S. *Royal Arthur*, was raided on February 17, 1941, when the sick quarters was damaged with the loss of sixty beds, and one air mechanic was killed.

Lowestoft Area. During nineteen air raids between April and July 1941, 213 high explosive bombs were dropped in or around H.M.S. *Europa*, the local naval base; 4 men were killed outright, 4 died of wounds, and there were 24 other casualties.

Further air raids in the last quarter of the year produced only 4 naval casualties.

Great Yarmouth Area. In 1941, the complement of the local naval base was 2,650, but air-raid casualties were only 1 killed and 22 injured.

Harwich Area. Many small ships were damaged and some were sunk by air attacks during 1941. These included H.M.S. *Marmion* which was bombed alongside the quay at Harwich. She had 12 casualties on board, 2 of them fatal.

OVERSEA

Suez Canal Zone. During 1941, air raids occurred with a steady frequency particularly during the period of full moon. The naval casualties were small in number and minor in degree.

Alexandria Area. A small number of naval casualties occurred following air attacks during 1941. Damage was caused, with the death of her Senior Medical Officer, to the Hospital Ship *Maine*. An account of this incident has already been given in Chapter 8 of the Navy, Volume I, (Administration).

Malta. The Island of Malta had sustained some air raids during 1940, following the entry of Italy into the war. The Royal Naval Hospital had been damaged and a sick berth attendant had been killed. But these early attacks had been too infrequent seriously to affect the life of the Island. However, in January 1941, as has been described earlier in this chapter, air attacks became intensified and concentrated following the arrival of H.M.Ss. *Illustrious, Bonaventure* and *Gallant*. The presence of H.M.A.S. *Perth* and the S.S. *Essex* carrying aircraft and ammunition also played a part in making the Grand Harbour an attractive target for enemy bombers.*

---

* The S.S. *Essex* was badly damaged and set on fire, while in harbour at Malta, on January 16, 1941. A surgeon commander, R.N., on the staff of Malta Dockyard was decorated for gallantry on this occasion, the citation reading: 'This officer was informed that casualties had occurred on board an ammunition ship. He immediately went on board the *Essex*, which was on fire, and descended to the engine room where he rendered first aid to casualties who were still alive. He had these men removed from the ship, and his coolness and calmness were a fine example to others.'

From this time onwards, Malta had little respite from air attack for a number of months. Material damage was steadily progressive but loss of life remained remarkably low. This can probably be attributed to the ample provision of tunnels in the local sandstone which could be quickly and easily bored and was very resilient to blast. A system of such branching tunnels was available inside the dockyard and all medical provision in the dockyard area was made under this type of protection. Casualties from ships in the harbour received attention in the reception and resuscitation centres which formed part of the tunnel system, and they were later evacuated by road to the military hospital thirteen miles away. Fortunately such casualties were infrequent because few ships remained in harbour for any length of time.

On March 21, H.M.S. *Defender* was dive bombed and 5 seamen were wounded by bomb splinters. On March 23, 2 seamen were wounded when H.M.S. *Griffin* was bombed and machine-gunned, and a third died later from burns.

In the same raid a Royal Marine on board H.M.S. *Calcutta* was injured by falling masonry. This was an example of a unique hazard which attended air raids on Malta, whereby masonry and large fragments of sandstone from the low cliffs surrounding the dockyard area were liable to become dislodged by bomb explosions and to strike the upper decks of ships close alongside.

On June 30, during a heavy raid on the dockyard area, an officer in H.M.S. *Jade* was killed by a gunshot wound of the lung. In the same raid a Royal Marine manning a gun was killed in Fort St. Angelo, the local naval base, and another rating was killed by blast. It will be appreciated how slight these casualties were in relation to the total number of personnel exposed to such air attacks.

During the second quarter of 1941, the activities of the Royal Naval Hospital were still further curtailed. Heavy air raids caused considerable damage to the hospital buildings and destroyed the water, electricity and gas mains. Telephone circuits were also destroyed, and the communications of the hospital with the outside world virtually ceased. Water had to be obtained from wells inside the hospital boundaries, and had to be boiled before use. Lighting was by candle, and cooking and sterilising could only be carried out on oil stoves for a limited period owing to shortage of paraffin. X-ray and other special departments requiring electric power were at a standstill. On the night of April 29–30, one ward block was demolished by a direct hit. Unfortunately this ward block contained a large consignment of surgical dressings which had only just been received. These dressings became ignited and a serious fire resulted in the total loss of these stores.

Some account of the function of the Royal Naval Hospital, Malta, at this time has already been given in Chapter 15 of the Navy, Vol. I (Administration).

REMARKS ON THE EFFECTS OF PARTICULAR WEAPONS, 1941

MINES

During 1941 small ships were the predominating victims of this weapon, and included barrage balloon tugs, auxiliary patrol trawlers, minesweepers, minelayers, harbour launches, anti-submarine craft, mooring vessels, motor torpedo boats and motor gunboats. Inevitably it was those vessels, designed to overcome the mine menace, which succumbed in the greatest numbers, and the heaviest losses occurred in the estuaries and harbours around the British Isles. During 1941, 67 vessels were damaged by mines and 48 were sunk. Out of this total of 115 ships, approximately one half were trawlers employed in minesweeping.

None of these small vessels carried medical officers, so little data exist concerning their casualties.

In the case of larger men-of-war damaged by mines, the clinical features were similar to those already remarked in 1940. The following report by the Medical Officer of H.M.S. *Kandahar* illustrates the difficulties of dealing with wounded in a destroyer following mine damage, and the report also gives an account of the end of H.M.S. *Neptune*, a cruiser lost in the same operation:

'The loss of H.M.S. *Kandahar* took place one week before Christmas 1941, the original damage being sustained at about 0400 and the final sinking occurring 25 hours later. The scene was some 20 miles off the coast of Tripoli.

'In company with some cruisers and other destroyers, H.M.S. *Kandahar* left Malta at 1800 and steamed to the southward, the object being to intercept an Italian force known to be at sea and bound for Tripoli carrying stores for the German Army in Libya.

'We left Malta at high speed and, shortly before making contact with the enemy near the African coast, H.M.S. *Neptune*, leading the force, touched off a mine with her "sweeps". Shortly afterwards there was another explosion of a mine touched off in the same way. The remainder of the British force was warned to steer away clear of the minefield while the *Neptune*, now endeavouring to get clear herself by going ahead and astern on her port and starboard engines, touched off yet another mine under her stern blowing a portion of it off and rendering her immobile.

'There was a west-north-west wind blowing causing the *Neptune* to drift to the eastward and it was hoped that she would eventually drift clear of the minefield. Meanwhile we were patrolling in deep water to the eastward and keeping in visual touch with her.

'Two hours later, when the *Neptune* considered herself clear of the mines, she signalled that she was now ready to be taken in tow. The *Kandahar* altered course at 0318 with the object of closing the *Neptune* so as to go alongside her and take off casualties. As the *Kandahar* was swinging to starboard a mine exploded and the detonation caused the *Kandahar's* after magazine to blow up. Forty minutes later the *Neptune* drifted into yet another mine which damaged her amidships, and she slowly turned over and sank.

'Meanwhile, the *Kandahar* was in the sorry position of being surrounded by friendly ships none of which could come to her assistance because of the dangers of the minefield. So with sinking hearts, we witnessed their departure and were left to the tender mercies of the enemy and the elements.

'As soon as I heard that wounded were to be embarked from the *Neptune*, I went aft to make sure that the wardroom had been properly cleared for the reception of casualties. I then returned to the sick bay. Immediately afterwards I felt a violent explosion, and all the lights went out, engine noises ceased and the ship listed slightly and settled down somewhat by the stern. I lit the emergency oil lamps in the sick bay and then went up to the bridge in response to an urgent call for a doctor.

'A large amount of debris had been exploded into the air and had come down on all parts of the ship's superstructure. This debris included a depth charge which landed on the binnacle and struck the 1st lieutenant on the shoulder. The shell hoist of No. 3 gun, weighing about $1\frac{1}{4}$ tons, was also thrown into the air and landed on the upper deck above No. 2 boiler room.

'I gave first aid to the 1st lieutenant and then went aft to deal with any other casualties. These proved to be remarkably few in number, because the explosion of the magazine had completely removed the after part of the ship and with it some 60 men lost their lives and disappeared. Two men in the after part of the ship had a remarkable escape, as they were blown out of the wardroom, and came down on the upper deck. Both were badly shocked and one had lacerations of the face while the other had severe injuries to one leg. One man was found crushed beneath a pom-pom gun which had been dismounted by the explosion. He was moribund when I saw him and soon died. Another man had a severe spinal injury and died before daybreak. Most of the other injuries were minor in degree, but the 1st lieutenant was suffering from concussion, contusions of face and a fractured scapula.

'It was soon apparent that the ship was not going to sink immediately. It also seemed likely that we would be observed and attacked by enemy forces after daybreak.

'At this time a long trail of oil stretched from our open stern and the ship rapidly took on a 16° list to starboard to the accompaniment of the siren which continued to wail until the steam was shut off.

'At dawn I assembled my small party of wounded on the warm plates by the funnel. I wrapped them up in blankets and made what arrangements I could for their transport in the event of our having to abandon ship either by further enemy action, or should the remaining watertight bulkhead give way. There was only one semi-serviceable boat, a dinghy, and this was split in several places. However, the engine was taken out of this boat to increase its weight carrying capacity and we filled the many splits in its planks with *adeps lanae, ung. zinci* and *paraffin molle*.* Over this we

---

* This is the only recorded instance in naval medical records of medical supplies being employed in this way for boat repairs.—Editor.

tacked strips of rubber cut from the legs of sea boots, and we improvised buoyancy tanks from empty oil drums sealed with jaconet. We also improvised several rafts from mess stools, tables, doors and any other removable wooden fittings.

'This work filled in most of the day, which was one of brilliant sunshine with a smooth sea. Tripoli could be seen on the horizon to the southward. German and Italian aircraft flew over us during the day, but no bombs were dropped. In the afternoon we got into wireless touch with Malta and were told that H.M.S. *Jaguar* would come to our help after dark.

'At sunset the weather deteriorated and we felt some anxiety about the strength of our remaining bulkhead. But it held out, and at about 2200 a British aircraft flew low over us as a guide to our rescuers. The *Jaguar* appeared at 0330. An attempt was made to lay her alongside, but the weather had become too rough, so she steamed a short distance up to windward and we were ordered to abandon ship and make our way to her. I placed the wounded on a float and we paddled away and were soon alongside the *Jaguar* plus a bunch of survivors hanging on to our life-lines whom we had collected on the way.

'On the return trip to Malta the Medical Officer of the *Jaguar* dealt with my casualties and 30 were sent to hospital suffering from wounds, exposure and shock.'*

On January 5, 1941, H.M.S. *Lowestoft* struck a mine and was extensively damaged in the engine and boiler rooms. Her Medical Officer's report describes a characteristic injury due to mine explosion as follows:

'A seaman sustained a "T" shaped fracture of femur. X-ray showed an oblique fracture through the lower third of the bone with a vertical fracture running down through the distal fragment and passing between the condyles. This appearance suggested a shearing strain on the bone, together with a sudden application of fairly great vertical force, as if the man had been blown into the air and had landed in a twisted position with all his weight on the left leg. The two halves of the distal fragment were splayed slightly outwards at their proximal ends.'

When H.M.S. *Pelican* was mined on February 19, 1941, her casualties included 5 cases of fractured *os calcis*, 2 fractured tibias, 2 fractured fibulas, 1 fractured femur, 5 badly sprained ankles and 3 twisted knee joints.

At this time the characteristic bone and joint injuries which were seen in mining disasters at sea led to the suggestion that such injuries might be minimised if all men serving in small ships in mined areas could be equipped with sorbo rubber heels to their footwear.†

---

* After this rescue H.M.S. *Kandahar* was sunk deliberately by our own forces. Of her ship's company 168 survived, 60 were killed, and 7 were lost during the rescue operations. Her Surgeon Lieutenant was subsequently decorated for his outstanding conduct on this occasion, and the citation records that, in addition to his professional skill, 'he proved himself as good a seaman and executive officer as he was a doctor'.

† There is no recorded evidence that this suggestion was ever proceeded with.—Editor.

BOMBING

During 1941 the medical aspects of aircraft attacks against ships at sea merely confirmed what had already been observed in 1939 and 1940. The danger of flash burns was stressed and attention directed to the protection afforded by anti-flash clothing. Splinter wounds continued to produce extensive injuries.

An interesting side effect was seen in the cases of asphyxia and blast effects which followed the bombing of H.M.S. *Puckeridge* on December 13, 1941. This ship was hit by a bomb which passed through the deck and exploded on the messdecks causing a large fire to break out immediately. The fire rapidly filled the crater and made it impossible for the men surviving to climb the only ladder which had been left intact. The few men rescued complained of having been gassed in addition to their burns and were suffering from acute dyspnoea and fits of coughing which persisted for several days. Five men showed copious blood-stained frothy sputum after two hours and died from pulmonary oedema. This picture would seem to have represented one of blast injuries complicated by the presence of flash, fire and hot gases in a confined space.

TORPEDOES

The small number of casualties inflicted by this weapon in 1940 was again confirmed in 1941. At this stage of the war it was obvious that the torpedo resembled the shell in this respect, whereas the mine might well be classed with the bomb as a cause of high mortality and morbidity.

During 1941, ships involved in successful torpedo attacks by U-boats included the battleship *Barham*, the aircraft carrier *Ark Royal*, and the cruisers *Bonaventure*, *Dunedin* and *Galatea* all of which were sunk. Similarly the destroyers *Exmoor*, *Fearless*, *Broadwater*, *Mohawk*, *Cossack* and *Stanley* were lost, as were the armed merchant cruisers *Salopian* and *Rajputana*. (Plate XIII illustrates the sinking of the *Ark Royal*.)

In all these ships the casualties were due to many extraneous causes apart from the explosion of the torpedo itself. They were in great measure the result of such incidents as abandoning ship, fire or secondary explosions of magazines. The total figures of losses among these ships' companies are thus misleading if, as would appear to be the case at first sight, they were all directly attributed to the torpedo.

For instance, when H.M.S. *Ark Royal* was sunk following a hit by a single torpedo on November 14, 1941, near Gibraltar, out of 1,700 personnel on board there were no casualties directly attributable to this weapon. But one man was drowned in a flooded compartment, while 22 men sprained or fractured their ankles in abandoning ship, when they slid down ropes or jumped some distance on to the deck of the rescuing destroyer.

In the same way, when H.M.S. *Springbank* was lost, her 32 fatalities were not due to the explosion of the torpedo, but were caused as follows:

Lost alongside H.M.S. *Coxwold* after attempting to swim from a raft	2
Lost in the propellers of H.M.S. *Coxwold* and S.S. *Starling*	8
Lost from a capsized whaler	4
Lost from a capsized dinghy	2
Lost by refusing to abandon ship	1
Lost by falling between the sinking ship and the rescuing ship	3
Lost from miscellaneous injuries such as striking wreckage in the sea and being crushed between ships, etc.	12

When H.M.S. *Phoebe* was torpedoed on August 27, 1941, only 2 men were killed by the explosion, though 6 were later drowned in oil fuel.

When H.M.S. *York* was torpedoed at Suda Bay on March 26, 1941, the majority of her ship's company were asleep between decks. Nevertheless, only 2 men out of 720 were killed as a direct result of the explosion.

An interesting account, which includes the rare circumstance of living men being left behind for dead in a sinking ship, is seen in the report of the Medical Officer of H.M.S. *Cossack* which was torpedoed on October 23, 1941:

'The order to abandon ship having been given I filled my pockets with morphia and syringes and put my first-aid pack over my shoulder. I then went round the decks with my torch looking for wounded. I found several dead and one seaman with a leg injury. I gave him morphia and lowered him on to a float. Then, as there were only three of us left on the quarter-deck, and as I could find no one else requiring attention, we abandoned ship. After $1\frac{1}{2}$ hours in the water I was picked up by H.M.S. *Carnation*. As the *Cossack* was still floating, though on fire, the *Carnation* went alongside her and sent a boarding party on board her to attempt to control the fire. I accompanied this party taking my sick berth attendant with me. Among the dead bodies we found 1 officer and 2 seamen who had been assumed dead but were actually alive. We subsequently transferred them to H.M.S. *Legion*. All these cases had severe head injuries. One seaman died on board the *Legion*, but the other seaman and the officer, the latter with a fractured skull, both made a complete recovery within a few months.'

Further interesting details of miscellaneous casualties are given in a report by the surviving Medical Officer of H.M.S. *Bonaventure*, whose Senior Medical Officer lost his life:

'H.M.S. *Bonaventure* was sunk at 0300 on March 31, 1941 100 miles north of Alexandria. She was hit by two torpedoes on her starboard side amidships. She immediately listed heavily to starboard. Shortly afterwards she heeled over still further, but then sank rapidly by the stern, righting herself as she went down. She sank in less than five minutes. The sea was calm, and sea temperature was 60° F.

'Seven of the officers missing were apparently asleep in their cabins, and 14 other officers are known to have been trapped in a lobby when the lid of a man-hole jammed. They were seen trying to open it, but were defeated by the list of the ship and the rapidity with which the stern went under water. Nearly all those who reached the upper deck were rescued.

'The injuries of surviving casualties fell into four classes:

'(1) *Concussion of the Explosion.* The remote effect of the explosions of the torpedoes caused remarkably few injuries, in spite of the fact that the ship was considerably distorted and buckled. The only severe injury was a man with a comminuted fracture of his humerus.

'(2) *Burns.* Three ratings had second degree burns of the face and arms which were either due to the flash of the explosion or else to a small fire which broke out.

'(3) *Bilge Keel Casualties.** It seems probable that the bilge keel was responsible for the numerous dislocated ankles, fractured forearms and nine cases of fractured spine. All these people slid down the ship's side with considerable speed, and they hit the bilge keel unexpectedly with various parts of their anatomy.

'The actual mechanism of causation of the fractured spines is obscure. Their distribution and formation was uniform, being the anterior part of the bodies of vertebrae D.12 to L.1 to 3. It has been suggested that these were due to depth charges which were being dropped by neighbouring destroyers, but I consider this unlikely as none of these cases had any evidence of chest or abdominal injury. It was also suggested that these spinal injuries were caused by the feet hitting the bilge keel unexpectedly with the result that the body became forcibly and violently doubled up. However, taking into consideration the angle of heel and the shape of the bilge keel, I think that the most likely mechanism that operated was that which is known as a "deceleration" fracture in circles of aviation medicine.'

DEPTH CHARGES

These caused one known fatal casualty, who died three days later following operation for a ruptured sigmo-rectal junction. When taken from the sea this man was severely shocked and in great pain. There was a small amount of anal haemorrhage present, but no other external sign of injury. Other persons felt the effects of exploding depth charges while in the water and subsequently suffered from generalised stiffness and muscle aches and pains which persisted for about one week.

---

* *See* the account of the sinking of H.M.Ss. *Prince of Wales* and *Repulse* earlier in this Chapter.

The presence of toxic gases following torpedo attack had already been noted during 1940, and is again referred to in the medical records of 1941 as in the case of H.M.Ss. *Manchester* and *Aurania*.

The *Aurania* was torpedoed on October 21, 1941, and a number of her survivors complained of the effects of inhaling fumes before escaping from the ship. These men showed pallor, dyspnoea, a dry cough, lassitude and vomiting. Two developed broncho-pneumonia and one died a month later with pulmonary oedema. It is of interest that these were the only casualties in this ship, despite the fact that she had been torpedoed.

A curious and unusual casualty sequence was recorded after the sinking of H.M.S. *Dunedin*. This ship was torpedoed in the South Atlantic at 1300 hours on November 24, 1941. She was struck by two torpedoes and sank in twenty minutes, and only 144 men appear to have abandoned her out of her total complement of 470. During the next three days 73 men died from exposure and particularly from the vicious attacks of what is described as 'a small fish about a foot long which was in the company of many sharks'. Of the 71 survivors rescued by the American S.S. *Mishmaha*, 4 died soon afterwards, and 43 were later landed and sent to hospital at Trinidad. The most serious cases among these were observed to be suffering from multiple 'punched out' ulcers caused by fish bites.

MISCELLANEOUS CAUSES

These include machine-gun, cannon and shell fire, and the records of 1941 show little which has not been observed during the previous year.

However, of some medical interest is the action between H.M. cruiser *Cornwall* and Raider No. 33 on May 8, 1941. This action was fought in the Indian Ocean, in the late afternoon, just north of the Equator and after a prolonged chase at high speed for some thirty-six hours. The action lasted only eleven minutes, at the end of which the enemy ship blew up. But, unfortunately, the *Cornwall* herself did not escape unscathed. Right at the beginning of the action the enemy raider seems to have scored a direct hit by gunfire on the *Cornwall*'s 'ring-main' with consequent failure of various of her electrical circuits. This had the effect not only of interrupting the control of the guns, but there was also a failure of the fans supplying ventilation to the engine rooms.

This short action therefore brought strenuous work to the ship's medical department. Apart from a number of wounded among the ship's company of the Cornwall, 21 British* and 57 German survivors were picked up of whom 14 were wounded. These British survivors included one Merchant Navy officer who had a penetrating wound of

---

* These British survivors were men from ships previously sunk by the raider.

the abdomen from which he died three days later. In addition, there were severe cases of heat stroke following the failure of the ventilation fans. These included an engineer officer who collapsed in the engine room. He was rescued and brought out by volunteers at a time when the temperature of the engine room had reached 200° F. By then the officer's own temperature was already 106·2° F. Despite the measures which were taken to resuscitate him, he died during the course of the following night, his last recorded temperature being 108° F. with a pulse rate of 140 and a respiration rate of 46.

CHAPTER 4
MEDICAL ASPECT OF THE CHIEF NAVAL EVENTS 1942-1943
Some Minor Naval Operations, 1942
NAVAL OPERATIONS OFF CEYLON,* APRIL 1942

FOLLOWING the disastrous Battle of the Java Sea, the surviving naval units in the Far East withdrew to Colombo or Australia and naval strategy was fraught with difficulties which were hard to surmount immediately. But by March 26, 1942, the Eastern Fleet was in process of gradually assembling and the British Commander-in-Chief had hoisted his Flag in H.M.S. *Warspite*. Within forty-eight hours reports were received that a Japanese carrier-borne force might be expected to attack Ceylon by air. On the evening of March 31, the Commander-in-Chief concentrated his Fleet in a position from which the enemy might be intercepted, and several sweeps were carried out by the British Force, but without encountering the enemy. At 2100 hours on April 2 therefore, course was shaped for Addu Atoll by the Third Battle Squadron and, during the forenoon, H.M.Ss. *Dorsetshire* and *Cornwall* were detached and ordered to proceed to Colombo. At the same time H.M.Ss. *Hermes* and *Vampire* were directed to proceed to Trincomalee where they were needed to take part in a special operation.

Soon after 1600 hours on April 4, a Catalina aircraft reported the approach towards Ceylon of a Japanese carrier-borne force. At this time the Eastern Fleet was some 600 miles away and short of water and fuel. Immediate steps were taken to disperse the merchant shipping in Colombo Harbour, and the same evening twenty-five merchantmen sailed to the westward accompanied by H.M.Ss. *Shoreham*, *Marguerite* and *Clive*.

This left in Colombo Harbour twenty-one merchant ships, the submarine depot ship *Lucia*, the armed merchant cruiser *Hector*, the destroyers *Tenedos* and *Decoy*, the submarine *Trusty* and H.M.Ss. *Dorsetshire* and *Cornwall* which had arrived at Colombo during the forenoon.† There was also present in Colombo Harbour a small number of Fleet Auxiliary vessels.

---

* Some account of the early naval operations associated with the outbreak of war with Japan have already been described in Chapters 2 and 3 of this Volume.
    See 'The Loss of H.M.S. *Exeter* and Subsequent Events', 'Escape from Singapore', 'The Fall of Hong Kong' and 'The Loss of H.M.Ss. *Prince of Wales* and *Repulse*'.

† H.M.Ss. *Tenedos*, *Decoy* and *Trusty* were unfit for sea owing to defects. H.M.S. *Hector* had only just undocked following refitting.

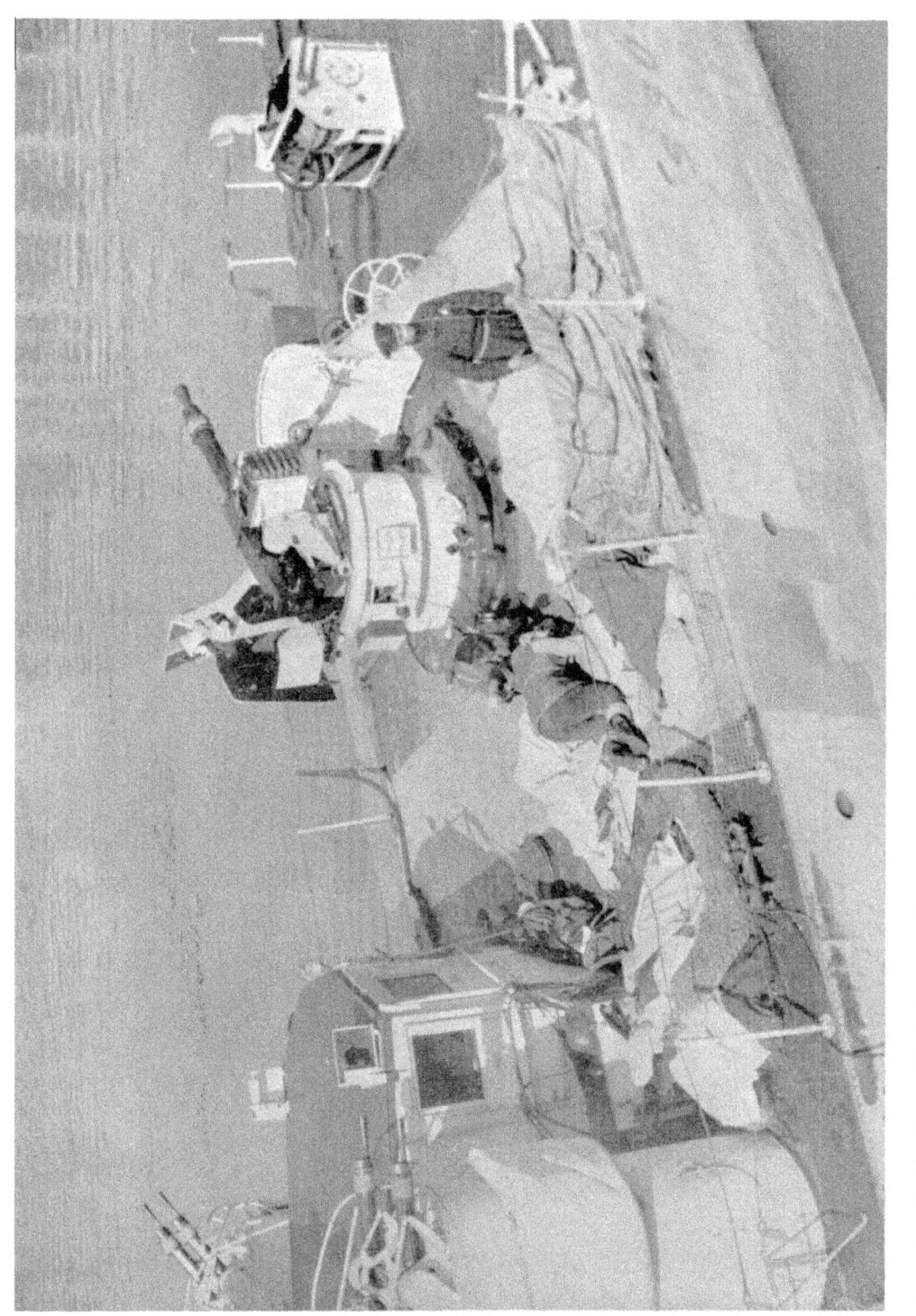

PLATE XIV. Boulogne–Le Touquet Area, June 3, 1942. Wounded Naval and Military personnel being removed from Naval Craft on return from the raid.

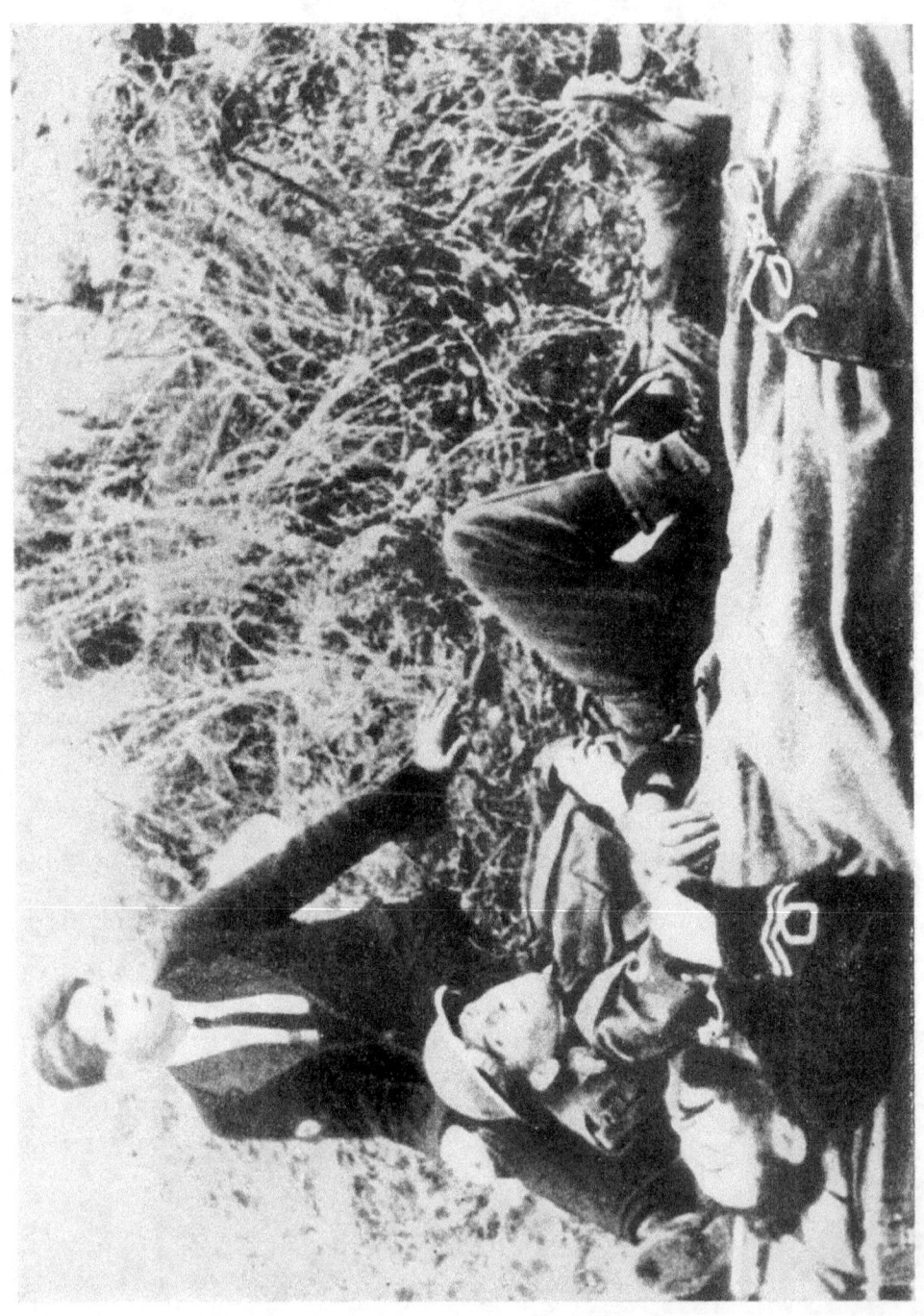

PLATE XV. Dieppe—A Sick Berth Attendant stays behind with two British wounded after the raid.

As a precautionary measure, albeit with tragic results, the *Dorsetshire* and *Cornwall* were ordered to leave Colombo, and they sailed for Addu Atoll at 2200 hours on April 4.

The expected Japanese air attack developed at 0800 hours on April 5. It was concentrated on the harbour area of Colombo and was carried out by some seventy Navy type dive-bombers which made both high- and low-level attacks on shipping. The attack lasted until 0930 hours.

The *Hector* was hit and set on fire by four bombs, and she sank at her mooring. Her casualties were 1 officer killed and 2 wounded, 2 British ratings killed and 8 wounded, and 11 Asiatic ratings killed and 3 wounded.

H.M.S. *Tenedos* was sunk by two direct hits aft, with the loss of 3 officers and 12 ratings.

H.M.S. *Lucia* was hit by one bomb and suffered 2 killed and 19 wounded.

The wounded from these ships were received at the R.N. Auxiliary Hospital, Colombo, where they made an uneventful recovery.

THE LOSS OF H.M.Ss. DORSETSHIRE AND CORNWALL

The *Dorsetshire* and *Cornwall* had left Colombo for Addu Atoll at 2200 hours on April 4. The following day was calm, with little or no cloud and the sun slightly obscured by haze. Single enemy aircraft were sighted at 1100 and 1300 hours. At 1340 hours three aircraft dived on the *Cornwall* and simultaneously three other aircraft attacked the *Dorsetshire* a mile away.

The *Dorsetshire* was immediately struck by three bombs which passed through the quarterdeck, disabled the steering gear and wrecked the port anti-aircraft armament. Attacks by other formations of aircraft followed immediately, and further hits were received which disabled other armament, damaged a boiler room and blew up a magazine. Within four minutes of the initial attack the ship listed to port and, within eight minutes, capsized and sank. Enemy aircraft then flew low over the water and machine-gunned groups of survivors.*

Meanwhile, H.M.S. *Cornwall* had fared no better, and after being repeatedly hit by bombs dropped by succeeding waves of enemy aircraft, she sank twelve minutes after the initial attack.

In H.M.S. *Cornwall* the medical staff were distributed as follows at the time of the attack:

The Senior Medical Officer had a 'roving commission'.
Main Dressing Station (sick bay), 1 surgeon lieutenant and 1 S.B.P.O.

---

* The *Dorsetshire's* Senior Medical Officer, a surgeon commander, R.N., was killed after abandoning ship.

After Dressing Station (wardroom bathroom flat), 1 surgeon lieutenant and 1 L.S.B.A.
No. 1 First-Aid Post (seamen's messdeck), 1 S.B.A.
No. 2 First-Aid Post (seamen's recreation space), 1 S.B.A.
No. 3 First-Aid Post (fore-cabin flat), 1 S.B.A.
In addition medical assistance was rendered by a surgeon lieutenant (D).

The sick bay received a direct hit early in the action and all its occupants were killed, including one medical officer. The three first-aid posts were badly damaged, and a sick berth rating killed in each case. The after dressing station was flooded, but the surgeon lieutenant and sick berth attendant managed to escape.

When the first bomb struck, the *Cornwall's* Senior Medical Officer was making his way from the sick bay to the after dressing station. He turned to go back to the sick bay, but was prevented from doing so by an explosion in the fore-cabin flat.

The ship had quickly taken a sharp list to port and this, together with the absence of light between decks and the violent concussion of rapidly consecutive explosions, made useful action almost impossible. However, a sick berth attendant returned to the flooded after dressing station against a stream of escaping men, and managed to retrieve a 2-oz. bottle of morphia, a hypodermic syringe and a small case of surgical instruments.

By now it was obvious that the *Cornwall* was sinking rapidly, and her captain gave the order to abandon ship. Nearby wounded were lowered into a whaler, the only boat which it was possible to launch, though five Carley floats were got into the sea. The ship then sank bows first, and as she sank one of her motor boats fortunately floated off and remained upright.

About two-thirds of the *Cornwall's* complement had been able to abandon ship, totalling over 500 officers and men. These survivors were scattered over an area of about one square mile and they included many injured. Morphia injections were given to those within swimming distance. Three of the ship's officers had been supplied with tubunic ampoules of omnopon. One of these officers survived, and his ampoules were made good use of.

Wreckage was gradually gathered together in the sea to make rafts, and the survivors formed themselves into about a dozen groups. The floating motor boat was reserved for those badly wounded, and bit by bit the floats and rafts were brought alongside it and the worst cases transferred. Those wounded who were able to sit or remain propped up were placed in the motor boat's engine room and after cabin. The remainder, most of them unconscious, were laid in the fore-peak and on the canopy. The number of persons in the motor boat was maintained at about 40 wounded, 3 medical staff, 3 men at the pump and 3 others baling. The boat's gunwale was within a few inches of the water, but, fortunately, the sea was calm and with care it was possible to keep the boat afloat and on an even keel.

Men with simple fractures were left on the Carley floats, and although lying in twelve inches of water they were surrounded and supported by uninjured men and were thus less liable to further injury than they would have been in the motor boat.

By the evening, the wounded had been catered for as far as possible and the various craft had been manœuvred into a 'snake', kept head to wind by the whaler, with the motor boat lying second.

The surviving Surgeon Lieutenant attended to the wounded in the after part of the motor boat, and the Senior Medical Officer and an L.S.B.A. attended to those in the fore part. This sick berth rating had done valuable work in hauling the wounded aboard, and his competence and cheerfulness were remarkable.* Two of the wounded had died during the afternoon and they were passed overboard. Three of those in the fore-peak were obviously dying, so they were hoisted out on to the boat's canopy, and three from the canopy were transferred to the shelter of the fore-peak.

During the night eight wounded died and were lowered over the side. Their clothing was retained to be used to make dressings and coverings for the others.

After sunrise on April 6, the heat began to be troublesome and the men in the water passed their clothing into the motor boat to be used as coverings for the wounded who were kept cool by repeatedly soaking the clothing in sea water. Those wounded who were able to do so were instructed to dip their burns and wounds into the sea at frequent intervals. Some of the serious cases of burns were lowered into the sea from time to time, and this gave them great relief.

Sharks were present in fair numbers. But, fortunately, the sea was clear, and the sharks could be easily spotted especially when preceded by pilot fish. Vigorous splashing in the water invariably made them turn away.

At 0800 hours the Senior Medical Officer made a 'round swimming tour' of the survivors. Many were suffering from blepharitis, due probably to a combination of blast, oily salt water and strong sunlight. A small quantity of clean cotton wool had been saved and this was used to wipe their eyes, and it gave an unexpected degree of relief. Attention was given to fractures, and a dislocated shoulder was reduced.

On the whole, those in the water and on the floats were much cooler and more comfortable than those in the motor boat. A large amount of wreckage had by now been collected and lashed together, and many men had slept 'strap hanging' on to these temporary rafts, supported in

---

* This sick berth rating was subsequently mentioned in dispatches for his devotion to duty on this occasion.

the water by their lifebelts. Suitable cases were selected to fill the vacancies in the motor boat, and these were brought alongside and hoisted aboard during the forenoon.

A ration of 3 drachms of water was issued to each survivor at 0900 hours, and at midday a further ration was issued to the wounded. The remainder were issued with a teaspoonful of corned beef. Many found that this made their mouths swell and it was difficult to swallow. But when rubbed on the lips, the fat greatly eased the dryness and cracking from which a large number were now suffering.

The Surgeon Lieutenant organised and supervised the issue of all rations in the motor boat. In addition, he had throughout been dealing, single handed, with the wounded in the after part of the boat. Many of these were in considerable pain and needed continual care. At about noon the Surgeon Lieutenant collapsed from exhaustion. He was made as comfortable as possible propped up against the legs of his patients. After half an hour he recovered and carried on with his work as before.*

At 1400 hours shouts were heard in the distance, and two men were seen swimming in the sea. The whaler was sent to pick them up, and it was revealed that they had swum from a point four miles away where there were thirty-three more *Cornwall* survivors on a home-made raft with the Surgeon Lieutenant (D) in charge.† There were wounded among these men who needed further attention, and the whaler set out to bring them in. In the meantime patients were transferred from the motor boat to the floats to make room for these new casualties. When the whaler returned, the six worst cases were taken into the motor boat, and the rest were distributed among the floats and rafts.

The whaler reported that there were more survivors who had been sighted even further afield, and she set out again to attend to them this time with the Surgeon Lieutenant aboard.

At 1500 hours a ration of peaches was issued, one-third of a peach to each man who could chew and the juice divided among the remainder.

At 1530 hours an aircraft was sighted, and as it came nearer it was seen to bear British markings. In the excitement of the next few minutes the motor boat almost capsized. Hopes of rescue now ran high, and a further ration of peaches was issued followed by a ration of water. However, the aircraft had made no signal, so it was thought unwise to issue more than a mere ration.

---

* This Surgeon Lieutenant, R.N.V.R., was made a Member of the Most Excellent Order of the British Empire for his devotion to duty on this occasion, his citation reading: 'When H.M.S. *Cornwall* was sunk by Japanese aircraft on April 5, 1942, this officer displayed wonderful endurance and devotion to duty. He worked on the wounded in the boats for thirty hours, and when picked up by H.M.S. *Enterprise* he continued to work on them for a further twenty-four hours. He went on working with undiminished zeal at Addu Atoll when the survivors were landed.'

† This dental officer was mentioned in dispatches for his courage and devotion to duty on this occasion.

At 1730 hours smoke was sighted on the horizon and once more the motor boat nearly capsized! Fruit was now issued as fast as the tins could be opened.

The smoke soon gave way to the outline of a British cruiser,* and as she approached she was signalled by semaphore that there were wounded in the motor boat and that Neil-Robertson stretchers would be needed for about twenty of them. Within a short time the survivors of H.M.S. *Cornwall* had been rescued and their long ordeal was at an end.†

In the case of H.M.S. *Dorsetshire*, only one medical officer survived‡ and records are less detailed. When the ship sank, it had not been possible to launch more than two whalers both of which were leaking, but a skiff floated off when the ship took her last plunge. In addition to these, a number of rafts, two Carley floats and one flotanet were released.

The surviving personnel soon collected together in the sea and those severely injured, which included the ship's commander, were placed either in the boats or on the rafts. Officers and men then collected odd pieces of wreckage and joined them up as rafts round the boats, so that soon more than 500 persons were gathered together in the water in one area under perfect discipline and control.

At about 1800 hours, two British aircraft circled the boats and passed them a message to hold on.

During the night ten men died from their wounds, and two more the following morning.

At 1830 hours the next evening the survivors were rescued by the destroyers *Paladin* and *Panther*.

As regards the rescue and subsequent treatment of the survivors from the *Cornwall* and *Dorsetshire* tribute has been paid to the seamanship displayed by H.M.Ss. *Enterprise*, *Paladin* and *Panther*, as within a matter of a little more than a few minutes these three ships picked up 1,120 exhausted men, many of whom were wounded, without the loss of a single life.

H.M.S. *Enterprise* had only one medical officer on board, a surgeon lieutenant.§ This meant that the bulk of the surgery carried out on casualties in this ship had to be performed by the Senior Medical Officer of H.M.S. *Cornwall* in spite of his exhaustion after his long

---

* H.M.S. *Enterprise*.

† The above account has been compiled from the official report of the Senior Medical Officer of H.M.S. *Cornwall* who was subsequently made an Officer of the Most Excellent Order of the British Empire for his endurance and devotion to duty on this occasion.

‡ This Medical Officer, a surgeon lieutenant, R.N.V.R., was made a Member of the Most Excellent Order of the British Empire for his devotion to duty on this occasion, the citation reading: 'This officer could only just swim, but while on a raft, he encouraged all around him. Later on he worked on the wounded in a whaler without rest for thirty hours.'

§ *Enterprise's* Senior Medical Officer was sick on shore.

period of ordeal. The medical arrangements made by the Surgeon Lieutenant of H.M.S. *Enterprise* for the reception and treatment of these survivors were of the highest order.

Similar tribute has been paid to the reception of casualties on board H.M.Ss. *Paladin* and *Panther*.

The disposal of casualties on reaching Addu Atoll presented something of a problem to the local Medical Authorities. On April 8 all the survivors from H.M.S. *Panther* were transferred as non-cot cases to H.M.S. *Royal Sovereign*, for onward passage to Mombasa. Serious cases were accommodated in H.M.S. *Haitan*, consisting of 6 officers and 49 ratings. One officer and 33 ratings were received in a tented hospital ashore supervised by the Indian Army Medical Corps. Three casualties had died on board the *Enterprise*, and 1 other was too ill to move for some days.

On April 11 160 survivors were embarked in H.M.Ss. *Guardian*, *Kirrimoor* and *Foxhound* and taken to Mombasa. During the journey a large number required treatment for minor wounds, burns, and the effects of oil fuel and exposure to the sun; 63 of these cases were eventually transferred to No. 6 African General Hospital for further treatment.

The situation at Addu Atoll was greatly eased by the arrival of the Hospital Ship *Vita* on April 16, and all the seriously wounded were placed on board her and taken to South Africa. They were eventually discharged, on May 2, to the Addington Hospital, Durban.

For the most part the experiences of the medical officers involved in the foregoing accounts serve merely to confirm lessons already learned though, since the actions took place in tropical waters, some interesting, if obvious, facts do emerge.

The higher temperature of the sea enhanced the chances of survival, the effects of exposure to the heat and tropical sun were less severe than might have been expected, the menace of sharks was easily countered, and the collection of survivors into groups undoubtedly boosted morale and reduced losses from exhaustion. The following report of the Senior Medical Officer of H.M.S. *Cornwall* is instructive:

'Certain steps taken before the action proved their value when the time came. About two months before, I had informed my captain that, in my opinion, ships' biscuits and corned beef were not suitable fare for survivors in the sea in the Tropics. Forthwith, tinned fruit was substituted for ships' biscuits.

'We had recently lashed provisions and water to all floats, enclosed in sail cloth. Previously it had been the custom to store these emergency rations in the quartermaster's lobby to be collected when required. It is certain that had this old plan been adhered to, no rations would have been saved when the ship sank as the quartermaster's lobby was very soon flooded.

'For some time it had been the practice at sea to wear shoes and socks, shorts and cap. Six weeks before our sinking a medical memorandum had been issued from the Admiralty advising men gradually to get used to staying in the sun without any head covering, it already having been proved that this was possible without untoward effects.* We had adopted the provisions of this memorandum in the *Cornwall*, and we had gone so far as to make special arrangements to enable engine room personnel to come up on deck and get their bodies used to the strong sun whenever possible. It was pointed out that this immunity to sunlight which would result might be a great asset to them in the unfortunate event of their being cast adrift in the Tropics. As events proved, these steps were amply justified, for during our ordeal there was not one single case of heatstroke or really severe sunburn.

'Six sealed packets had been prepared, each containing a 2-oz. bottle of morphia and a hypodermic syringe. Each medical officer had one, the chaplain had one, one was issued to the bridge and one to the hangar deck. But in the end only two of these bottles were saved, and this was not nearly enough to meet requirements.

'As regards the treatment of our cases of burns, saline or bicarbonate solution proved very satisfactory. No cleaning up of tissues was necessary before applying dressings, and the whole treatment was carried out by non-medical personnel.

'Incidentally I continued to débride wounds up to 72 hours. No undue reaction followed, and I think the safety period for débridement could be extended for naval cases as there is so much less risk of infection than in the case of casualties caused upon land.'

Some interesting views on the rescue of survivors and survival at sea were also recorded by the Medical Officer of H.M.S. *Paladin* who wrote:

'There was too little insight into the organisation necessary to cope with such numbers as were encountered; 500 men clambering or being hoisted into a small ship has to be seen to be appreciated. There were not sufficient disciplinary measures to keep the wounded from mixing with the non-wounded and disappearing to various parts of the ship. An organisation should exist in the rescue ship which would control this influx. Sentries should be posted to guard against ingress to the messdecks and the wounded should be separated from the non-wounded at once in order to stop the two groups becoming mixed.'†

---

* *See* Volume I, Chapter 12.

† Though naturally easier in the larger class of ship, few men-of-war who had had experience of picking up survivors were lacking in a very adequate organisation for their reception. It was the practice for every survivor to be seen by a medical officer immediately he arrived in the rescuing ship, whether wounded or not, and after obvious casualties had been left in the hands of the medical department those apparently not requiring medical attention were cleansed, fed, clothed, etc., by the non-medical part of the reception organisation. Nevertheless, such a reception organisation, no matter how efficiently planned, cannot always control human emotional factors which are bound to be present. This is something which is very understandable as a man taken from the sea is an object of pity, be he even an enemy, and there is an instinctive urge in the sailor who rescues him personally to take him away and nourish him, thus displaying that bond of friendship which exists between seafaring men of

THE LOSS OF H.M.Ss. HERMES, VAMPIRE AND HOLLYHOCK, AND THE R.F.A. ATHELSTONE

While the above incidents had been occurring there had been concurrent sea and air activities off the east coast of Ceylon.

Early on April 9, the naval port of Trincomalee suffered a heavy air raid by a carrier-borne force of aircraft. The first warning was received on April 8, when a Catalina aircraft sighted Japanese surface vessels some 550 miles away. Since there was little air cover in Trincomalee, the Commander-in-Chief ordered the harbour to be cleared. That night H.M.Ss. *Hermes* and *Vampire* in company, the minelayer *Teviot Bank*, the corvette *Hollyhock*, the S.S. *British Sergeant*, and the auxiliary vessels *Pearleaf* and *Athelstone* all sailed with orders to keep close inshore and to be at least forty miles from Trincomalee by daybreak on April 9.

At 0725 hours, on April 9, approximately ninety enemy aircraft attacked the harbour area of Trincomalee. Several dockyard buildings received direct hits, and H.M.S. *Erebus* was slightly damaged by a near miss which caused casualties. One rating was killed and seventeen severely wounded, five of whom died in the Military Hospital, Trincomalee, within the next few days.

At daybreak on April 9, H.M.Ss. *Hermes* and *Vampire* were sixty-five miles from Trincomalee and about five miles off shore. At 0900 hours they altered course to the northward with the object of returning to harbour by late afternoon. The weather was fine, the sea calm and visibility good.

A report sent out by a Japanese aircraft was intercepted by the wireless station in Colombo, and on interpretation this proved to be a sighting report of the *Hermes*. As a result the Commander-in-Chief ordered the *Hermes* to return to Trincomalee forthwith.

The *Hermes* and *Vampire* increased to full speed and by 1025 hours were level with the port of Batticaloa. Ten minutes later Japanese aircraft were sighted diving out of the sun from a height of 10,000 ft. The air attack was carried out skilfully and fearlessly and direct hits were scored almost at once. During the next ten minutes attacks developed from every angle and bombs fell almost continuously with devastating effects. The *Hermes* was quickly sunk and the enemy aircraft at once turned their attention to the *Vampire*. The latter ship received a rapid series of hits and broke in two, the foremost end sinking immediately. The after magazine exploded shortly afterwards and her

---

all nations. No reception organisation can be perfect in the surge of excitement and joy which arises when shipwrecked men are found and rescued, and mistakes can never be completely avoided. In my own ship, after 200-odd survivors had been rescued, I was quite certain that all the casualties were under my care. Nevertheless, it was some days later before I discovered a man on the messdecks with a badly fractured radius and ulna which we had overlooked and he had not bothered about!—Editor.

stern sank at 1105 hours. Two minutes later there was a heavy underwater explosion, possibly due to the detonation of the *Vampire's* depth charges.

When the air attack developed the medical personnel in H.M.S. *Hermes* were at their action stations.

The Junior Medical Officer was employed in a first-aid post on the ship's flight deck, where he was assisted by a sick berth attendant and the ship's Master-at-Arms. The first three bombs dropped were near misses on the port side amidships, but quickly afterwards there was a heavy explosion and a huge mass of metal was thrown across the flight deck and ended up outside the entrance to the first-aid post.*

The Medical Officer filled a syringe with morphia in preparation for casualties, and instructed the S.B.A. to do likewise. Almost at once, the first casualty appeared, a seaman with a lacerated wound of his foot. This man was given morphia and his wound was dressed to the accompaniment of a series of explosions in various parts of the ship. The Medical Officer removed the casualty from the first-aid post and at once saw that the port side of the flight deck was awash and that the ship was heeling over rapidly with large numbers of men already jumping into the sea. The Medical Officer inflated the patient's lifebelt as well as his own and they entered the sea together.

The Medical Officer himself was caught and carried under water by the ship's boom and the ropes hanging from it, but, fortunately, he was able to wriggle free and reach the surface. He found his patient still there and together they swam away from the ship. Bombs were still exploding in the water, and the Medical Officer has recorded that each explosion gave him the impression of a severe blow in the abdomen.

After the *Hermes* had sunk, bombs still continued to drop and one exploded about twenty-five yards from the Medical Officer. Aircraft now opened fire on survivors in the water and several were killed including a sick berth attendant.

The Medical Officer still had his patient with him but he eventually left him in the care of some survivors on a raft. He then swam to an officer who was suffering from severe burns and managed to bring him to the comparative safety of a float. He then swam to two other casualties both of whom were in obvious difficulties, one being a non-swimmer. One of these men was not being supported very adequately by his lifebelt, so the Medical Officer removed his own lifebelt and placed it around the casualty. He then conveyed these men to a float.

On this float the Medical Officer attended to several seriously wounded men, and he then swam to other floats and rafts and dealt with such casualties as he discovered. Some of the rafts had fresh water but others

---

* This mass of metal is believed to have been the platform of the lift by which aircraft were raised from the hangar below up to the flight deck.

had none. On each raft survivors were instructed to remove their overalls and to use them as shades to protect men suffering from burns against the rays of the sun. No sharks were seen.*

The sinkings of the *Hermes* and *Vampire* were witnessed by the Hospital Ship *Vita*, which rescued and treated the survivors.†

About one hour after the sinking of the *Hermes* and *Vampire*, H.M.S. *Hollyhock* and R.F.A. *Athelstone*, proceeding south in company, were attacked by nine Japanese aircraft. Five direct hits were scored on the *Athelstone* which sank almost immediately. The *Hollyhock* attempted to close the *Athelstone* in order to rescue survivors, but she herself was hit and sank in a matter of seconds. The *Hollyhock* carried no medical officer. She had 16 survivors rescued by one of the *Athelstone's* boats, but 2 officers and 46 ratings lost their lives.

NAVAL OPERATIONS AT THE CAPTURE OF DIEGO SUAREZ MAY 1942

By April 1942, the advance of the Japanese enemy towards the south and west had been sufficient to constitute a grave menace to Ceylon and India.‡ It must also be remembered that at this time the siege of Malta was still at its height and the Mediterranean virtually closed to the free passage of shipping. All troops and supplies for the Army in Egypt and North Africa had already had to be transported *via* the Cape. This route had now to be employed as part of the building up of the future offensive which was being planned, albeit in its infancy, against the Japanese in the East.

A fleet anchorage had already been established at Addu Atoll in the Maldive Islands, and the island of Diego Garcia in the Chagos Archipelago, the Seychelles and Mauritius became of strategical value. In particular, it was considered that Madagascar, with its excellent harbour facilities at Diego Suarez, should be protected against possible occupation by the Japanese, such protection being vital to the safety of shipping journeying by the Cape route.

This extension of the operations of the war to Madagascar brought another island with a picturesque past to the public notice. It is of some historical interest that on a previous occasion, in 1811, it had become necessary for a British Force to occupy a port in Madagascar in order to

---

* There were 3 medical officers in H.M.S. *Hermes*, a surgeon commander, R.N., and a surgeon lieutenant commander and surgeon lieutenant, R.N.V.R. Only the surgeon lieutenant, R.N.V.R., survived, from whose report the above details have been compiled. This medical officer was subsequently made an Officer of the Most Excellent Order of the British Empire for his outstanding conduct on this occasion, the citation reading: 'When H.M.S. *Hermes* was sunk by Japanese aircraft on April 9, 1942, the surgeon lieutenant treated and encouraged the wounded on rafts and in the water. His devotion to duty was the more commendable in that he is not a strong swimmer.'

† *See* Volume I, Chapter 8.

‡ *See* Volume I, Chapter 15.

put an end to the activities of French men-of-war and privateers which were operating from Tamatave.

The capture and occupation of the Naval and Air Bases at Diego Suarez was a combined operation which involved the Royal Navy, the Army and, later, the South African Air Force. The invasion force was trained in the United Kingdom and was assembled at Durban where final plans and preparations were made.

The ships engaged in the operation were divided into two main groups, a slow convoy carrying supplies (Force 'Y') and a fast convoy carrying personnel (Force 'X'). The slow convoy sailed from Durban on April 25, and the fast convoy followed three days later. After passage through the Mozambique Channel, the two forces combined on the afternoon of May 2, 1942. They were now joined by two destroyers from the Eastern Fleet, and the striking power of the Naval Air Arm already provided by H.M.S. *Illustrious* was augmented by the addition of H.M.S. *Indomitable*.

For the final approach towards Madagascar, the Allied ships were organised in four groups:

- Group 1: H.M.Ss. *Ramillies* (Flagship), *Indomitable, Illustrious, Hermione* and eight destroyers.
- Group 2: H.M.S. *Laforey* and six minesweepers.
- Group 3: H.M.Ss. *Devonshire, Winchester Castle* and *Royal Ulsterman* with one destroyer.
- Group 4: S.Ss. *Karanja, Sobieski* (Polish) and *Bachaquero*.
- Group 5: H.M.S. *Pakenham* with two corvettes, and transports, store ships and auxiliary vessels totalling ten in number.*

Zero hour was 0430 hours on May 5 so that the moon would silhouette the land to the assault forces approaching from the west. The navigational hazards of the final approach under cover of darkness were very considerable and H.M.S. *Devonshire* acted as a guide while destroyers buoyed the route and the minesweepers swept ahead.

Broadly speaking, the tasks of this combined force were:

(1) To disembark the assault forces at selected points of the coast, under cover of bombardment if necessary.
(2) To establish command of the area.
(3) To immobilise any French naval units.
(4) To meet possible interference by Japanese naval forces.†

Although there was some slight delay in minesweeping operations, the final assault was accomplished according to plan, and beaches were

---

* In addition to the above groups the Hospital Ship *Atlantis* was to be standing by during the operation.

† This commitment was made by the ships of Group 1, which took up a suitable covering position to the westward of Cape Amber.

successfully occupied by troops from the *Winchester Castle*, *Royal Ulsterman*, *Keren* and *Karanja*.

The duties of naval medical officers taking part in this operation were primarily the care of their own ships' companies with the exception of those who were serving in personnel ships in which case casualties had to be allowed for in returning assault craft.

In the troop carriers medical officers had been provided by both the Navy and the Army and, although during the voyage each had cared for the medical needs of his own Service personnel, a close liaison was established as regards the care of casualties for the forthcoming operation. Casualties ashore were to be the responsibility of the 154th Field Ambulance and the 5th Field Hospital, and the more serious cases were to be sent on board the Hospital Ship *Atlantis*.

During the journey from Durban the troopships completed their medical arrangements. In H.M.S. *Keren* these arrangements included the following details:

In the case of all naval personnel:

(1) The issue of one first field dressing to each officer and rating.
(2) A personal issue of two tubunic ampoules of omnopon to each officer.
(3) T.A.B. inoculations had been brought up-to-date.*
(4) The blood groups of all personnel were recorded, totalling approximately 95 per cent. of officers and ratings.

To Beach Party, Beach Signals personnel and Assault Craft crews:

(1) Lectures were given on first aid with special reference to the Tropics.
(2) Sufficient chloride of lime solution to chlorinate ten gallons of water was placed in each assault craft.
(3) Ten benzedrine tablets were issued to each officer.†
(4) Each officer and rating was supplied with a water sterilising outfit and a tin of anti-mosquito cream.

---

* The reader is referred to Chapter 12 of Volume I (Administration) of the Royal Naval Medical History and also to that part of Chapter 1 of the present volume which gives daily details from the official journals of a naval medical officer afloat.

It will be seen that reference is frequently made to T.A.B. inoculations which presented constant difficulties. There is no doubt that there were times when the inoculations of both ratings and officers were not up-to-date. Alternatively, absence or delay of medical records made it impossible for a ship's medical officer to ascertain the precise state of inoculation of his ship's company. Naturally his own inclination was that the personnel under his medical care should be in a proper state of inoculation, particularly in circumstances where men were likely to be sent ashore in areas where the enteric diseases were endemic. Nevertheless, the medical officer could do no more than advise his commanding officer at such a time, and the latter was frequently and understandably reluctant to run the risk of a proportion of his complement being incapacitated by the effects of inoculation at a time when action was imminent and they were required to be in a high state of operational efficiency.

In essence, a happy medium had to be found between what was desirable from the viewpoint of preventive medicine and the man's fitness to fight, and this was not always easy.—Editor.

† The reader is referred to Chapter 3 of this Volume under 'The Sinking of the Bismarck'.

(5) A prophylactic course of quinine was given to each officer and rating.*
(6) One first-aid tin was placed in each assault craft, with a more elaborate first-aid box to be shared between each two craft.
(7) Three first-aid boxes were supplied to each Beach Party.
(8) Two tubunic ampoules of omnopon were issued to each assault craft officer and four ampoules to each Beach Party.

As regards medical stores and equipment for this operation, the reports of medical officers are variable and the position would not seem to have been wholly satisfactory. For example, the Medical Officer of the *Keren* recorded that on leaving the United Kingdom his medical stores were well below requirements as those on order were never received. In his opinion this matter could have been serious had casualties been heavy and had it not been possible subsequently to obtain small quantities of stores at various ports of call.

On the other hand, the Medical Officer of the *Winchester Castle* has commented most favourably on the quantity and quality of stores with which he was supplied. In this respect he also emphasised the close degree of harmony and co-operation which existed between the Naval and Army Medical Services on board, the resources of each being pooled.

The landing in Madagascar began at 0215 hours on May 5, little opposition was encountered and there were few casualties. By 1100 hours the leading troops were four miles from Diego Suarez and by 1615 hours this town had been captured.

Naval medical records give little in the way of interest, Service casualties being negligible. The *Keren* received a small number of French Army wounded, and 12 survivors from a minesweeper which had struck a mine.

THE ATTACK ON ST. NAZAIRE
MARCH 1942

The epic story of the combined operation, the object of which was to destroy the main lock in the docks, is well known. The operation was carried out on March 28, 1942 by a force of motor launches and motor gunboats escorting the destroyer *Campbeltown* which acted successfully as a block ship. The force of small ships was itself escorted by the destroyers *Atherstone* and *Tynedale*.

As has been recorded in various publications elsewhere, this operation was completely successful and incidents occurred in which the greatest gallantry was displayed by all grades and qualities of the personnel involved. The Commanding Officer of the naval side of the operation later

---

* Mepacrine prophylaxis was not yet in vogue generally.

spoke highly of the courage and devotion to duty of the medical personnel, and further tribute was paid them by the Commanding Officer of H.M.S. *Campbeltown* and by the Military Commander, both of whom became prisoners-of-war.* But, unfortunately, the necessary security measures attached to this operation had to be so rigid that the Medical Department of the Admiralty itself had little knowledge of the medical organisation, which seems largely to have been built up from local resources. The result is that though the official St. Nazaire story is an accurate and comprehensive one, medical details are sadly lacking and such medical records as were set down after the operation are scanty and therefore of little use in this History.

For the purpose of this History, post-war research aimed at building up some picture of the actual pre-operational planning which it was assumed had been effected. This research was not fruitful, and perhaps the most revealing result of these investigations is given in the words of the Commanding Officer of the naval side of the operation:

> 'On the naval side each M.L. had its normal store, plus, I think, extra issues of morphia. We had agreed, I think, at our briefing meeting, that we would try to pick up casualties with the two Hunt Class destroyers, and in fact did so.... But, in general, I do not think I issued any orders regarding medical arrangements. It was always my intention to try to keep the written orders to a minimum.'†

The most valuable record is that of the Medical Officer of H.M.S. *Atherstone*,‡ which states that at the close of the St. Nazaire operation, at 0630 hours on March 28, 1942, casualties were taken on board the *Atherstone* from two of the surviving motor launches and motor gunboats. The casualties numbered 23, one of whom died within half an hour of being received following multiple gunshot wounds with a traumatic amputation of the right leg. Three of these casualties were officers and the remainder naval ratings and commandos. Seven of the naval ratings were from H.M.S. *Campbeltown*. The wounds treated were widespread and caused by shrapnel.

---

* Captain R. E. D. Ryder, V.C., R.N. (Retd.), M.P.; Captain S. H. Beattie, V.C., R.N.; Lieut. Colonel A. C. Newman, V.C.

† Extract from a personal letter to the Editor. *See* second footnote to The Raid on Dieppe, *post*.

‡ This medical officer, a surgeon lieutenant, R.N.V.R., was decorated with the Distinguished Service Cross for his gallantry and devotion to duty on this occasion. His citation read: 'As Medical Officer of H.M.S. *Atherstone*, while returning from the St. Nazaire operation, and while the ship was being heavily attacked by enemy aircraft, he was responsible for the handling and care of casualties received from small craft. Eight men were critical cases and he is considered to have been responsible for saving their lives by his skill in giving them blood transfusions under conditions of action and bad weather. He was personally engaged in this work of saving life for 22 hours continually, and his skill and devotion to duty are worthy of high praise.'

The sick berth attendant of the *Atherstone* was mentioned in dispatches for the part which he played on this occasion, and the record states: 'His intelligent anticipation of the requirements of the medical officer did much towards the excellent results achieved and the saving of the lives of those critically wounded.'

These cases were discharged to the Royal Naval Hospital, Plymouth, at 0200 hours on March 29.

THE RAID ON DIEPPE
AUGUST 1942

As in the case of the raid on St. Nazaire, the operation against Dieppe on August 19, 1942 has already been widely publicised. But here again, although the naval losses totalled 550,* the available official documents give little assistance in compiling any accurate record or in giving any conception of either the basic medical organisation for the operation or details of the medical incidents involved during its course.†

Nevertheless, study of the scanty records which are available does at least confirm that naval medical officers and sick berth staff carried out strenuous duties in this operation, and displayed the greatest gallantry.

---

* Naval casualties, including Royal Marines, amounted to:

	Officers	Other Ranks	Totals
Killed and died of wounds	11	64	75
Missing or prisoners-of-war	39	230	269
Wounded	31	175	206
			550

Material losses were one destroyer (H.M.S. *Berkeley*) and 33 assorted landing craft.

† There is no doubt that whenever small-scale combined operations were planned, the Department of the Medical Director-General of the Navy, more often than not, had no knowledge of them or of their suggested medical requirements until the last possible moment. This was partly due to reasons of rigid security and partly to the early 'teething troubles' attached to the gradual development of the combined operations organisation.

In addition, such requirements always meant sudden demands upon the Medical Director-General which he had to view against the background of constant insufficiency of medical officers and sick berth staff from which his wide commitments had to be fulfilled. (*See* Volume I, Chapter 2.)

Although, by May 1942, a senior medical officer had been appointed to the permanent staff of the Combined Operations Headquarters, the medical organisation which he planned, most efficiently, could never include the training of medical officers and nursing staff during periods of preparation. This was because the necessary personnel could not be spared from other essential Service medical commitments. The result was that when a combined operation was planned in advance, the intended disposition of medical officers and staff was forecast, but could not be put into actual practice until virtually the last moment. The Medical Director-General's Department would merely be informed that a specific number of medical officers and sick berth ratings was required to report to a particular place for special duty forthwith. For example, in the case of the Dieppe raid, sick berth staff were sent from the Royal Naval Hospital, Haslar, only a few hours before the operation commenced.

Naturally, this sporadic type of commitment militated against accurate medical records, and in any case the medical officers involved were frequently young, and lacking in that administrative training which would have prompted them to make adequate official reports of their experiences.

It was not, in fact, until the liberation of North Africa (Operation 'Torch') and the liberation of Normandy (Operation 'Overlord') that the Department of the Medical Director-General of the Navy was involved in the original medical planning from the beginning. But even so, circumstances still did not permit the necessary medical personnel to be drafted until a few days before the operations were due to begin.
—Editor.

The Staff Medical Officer of Combined Operations Headquarters organised the medical arrangements afloat with the greatest efficiency. During the operation he took passage in H.M.S. *Fernie* and was most energetic and untiring in his efforts to deal with the large number of casualties for whom arrangements had to be improvised owing to change of plan. Likewise, the Medical Officer of H.M.S. *Fernie* displayed great coolness and devotion to duty in dealing with the many wounded who came under his care, and his work was worthy of high praise.*

H.M.S. *Calpe* had 306 casualties on board, and many lives were saved through the cool efficiency and ceaseless energy of her Medical Officer and sick berth attendant.† At one time the sick berth attendant was blown across the ship by blast, but he contrived to carry on work without rest.

In H.M.S. *Garth* only 21 casualties were dealt with, all of them shrapnel wounds. There were no burns or fractures. In this ship it was found that the Army type of stretcher was much more convenient than the Naval Neil-Robertson pattern when it came to taking cases aboard from small craft.‡ Her Medical Officer also complained that the number of blood transfusion sets with which he had been supplied was inadequate.

H.M.S. *Albrighton* formed part of the escorting force to Dieppe. She remained from one to two miles off the coast from 0500 until 1400 hours, bombarding targets ashore. Eventually she withdrew successfully and arrived at Portsmouth at 0100 hours on August 20. She had on board 30 unwounded survivors who had been rescued from the sea, 68 casualties from shore parties and landing craft and 7 other casualties which occurred on board.

The casualties on board the *Albrighton* were as follows:

(1) A 4-in. shell exploded on the ship's side at deck level opposite one of the guns and burst into the forward messdeck. Three members of the gun's crew were wounded in the shoulder and legs, and one rating on the messdeck received a scalp wound.
(2) A projectile from an anti-tank rifle pierced some armour plating and caused a through-and-through wound of the thigh of a rating.

---

* The Staff Medical Officer was an acting surgeon commander, R.N.V.R. He had previously been mentioned in dispatches, and was decorated with the Distinguished Service Cross for gallantry on this occasion.
The Medical Officer of H.M.S. *Fernie*, a surgeon lieutenant, R.N.V.R., was mentioned in dispatches.

† The Medical Officer of H.M.S. *Calpe*, a surgeon lieutenant, R.N.V.R., was decorated with the Distinguished Service Cross for his gallantry on this occasion.
The ship's sick berth attendant was decorated with the Distinguished Service Medal.

‡ This somewhat surprising view of *Garth's* Medical Officer is probably associated with the fact that the freeboard of the *Garth* was about the same as that of most of the small craft which brought casualties alongside her. But this opinion could not be accepted as a general rule in the case of any other type of vessel, e.g. H.M.S. *Albrighton*.—Editor.

(3) A rifle bullet lodged in the hand of an officer on the bridge.
(4) A small bore shell entered the ship on the starboard side and passed out on the port side without exploding. But on its passage it amputated both legs of a Canadian soldier below the knees, and he died about three hours later.

Tank landing and other small craft began to arrive alongside the *Albrighton* with wounded and survivors by about 0530 hours, and continued to do so until the withdrawal was completed. Casualties had to be lifted about 4 ft. from the well of each craft on to its deck and another 4 ft. on to the deck of the destroyer. Fortunately the sea was completely calm, but even so Army pattern stretchers could not be used on account of the difference in height between the vessels.

All the wounded received were suffering from shock and many were wet, but their morale was high even during the heavy bombing attacks on the return journey. The majority were Canadian army casualties all suffering from gunshot wounds.

During the cross Channel journey the ship's medical officer was assisted by the Medical Officer of the South Saskatchewan Regiment and a medical officer and two sick berth attendants who had been transferred from H.M.S. *Fernie*.

All these casualties were transferred to the Royal Naval Hospital, Haslar, on arrival at Portsmouth.

An interesting feature of the Dieppe operation which has not appeared in official records is the severe and almost paralysing effects of shingle thrown about by exploding bombs and shells. There is reason to believe that a number of men who landed on the beaches might have been able to make an effort to withdraw had it not been for their severely contused state caused by repeated blows from flying shingle.*

(Plate XIV illustrates the removal of rescued wounded from naval craft after a raid. Plate XV shows a sick berth attendant staying behind with wounded after the raid on Dieppe.)

Convoys to North Russia
1942 – 1943

The first Arctic Convoy sailed in August 1941, and this began a regular service of military supplies to North Russia, delivery being made at either Archangel or Murmansk, depending on the time of year. Between mid-December and mid-July the long journey across the Barents Sea ended at the Kola Inlet, but in the summer months the recession of the ice edge allowed the merchant ships and their naval escorts to travel on over the White Sea to Archangel.

---

* Based on the opinion, given me after the war, by a senior naval officer who was himself so contused and taken prisoner-of-war at Dieppe.—Editor.

From the beginning of 1942 there was strong opposition to the passage of these convoys. A number of heavy enemy surface vessels was stationed in the Norwegian Fjords, and a formidable force of U-boats and aircraft, including long range torpedo bombers, was based in the north of Norway at Bardufoss and Banka.

The convoy escorts of the Royal Navy varied, depending on what could be spared from the diminished resources of the Fleet at the time. For some months however, there was an alarming slaughter of shipping and grave loss of life, as in the case of Convoy P.Q.17 in July 1942, when of the 35 ships which started out, only 11 survived.

The route taken by these convoys depended on the time of year and the position of the ice edge. In the summer it was possible to pass between Iceland and Greenland, past Jan Mayen Island, and then to the region of Bell Sound in Spitzbergen, 78° N; down the coast of Spitzbergen, north of Bear Island, straight across the Barents Sea almost to Nova Zemlya, and then down and back to Archangel. This was a long journey and a very slow one as the speed of the Arctic Convoys averaged little more than 6 or 7 knots.* Its value was that of avoiding detection and keeping out of range of aircraft for as long as possible, but this advantage was offset by the long Arctic day, which meant exposure to attack for as much as 22 out of every 24 hours.

In the winter the route lay well south of Bear Island and much nearer to sources of enemy attack. At the same time, the long Arctic night, rough weather and bitterest cold were themselves a protection against the enemy. On the other hand, the Aurora Borealis was at times recorded as 'an absolute pest which could render the ship's blackout a farce.' (*See* Map opposite.)

MEDICAL ORGANISATION AFLOAT

Naturally, the first question which comes to mind concerns the subject of preventive medicine, and asks what steps were able to be taken as regards habitability so as to make life reasonably tolerable under Arctic conditions afloat. Study of the available records suggests that in 1941, 1942 and even in 1943 very little could be achieved in this way.†

By 1941, men-of-war were suffering badly from those changes which always occur as a result of modern developments, that is to say the

---

* Comparison between the vicissitudes and dangers of Arctic Convoys and Malta Convoys was a constant topic of friendly argument in the Navy at this stage of the war. The convoys to Malta had the advantage of speed, short duration and warmth with a better chance of survival in the sea. The Arctic Convoys were slow, of long duration and attended by hazards of cold weather which gave little hope of survival following immersion for more than a few minutes. Nevertheless, although Arctic Convoys were exposed to attack, and even served as bait for German men-of-war, the convoys to Malta had to face the menace of packs of E-boats by night and the accurate dive-bombing attacks of Stuka aircraft by day.—Editor.

† *See* Volume I, Chapter 12.

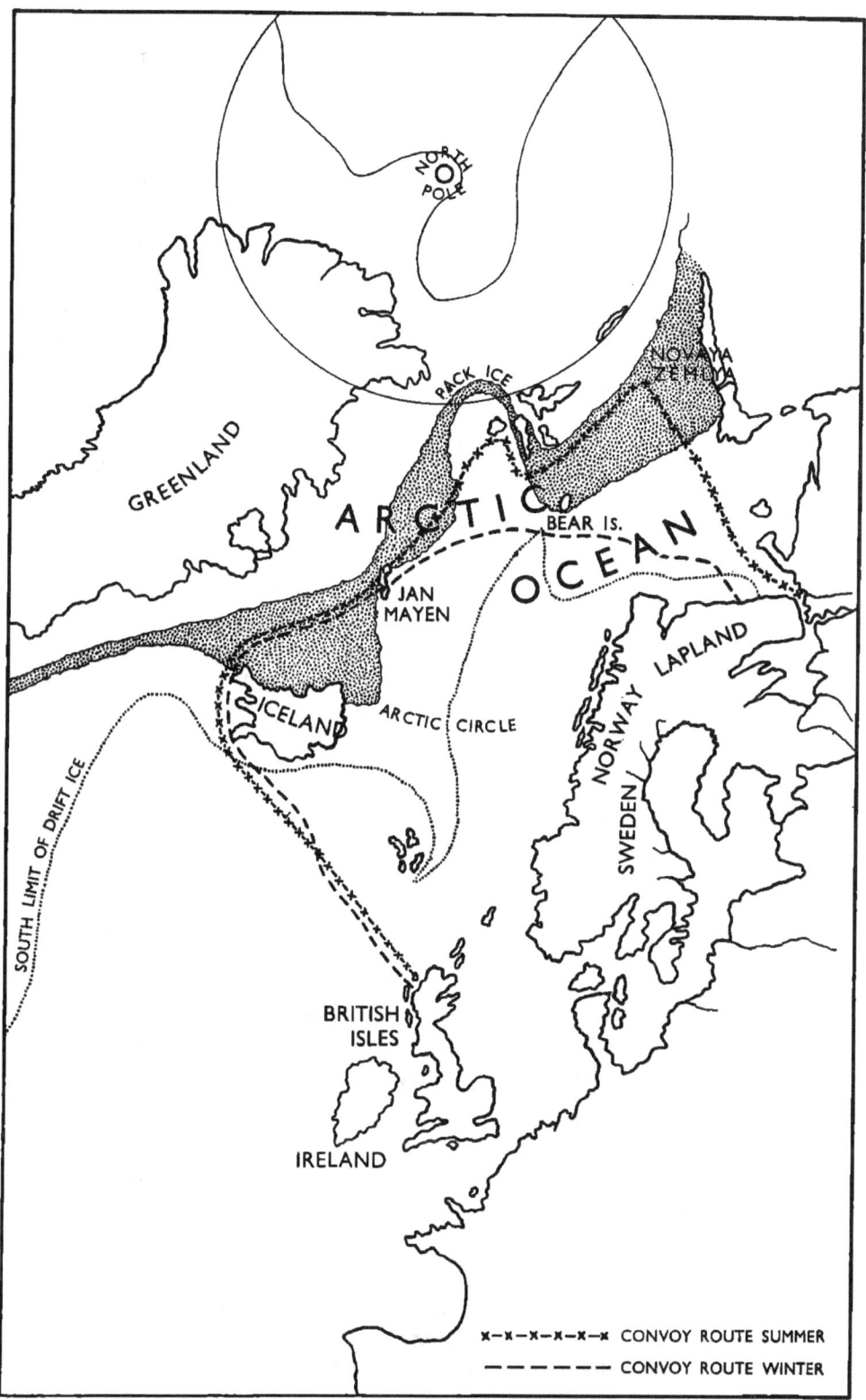

Map showing routes taken by convoys to North Russia.

introduction of modern technical machinery and equipment and extra men to work and maintain them. As has been explained earlier in this History, this entailed insidious encroachment on, and overcrowding of, living and working spaces which in any case were already very confined. Also, it had always to be borne in mind that the whole essence of the versatility of a man-of-war aims at suitability for active service in any part of the world, and in any extreme of climate at short notice.

One senior medical officer, describing his experiences of Arctic warfare afloat during 1942 and 1943 recorded:

'As far as my own ship was concerned, apart from switching off the overhead fans and, so to speak, keeping the doors and windows shut, there was no difference in the ship itself between operating inside the Arctic Circle and operating on the Equator. Such measures as were taken were aimed not at habitability, but at preventing the freezing up of gun mechanism, technical machinery, and the navigational instruments on which the ship's life depended. On one occasion we went from Algiers to Murmansk in three weeks, in the middle of January, which meant being transferred from a mean temperature of 70° F., to one varying between 18° and minus 30° F.'

Continuing his description, this medical officer states:

'There was usually a film of ice on the inside of the bulkheads of living spaces. You could get used to this, but one of the curses of the Arctic is the rapid variation in temperature due mainly to wind. There can be a rise or fall of 20° in as many minutes, particularly if the ship alters course or speed. This means that the film of ice may thaw, in which case you and your surroundings get saturated with water, after which everything freezes again. The same state of affairs prevailed even in the engine and boiler rooms, which presented a most attractive appearance with enormous icicles hanging down from the air supply trunks.

'So much for between decks. But these ships weren't just travelling quietly to Russia. In the bad convoys they were fighting their way there almost mile by mile. This meant a large number of the crew being at action stations, out in the open, for days on end. We soon found that the watchkeeping system had to be drastically modified, and that a four hour watch on deck had to be reduced to a half-hour watch, which was as much as most men could endure.'

(Plates XVI and XVII illustrate Arctic conditions on deck.)

At a later stage, steps were taken to introduce into men-of-war an elaborate heating system, a process which was known as 'arcticising'. Although greatly improved as the war progressed, to begin with these measures were largely emergency in nature and their efficacy was regarded with disappointment by some medical officers, whose outlook was expressed by one senior medical officer as follows:

'After some months we went to Newcastle and were "arcticised". This turned out to be a disappointing procedure which consisted of diverting the ship's steam supply through a vast number of new pipes which were installed throughout all living and working spaces, and at all kinds of places out in the open, both expected and unexpected. The consequence was that the temperature between decks was tropical, with water, ice-slush and steam everywhere. A man with a few minutes to spare for rest had to strip his clothes off in order to tolerate the heat, otherwise he got soaking with sweat, and started to freeze when he went outside again. Out-of-doors you were always liable to burn yourself on a hot pipe which you failed to recognise.'

Another medical officer recorded, with some indignation, that in his ship, steam pipes were installed behind the seats of the officers' W.Cs., the result being that performance of the intimate personal functions was always attended, particularly if the ship happened to be rolling, by the hazard of possibly 'seating the posterior on one of the things.'

As regards clothing in the Arctic, certainly to begin with, much depended upon local improvisation.* One senior medical officer recorded:

'Naturally our thoughts turned towards adequate clothing, and at that time our efforts depended much on individual enterprise.

'The ship's stores could supply long, thick underpants and thick vests, a limited number of pairs of sea boots for wear by upper deck personnel, and a small number of duffel coats which men coming off watch had to exchange with men going on watch.

'A certain number of officers provided themselves privately with "kapok" suits, but they were expensive and I myself could not afford one. I therefore, in company with most of my shipmates, had to depend on a vast quantity of "woollies". Some of these had labels attached on which were printed the words "Knitted by a grateful reader of the Daily Sketch", and very useful they were. We were thus clothed in a variety of garbs.'

Another medical officer humorously recorded that he was issued with a unique balaclava helmet which had obviously been knitted by a lady whose enthusiasm to help the war effort was greater than her skill with her needles. The garment had a large triangular aperture intended for the face, the apex of which was the point of the chin with the base extending between the nipples!

Naturally, later experimental trials and research went far towards solving the problem of scientific clothing afloat. But the difficulty of the research teams is well expressed in the journal of one medical officer where he states:

'Our problem in the Arctic was never the same as that of the explorer. Our problem was to find something which a man could wear in the open sitting still for long periods, not pulling a sledge or following a dog-team'.

Records show that during the early Arctic Convoys, the personnel of men-of-war soon trained themselves in the basic precautions

---

* *See* Volume I, Chapter 12.

necessary in the Arctic, mainly as the result of bitter experience. They learned not to touch metal with the bare hands or the lips with a tin mug for fear of freezing on to them. They acquired the habit of remaining constipated, and they went about making faces at each other, so as to feel whether or not they were getting frost-bitten on the cheeks, lips or nose.

Ship's companies in the Arctic were liberally dieted with ample supplies of fat pork and butter. Nevertheless, 'Action Messing' was a big feeding problem, when the men had to be fed at the guns during such lulls as did occur. The extinguishing of galley fires when action was imminent also meant that hot drinks had to be provided by steam heating.

Ships working on the Arctic route have described numerous physical ailments among personnel, but nothing, apart from frost-bite, which could be specifically attributed to the climate alone. The numerous ailments common among seamen were aggravated by the cold conditions. Pediculosis was prevalent in some ships and was undoubtedly related to wearing clothing for long periods. Foot trouble, such as mere sore feet, eczema and exacerbations of epidermophytosis, was aggravated by wearing sea boots and coarse sea boot stockings for many days, or even weeks on end without taking them off. In the same way, it was hard for both officers and men to keep themselves bodily clean. Naturally, chronic sufferers from sinus and antrum infections were worried, and a carious tooth was soon likely to make its presence known.

The senior medical officer of one cruiser recorded:

'During one winter convoy, we had an outbreak of what we called "Arctic Eye". Though it mainly affected men whose duties required them to spend long periods staring through binoculars and the eye-pieces of technical instruments, many others were also involved. The condition was not "snow-blindness", though it did seem to start suddenly out-of-doors. It took the form of an acute conjunctivitis and blepharitis which was most painful and incapacitating. Pus would soon freeze the lids together, or would pour on to the face and freeze there, and so a widespread and most resistant impetigo would start. But I think that this sort of thing was largely due to the fact of our lowered resistance to any kind of infection by this time.'

Many interesting views have been given by naval medical officers on the care of casualties and survivors on these Arctic Convoys. It is perhaps fair to summarise their opinions by a general statement that the climate tended merely to upset all previous experience of resuscitation and war surgery, and to aggravate the difficulties already formidable enough under the best possible conditions of action at sea.

Among other matters, the use of morphia came under review, and a senior medical officer recorded:

'In the Arctic I found that people seemed not only to die more quickly, but also to give up more quickly. This made me regard morphia with much respect, and to this day I feel, that under conditions of extreme cold, morphia should not be given indiscriminately to shocked casualties, particularly men who have been pulled out of the sea. Pain or distress must be the criterion. Where a man is quiet, I am convinced that to give him morphia is quite unnecessary and reduces his will to live. In a ship in action afloat, this is of some great importance, because it means that the man's will to save himself is also reduced should his ship be hit and start to sink.'*

While confirming the life-saving value of dried plasma, it was suggested by some ships that the solution took longer to run in the Arctic. It was also suggested that in a very cold climate the bottles tended to become brittle, and that near explosions of depth charges, bombs and the ship's own guns would cause them to burst, which was frightening to the patient and exasperating to the doctor. It is difficult to reconcile this view with the standard theories of manufacture, and it seems likely that the circumstances of action and general turmoil were more responsible for such breakages than the climate. On the other hand, there is no record of such breakages having occurred under action conditions in other climates.

One senior medical officer's official journal describes how, in the course of one Arctic Convoy, he and his junior did their best to deal surgically with all the commoner action catastrophes, including penetrating wounds of abdomen. But he is careful to emphasise the fact that they really did little good, and he denies that anyone's life was ever saved by surgery under Arctic conditions in his particular ship. He points out that the fingers of the surgeon would not work properly, that sterilisation and asepsis were unreliable, that things used to break, that the lights were always failing, that there was always the noise of explosions, and that he and his assistant used to be thrown about so much and tended so to slither about on their feet that most of their work they did kneeling down, on patients placed in a lower bunk. In his opinion a knee-high operating table, clamped to the deck, would have served a useful purpose.

Another medical officer recorded:

'After one experience of applying a tourniquet with numbed fingers, on a heaving deck covered with ice, I took pains to train my first-aid parties

---

* Acceptance of these views on morphia is reflected by Admiralty Fleet Order issued as recently as January 1951, in which it is laid down that:
 'The use of morphia is to be reserved entirely for the relief of pain and distress in the case of persons wounded or injured, including burning and scalding. It is on no account to be given to anyone suffering from pain not due to these causes. It should be avoided, if possible:
 (a) In cases of head injuries, unless the patient is violent.
 (b) *In very cold climates.*
It should be borne in mind that though wounds and injuries frequently cause shock, morphia should not be given where the shock exists without pain or unrest. A shocked patient may be abnormally quiet, and may not complain of pain, in which case morphia is not necessary, and may even do more harm than good.'

in tourniquet drill in the open and with bare hands, just in case. It takes some doing, even if you can get at the limb inside the layers of clothing which cover it.'

In general, battle casualties on Arctic Convoys showed the same types of wounds which had come to be expected afloat in any other theatre of war at sea. But that there does seem to have been a difference of mental trauma is illustrated in the following account of a senior medical officer after one of the worst Arctic Convoys of the war:

'In my opinion, the greatest danger of the Arctic in time of war afloat is the mental effect of the climate. I have no doubt at all, that fear against an Arctic background is a far more difficult thing to control than fear in other theatres of war.

'The average speed of our convoy was about 7 knots, and the round journey took about three weeks. The naval escort had to turn round at sea at the end of the outward voyage and bring back another slow homeward bound convoy. This meant a nasty battle for some days at least, going and coming.

'On the way out, U-boats were met off Jan Mayen Island, and from then on accompanied the convoy in packs. Shadowing aircraft now soon took a part, and remained in sight day after day, reporting the convoy's movements. The result was that by the time the convoy reached the seas north of Norway, the enemy was well prepared to receive it, and a four-day battle followed.

'Attacks by U-boats were synchronised with those of high level, low level and torpedo bombers, and with the launching of mines and circling torpedoes dead ahead of the convoy's course. The first wave of torpedo bombers to attack us consisted of 47 aircraft, which meant a lot of torpedoes to be avoided. I think we lost 8 ships in about twenty minutes. Some of these were carrying aviation spirit, and I watched one blow up close to us, which was a terrifying sight.

'The noise was dementing, and behind it all was the awe-inspiring beauty of the Arctic, with its cruel cold, its dreadful loneliness, and what seemed to be the utter hopelessness of survival if the worst should happen.

'My own mental attitude had always been different in the Mediterranean and the Tropics where I knew that the water was warm and that most of the surrounding lands would at least be populated, even if you were taken prisoner. But here in the Arctic there was just nothing.

'Our men seemed to get hyper-emotional and disorientated on this convoy, and I must admit that a lot of it is a mental blur to me. But one thing I do remember is that in the Arctic men seemed to be less philosophical than in warmer climates.

'As the days passed and we became more weary, my office became a sort of focal point for visitors whenever there was a lull in the action, and here I used to dispense teaspoonfuls of whiskey in hot tea to the most exhausted of my combatant colleagues. I found it common enough for a responsible officer or rating to sit alone with me and weep a little, and dry his eyes, and go back to his job.

'At one time, I can't remember on which day, I saw a seaman aiming at an aircraft, and he broke down and sobbed because his hands were too coldly clumsy to work his gun.

'After the first few days we had over 200 survivors on board from sunken merchantmen, and the worst of them in bunks and hammocks in the sick bay. During a subsequent attack, we were near missed several times, and the lights went out. One man's nerve went and he started screaming, and the rest joined in. One had a puppy which he had rescued and refused to be parted from, and that too gave tongue. I was strongly tempted to join the chorus myself!'

This latter incident has been even more vividly described by one of the survivors concerned, an American Merchant Navy seaman, who wrote:

'I thought surely we had been hit. Sound seemed to belch at us. The ship shuddered as though she would shake the steel plates off her frame. The walls round us swayed and the deck lifted under us, and then sickeningly dropped. We could feel it in our stomachs. Then the lights went out and we were in darkness except for a shaft of light through the open man-hole. The concussion echoed and echoed until my head felt like an iron bell that someone was beating with a hammer.

'The ship then recovered and came, more or less, on an even keel again, and now shaking with the steady recoil of her own armament. Then the guns directly over our heads exploded with a thunder which swallowed everything else. The ship lurched and through the man-hole we could feel the hot draught of their recoil. The air grew thick to breathe and we began to cough, and when the lights abruptly flashed on again we saw that the space was filled with dust and paint was stripping from the bulkheads, shaken loose by the ship's terrible shivering.

'I sat up, as I was damned if I was going to be killed lying down. I preferred to be sitting up. Some of the others had the same thought. My hands were clammy. I sat staring at the man-hole opening, and I was frightened and awed as I have never been before in my life. It was one thing to be on deck, and taking part in what was going on, but another thing to be below like rats in a trap.

'The infernal cacophony of exploding bombs went on, with the massive thunder of the ship's own guns beating through the other waves of sound again and again.

'One man began to pound on a table with his fist. A coloured man sat up cross-legged, swaying to and fro, holding his ears and rolling his eyes at the deck above. Under the impact of sound alone men seemed to go to pieces. Some tried to talk but could only stammer. One crawled under a table and curled up there. Even among the quieter, self-controlled men you could watch the tension increasing like a coiled spring. It showed in the nervous way they drew back their lips. It came into their eyes and into their drained, white faces.

'Hour after hour it continued, the beat and roar and thunder of the explosions, the warm breathing of the man-hole, the shuddering and swaying of the deck and bulkheads and the shouting and yelling of men.

'I don't know how long I could have taken it, when suddenly it ceased.

'The shock of sudden silence was almost as unnerving as the shock of the sound had been. We stared at each other with our mouths and eyes agape. Then gradually spread the noise, growing louder, of men talking, men delivering judgments, men arguing, men swearing and men laughing with relief.

'A voice on the loudspeaker announced:

"The enemy appears to have withdrawn. The Captain wants me to congratulate the crew and everyone else below. It has been a very difficult day, and everyone has conducted himself admirably".

'. . . I put my head on the pillow. I had no certain knowledge that we were anywhere near our destination. I had no idea how far the enemy would carry his attacks into the White Sea. I put out of my mind the necessity of running the same gauntlet from East to West on our return trip. I just warmed myself with the conviction that the worst was over. . . . I dropped off to sleep, and slept like a stone.'*

In a later assessment of the effects of Arctic warfare afloat, a medical officer considered that mental stress in the Arctic tended to bring about physical deterioration which eventually made it a major problem of energy to climb a ladder or even to brush the hair. His view is confirmed by the records which show that 9 officers were invalided from his ship at the end of one year in commission. The diagnosis was 'fatigue', with the statement that 'there was nothing wrong with the morale of these officers, all of whom had fought magnificently, and did so again'.

As regards these mental effects, the records suggest that they tended to be worse with repeated journeys, and one medical officer, writing his impressions during a winter convoy to Murmansk said:

'I am finding the apprehension much worse, even though things are quieter than on my other trips. But I have never felt so tired.'

Study of the copious records available in the Admiralty shows repeated reference to mental stress in the Arctic, and medical officers have frequently been frank enough to confess that they themselves were far from being unaffected.

One set of records, which is most enlightening, is concerned with communications which passed between a member of the Medical Director-General's staff and a medical officer of one of H.M. ships engaged on Arctic Convoy work. At the end of one convoy, the latter forwarded his official action report to the Admiralty. The staff officer acknowledged the report in what he himself later described as 'rather an officious letter, rebuking him for the brevity of his action report and suggesting that the Admiralty would welcome something more detailed with particular reference to research into a number of scientific matters for which great opportunity must have existed on his recent Arctic Convoy.'

---

* Extract from *Dynamite Cargo—Convoy to Russia*, by Fred Herman, published by Cassell & Co., Ltd., 1943.

Some weeks later the staff officer received a letter from the medical officer concerned. The staff officer, to his credit, has recorded that 'I found his reply rather shaming'.*

The letter concerned, which is considered worthy of a place in this History, reads as follows:

'... There is a lot of truth in what you say and I think that the questions you raise are of great importance. Naturally, during our last period up North there was a lot to be observed, and I suppose, looking back, I could have written a lot more. But let me just try to explain why I narrowed my report down to the bare facts. Here are the reasons, each or all of which had a bearing on its brevity:

'*A*. Owing to possible movements, Fleet policy, etc., our reports had to be forwarded quickly. At the time of writing there was very little time to do any very careful thinking.

'*B*. During the week or so following the kind of fun and games we had up North, even those who possess the highest form of morale confirmed the findings of those with lower morale, such as myself. That is, one is inclined to be irritable, disorientated, with a loss of sense of proportion to some extent, and more tired than I ever remember feeling before. There is a disinclination to revive incidents in one's own mind again owing to certain more horrific happenings which were a bit unpleasant and best forgotten. Also, I was very deaf for a time, not that that should have affected my report, but I was, and felt very "punch drunk."

'You will realise therefore that reports probably would be better written a month or so after the event, rather than a few days later. I mean to say that now I am absolutely fighting fit, and completely normal, and ready for the next convoy, which is more than I was when I wrote my report.

'All the above things are purely transitory, but are not conducive to clear thinking just for a week or so. In this relation it might be a good thing if the governing Admiralty Fleet Order on Action Reports demanded a preliminary report to be concerned with matter noted which warrants immediate attention. This could be followed by a later detailed report to be prepared after the unfortunate medical officer has had time to put his house in order, tot up his stores, finish writing his Quarterly Journal, do some 400 inoculations which have had to be put off for operational reasons, get some sleep, censor the biggest series of mails on record, and write to tell his wife he is safe!

'*C*. This is, I think, my most important reason, and one which I do hope you will understand. The writing of official reports after such an action coincided, quite naturally, with the usual "Bill of Recognition". In the case of my ship things were very much influenced by the sudden tremendous press publicity which we received.

---

* This same Staff Officer later himself performed gallant service on Arctic Convoys. He eventually lost his life in the sinking of H.M.S. *Charybdis*.

When this publicity broke out, my captain was very perturbed, and I think his attitude was good and sound as he is no self-advertiser. He was careful to broadcast to the ship's company that no more than a normal job of work had been done, no matter what had appeared in the press, and the less said about it the better. Then, when calling for action reports his orders were that they were to be brief, and he took pains to point out that names for recognition should not be included save in the case of outstanding zeal of such a degree as to be considered outside the limit of normal duty. In this respect his view, which I personally think is right, is that no person is entitled to recognition for doing his best in action, because to do your best is no more than you are expected to do.

'Naturally therefore, it became of supreme importance to those of us who had to write reports that we should be concise, and that our reports should be minimised as much as possible and should contain nothing in any way tending to savour of advertisement of either ourselves or our departments.

'However, looking back now, I am not so certain that I was really right to adopt this attitude of reticence to the extent which I did. What I am getting at is that my small sick berth staff on board were not much mentioned by report, and I feel that by being reticent I possibly have not done as much to publicise them as I should have done. The Sick Berth Branch got few of the plums of life and I might have pushed them into the limelight a bit after this convoy. This is a difficult thing to assess, of course. On the face of it they merely had a few casualties and survivors to look after, and miraculously the ship herself was not hit. But looking at it from another angle they had their work cut out. In the first place both my S.B.As. are martyrs to seasickness, which they just had to put up with. Regarding the operations we had to do on board, which are rare things at sea at the best of times, it was the first experience of any kind of surgical operative work at all for the two S.B.As. They would probably have felt green therefore in a peaceful hospital on shore. But on board here their greenness was much worse as it was also very noisy at the time! The S.B.P.O. once saw an operation performed while training at Haslar, but until this convoy, had never been invited to take part in one! By the way, there was enough movement of the ship to make it necessary to tie the chaps on to the table pretty firmly. Also any cutting had to be done between depth charges!

'I know that six serious cases, minus one who died after 48 hours, leaving five, does not sound much work for three staff under normal conditions. But these few, under the prevailing conditions, were more trouble than a whole wardful on shore. For the first six days there was always a flap of some kind going on in the vicinity. The noise of course was quite frightful, both friendly and unfriendly, and there was always somebody screaming his guts out, and once one started, the others got infected. You see, you can't fill chaps with morphia for ever.

'One of the curses of the Northern Convoy route is that, at the moment, there is nowhere to dump your casualties at the Russian end, so you have to bring them all the way home again. On the way back this last time, the weather conditions were the worst possible, and the nursing of strict bed cases was the very devil. Incidentally, there were no bedpans in my stores so I got the blacksmith to make one or two metal ones on board. These were absolutely grand, far better than those normally supplied, being large enough to receive the sailor's bottom in comfort!

'Therefore, what with looking after these casualties, which they did very well, and contriving to keep the place clean, and maintaining their action stations as well, my little staff got no rest at all and they did a fine job of work. I suppose one should say "in accordance with the highest standard of nursing tradition." From one point of view I suppose they just did their normal duty, but My God, they certainly did it.

'I hope that you chaps at headquarters are going into a lot of this Arctic stuff, i.e. clothing, etc. Also, I hope that the Supply Branch are looking into the messing situation during action. This latter obviously involves the question of complement, as with the chaps at action stations for many days on end, meals must be cooked and served hot somehow. In other words, if there is a brief lull, guns' crews, etc., get a chance for a short sleep. But the cooks, who have been on duty down in the magazines, etc., must now go and do some cooking. Likewise, supply ratings invariably have to start serving out bedding and clothing to the survivors we have picked up and who have to be cared for by somebody.

'Even nowadays the ships' complements seem still to be based on the assumption that being in action at sea means that smoke is seen on the horizon, after which the enemy goes "bang" and you go "bang", after which the incident is closed. But we find that the "bangs" go on for days on end, and lulls are few. In our case the cooking was done by a handful of chaps relieved from their action stations, who never could have got a rest of any kind, and who did absolute miracles.

'I hope I have made things clear, and I am sorry that my original report was not more detailed. I will try to do better next time. But, I repeat, I am still rather deaf, and I am not sure that I am even yet quite mentally re-adjusted since we got back safely.'

MEDICAL ORGANISATION ASHORE IN NORTH RUSSIA

It will be noted that the writer of this letter has stressed the nursing difficulties which arose due to the fact that casualties which were suffered on the outward journey had to be retained on board for the homeward journey. This was a state of affairs which became progressively worse during 1942, and eventually led to the opening, at the end of that year, of the Royal Naval Auxiliary Hospital, Vaenga, North Russia. Some account of this hospital has already been given in Chapter 15 of Volume I (Administration) of the Royal Naval Medical History.

Towards the end of 1941, a small Royal Naval base had been established at Kola Inlet by a party consisting of 12 officers and 38 ratings, who made the journey to Murmansk in two submarines. As part of this local British naval shore organisation, there were two sick bays each in the care of a sick berth attendant. At this time, when enemy attacks on the convoy route had not yet got into their stride, the reception of British patients into hospitals in Murmansk was described as adequate and the attitude of the local Medical Authorities as very helpful.

At Polyarnoe, the headquarters of the British Naval Base, the local hospital, though now serving the U.S.S.R. Northern Fleet, and though equipped with 350 beds, possessed accommodation of a somewhat simple nature. Though regarded by the Russians as a general hospital designed for all purposes, it appeared really to be more of a casualty clearing station and nothing more than might have been expected at a small and normally unfrequented port in this remote part of Lapland in time of peace. The absence of adequate sanitation and washing facilities, the lack of privacy, the overcrowding, and the absence of segregation of clean and septic cases caused a most unfavourable impression among naval patients who were admitted to this hospital.

These reports were confirmed by several naval medical officers who visited it, one of whom recorded:

'On entering the place, I was assailed with a strong smell which necessitated the smoking of a cigarette, and I was forced to put on a white gown which might well have been used for cleaning the windows. The sanitation was shocking with grossly inadequate lavatory accommodation.

'The operating theatre was 36 ft. $\times$ 15 ft., but it contained no sink and there were no facilities for scrubbing up.

'There were three surgeons operating at the time at three wooden operating tables. On the first of these a negro was having radiant heat treatment for frost-bitten feet. On the second a blood transfusion was being given to a Russian soldier who had a compound fracture of the thigh. On the third table a supra-pubic cystotomy was in progress.'

Another report reads:

'There is one surgical ward into which clean and dirty cases are received indiscriminately. It is very overcrowded and there is no ventilation as all the windows are permanently boarded up.

'The food supplied is quite unsuitable for British personnel who are seriously ill, the routine diet being:

7 a.m.	Tea, bread and butter.
12 a.m.	Rice or macaroni soup, fruit juice, bread and butter.
6 p.m.	Rice or macaroni soup, raw fish, bread and butter, coffee.
8 p.m.	Tea, bread and butter.'

Of the same hospital another report noted that:

'The hospital itself is far from clean, the wards are very large, accommodating between 50 and 60 beds which are crowded close together.

'A constant noise goes on from a radio, mostly broadcasting propaganda talks, while each day a talking war film, usually horrific in type, is exhibited in every ward.'

Nevertheless, a number of reports do record other matters of interest which were of credit to the local Russian medical administration. In particular, mention is made of the fact that at this time the Russians had their hands full in dealing with their own casualties. But, in spite of this, there were many occasions when British patients were given preferential treatment. For example, one naval medical officer who landed Russian and British casualties from his ship after a convoy battle wrote:

'The British naval survivors were admitted at once, and the largest ward was put at my disposal. The Russian survivors were laid on stretchers in the corridors outside.'

It has also been recorded that the Russian doctors were helpful and competent within the limits of their supplies, the latter always being short. It seems too that the Russian nursing staff, although badly trained and inexperienced, particularly in dealing with wounds, were at least willing and sympathetic.

Meanwhile, at this early stage, the British naval medical organisation ashore was not above reproach. There was a small Royal Naval sick bay at Polyarnoe but it lacked equipment and could only deal with minor cases. For medical stores it was, at this time, dependent on what it could obtain from visiting men-of-war. Its accommodation consisted of one large room containing twenty beds, and a smaller room for dispensing and for keeping stores. It was staffed by one naval medical officer and one sick berth attendant.

This small sick bay had to serve the needs of 25 naval officers and 78 naval ratings by mid 1942. These persons were scattered over a wide area locally, being based on Vaenga 9 miles away, Grayaznaya 13 miles, and Murmansk 23 miles distant. The mileage in each case is that of water transport. In addition provision had to be made for the needs of survivors landed locally after convoy battles. These numbered as many as 800 at one time, and they were accommodated in camps at Vaenga and Grayaznaya.

Up to mid 1942, the local accommodation of British survivors and casualties after the convoy battles had become progressively more difficult, and during the fourteen weeks prior to the end of July, 54 wounded had been landed at Kola from a cruiser, 35 from a destroyer, while other batches of survivors had numbered 47, 35 and 33, most of them belonging to the Merchant Navy.

As regards Vaenga and Grayaznaya, to which reference has already been made above, local hospital resources were essentially improvised and only intended as an overflow from those of Murmansk and Polyarnoe. At Vaenga the hospital was in the lower floor of a barracks, and at Grayaznaya a converted school was used. But in spite of their difficulties and limitations, both these hospitals contrived to care for

British cases, and both received wounded from H.M.S. *Gossamer* at the end of June 1942.

At Murmansk itself, some 30 miles up the Kola Inlet, a Royal Naval medical officer acted as base medical officer. The only hospital available for British wounded was a former school in which the Russians had accommodated 400 beds.

This hospital had the added disadvantage of unsuitable buildings superimposed upon the usual limitations of all the regular hospitals in the vicinity. Among these limitations were a lack of sulphonamides, a scarcity of plaster, narcotics and antiseptics and a complete absence of inhalation or intravenous anaesthetics. The only type of anaesthesia available was novocaine. Sanitary provision was inadequate and the hospital suffered badly from an absence of lifts.

Nevertheless, until it had to be evacuated on account of intensive bombing, this hospital did useful work, and many of its obvious disadvantages were overcome by international goodwill. When wounded from H.M. destroyers *Foresight* and *Forester* were admitted on May 3, 1942, everything possible was done for them. Also, permission was given for medical officers of these ships to visit the hospital and attend to their own cases, and to use their own medical supplies which they brought ashore with them.

Although the nursing sisters of this hospital were well trained, competent and hard working, there was a great scarcity of them and the nursing was chiefly done by women of little experience. Nearly every surgical case became septic. The Russian wards were desperately crowded, and every available passage, hall or corridor was filled with beds, or with cases still on stretchers waiting for a bed to become vacant. It was not uncommon to see two Russian casualties sharing a single bed between them. Bedpans were scarce, urine bottles were non-existent, their place being taken by tobacco tins.

The Medical Officer of H.M.S. *Forester*, who made these observations, had many more opportunities to become familar with Murmansk and with the difficulties under which this particular hospital was working. Therefore, for the purposes of this History, it is considered that his remarks carry more weight and authority than those adverse reports made by numerous other naval officers, both medical and executive, whose visits were briefer.

The Medical Officer of H.M.S. *Forester* recorded:

> 'On admission every patient was put through a regular routine. The wounded were collected in a casualty room on the ground floor, where their names and numbers were taken. Every patient, no matter from what he was suffering, was then stripped in preparation for a shower-bath which was given with the greatest energy and diligence by a nurse. The patients were then seen by two admitting medical officers, one of whom was a woman whose duty was to make a rapid preliminary examination and diagnosis,

and to divide the patients up into their various types and to distribute them to the various departments of the hospital. All cases of splinter wounds, fractures or suspected fractures had X-rays taken at once before being sent off to the operating theatres or fracture wards. The whole system seemed to work very smoothly and a large number of patients was got through in quite a short time.'

This Medical Officer remarked that local travelling in Murmansk was extremely difficult there being no buses and no dependable train service. Motor cars were all state owned and only available for official business of high priority. The Medical Officer found that the only modes of transport between Kola Inlet and the hospital in Murmansk were by steamer, walking or 'hitch-hiking'. By one of these methods he contrived to arrive at the hospital by 0900 hours daily, ending his journey with a 'seemingly endless walk uphill against biting wind and driving snow'. He then did a round of patients and decided which were in need of special attention. He then set to work on dressings which he continued doing each day until approximately 1800 hours. The only place where he could get food was the British Mission, which he had to reach on foot a mile and a quarter away.

This Medical Officer assessed the position at that time very fairly when he wrote:

'Everything in the hospital is less than twenty years old, but is as yet only partly completed. It is therefore impossible to form a true judgment on anything one sees. The future only can tell what will happen or how development will proceed.

'Everyone seems happy and very confident and hopeful as to the outcome of the war.

'There is a desperate shortage of instruments and anaesthetics and medical supplies. But in spite of this the Russians give us of their best, and our patients receive preferential treatment over their own wounded.'

This measured estimate is of particular value since it was written at a time when daily air raids on Murmansk were being intensified and conditions were such as to magnify any causes for criticism.

One of the great difficulties encountered in preparing this particular section of this History has been to give a fair and accurate report of the attitude of the Russian medical authorities in their hospitals at this time. This task has been far from easy, and the many official reports which have been studied in the Medical Department of the Admiralty, and which cover the particular period, have had to be sifted with very great care. For example, one naval medical officer recorded that:

'Conditions were appalling in the hospitals of Murmansk, and British naval patients were taken completely out of the control of their own medical officer. The food consisted entirely of black bread, which caused patients to develop a chronic diarrhoea.'

In point of fact investigation of this statement showed that the medical officer himself had never visited any of the hospitals, and that his report, though made in good faith, had been founded on what had been told him by other people with whom he had talked.

Apart from false impressions due to hearsay evidence, other factors tended to cause divergencies in the reports which were made. These factors included the frame of mind of the writer who had either been subjected to the ordeal of the northern convoy battle, or else had spent months of monotony and boredom in a community whose language and culture he was unable to share. Other variable factors which influenced the reports were the degree and effectiveness of enemy air attack which at one time almost paralysed the life of Murmansk. There were also periods of great activity on the North Russian front, when casualties would arrive in Murmansk faster than the hospitals could deal with them. It was during such a period as this that the Medical Officer of H.M.S. *Eclipse* landed British casualties from his own ship and transported them to one of the Murmansk hospitals. He wrote:

> 'The arrangements for the transport of my patients to hospital were excellent. Three ambulances arrived within ten minutes, and I was pleased to notice that there were two medical officers with them. I went to the hospital with my casualties, and during the short time at my disposal I found that the arrangements, in all respects, appeared very satisfactory indeed. There were numerous surgeons in attendance. I noticed that nobody was allowed inside a ward unless wearing a clean white gown.
>
> 'Unfortunately, owing to the movements of my ship, I was unable to stay and watch the surgeons operate on my cases. However, the naval base medical officer was in attendance.
>
> 'But I had one other opportunity to visit the hospital, and I found that the treatment given seemed good and that my patients were quite satisfied. My own sick berth attendant was a patient and, that day, had complained of a sore throat. Immediately the Russian throat specialist for the Northern Area had been sent for in consultation.
>
> 'My only complaints were that the beds seemed rather close together and the food was far below our standard. But I talked to some 60 survivors from British merchant ships who said that they were well looked after and were pleased with the attention which they had received. Their chief difficulty was lack of interpreters.'

In similar circumstances, after landing casualties, the Medical Officer of H.M.S. *Niger* recorded:

> 'I found the staffs of the hospitals at Polyarnoe and Murmansk most anxious to help and ready to go to extreme lengths to carry out any of my suggestions with regard to the treatment of British patients.'

In contrast to the many favourable reports made on Russian hospitals in the area around Kola Inlet, the corresponding reports of the medical and surgical facilities in the Archangel area seem to have been generally adverse.

Archangel was not regarded as an agreeable place in which to arrive after running the gauntlet of the Arctic Convoy route. To the all-pervading smell of sewage was added, in summer, the annoyance of mosquitoes and other biting insects, while bed-bugs were a perpetual source of complaint.

The countryside was uninteresting, consisting of pine forests as far as the horizon, and the custom of constructing houses, roads and wharves of unpainted wood made for a drab environment which the local dress of the people did nothing to relieve.

Transport from the various jetties where our ships lay was at all times difficult, and such medical organisation as did exist ashore was not always easy to discover, because so often all the available interpreters were engaged elsewhere.

In the early months of 1942, the position of a naval medical officer arriving at Archangel with wounded was not enviable. One medical officer recorded:

> 'There is a complete lack of organisation and even interest in medical affairs. No information is available regarding hospital or dental facilities. A Captain R.A.M.C. does his best to deal with naval cases, but there is no liaison with the Russians.'

A naval medical organisation ashore had in fact been improvised at this time, but from its very nature it was ineffectual, since it consisted of installing at the small local Royal Naval Base a medical officer from one of the ships due to return to the United Kingdom, or a surviving medical officer from some ship which had been lost, who was awaiting passage home in due course. These medical officers were never there long enough to get their bearings, and the constant change of doctor did little towards establishing a sound understanding with the local medical authorities. There was a great need for a permanent naval base medical officer, and also for a small sick quarters of some kind for the reception of British patients.

Archangel itself was ill-prepared for the strain which was to be placed upon its resources, and which would have proved exacting even to a highly organised community provided with modern amenities. These latter were completely absent, and one report reads:

> 'The sanitary conditions of this town are almost unbelievably bad, sewage lying in open cesspools. Few forms of water closet exist, and public lavatories consist of a small shed where the needs of humanity are simply relieved on the floor. It is the same even in some of the houses where a special room is set aside as a lavatory with no plumbing arrangements at all.'

Crude untreated sewage from the town was discharged into the river from which the water supply was drawn and, though naval medical officers gave instructions for the boiling of all drinking water used by sailors, this, when combined with the millions of flies, was probably the cause of a severe outbreak of enteritis which complicated the already difficult local medical problems.

The local Russian hospitals did their best for British sick, but their beds were crowded and they suffered from severe lack of supplies. Absence of anaesthetics and occasional lack of skill is regarded as having been responsible for much suffering among patients, especially where burns and fractures were combined.* Regarding the unsuccessful attempt of a Russian hospital to reduce the fracture of a naval rating also suffering from burns, a naval medical officer recorded:

> 'Throughout the entire operation the patient was conscious and suffered acutely. The next day he was extremely ill and the affected areas were obviously septic. Three times in the next fortnight his plaster was altered, and finally abandoned. His pulse was irregular and weak and his temperature soaring. By this time his condition was extremely grave, he was emaciated, unable to digest food and covered in bed sores.'

If the strain on local resources at Archangel was already great in the early months of 1942, the demands which arose in July of that year following the arrival of survivors from Convoy P.Q.17 were incalculably more exacting. Reference has already been made to the Russian aspects of the situation, but the local British medical organisation must now be considered in greater detail.

The medical facilities ashore at this time were the nucleus of what had originally been a British Army Field Ambulance Unit for 18 beds, but from which the major in charge and his nursing orderlies had since been withdrawn. This left the following:

> 1 Captain R.A.M.C.,
> 1 Sergeant Dispenser,
> 1 Corporal R.A.M.C.,
> 1 Lance-corporal,
> 2 Orderlies,
> 1 Cook R.A.M.C.,
> 1 Plumber/Carpenter.

A Sanitary Assistant and a Disinfector Operator were also available from the local detachment of the Royal Pioneer Corps.

This small number of army men, together with such naval medical officers and sick berth staff as might be available, was confronted with a task on the arrival of Convoy P.Q.17 which was so enormous as to become almost chaotic. The senior naval medical officer present, who had historical leanings, described the medical situation ashore as only comparable with that at Dover during the days of the Dunkirk

---

* The combination of fractures and severe burns was a common feature in casualties from the early Arctic Convoys.

evacuation. But he pointed out that, though at Dover there had existed all the resources of British hospitals and transport, at Archangel there were only the heavily strained local Russian medical facilities which could not meet a huge commitment. Every hospital, school and adaptable building was already occupied by Russian casualties who were being nursed under conditions which, this medical officer considered, resembled those at Scutari during the Crimean War.

The equipment of the army personnel consisted chiefly of consumable stores most of which at this time had already been used. The unit maintained and manned two medical inspection rooms at nearby ports, and it was responsible for the medical care of a total of 90 Royal Navy, Army and R.A.F. personnel scattered throughout the district.

It will be remembered that Convoy P.Q.17, in July 1942, had originally consisted of 35 ships, of which only 11 completed the voyage safely. Under the threat of attack by German surface vessels, this convoy had split up, and the surviving ships were stragglers which made their way to Archangel largely independently and unescorted.

During the first week in which these ships arrived, the total of survivors landed at Archangel reached 1,245, of whom 688 were British and Dutch, and 557 American. They included 179 cases of immersion foot.

These ships staggered into port at indefinite times, and could send no signals stating the number of cases to be catered for. Although many of the survivors landed were uninjured, about 90 per cent. of them developed complaints of some kind or other. For the hospital cases such arrangements as were possible were made by the Medical Officer of the Rescue Ship *Zaafaran*, himself a survivor, who was temporarily appointed Base Medical Officer, Archangel, on landing.

In preparation for the first batch of survivors, Sevroless Hospital had been made into a hostel with two wards left for the sick. This hospital offered little comfort. Not only was there the usual absence of adequate sanitary provision, but the presence of sick aggravated this lack of hygiene. Soap was very scarce, and the atmosphere soon became one in which were mingled the odours of cooking, smoke, gangrene and stale urine. Beds were small, with mattresses and linen of poor quality.

British survivors remained in this hospital for only two weeks. The fit were then accommodated in a large school building, and the sick were transferred to Military Hospital No. 2524. Sanitation in the school building was difficult owing to lack of water pressure, which prevented the flow of any water above the level of the ground floor.

As more survivors arrived, they were accommodated in the upper two floors of the Intourist Hotel which had previously been a Russian military hospital. Bedding in this building was provided by the Russian

Authorities. This batch of survivors arrived, exhausted, in the late evening. The following morning it was apparent that there was a gross infestation by bed-bugs, and every man had been severely bitten without exception. The rooms were cleared and the bedding condemned. The iron bedsteads were scrubbed and all possible crevices were stoved with burning newspaper.

As these and many other obstacles were overcome, it was possible for the base medical officer to organise a more regular routine and to hold definite hours for visiting buildings in which survivors were accommodated. These buildings included schools and General, Mental, Fever and Skin Hospitals. These centres of accommodation varied chiefly as regards the extent to which deficiencies were admitted and help offered. In course of time, as survivors accumulated, they became widely distributed. Meanwhile, further survivors landed at Murmansk were evacuated to Archangel as a result of the increasing enemy air attacks against the former port.

The problems of ministering to the medical needs of this widely dispersed community were aggravated by lack of transport. The base medical officer had to contrive to keep an accurate record of his elusive patients. He had to maintain liaison with many Russian medical staffs and to attempt to influence them when their treatment was not in accordance with accepted British practice or caused discontent among British patients. He had to hold consultations with other naval medical officers, and he had to arrange for his stores to be dispersed owing to enemy air raids. One of his most difficult tasks was that of assuming responsibility for the medical care of British ships at anchor in the harbour. Here the chief impediment was concerned with the rigid Russian civil and political administration locally. In one of his reports he has recorded:

'A visit to a ship meant arranging transport to her in a Russian launch. To do this through an interpreter, and to obtain the necessary permit to visit the ship usually occupied a whole forenoon. It was a complicated procedure, as every American and British merchant ship was guarded by a Russian sentry. Despite the fact that I was a British naval doctor I was unable to proceed on board any British ship without a special pass from the Customs Office, and my pass had to be renewed every day.'

In the midst of these activities an epidemic of enteritis broke out locally which was acute although its course was brief. The cases were shocked, collapsed and incontinent, and the position was aggravated by them being scattered in so many buildings in circumstances in which dieting, nursing and sanitation were almost impossible.

By now it was more than obvious that the medical situation ashore in Archangel merited an adequate British hospital unit locally, and representations to this effect were made to the Senior Base Naval Officer, Archangel.

Signals to this effect were made to the Admiralty in London and to the Ministry of War Transport, while at the same time a similar approach was made to the Russian Government through diplomatic channels in Moscow. But, in spite of these representations, by the time of the arrival of Convoy P.Q.18, in September 1942, following a severe period of action at sea, no further result had been achieved.

It had been known that Convoy P.Q.18 would be involved in heavy enemy opposition during its passage to Archangel in September 1942, and heavy casualties were anticipated. With this contingency in view, a medical officer and 8 sick berth ratings, with stores and equipment, were sent to Archangel during August in H.M.Ss. *Blankney* and *Middleton*. On August 29, these personnel and stores were still embarked at Archangel and had not been permitted to land. On September 12,* the British Ambassador in Moscow was refused permission, by the Russian Government, for the disembarkation of this hospital unit. On September 14, permission was given for the stores and equipment to be landed, but the personnel had to be transferred to H.M.S. *Palomares*, on September 14, and returned to the United Kingdom. Fortunately the medical officers of the naval escort of P.Q.18 were able to arrange for survivors and casualties to be cared for afloat, and to be nursed somehow until arriving back at Scapa Flow.

Thus the year 1942 closed at Archangel without any change in the position which had provoked such criticism among wounded and survivors from the Arctic Convoys.

At this point, it is of some interest to view the medical organisation and facilities at Murmansk and Archangel through the eyes of the Admiralty in London. By July 1942 the British Naval Authorities ashore in North Russia had become firmly aware of the need for some form of established British Service Hospital for the reception and treatment of casualties and survivors from the convoys. Their complaints of what appeared to them to be Admiralty procrastination are more than reflected in their numerous official reports. But these local authorities in North Russia were not aware of the many conflicting reports which the Admiralty had received up to this time, and which, combined with the repeated difficulties at diplomatic level which accrued during the remainder of the year, build up an administrative chain of events which is somewhat bewildering to follow in sequence.

To begin with, during the winter of 1941-2, in response to urgent appeals, the Admiralty had already sent two medical officers for duty ashore in North Russia. These medical officers had promptly been returned to the United Kingdom on the grounds that there was insufficient work ashore to occupy them.

---

* On September 12, the P.Q.18 convoy battle was approaching its height, and casualties were already known to be severe.

In February 1942, the Admiralty had been officially informed that the combined medical work at Archangel was insufficient to occupy the time of more than one naval medical officer ashore. This report also commented favourably upon local hospital accommodation and treatment.

In May 1942, the Senior Naval Officer, North Russia, requested either a hospital unit ashore or a hospital ship, but failed to indicate where he required either to be. In response to this request, the Admiralty immediately arranged to dispatch 4 medical officers and 31 sick berth staff as a hospital unit, and at the same time asked whether this unit was required for duty at Kola Inlet or at Archangel. On June 7, the Senior Naval Officer, North Russia, indicated the need for the unit at Archangel, but on June 11 he signalled to Admiralty that the personnel for the unit were not necessary, and that local Russian hospital resources were adequate for British requirements, provided instruments and medicines could be supplemented.

Meanwhile, the position ashore at Kola Inlet remained vague so, on June 15, the Admiralty asked whether a hospital unit was required at Murmansk. In his reply, on June 16, the Senior Naval Officer, North Russia, stated that this was not the case but that he wanted one at Archangel. A further signal from Archangel, on June 19, requested a medical officer ashore, but no medical stores or equipment!

In view of this confusing series of communications, the Admiralty in London can hardly be blamed for abandoning its plans and preparations to send the personnel and stores for a hospital unit in North Russia at this particular time.

The whole project seems now to have remained in abeyance until July 30, on which date the Commander-in-Chief of the Home Fleet expressed his great concern on the reports of the wounded reaching him from Russia. The Admiralty shared his anxiety, and simultaneously the Senior Naval Officer, North Russia, asked for a hospital unit to be sent to Polyarnoe, in a signal dated August 1.

On August 17, the medical stores and equipment, so long assembled and so much needed, and the equally long anticipated medical staff were embarked in the U.S. cruiser *Tuscaloosa*; 4 medical officers, a dental officer and a warrant wardmaster took passage, and some 30 sick berth ratings were provided, in miscellaneous ships, for duty in North Russia by the end of this month. It was now the intention that this medical party should establish a Royal Naval Auxiliary Hospital at Vaenga Bay, an anchorage on the east of the Kola Inlet which was much used by H.M. ships.

The unit arrived at Kola Inlet on August 23, 1942. But immediately the divergent needs and alternating periods of activity between the Murmansk and Archangel administrations were revealed.

The Senior Naval Officer, North Russia, decided to send two-thirds of the unit to Archangel at once, keeping the remainder for duty at

THE CHIEF NAVAL EVENTS, 1942-1943

Vaenga. The two-thirds of the unit arrived at Archangel but was never permitted to land, the result being that the unit returned to England forthwith, thus depleting the needs of Murmansk without any benefit to Archangel.

Meanwhile, the residual one-third of the unit which had remained behind at Kola Inlet, continued its preparations to set up a naval auxiliary hospital at Vaenga Bay. But on September 21, the Commander-in-Chief of the Soviet Northern Fleet received orders from Moscow that the arrangements for this hospital were suspended and that the unit was to be returned to England in Convoy Q.P.15. Steps were taken to implement these instructions to withdraw, but on September 25, negotiations for the retention of this hospital were reopened at diplomatic level. These negotiations continued until October 2, when the Russian Government gave permission for 'a certain number of British medical collaborators' to work in Soviet hospitals, but refused permission for a separate British Service medical establishment to be set up on shore.

The Admiralty now decided to provision, staff and equip one of the Arctic Convoy rescue ships as a small hospital ship, for permanent service as base hospital at Kola Inlet. But barely had this project been raised when, on October 5, the Russian Government approved the establishment of a Royal Naval Auxiliary Hospital ashore at Vaenga Bay.

An account of this hospital, which was completed by the end of 1942, has already been given in Chapter 15 of the Administration Volume of the Official Naval Medical History of the War. There were hopes of a similar hospital at Archangel, the need for such an establishment being beyond dispute. However, protracted negotiations met with no success in the case of this port.

ARCTIC CONVOY BATTLES

The convoys to North Russia were given the distinguishing letters P.Q., while those returning to the United Kingdom were known as Q.P. Convoys. The following table shows the chief events when casualties occurred, or which had some other medical significance.

Of the earliest loss shown in this table, that of H.M.S. *Matabele*, few medical details are available. Three seamen were recovered by H.M.S. *Harrier* after half an hour in the water. The survival of two of these men was attributed to the fact that they were wearing clothes and were saturated with oil fuel.

At first the size of these convoys was small, varying from 9 to 12 ships only. But by the spring the number had increased as had the amount of supplies carried to Russia. Naval escorts had to be increased proportionately and at the same time the enemy developed his provision for interfering with the safe progress of these convoys.

Date	Convoy	Incident
1942:		
January 17	P.Q.8	H.M.S. *Matabele* lost
March 28	P.Q.13	Attacks by enemy aircraft
March 29	P.Q.13	H.M.S. *Trinidad* torpedoed
April 11	Q.P.10	Attacks by enemy aircraft
April 12	P.Q.14	Scattered and damaged by ice
April 13	P.Q.14	Attacks by U-boats
April 30	Q.P.11	H.M.S. *Edinburgh* torpedoed
May 1	Q.P.11	Attacks by enemy destroyers
May 2	P.Q.15	Attacks by enemy aircraft
May 2	Q.P.11	H.M.S. *Edinburgh* sunk
May 14	Q.P.11	H.M.S. *Trinidad* damaged by enemy aircraft
May 15	Q.P.11	H.M.S. *Trinidad* sunk
May 25	P.Q.16	Attacks by enemy aircraft and U-boats
May 30	P.Q.16	27 out of 35 ships reached Murmansk during heavy enemy air attacks
July 4	P.Q.17	Attacks by enemy aircraft and U-boats, 22 ships sunk. Threat of surface action by *Tirpitz* and *Hipper*
August 5	Q.P.13	5 ships and H.M.S. *Niger* lost in minefield during fog
September 13	P.Q.18	12 ships sunk
September 19	P.Q.18	27 ships out of 40 reach Archangel
September 20	Q.P.14	H.M.S. *Leda* torpedoed and sunk
September 24	Q.P.14	H.M.S. *Somali* torpedoed and sunk

N.B.—H.M.S. *Achates* was sunk on the last day of 1942, in Convoy J.W.51B, the distinguishing letters having been changed for the 1943 convoys.

On March 29, H.M.S. *Eclipse* was in action with German surface craft and sustained 10 casualties by shellfire. The foot of one casualty was amputated on board, and another died of a rapid pneumonia following the inhalation of fumes from burning cordite. These casualties were landed at Murmansk.

On the same date Convoy P.Q.13 was intercepted by German destroyers, and H.M.S. *Trinidad* was damaged by a torpedo. She suffered 6 officers and 25 ratings killed, and 10 other casualties due to flash burns, shock and bruising. These casualties were treated and retained on board. The fatalities were due to multiple injuries from the explosion of the torpedo combined with drowning from being trapped in flooded compartments.

The conditions in the ship's sick bay after damage, and with inadequate heating and water supply, were very bad.

H.M.S. *Trinidad* received temporary repairs at Murmansk and then attempted to return to England in Q.P.11. She met with prolonged enemy air attacks for 48 hours, and then received direct hits by bombs on May 14. In addition to her own complement, she had on board survivors from H.M.S. *Edinburgh*, a wounded British officer from the Polish submarine P.551, and survivors from the S.S. *Botavon*. Her Senior Medical Officer recorded:

'After we were hit by bombs there was no further attack that day. As the sick bay was out of action and the medical officer there wounded, all casualties were taken aft to my first-aid post. There were 50 men killed outright and 25 other casualties. To these it was only possible to give first-aid treatment and morphia and nothing more elaborate was attempted. When the ship had to be abandoned, the captain ordered all wounded first to be transferred to one of the destroyers, and I myself transferred to the same destroyer before the ship sank the following day.'

These casualties were dealt with most efficiently in H.M.S. *Forester* and were eventually disembarked safely at Scapa Flow and transferred to hospital ships. This medical achievement of H.M.S. *Forester* is notable in that she had herself been heavily in action on May 2, when she had sustained 25 casualties, including her sick berth attendant,* of which 13 had been killed. In the interval she had evacuated her own wounded at Murmansk, but had there shipped 5 wounded seamen for passage to the United Kingdom. She eventually had 41 seriously wounded men on board all of whom she carried back to Iceland, where 11 were landed, and the remainder to Scapa Flow.

As in the case of H.M.S. *Trinidad*, H.M.S. *Edinburgh* was also damaged in two different engagements before she was finally sunk. While escorting Convoy Q.P.11, she was torpedoed at 1613 hours on April 30, 1942. This incident occurred a few miles outside Kola Inlet. Enemy attacks were now concentrated against this ship, until she was again hit at 0652 hours on May 2 and had to be abandoned. Medically, her position was complicated by the presence of a number of gravely incapacitated patients who had been embarked for passage to the United Kingdom. A further handicap was the loss of her main medical store during the first attack. The Senior Medical Officer of H.M.S. *Edinburgh* recorded:

'On April 26, 1942 H.M.S. *Edinburgh* embarked 28 British patients from the Russian Naval Hospital, Murmansk; 24 were cot cases and 4 non-cot. Of the 24 cot cases, 4 were fractures and the remainder were cases of gangrenous frost-bite of varying severity. Of the 4 non-cot patients, 3 were cases of mild frost-bite and the other was suffering from cholecystitis. In the sick bay there were already 4 other sick of our own.

'The accommodation of the sick bay was fully occupied by the worst of these cases, while the remainder were slung in stretchers in the ship's recreation spaces.

'All the frost-bite cases required immediate dressing, and further daily dressings and treatment. One case with frost-bite of both feet and hands was given one pint of fresh blood transfusion, after which amputation was

---

* The Medical Officer of H.M.S. *Forester*, a surgeon lieutenant, R.N.V.R., was mentioned in dispatches for his devotion to duty on this occasion. The ship's sick berth attendant was decorated with the Distinguished Service Medal, the citation reading:
'This rating, although wounded, continued throughout the action and the remainder of the day to assist his medical officer to his utmost.'

performed through the lower third of the right leg. It would have been necessary to perform further amputations in the course of the next few days.

'On April 30, the ship received two hits with torpedoes. The forward hit was below the after end of the sick bay which had to be evacuated in order to permit the shoring up of adjacent compartments. The second torpedo struck the starboard side of the steering compartment and did not affect any medical aid station or equipment. The damage done by the forward torpedo rendered two of the first-aid stations unusable, and destroyed the medical stores distributed there. Therefore two fresh stations were established in the port hangar and the upper cabin flat.

'The injuries caused by the forward torpedo were chiefly in the nature of multiple lacerations and fractures. All were suffering from shock and oil immersion. One officer was injured by the after torpedo.

'Initial treatment was given to 50 cases in the eight hours immediately following the disaster, and 27 of these men were able to carry on working.

'During the next 24 hours further treatment was carried out, but began to be embarrassed by the low temperature which at this time was some 20° below freezing point.

'Attempts were made to transfer a number of the sick and wounded to a minesweeper, but the sea was too rough to permit this to be carried out safely.

'The ship was again torpedoed 38 hours after the initial attack, and at once listed 12° to port. This list gradually increased to 17°. Fortunately this second attack resulted in only a few additional minor casualties. All the casualties and sick were now safely transferred to two minesweepers, in spite of the decks being covered with oil and ice. These cases were eventually landed at Murmansk.'*

The minesweepers which gave this assistance were H.M.Ss. *Harrier* and *Gossamer*,† and between them they took on board some 800 survivors.

Altogether 2 officers and 55 men were killed in the *Edinburgh*, and a further 23 were badly wounded. This casualty list was typical of torpedo attacks, a number of men being killed outright and a relatively small number being wounded.

On May 1, 1942, H.M.S. *Amazon* suffered casualties by enemy shellfire on the Arctic Convoy route. In all there were 19 cases of shell

---

* The Senior Medical Officer of H.M.S. *Edinburgh* was mentioned in dispatches for his devotion to duty on this occasion.

† These two ships performed most valuable services on the Arctic Convoy route during 1942.
The Medical Officer of H.M.S. *Harrier*, a surgeon lieutenant, R.N.V.R., was decorated with the Distinguished Service Cross, and his sick berth attendant with the Distinguished Service Medal.
A later Medical Officer of H.M.S. *Harrier* was awarded the Order of the Red Star by the Soviet Authorities.
H.M.S. *Gossamer* was herself sunk in July 1942. Her sick berth attendant was awarded the British Empire Medal for gallantry on this occasion, the citation reading:
'This man, at great personal risk, extricated a badly wounded seaman from the debris in the after part of the ship, just before this part of the ship became submerged, and got him safely into a boat.'

splinter wounding, 2 proving immediately fatal and 2 dying forty-four hours after injury. The air temperature at the time was 14° F. The cramped quarters on board made attention to these wounded very difficult. At first it was hoped to transfer them to a larger ship, but this was impossible, and they had to be retained on board. Débridement of wounds was effected under 2 per cent. novutox. The cases were given anti-gas gangrene serum, and a course of sulphonamide therapy was begun. Four days later these cases were landed at the R.A.M.C. Hospital, Seydisfjord, Iceland.*

In her action with surface forces on August 25, when returning to the United Kingdom with survivors from H.M.Ss. *Edinburgh* and *Gossamer*, H.M.S. *Marne* suffered 3 men killed and 5 wounded by shell splinters. These wounded had to be kept on board. The report of her Medical Officer recorded that:

'It was necessary to excise major wounds under local anaesthesia as they were very dirty with clothing, splinters and pieces of skin carried deep into the tissues. Dressings were sterilised by baking them in cigarette tins in the galley oven, and they proved very satisfactory. As the ship was rolling considerably, the deck itself proved to be the best instrument table. Operating was carried on at speed as the ship was still in very dangerous waters.'

The conditions on board the *Marne* were even more complicated by the twin guns which were mounted above the sick bay, so that much dust and smoke found its way into the atmosphere during the course of any surgical procedure. This ship had also been short of food for the preceding fortnight, and this fact also made her Medical Officer fear that the resistance to infection of his casualties might be lowered. However, this did not prove to be the case, and all these men were apyrexial with their wounds clean, when transferred to the Hospital Ship *Amarapoora* at Scapa Flow.

H.M.S. *Somali* was another of the escorting naval vessels which experienced long periods of action on the Arctic Convoy route, before her final loss in September 1942. Her last voyage was made with Convoys P.Q.18 to Russia, and Q.P.14 homeward bound, in the face of the most determined enemy attacks recorded against these convoys. Her Medical Officer recorded:

'H.M.S. *Somali*, in company with 7 Fleet destroyers, left Akureyrie, Iceland, during the evening of September 8, 1942. She arrived in Lowe Fjord, Spitzbergen, on September 11. After refuelling, the destroyers put

---

* The Medical Officer of H.M.S. *Amazon*, a surgeon lieutenant, R.N.V.R., was mentioned in dispatches for his devotion to duty on this occasion. The citation emphasised that:
'This was this surgeon lieutenant's first convoy trip. He joined H.M.S. *Amazon* in February 1942, having only completed his qualifying medical examinations at the end of 1941. Inexperience was more than offset by this officer's endurance and devotion to duty.'

to sea the following morning and joined Convoy P.Q.18 during the early hours of Sunday, September 13.

'The first call on the medical department came on Monday 14 when, during an attack on the convoy by torpedo bombers, a damaged enemy aircraft passed *Somali* 50 yards away on the starboard beam. This aircraft, flying just above the water, machine-gunned the ship, the bullets used being about $\frac{1}{4}$ in. diameter and armour piercing. Bullets were subsequently found in the canteen, in the captain's cabin and in the wardroom. Three members of a gun's crew were wounded.

'Though in action almost continuously, *Somali* herself was not damaged again during the remainder of the voyage of P.Q.18. She then formed part of the escort of the returning Convoy Q.P.14.

'On September 20 H.M.S. *Leda* was torpedoed and sunk. Her survivors were picked up by H.M.S. *Seagull*, and included 6 casualties who had been immersed in the sea for thirty minutes. Fortunately the air temperature at the time was as high as 31° F., and sea temperature 40° F.

'As the *Seagull* had no medical officer on board, *Somali* was ordered to close her and render medical assistance. A whaler was lowered and I was transferred to *Seagull*.

'On board her I found that one casualty from the *Leda* was already dead. I could see no sign of injury on him and concluded that he must have died of exposure. Two other men without obvious injuries were receiving artificial respiration, but they too died shortly afterwards. One other casualty had a fractured femur and burns, and there was a second case of extensive burns which proved fatal.

'I remained on board H.M.S. *Seagull*, and the following day we picked up a number of survivors from a torpedoed merchant ship.

'There were no further incidents, and we arrived at Scapa Flow on September 26 and transferred the casualties to the Hospital Ship *Amarapoora*.'

This transfer of the Medical Officer of the *Somali* to the *Seagull* was unfortunate in that his absence was soon keenly felt in his own ship. Nevertheless, the transfer may well have saved the medical officer's life because H.M.S. *Somali* was herself torpedoed later on September 20. For three days the *Somali* was towed by another destroyer. Fortunately most of her wounded had been removed to H.M.S. *Opportune*. There is no doubt that, given reasonable weather, the damaged *Somali* might well have been brought safely into port. Unfortunately conditions deteriorated, and after being towed in the teeth of a high gale, she eventually broke in two and sank.

The last Arctic Convoy action in the year 1942 in which there were medical incidents of note is best described in the words of the Medical Officer of H.M.S. *Onslow*:

'Our destroyers sailed from Seydisfjord at 2300 on December 24, and we joined the convoy at 1430 on Christmas Day. From then until December 30, there was little of note to record. The hours of daylight were decreasing while the cold was increasing, and ice and snow were collecting on the superstructure and making the ship appear to roll more than usual.

'At 2020 on December 30, an enemy submarine was sighted on the surface and was attacked, but the result was unknown.

'Early on December 31, enemy surface craft were suspected to be in the vicinity, and at 0825 two unidentified destroyers had been sighted. At 0928 H.M.S. *Onslow* went to action stations and gun flashes could be seen in the distance. The weather was moderate with a fair breeze, and the thermometer registered 12° of frost.

'At 0942, the *Onslow* engaged an enemy cruiser which had opened fire on the convoy. I did not realise that the ship had been hit until three casualties were brought up to the sick bay flat. Actually we had been hit three times at 1018, in the funnel, in the superstructure under "B" gun and on the forecastle under "A" gun. The second and third hits caused fires to break out on the messdecks.

'I put the three casualties into the sick bay and controlled the haemorrhage, administered morphia and applied dressings. By this time several other casualties had arrived as the forward first-aid post was untenable due to smoke.

'At about this time I received a message from the bridge to say that the captain* had been wounded. I left the sick berth attendant to carry on in the sick bay and went up on to the bridge. I found that the captain had sustained a severe gunshot wound. It was possible to get him down to his sea cabin without delay where I gave him morphia, controlled the haemorrhage and applied dressings. I made him as comfortable as possible on his bunk and left a seaman to watch for further haemorrhage and to act as a messenger.

'On returning to the sick bay flat I found it full of casualties and thick with smoke from nearby messes which were on fire and untenable. Fire parties were dragging hoses over the casualties and inevitably soaking some of them with water as they pushed through the smoke to get at the fires.

'I found that the after end of the ship was clear and relatively undamaged, so I managed to transfer the wounded there. The sick berth attendant went aft and saw that the more seriously injured were placed in cabins, either in bunks or on the deck with pillows and blankets. The less seriously injured and the walking cases were put into the wardroom. There was no panic and the wounded quietly waited their turn to be moved.

'By this time 14 men had been killed.

'I was called to the bridge again and found that a seaman had sustained a compound fracture of the left leg just above the ankle. Dressings were applied, the leg splinted, haemorrhage controlled and morphia given. He was made as comfortable as possible on the deck with duffel and sheepskin coats wrapped around him. It was impossible to move him at the time owing to the movement of the ship which was listing and proceeding at more than 20 knots. We continued to nurse this man where he was for the

---

* Captain, now Rear Admiral, Robert St. Vincent Sherbrooke, V.C., D.S.O. Captain Sherbrooke lost an eye as the result of his wounds. He received the Victoria Cross for his part in this gallant action.

next 24 hours, and did not finally move him until the ship was approaching harbour.

'From now onwards I find it difficult to record exact events in any relation to time. It seems that all fires were extinguished by 1430, and by 1930 it had been decided that in view of the damage sustained and the likelihood of bad weather, *Onslow* should proceed independently to Kola Inlet.

'By now three of the casualties were moribund and required constant attention. They had suffered from severe shock aggravated by exposure in the extreme cold. They had been drenched with water during the course of the action. A number of other casualties appeared to be suffering from the effects of blast and complained of difficulty in breathing and pains in the chest. All were extremely restless and despite morphia kept sitting up and tugging at their bandages.

'Those wounded who survived had mostly received injury from shell splinters which varied in size from pin-head to pieces 4 to 5 inches in diameter. Some had also been wounded by fragments of metal from the ship herself. The injuries were mostly to the limbs and head. Those who were killed instantly had received multiple injuries of all kinds and many of the bodies had been disintegrated by explosions. Others were so charred from fire as to be practically unrecognisable.

'Once the patients had been settled, the sick berth attendant kept a constant patrol, administering fluids, refilling hot water bottles, attending to sanitary needs, and slackening tourniquets every twenty minutes. I myself gave morphia as necessary and periodically removed tourniquets and inspected dressings for further haemorrhages. The captain was cared for by his steward, and the fracture case on deck was watched by a seaman. All the dead were buried at sea.

'The ship berthed alongside at Kola Inlet at 1155 on January 1, 1943 and a medical officer with three ambulances was awaiting the arrival of our 23 casualties. These were transferred forthwith to the Royal Naval Auxiliary Hospital, Vaenga. Fortunately the journey only took a very short time, as by then the local temperature had fallen very low and 32° of frost were registered.'*

---

* The Medical Officer of H.M.S. *Onslow*, a surgeon lieutenant, R.N.V.R., was decorated with the Distinguished Service Cross for his gallantry on this occasion, the citation reading:

'This surgeon lieutenant rendered a very great service to his shipmates. Casualties were heavy, a total of 30 being seriously wounded within a few minutes. While still under enemy fire, the surgeon lieutenant set about his task with complete calm. No sooner had he collected the wounded in one place, when fire broke out nearby. He rightly made the immediate decision to transfer all his casualties aft. Their removal and the setting up of an expanded organisation were carried out most expeditiously and efficiently, although he had only the services of a single small first-aid party.

'Greatly hampered by the confined quarters in which he had to work, he dressed wounds, administered morphia and made his patients comfortable in a remarkably short time. He then kept a constant vigil over his patients, tending to their needs throughout the day, the following night and the next day, not resting for one moment until his charges were safely in hospital.

'He has the complete confidence of the officers and men of his ship, and they would like to see his services to them rewarded.'

THE CHIEF NAVAL EVENTS, 1942-1943

RESCUE ORGANISATION

In spite of the intensive attacks to which the Arctic Convoys were exposed, relatively few men-of-war were lost or damaged. On the other hand the mercantile losses in some of the convoys were very high indeed. Consequently any account of the rescue and care of survivors on these convoys must include the organisations on board H.M. ships and Merchant Navy ships which worked jointly towards this common purpose.

Much of this work was performed by the official Merchant Navy Rescue Ships carrying R.N. medical officers, of which some account has already been given in Chapter 7, Volume I (Administration) of the Royal Naval Medical History.

By this stage of the war most men-of-war had themselves evolved an organisation on board for the rescue, resuscitation and after-care of survivors from other ships.

In January 1942, H.M.S. *Harrier* rescued 16 survivors from a lifeboat belonging to the S.S. *Effingham* (U.S.A.). On February 3, the same ship took on board 17 survivors from the torpedoed S.S. *Greylock*; 58 other survivors from this ship were picked up by the S.Ss. *Northern Wave*, *Oxlip* and *Lady Madeline*. The air temperature on these occasions was 15° F., and sea temperature 36° F.

Between August 13 and 15, H.M.S. *Sharpshooter*, acting as a rescue ship, picked up 101 survivors, of whom 20 were suffering from immersion.

Before the end of 1942, H.M.S. *Harrier* had had many such experiences. The organisation on board this ship was based on the principle which aimed at the least movement of injured survivors. The ship's wardroom and the captain's cabin were used for resuscitation because of their easy access. The sick bay was used for walking casualties and for nursing those badly injured. The positions chosen were such that, having been dealt with and resuscitated, survivors could pass to the messdecks where they would be fed and warmed.

It is of interest to note in the record of this ship's organisation that no attempt was made to arrange sleeping accommodation for uninjured survivors. This was a deliberate policy, it being considered essential that the ship's company, upon whom the lives of these survivors depended, should retain their own customary sleeping billets for such short periods in which they could enjoy rest.* Uninjured survivors had to make use of what space they could find elsewhere on board.

The ship's sick berth attendant was decorated with the Distinguished Service Medal, the citation in his case reading:

'This man, the only sick berth attendant on board, carried out his arduous duties with skill and determination during and after the action. Throughout he was of the greatest assistance to his medical officer, being entirely dependable, and doing much on his own initiative.'

* Some reference to this policy has already been made in Chapter 1 of this Volume.

This experienced organisation of H.M.S. *Harrier* was particularly tested in September 1942, when in company with Convoy P.Q.18 to Archangel. Her Medical Officer recorded:

'Although the convoy had been spotted and shadowed for three days, all was well until the morning of September 13. Then, at about 0900, the S.Ss. *Stalingrad* and *Oliver Ellsworthy* were hit by torpedoes during a torpedo attack. Although the *Stalingrad* sank in about four minutes, 72 survivors were picked up.

'At 1500, eight ships were sunk during a heavy torpedo bomber attack. We picked up about 100 survivors, most of whom were transferred to the Rescue Ship *Copeland*.*

'A quiet few hours followed until the S.S. *Athel Templar* was torpedoed at 0400 on September 14; 35 survivors were rescued, including two badly injured cases from the ship's engine room, who were transferred by Neil-Robertson stretchers.

'During the afternoon the S.S. *Mary Luchenbach* blew up during another torpedo bomber attack.

'On September 15, we transferred all our survivors to H.M.S. *Scylla*, with the exception of a number of Russians from the *Stalingrad*.

'Although bombing and U-boat attacks continued, there were no further casualties until September 18, when the S.S. *Kentucky* was torpedoed and bombed; 33 of her survivors were picked up.'

The report of this Medical Officer gives an interesting insight into the state and care of some of these survivors. In the case of the Russian ship *Stalingrad*, some 25 survivors had been in the sea for as long as forty-five minutes. They were received in the *Harrier* in two batches. The first batch were in fairly good condition and recovered rapidly.

The second batch were in poor condition and comprised six women and eleven men. Among the latter was the ship's third mate who was unconscious and shocked and had been in the sea wearing only a thin set of underclothing. Although artificial respiration and oxygen were administered for 1½ hours, the patient died suddenly and his death was presumed to be due to cardiac failure.

All the women responded well to treatment. One woman had given birth to a child two days before. She had been crushed when her ship sank and had suffered four fractured ribs. Her chest was strapped and she was made comfortable. During the subsequent seven days the lochia appeared normal and there was no sign of uterine infection. This woman's child had been lost with the ship, and this, coupled with the fractured ribs, resulted in some difficulty with lactation. But she was relieved by drawing off the excess milk from time to time.

---

* The Medical Officer of the *Copeland*, a surgeon lieutenant commander, R.N., was mentioned in dispatches for his devotion to duty in the care of survivors on the Arctic Convoy route.

Another Russian woman was eight months' pregnant, but reached Archangel without any mishap.*

Survivors from the S.S. *Oliver Ellsworthy* were in good physical and mental condition, having taken to lifeboats and rafts. One man had some fractured ribs and another injuries to ankle and spine as a result of the explosion.

Of the survivors rescued from the S.S. *Athel Templar*, two were men who had been trapped in the ship's engine room, which was flooded with sea water and oil. Both were very shocked and one was badly injured. The latter had to be rescued by a rope passed over his oily body. Unfortunately, in the speed of the moment, this rope slipped so that the man fell and struck his head. He already had multiple lacerations, a fractured humerus and a deep gash over the left eye. Within two hours he had exhibited typical signs of an intra-cranial haemorrhage from which he died. The other man was transferred to H.M.S. *Scylla* by Neil-Robertson stretcher.

H.M.S. *Harrier* also picked up survivors from S.Ss. *Waicosta* and *John Penn*. These numbered about 50, and were all in good condition with the exception of one man suffering from a fractured pelvis involving the right sacro-iliac joint. A local injection of 6 c.c. of novocaine relieved his pain and he was later transferred to H.M.S. *Scylla* by Neil-Robertson stretcher. The Captain of the *Waicosta* had dived from his ship into the sea as she sank. He was picked up after ten minutes and, although an oldish man, his condition was fairly good. But he deteriorated as time passed, and was in an unfit state when later transferred to H.M.S. *Scylla*.

Without exception, medical officers responsible for the care of rescued survivors on P.Q.18 have commented on the relatively small number of injured who had to be treated. This differs greatly from what was seen when survivors were rescued in warmer climates, and it is possible to set down a series of reasons which were common in the case of the Arctic Convoys:

(1) A large number of deaths occurred instantaneously, probably due to the fact that a number of ammunition ships blew up when hit, leaving few if any survivors at all.

(2) Most ships sank very quickly, so that they were abandoned rapidly. There seems no doubt that in some cases this meant that injured men were not removed, but were left on board.

(3) Such injured and shocked casualties as did manage to escape did not survive the low temperature of the water. A number of ships reported that bodies, obviously badly injured, were seen floating about in the sea.

---

* This woman gave birth to a living male child 24 hours after landing at Archangel.

(4) In any case, the very nature of the weapons employed by the enemy, i.e., U-boat and torpedo bomber attacks predominating, meant that on the whole, casualty rates were in any case fairly small. On this convoy, high level and dive bombing attacks only accounted for one ship.

Nevertheless, although wounds were relatively few in number, exposure proved a formidable problem, about 30 per cent. of all survivors needing strenuous medical attention for this reason. It is also of interest that exposure was marked in spite of the fact that rescue from the sea was invariably reasonably prompt.

It was found that the following degrees of exposure were met with:

(1) Cold but dry.
(2) Wet, slightly shocked but conscious.
(3) Grossly shocked, pupils widely dilated, limbs rigid, unconscious, and stomach and lungs containing oil fuel.

Those in the first category came usually from lifeboats and commonly responded quickly to warmth and hot drinks.

The majority of cases fell into the second category. They had usually been in the sea up to about twenty minutes and their condition seemed to depend mainly upon the clothing which they happened to be wearing at the time. Treatment consisted of removing their wet clothes and wrapping them in blankets. When their shivering had stopped they were usually fit to be given clothing and to join their companions.

Navy rum was of great value in dealing with these two first categories.

The third degree presented a more difficult problem. These men had usually been in the sea for half an hour or more in different states of undress. When brought on board they were taken into a warm compartment, their clothes removed and they were wrapped in blankets. Artificial respiration was started immediately and intramuscular injections of camphor in oil were considered to be of benefit. The mouth, nostrils and eyes were cleansed of oil fuel.

As soon as breathing became deeper and more regular these patients were not interfered with further until the pulse became palpable and the pupils began to contract. A prolonged bout of shivering usually followed after which consciousness would return. The patient would then be moved gently to a warm billet and sleep would be induced with morphia if necessary.

It was found that in the third category hot drinks were of no value as they invariably resulted in vomiting of blood-stained froth mixed with oil fuel.

These men commonly took forty-eight hours to recover provided that no complications occurred meanwhile.

The reports of Convoy P.Q.18 make frequent reference to the transfer of survivors to H.M.S. *Scylla*. Such transfer was part of a deliberate policy, in the absence of a hospital ship in convoy. This policy, which had in mind the transference of survivors to larger vessels of the escort which would be returning to the United Kingdom in due course, aimed at relieving the strain on accommodation ashore at Archangel and at avoiding the confusion which had followed the influx of large numbers of survivors ashore after previous convoys.

It is therefore of some interest to study the official report of the Senior Medical Officer of H.M.S. *Scylla*:

'Between 1.9.42 and 22.9.42 H.M.S. *Scylla* was employed as Flagship to the Rear Admiral (Destroyers), directing the naval escort of Convoy P.Q.18 to and Convoy Q.P.14 from North Russia. During some part of this period the convoys and escort were subjected to intense enemy attack by aircraft and submarine.

'*General Health of Ship's Company*

'Physical—excellent. Arctic conditions were faced with no adverse effect on the physical well-being of any man.

'Mental—excellent. The highest standard of morale was maintained. This is considered of some importance as, since commissioning, some 60 ratings have pleaded their inability to stand up to action conditions owing to various imaginary or exaggerated ills, summed up as "nerves". Previous experience had suggested that if such men were seen by a neuropsychiatrist, they would undoubtedly have been regarded as potential "anxiety states" and found unfit for sea service as a routine, in which case it was felt that the "infection" might spread to others.

'It was therefore decided to institute elementary methods of psychiatry on board, and over a long period these ratings were trained to take a grip on themselves.

'During all phases of these operations, care was taken to observe the reactions of each of these men at his action station. In not one single case was there any sign of mental breakdown, and each performed his task efficiently.

'Of two other cases who did break down during action, one had been treated in H.M.S. *Standard*, but obviously without success.* The other was a frank case of panic.

'There were no casualties among the personnel of H.M.S. *Scylla*.

'*Survivors*

'Approximately 300 survivors were received on board, either by transfer from smaller ships of the escort or rescued directly from the sea.

'Minor Casualties—of the survivors taken on board some 40 were treated for minor effects of exposure, cuts, contusions, etc.

'Major Casualties—received from H.M.S. *Harrier*:

(1) A Gunner, U.S. Navy, aged 21, ex S.S. *Oliver Ellsworthy*.
    One hour in water.
    Exposure.
    Injury to Ankle.

---

* *See* Volume I, Chapter 10.

Severe pains in loins, with frequency of micturition and slight pyuria for 24 hours.
Progress satisfactory.
Finally discharged to H.M.H.S. *Amarapoora* on return to Scapa Flow.

(2) U.S. Merchant Seaman, aged 31, ex S.S. *John Penn*.
Exposure and shock.
Fractured pelvis.
Contused right kidney.
Acute retention with strangury for 48 hours.
Catheterisation showed marked pyuria. After 48 hours condition clear.
This patient's condition caused some anxiety for a few days, and progress was somewhat retarded by outbursts of acute hysteria during the course of subsequent enemy attacks.
Eventual progress was satisfactory.
Discharged to H.M.H.S. *Amarapoora* on arrival at Scapa Flow.

(3) U.S. Engineer, aged 44, ex S.S. *Oliver Ellsworthy*.
Exposure and shock.
Fractured ribs.
Burns of chest.
Progress satisfactory.
Discharged to H.M.H.S. *Amarapoora* on arrival at Scapa Flow.

(4) British Merchant Navy Engineer, aged 20, ex S.S. *Athel Templar*.
Severe exposure.
Severe oil fuel poisoning with haematemesis for 24 hours.
Broncho-pneumonia.
Condition caused anxiety for some days.
Subsequent progress satisfactory.
Discharged to H.M.H.S. *Amarapoora* on arrival at Scapa Flow.'

'Received from H.M.S. *Impulsive* :

'P.m. 14.9.42, two serious cases were transferred to Scylla, having been injured in the S.S. *Empire Baffin* by an explosion during enemy air attack 8 hours earlier. When received the condition of both was grave.

'A British Merchant Navy Steward.
Exposure and severe shock.
Multiple shrapnel wounds over the whole body.
Lacerations of both arms.
Partial traumatic amputation of both hands.
Penetrating wound of abdomen.

'An Able Seaman, Royal Navy, who had been acting as an oerlikon gunner in the *Empire Baffin*.
Exposure and severe shock.
Shrapnel wounds of body.
Partial traumatic amputation of the right hand.
Multiple bullet wounds of both legs.
Compound fracture of right tibia.
Penetrating wound of right ankle-joint.

'It was at once apparent that the former patient must take preference for the moment. The latter patient was therefore morphinised, placed at rest, and watch kept for increase of haemorrhage.

'The former case was moribund. Transfusion of 500 c.c. dried plasma was given at once, and surprisingly there was some slight recovery. A further 500 c.c. was transfused, and there was a further slight recovery.

'Brief examination then showed signs of internal haemorrhage and intra-abdominal injury.

'By 0100 on 15.9.42, it was obvious that death was impending, and that any further recovery was impossible in the way of resuscitation. Operation was therefore decided upon as a last resort.

'By 0130, the necessary instruments had been collected from the distribution centres, and the sick bay prepared.

'Under intravenous pentothal anaesthesia, the abdomen was opened. A small penetrating wound over the right iliac fossa was traced through the right anterior abdominal muscles and through a small hole in the peritoneum. This hole was found to be plugged with a large piece of omentum. The peritoneal cavity was full of blood, and a small piece of metal was found towards the posterior abdominal wall, which had torn the small intestine in three places.

'The intestinal tears were closed with catgut, bleeding was arrested, and the abdomen quickly closed, a drainage tube being left *in situ*.

'With depth charges exploding frequently, conditions for an operation of such magnitude were far from ideal, and the patient was again moribund at its close.

'There was again some recovery following transfusion of a further 500 c.c. of blood, and by 0700 the patient was fit to be transferred to a cot.

'During the rest of the day the man recovered quickly and responded to nursing until, in the afternoon, he became alarmed and restless by the intense noise and concussion of further enemy air attacks. During these attacks a further transfusion of 500 c.c. blood was given with some difficulty, and though his life was despaired of he rallied again towards the evening and was nursed throughout the night.

'On the morning of 16.9.42, his condition had greatly improved, but in late afternoon, following further enemy attacks, he collapsed again and died at 1745.

'The ship's chaplain was in attendance at the time of his death, and burial at sea was carried out during the following night.

'Meanwhile, the general condition of the other patient had improved considerably, but it was obvious that if the right leg was to be saved early operation must be carried out.

'At nightfall on 15.9.42 a prolonged surgical procedure was carried out on both legs and on the right hand. Compound fractures of the upper and lower ends of the right tibia were cleaned. Numerous wounds were excised, treated with sulphonamide powder and packed with gauze soaked in flavine emulsion. The wounds were left open, and there was no attempt at primary suture.

'During the days which followed the dressings were not disturbed, and streptocide was given by mouth.

'Apart from a very slight evening pyrexia there was nothing to suggest any dangerous degree of infection.

'Nursing was somewhat difficult owing to further enemy action, and became almost impossible during the very rough weather experienced over the final 48 hours of the return journey. Nevertheless this man had made very satisfactory progress by the time of his discharge to H.M.H.S. *Amarapoora* on arrival at Scapa Flow.'

'*Experience of these cases has proved*:

(1) That transfusion of dried blood is a life-saving measure which can and must be undertaken under actual action conditions. There is no justification in waiting for a lull in the action which, under modern conditions of war, may not occur for many hours or even days.

(2) That under such conditions, for surgical purposes, an intravenous form of anaesthetic is the one of choice. Quite apart from the danger of fire or explosion, ether would be unwise unless used with discretion on the air passages of patients suffering from Arctic exposure.

(3) That in a destroyer Flagship, where surgical cases may be expected from smaller ships during Operations extending over a long period and where hospital assistance cannot be obtained, a third medical officer should be carried on loan for the period. With the ship's two medical officers engaged on any surgical procedure, it is essential for a third to be available to deal with medical action duties in other parts of the ship. This necessity is raised quite apart from the danger of depletion by one medical officer himself becoming a casualty!'

'*Further observations of importance*:

(1) It was observed among casualties and survivors that few identity discs were being worn.

(2) It was also observed that such anti-flash gear as was worn gave no protection to the eyes. One member of a damage control party was exposed to the flash of an electric short circuit for a fraction of a second. He suffered from some swelling of his eyelids and photophobia for several days afterwards. Following this I have advised damage control parties on board to wear anti-gas goggles with their anti-flash gear. There was some doubt as to the combustibility of these goggles themselves. However, trial with a naked flame showed that the material tended to smoulder and melt rather than to burn. It was therefore considered that these goggles would be safer than nothing at all and should give a fair measure of protection to the eyes.

'During the course of these Convoy Opérations the work of my sick berth staff reached a high peak of efficiency under most trying conditions. Their morale remained high in the face of heavy enemy attacks which were at times concentrated against *Scylla* herself. A good standard of nursing was maintained, and the death recorded was no fault of theirs.

'My surgeon lieutenant, R.N.V.R., was on loan and it was this officer's first trip to sea, and his first experience of war casualties. His anaesthetics were most efficiently given and his bearing and personal conduct in action were of the highest order.

'In completing this report I trust I may be forgiven for making some reference to the wide Press Publicity which has revolved around H.M.S. *Scylla* as a result of these Convoy Operations. A measure of this publicity was applied to the medical department on board, and in at least one newspaper my own name was given.

'This publicity was most unsought by my department and is deeply regretted. I indeed trust that it will be understood how difficult it has been to avoid, in view of the fact that Reuter's Correspondent was accommodated on board for the whole period of these Operations.'

A further account of the survival problem in the Arctic is given by the Medical Officer of the Rescue Ship *Zaafaran* who joined her for service on the Arctic Convoy route in April 1942. The personnel of this ship were all Merchant Navy with the exception of her medical officer and sick berth staff and her seamen gunners. The youngest member of the crew was 14 years of age and the eldest 62. The medical officer recorded:

'In spite of our destination being supposedly secret, it was well known to all hands. This early produced a state of tension which had a noticeable effect on some members of the crew. No actual case of sickness resulted, but note was made of those likely to require medical aid for psychological weakness.'*

The recorded action history of the *Zaafaran* is that of Convoy P.Q.17, which began to be heavily attacked from the air on July 4, 1942. On this day survivors totalling 49 were picked up. Eight of these were suffering from immersion, but none was seriously injured. Three were very shocked and cold. The sea temperature on this day was 38° F.

It is of interest that the *Zaafaran's* Medical Officer instituted a reception system whereby the natural inclination to resuscitate survivors with rum was prohibited until the men had been dried, warmed and reclothed. This decision was made in the light of experience, in order to deprive survivors of the temptation to dawdle and sleep in the same state as when removed from the sea.

Zaafaran's Medical Officer was on deck dealing with 8 Russian survivors when the signal from the Admiralty was received which ordered Convoy P.Q.17 to scatter owing to the imminent arrival of German heavy surface craft. He recorded:

'As our ship was 4 miles astern after picking up survivors, we had an excellent view of the situation. The signal to scatter had been received about half an hour previously. To port and ahead, the merchant ships were

---

* Similar views are implied in the record of the Senior Medical Officer of H.M.S. *Scylla, ante.*—Editor.

spreading out fan-wise, full steam ahead and belching smoke. To starboard, the destroyers were in line ahead and disappearing at top speed. On either beam was a sinking ship, and astern could be seen the wreckage of two enemy aircraft. The smoke of the battle was drifting away over the quarter.

'The prospect of early surface action with the enemy meant great mental strain for our crew, which was borne well by everyone.

'In view of the possibility of sinking, emergency medical stores were split up between the boats. A secondary temporary dressing station was established aft, and my S.B.A. and the first mate were each given some tubunic ampoules of omnopon with instructions for their use.

'In spite of the constant presence of hostile aircraft a meal was served. To any man showing loss of appetite, infusion of gentian and a stiff dose of bromide were issued. Though less acceptable than rum, this was found to be more efficacious to those whose morale was wearing thin.

'During the next 24 hours, the difference between the few British survivors on board and the remainder was most noticeable. The former were well disciplined and maintained a higher standard of morale as a body of men, whereas the latter degenerated according to their own character and that of their leaders. The majority of these survivors were Russian and Arab firemen all of whom were mentally exhausted and on the verge of hysteria.

'On the evening of July 5 a bomb struck the ship and she sank in eight minutes. No one was killed, but the personnel of the after guns' crew were shaken severely and they were all quickly questioned and examined to see if they were fit to proceed to the boats unaided. All were sent to the boat deck. An attempt was made to see if there were any injured in the engine room, but it was impossible to be certain owing to steam, darkness and damage to ladders. However, no response could be obtained to our shouting and as the bed-plates were seen to be awash, no further investigation could be contemplated.*

'Meanwhile, my S.B.A. went round with the boatswain and helped to launch rafts, leaving in the last one himself when the lee rail was awash. He carried his first-aid bag throughout, and it was still dry with its contents complete when we were picked up.

'Only two lifeboats survived the action and when the ship sank they were well away from her, filled chiefly with the original survivors whom we had picked up. I had heard no orders at all since the explosion and now, since I could find no injured and nobody but two ratings left on board, I abandoned ship with them.

'Once in the sea, I was interested to note that although the water temperature was 32° F. by the last recording, the shock of immersion was not very great. Presumably this was because I was fully clothed and because the temperature of the air which I had left was much lower than that of the sea.

'I was fifteen minutes in the water before being able to get on board a raft which had floated up from the wreck. I regret having to refer to my own

---

* It was subsequently found that all the engine room personnel had escaped unhurt. —Editor.

condition at this time but, as I was the only one swimming, I had no other cases on which to make observations. When I boarded the raft my skin was completely anaesthetic to the neck. My joint sense was very impaired and there was a well marked ischaemia of my hands and feet. Massage and exercise pulling an oar restored sensation rapidly and painlessly except in the case of my fingers.*

'A ship was sighted and once she was seen to alter course towards us, a bottle of gin and a box of cigarettes were passed round. Chocolates and biscuits from containers were eaten and clothing was shared. The mental and physical effects were immediate and what could only be described as a holiday spirit prevailed with much singing. After fifty minutes we were picked up by the Rescue Ship *Zamalek* and were all in fairly good condition after being warmed, dried and reclothed.'

Though touched on in Volume I (Administration), Chapter 7 of the Royal Naval Medical History, a more detailed account of these rescue ships and their mode of operation is given in the records of the Medical Officer of the Rescue Ship *Rathlin*, who served in this ship from the autumn of 1941 until the spring of 1943, seeing action on both the Atlantic and Arctic Convoy routes. He describes a rescue ship as:

'A small converted merchant ship of some 1,500 tons fitted with life-saving apparatus, accommodation for survivors and a small hospital. In peace-time, the *Rathlin* was employed on the carriage of cattle from the Clyde to Northern Ireland.

'Our duties were to pick up and resuscitate survivors, and our most important rôle was that of maintaining the morale in merchant ships of a convoy in the knowledge that there was a ship in company whose specific duty was to pick them up at all costs. Our cattle deck had been converted into survivor accommodation which consisted of a large compartment amidships fitted with about forty bunks, benches and mess tables. There were a further fifty bunks fore and aft on the same deck around the sides of the engine room. The total bunk accommodation was augmented by large numbers of mattresses and bedding which could accommodate additional survivors on the deck.

'We were actually fitted and provisioned to carry 150 survivors in all. But we could carry more, as indeed we did when necessity arose.

'Under my charge was a large store of clothing and comforts provided by the British Red Cross Society, the Women's Voluntary Services and the National Sailors' Society. This store included complete outfits of shoes, underclothing, trousers, sweaters, caps and coats, knitted comforts, toothbrushes, shaving gear, towels, etc. There was also a very adequate supply of cigarettes and naval rum. There were two cranes forward in the well-deck from which could be swung large baskets capable of lifting two men at a time. Rescue nets were fitted along the ship's sides over which survivors could scramble on board from the sea. We also had other rescue nets fitted

---

* This Medical Officer later recorded that he felt no ill effects from his immersion except some general muscular stiffness. But he still had some loss of sensation in his fingers as long as eight weeks afterwards.

to booms near the bows of the ship. These could be swung out well clear of the ship's side so that the nets were at right angles to the ship itself. These proved most successful as, before they were fitted, men or boats in the water ahead of the ship were washed out away from the ship's side by the bow wave, which is very powerful when steaming even dead slow ahead. I am sure that quite a number of survivors was lost in this way.

'We also had large numbers of lifebelts, heaving lines and ropes which could be thrown to men in the sea.

'An adequate number of lifeboats and rafts was carried to accommodate 150 survivors as well as our own ship's company should we in turn be unlucky enough to be sunk ourselves. We also had a 22 ft. motor lifeboat which could be sent away to pick up men in the sea. Occasionally we had to let go a raft as we passed a group of survivors in the sea so that they could hang on to it before we returned later to pick them up. But this practice was not encouraged as it meant depleting our total life-saving equipment.

'The ship was manned by Merchant Navy seamen and officers, numbering about 50. These were mostly expert seamen from the Hebrides. In addition there were 20 naval and army gunners under the command of a naval Gunnery Officer. There was one sick berth attendant and myself.

'The hospital compartment had six fixed cots and was situated just beneath the bridge and was originally the passengers' lounge. It was quite adequate and well equipped. The operating theatre consisted of a small cabin built alongside the hospital on the boat deck. It was fitted with a wooden fixed operating table to which straps were attached, so that the operator and assistant could strap themselves and so avoid being thrown about by the ship's roll.

'At sea the rescue ship took up a strategic position at the stern of the convoy. There was nothing to distinguish her from the other merchant ships in convoy. No Red Cross signs were displayed. For protection she relied upon her own armament.

'When a ship was torpedoed or bombed in daylight, we steamed out of line, hoisting a special signal so that other ships steered clear of us, and we closed with the sinking ship as fast as possible. This usually took only a few minutes. Meanwhile the convoy and escort steamed on ahead leaving, if possible, one escort vessel to afford protection for the rescue craft.

'When the rescue ship had closed the sinking ship as near as possible, it stopped with its scrambling nets down and picked up survivors from lifeboats and rafts. There was an electric microphone and loud hailer on the bridge through which instructions could be given to men in the sea to get alongside as soon as possible.

'Naturally, while stopped, the rescue ship itself presented a tempting target. But in our case enemy U-boats did not attempt to molest us, though we sometimes saw them for a brief moment on the surface, especially at night time in moonlight. But enemy aircraft behaved very differently and commonly continued their attacks while rescue work was in progress.

'If there were many survivors in the sea who had not managed to get into lifeboats or on to rafts, we had to lower our own motor lifeboat in order to pick them up. We did this on numerous occasions and sometimes in terrible weather, a feat which will be appreciated by all who know the North Atlantic and the Arctic in winter time.

'Once having received men from rafts and boats, our custom was to steam very slowly among the wreckage, making a thorough search for any remaining survivors. One of our chief difficulties now was attempting to get on board from the sea men who were covered with oil fuel. It was necessary for some of us to climb down the rescue netting with heaving lines and to try to pass the line round their chests. But even so, the line was inclined to slip and allow them to be precipitated back into the water.*

'At night time our rescue work was much more difficult. Most merchant seamen carried a small electric torch with a red bulb which clipped on to the shoulder of their life-jackets and helped to show where they were on a dark night. But often this bulb became obscured by oil fuel and could not be seen, and I am afraid that many men succumbed to exposure in the icy seas before we managed to reach them. It was obviously asking for trouble to turn on a searchlight but occasionally this risk had to be taken.

'We estimated that our rescue work usually took about two hours in the case of each ship, and once we were satisfied that no more survivors were in the sea, we steamed at full speed to rejoin the convoy which by this time would be a considerable distance ahead of us.

'It was at this stage that the medical officer's real work began. The survivors were all mustered in the saloon, and the injured were kept there until they had been sorted out and dealt with. The remainder were taken below and issued with full sets of clothing and comforts, and allocated a sleeping billet.

'For the good of their morale these survivors were organised into working parties under the charge of one of their own officers. Among some of them a great tendency was found to rush up on deck at the least explosion, and this had to be discouraged as much as possible as they were likely to impede the ship's company in the performance of their own action duties. But some survivors emphatically refused to go below at any cost, and in one particular homeward bound convoy, some 50 survivors never used their bunks at all and, even on the coldest nights, were to be found huddled together on the boat deck where they remained until arriving back in the United Kingdom.

'On one occasion we had on board 220 survivors whose morale was very low indeed. They included some 30 stretcher cases and my fear was that should we ourselves be hit, the survivors on the boat deck would panic and rush the boats before I was able to get my patients into them.†

'The commonest injuries treated on board the *Rathlin* were compound fractures, head injuries, burns and scalds. Plasma transfusions were given

---

* Later in the war a life-jacket was devised which had a rope loop attached to its back, through which a hook could be inserted in order to hoist a man out of the water.

† In one rescue ship survivors were so hysterical as to need the administration of morphia at once with liberal doses of potassium bromide during subsequent days. When there was an explosion in the vicinity of the ship one of these survivors let go a raft, while others began to lower one of the ship's boats. It became necessary to train a machine-gun on the boats supplemented with a guard of armed sentries.

when necessary, but frequently with some difficulty as the ship might well be rolling 20 or 30 degrees.

'Surgical operations required rather a complicated co-operative procedure between my sick berth attendant and myself. After inducing the patient with his anaesthetic, I handed over to my assistant* and scrubbed up to undertake my other rôle of surgeon.

'Fracture work was the easiest with which I had to deal on board as there was a plentiful supply of plaster-of-paris. I was not as greatly hampered by lack of an X-ray apparatus as I had expected. The Winnett Orr or Trueta method was used for treating compound fractures. We were fortunate too in having adequate supplies of sulphonamide powder. In my fracture work I was greatly assisted by the co-operation of various members of the Merchant Navy crew. In one case the engineers welded a piece of iron into the sole of a man's boot for purposes of extension. In another case the chief engineer fashioned an excellent Steinman's pin from a length of steel packing metal.

'Burns and scalds were always troublesome as it was very difficult to maintain asepsis. I treated second degree burns by cleaning them thoroughly with soap and water and applying triofax jelly. Third degree burns I treated with sulphanilamide powder and *tulle gras* dressings, soaking them off daily in saline baths. These methods seemed to give good results.

'One of my casualties was a petty officer from one of H.M. ships which was torpedoed in the engine room. He had second degree scalds to his face, trunk, arms and third degree scalds of his hands. The explosion had blown him into the sea, at a temperature of 29° F., and he swam one mile to a trawler. He was naturally severely shocked but responded on board my ship to large plasma transfusions.†

'Our second duty as a rescue ship, namely the routine medical care of ships in convoy, provided some interest. Naturally, with 30 or 40 ships in convoy, there was usually some sickness to be dealt with. On an average there was an acute abdominal emergency on every other trip.

'On receiving a signal that a ship had a sick man on board, we used to steam up alongside as near as possible and then, using the loud hailer, I would attempt to get some kind of a verbal history of the case. Should the clinical details not appear serious, merely requiring medicine of some kind, this would be fired across to the ship with a rocket and line apparatus. But if the case did not sound straightforward, I would be transferred to the ship by our motor lifeboat, weather permitting, and would go on board and examine the patient.

'The cases were varied. For example, there was the Master of a Greek ship suffering from bacterial endocarditis, for whom I could do little and who died. On another occasion assistance was required by a merchant ship with a madman on board. He was armed and was attempting to set

---

* This Medical Officer describes how he had:
'Two assistants for anaesthetic duties. The Second Mate had been a medical student at one time. The Third Mate claimed to be qualified as an anaesthetist by virtue of having sold patent medicines before the war. Both were ready pupils.'

† This man survived and was subsequently treated in the Royal Naval Hospital, Chatham, from where he was discharged to full duty about twelve months later.

fire to his ship. Fortunately I was assisted in controlling him by an armed guard provided by one of our escorting destroyers.

'I frequently had to undertake dental emergencies, and here again our chief engineer made for me a most effective pair of elevators which I found most useful in extracting the buried carious molars of Merchant Navy seamen.'

This general picture of the Medical Officer of H.M.S. *Rathlin* may be supplemented by one of his more detailed reports covering his activities over forty-eight hours at the height of the battle which occurred during the course of the passage of Convoy P.Q.18. Not only was it the duty of the *Rathlin* to be readily available in the course of enemy attacks, but she was faced with periods of rescue work when she herself was quite unprotected. She soon became overloaded with apprehensive survivors, many of them seriously wounded, on whom major operations had to be carried out whatever the ultimate outcome of the voyage. Recording these events this Medical Officer wrote:

'Early on September 20, H.M.S. *Leda* was torpedoed and quickly sank. We went to pick up her survivors, but were forestalled by H.M.Ss. *Northern Gem* and *Seagull*. At noon we were instructed to remove some of the survivors from the *Northern Gem* after she had buried her dead, and at the same time we received a signal that the Captain of the S.S. *Samuel Chase* had acute appendicitis.

'We lowered the motor boat which removed 33 survivors from the *Northern Gem* in three trips. There was a heavy swell running at the time. One case was very badly burned, and a Neil-Robertson stretcher could not be used as it caused him too much pain.

'We then proceeded to the *Samuel Chase* and took off the Captain. Incidentally, we also obtained some flour from her, as we were very short and down to a ration of one slice of bread twice a day.

'No sooner had we hoisted the motor boat back on board when the S.S. *Silver Sword* was torpedoed fore and aft. We went about and picked up 56 survivors from boats and rafts. One man was very seriously injured with multiple lacerations of his scalp and face and obviously an intra-cranial haemorrhage.

'On September 22, at dawn, the S.Ss. *Grey Ranger*, *Bellingham* and *Ocean Voice* were torpedoed and sunk.* We dropped astern and picked up 59 survivors from open boats and out of the sea. Altogether, after 48 hours, we had 281 survivors on board.'

REPATRIATION OF SURVIVORS

There were many variable circumstances which governed the repatriation of survivors whose ships had been sunk on the Arctic

---

* This report is at variance with the official Admiralty record which makes no mention of the S.S. *Bellingham*, and which gives September 20 as the date on which the *Grey Ranger* was lost.

However, this discrepancy may well be yet a further example of the inaccurate and disorientiated reports which were framed too quickly against an environment of prolonged enemy action at sea.—Editor.

Convoy route. The time which might elapse between the loss of a man's ship and his return to the United Kingdom, his accommodation in the interval, and the degree of risk encountered on the voyage home all made for a general trend of uncertainty. The circumstances might differ in almost every case. One man might be rescued by a ship in homeward bound convoy, in which case his ordeal was brief. But another man might be rescued and landed at Murmansk or Archangel, there to endure a long waiting period under conditions of poor accommodation.

In the case of men landed in North Russia, the majority were moderately or wholly fit by the time that a chance to return to the United Kingdom was presented. But the physical state of others was sometimes so low, following wounds and exposure, that the hazards of the return sea voyage had to be balanced against the steady deterioration which accompanied a prolonged stay in a Russian hospital with its limited facilities. Many of these survivors had to wait weeks or even months before they could be brought back to England, and consequently became depressed mentally in addition to their physical disabilities.

The vicissitudes of survivors and the uncertainties of their repatriation are well illustrated following Convoy P.Q.17. Ten merchant seamen, frost-bitten and wounded, made their way to a small settlement on Nova Zemlya. Attempts to rescue them by air did not succeed and an American merchantman which visited the area, ran aground. In due course, these men were fortunate to be rescued by a British merchant ship which herself took temporary refuge in a bay near to the settlement.

That opportunities for passage back to the United Kingdom were rare and hazardous is shown in the case of survivors from H.M.S. *Edinburgh*, who were then wounded and rescued while attempting passage in H.M.S. *Trinidad*, and were lastly transferred to H.M.S. *Forester* before finally reaching the United Kingdom. Other survivors from H.M.S. *Edinburgh* took passage home in H.M.S. *Marne* but soon found themselves in action again off the North of Norway, a small number being killed and others wounded.

MORALE

Some reference has already been made to the mental effects which were observed among personnel employed on the Arctic Convoy route. In addition, the question of morale is considered worthy of a place in this History in some detail. Study of the available records shows that it is possible to classify those persons who showed deficiencies of morale into two main groups:

A. Survivors of ships which were lost.
B. Personnel whose ships were not lost.

As regards the former group, in general the morale of survivors was considered to be low. But this appeared to be due not so much to lack of personal courage, as to a combination of several factors which may be set out in the following order:

(1) Having been resuscitated on board the ship which rescued them, most survivors then were unoccupied, which was bad for their morale, particularly during ensuing enemy action.

(2) Most officers and men rescued were professional seamen of either the Royal or Merchant Navy. They now found themselves travelling as 'passengers' in the ship which rescued them, and they found the unaccustomed status an irksome one, and, being themselves unoccupied and concurrently disorientated, they were not slow to shower adverse criticism on the seamanship qualities of their 'hosts'.

(3) Many survivors were 'lifeboat and raft conscious' for a considerable time after being rescued. They were apprehensive during subsequent enemy action, and found it difficult to remain below decks.

(4) After rescue, in a crowded ship, it was more than obvious to survivors that there was inadequate boat or raft accommodation to fit the large numbers on board should the rescuing ship be sunk herself.

(5) Where possible, British Royal Navy and Merchant Navy survivors were absorbed into the organisation of the ship which had rescued them. But this was not always possible in the case of survivors of other nations. In the latter case an interesting contrast was observed in that lower deck survivors frequently assumed that their officers no longer had authority over them, and the morale of both officers and men suffered in consequence.

So much for the morale of survivors afloat. Once landed in North Russia every factor which might have assisted the morale of these men was lacking from that time onwards. Their homes, corporate ship-life, discipline, occupation, even their uniforms and to some extent their identities disappeared. The result was seen in large numbers of men whose ships had been lost, loitering in the streets of Archangel and Murmansk, or hanging about gloomy hospitals, with shaved heads and dressed in a miscellaneous assortment of garments which themselves went far to remove the last supports of a crumbling self-respect. Boredom, vodka and hope deferred were usually added to the initial trials until such time as they could be accommodated in homeward bound ships which had yet to run the gauntlet of further severe enemy action before safety was reached.

As regards personnel in the second group, i.e. men whose ships were not lost, morale was found to be extremely high during the course of operations. But the constant strain of action left its mark on many and manifested itself in various forms after the experience was over. Some indication of the demands which were made on the endurance of a ship's company is given in the records of the Medical Officer of H.M.S. *Leamington*, after escorting the ill-fated Convoy P.Q.17 in July 1942:

'During this time the period between any two air attacks was never longer than two hours. For five days this imposed a strain on all, particularly as the enemy was achieving success and everyone felt the necessity for being constantly on the alert. The ship was not fitted for Arctic conditions, and it was just as cold between decks as it was out in the open. Food became less interesting and appetites went and finally disappeared.'

The Medical Officer of H.M.S. *Leda* also recorded:

'It has been rather interesting to observe the reactions of people to the abnormal stress and strain which action in this climate has imposed upon them. The immediate effect of air attack is one of nervous stimulation coupled with fear or acute apprehension. This apprehension is minimised for those whose minds are occupied with a particular job. But for those whose task it is to watch and wait, it is at a maximum. When a particular incident is over a variety of reactions are seen. Some men laugh hilariously and hurl illustrated epithets after the departing enemy. By contrast, other men reflect despondency. Following a prolonged period of attacks, there may be a period during which everyone outwardly appears normal apart from obvious weariness from lack of sleep. Then the glimmerings of psychoneurosis begin to appear. Most of those affected are normally of a nervous or anxious disposition, but a few ostensibly phlegmatic individuals also exhibit signs.

'There are roughly three classes:

(1) The man who comes and says outright that he is afraid and cannot stand up to things any longer.
(2) The man who veils his mental state by assuming a physical malady.
(3) The person who seeks a means of escape in alcoholic intoxication.

'As an example of the first group may be quoted the case of a leading seaman, a member of a gun's crew. This man came to me in great distress and stated that he could not carry out his duty any longer, as he was so frightened by enemy air attacks that he feared he might run from his post and seek cover. It was obvious from the man's general behaviour that he was carrying a heavy mental burden. His previous record showed that he had experienced heavy enemy action in other ships.

'In his case suggestion was employed and he was shown other aspects of his own position and was assisted to redirect his thoughts from himself and his own personal safety to the wider implications of his duty as a leading seaman and a gunner. This suggestion, together with the sedative effects of potassium bromide, produced marked improvement and he subsequently performed his duties in action and showed no signs of collapse.

'In cases of the second group there was a rating who complained that he had a pain in the region of his heart. He later produced abdominal pains and vomiting, continuously present and unrelated to meals. Improvement followed the suggestion and assurance that he was suffering from no organic disease.

'The third group requires no amplification.

'I have formed the opinion that no one, except those who desire to stay, should remain in a ship of this size under the conditions which we have experienced for a period longer than eighteen months, because:

(1) It appears to me that reactions are bound to occur, but in many cases will not manifest themselves until later by which time the environment associated with unpleasant experience has become the ship itself from which there is no escape. A period of rest ashore, or even transfer to a new ship, would mean a change of environment which would bring forth new mental and psychological adjustment.

(2) Despite the fact that sport and entertainment are organised when opportunity arises, I have yet observed that there is a general listlessness and apathy of late which is quite foreign to the nature of our ship's company. This has increased to a marked degree after the rigorous and exacting winter months spent on the Northern convoy route, and it certainly militates against the happiness and efficiency of the ship as a whole. I am not suggesting that anyone has failed to do his particular duty or that there is even any tendency for that to happen, but after living in the ship for eighteen months, I now observe that the zeal, adventurous spirit, general comradeship and harmony which once existed among us appear less keen.

(3) Mental and physical stress are severe. This in turn tends to upset the equilibrium of normal bodily functions, and lack of fresh food does little to improve this state of affairs. I feel that we shall soon once more be facing a rigorous winter in the knowledge that we have not been fortified by the fruits of summer to overcome its ills.'

The more delayed effects of strain of Arctic Convoys were frequently to be observed on return to the United Kingdom. The Medical Officer of H.M.S. *Eclipse* reported:

'Since our visit to North Russia, with its action with enemy surface craft and the unrest of daily bombing attacks, there has been a marked increase in the sick parade. On one day recently I have had to send twelve men for medical and surgical consultations. Of these twelve, eight have already been discharged to hospital and the other four are awaiting relief. The important point is that these men had been suffering from their complaints for months, and in some cases for years without reporting sick. The reasons given were that they desired to remain on duty, on war service, and they were afraid that their complaints, if reported, might mean that they would have to leave the ship.

'The extreme cold off North Russia, combined with prolonged action conditions had a most marked effect on our crew. In action, two guns were frozen solid, spray froze on the men, and the leather sea-boots of one officer were literally frozen to his feet.

'These conditions greatly affected the nerves of the crew, with the consequent results that complaints which they previously hid have become aggravated, and are now disclosed.

'These twelve men were good, conscientious workers who had been in the ship since before the outbreak of war. It is only now that they feel the strain on their nervous systems to such an extent that they must report sick with a long standing physical disability.

'In any case I feel that when officers and men have completed eighteen months to two years under these conditions, their efficiency becomes impaired and this tends to get worse as time goes on.'

Intermittent strain operated more often than that of continuous and prolonged action. But it proved equally exacting and was held by some to be harder to endure.

The Occupation of North Africa*
Operation 'Torch'

The assaults on Algeria and French Morocco by British and United States seaborne forces commenced on Sunday, November 8, 1942, and resulted in landings being effected in the vicinities of Algiers, Oran and Casablanca. There was little in the way of sustained resistance to this operation, and the successful occupation of all three areas had been completed, and an Armistice signed, by November 11. On the same day Allied troops were landed east of Algiers, at Bougie, and on November 12 a force was also successfully landed even further east, at Bone. But the eastward advance from this point onwards was fiercely contested by the enemy and, as is well known, many months were yet to pass before the ultimate object of this operation was achieved with the capture of Bizerta and Tunis, and the elimination of all the enemy forces in North Africa.

THE PLAN

The planning of Operation 'Torch,' being the largest Allied amphibious operation of its kind to date, was carried out under conditions of extreme secrecy for a number of months beforehand. As has been written elsewhere, this secrecy was maintained until the assaults were actually commenced, and the enemy was deluded into the assumption that the large convoy of shipping passing into the Mediterranean was merely a further attempt to pass supplies to the beleaguered island of Malta.

The actual operation envisaged a simultaneous assault in three areas by forces which were designated Western, Centre and Eastern Task Forces. The assaults were carried out from infantry and vehicle landing ships over beaches, with the intention of occupying the local ports and opening them for shipping within a few days.

The Western Task Force was to be entirely American, and no British organisation was called for. The Centre Task Force was also an

---

* Compiled largely from the records of Surgeon Captain C. B. Nicholson, R.N.

American commitment, but troops were to be carried in British ships and British beach parties were to be employed. Similarly, the Eastern Task Force involved British naval direction in its initial stages, with Algiers as its immediate objective and subsequent occupation of the ports further east.

The British Naval Commander (C. in C. X.F.)* had a very large force of naval ships, and his command also included a large number of Merchant Navy ships to be used in the assault phase as troop carriers. The Naval Commander and his immediate staff left Plymouth at 1730 hours on Thursday, October 29, taking passage in H.M.S. *Scylla*, and arrived at Gibraltar at daybreak on Sunday, November 1. During the assault phases his headquarters were at Gibraltar.

Within his command were the forces taking part in the assaults, each under the command of a Rear Admiral. Each separate landing was under the command of a Captain, R.N. (S.N.O.L.).

On a port being captured, it was arranged that a Flag Officer (F.O.I.C.) or Naval Officer in Charge (N.O.I.C.) should set up a port organisation. Algiers was to be a F.O.I.C. port, while those smaller harbours further east were to be N.O.I.C. ports.

The medical organisation for Operation 'Torch' was efficiently directed by an Acting Surgeon Captain, R.N., who had been appointed some time previously to the staff of the Naval Commander. This officer became Fleet Medical Officer, Mediterranean, consistently with the assumption of the office of Commander-in-Chief, Mediterranean, by the Naval Commander. Initially, before leaving England, he had the assistance of a sick berth petty officer for clerical duties.

The Fleet Medical Officer took passage from Scapa Flow in H.M.S. *Rodney* on October 22.† He arrived at Gibraltar on October 25, where he remained for ten days. He then took passage in H.M.S. *Charybdis* from Gibraltar to Algiers, where he set up his headquarters locally in the St. George's Hotel.

MEDICAL ORGANISATION

The medical organisation for Operation 'Torch' was broadly planned on the following lines:

(1) *Operational Phases*

(a) During the assault

A naval medical staff of 2 surgeon lieutenants and 6 sick berth ratings was to be carried for the round trip in each assault craft. Each

---

* Admiral Sir Andrew Cunningham, now Admiral of the Fleet, Viscount Cunningham of Hyndhope, K.T., G.C.B., O.M., D.S.O.

† Official records suggest that the Fleet Medical Officer arrived at Scapa Flow after leaving London 'from a little used station', in the greatest secrecy. But, in point of fact, he caught 'the ordinary 10 a.m. train from Euston'!—Editor.

personnel ship was to carry one Army doctor and 4 medical orderlies, and a Company doctor was to be in each merchantman.

The duty of the medical staff was the reception of casualties during the assault phase. It was expected that casualties occurring in the assault craft themselves would be returned to their parent ships, while casualties occurring on the beaches would probably be held there by Army medical staff landed for the particular purpose.

From the outset it was urged that the operation as a whole demanded the speediest possible unloading of ships with their rapid turn around. It was therefore considered impossible to provide for casualty evacuation directly from beach to ships, nor was such a procedure considered desirable as medical facilities afloat were not meant to be extensive and the subsequent disposal of casualties was not catered for in large numbers. It was emphasised that should casualties occur the actual beach conditions at the time would be the deciding factor, and should it be clearly impossible to deal with casualties ashore, facilities would then be provided for their removal to ships, and local conditions would also decide whether patients or medical staff should be moved from one ship to another.

The plan thus visualised a large number of ships each with comparatively few casualties, and covered the paramount consideration that the operational work must be interfered with to a bare minimum and ships retained in potentially dangerous areas for as short a time as possible. Subsequently these ships would join a homeward bound convoy, and it would be the duty of their medical staffs to retain and care for their casualties themselves. However, should this clearly become beyond their powers, orders would be given for such ships as necessary to proceed to Gibraltar where hospital and hospital ship facilities would be available.

(b) On the beaches and beyond

Military and naval casualties would receive their early treatment from field ambulances landed during the assaults. Within twenty-four hours of occupation of the beaches, casualty clearing stations would be landed and the ultimate embarkation of casualties was expected to be effected through the medium of the ports themselves as soon as they became opened up to traffic.

(c) In occupied ports

The responsibility for hospital and specialist facilities for all personnel in occupied ports would be accepted by the Army. Naval responsibility would be confined merely to setting up sick bays as required in naval headquarters establishments.

(2) *Naval Beach Parties*

As these parties would be out of touch with naval medical staff, they would become an Army medical responsibility.

(3) Hospital Ships

It was intended that three British hospital ships would be made available and their early disposition was to be as follows:

(a) H.M.H.S. *Oxfordshire* was to be at Gibraltar 24 hours after the assaults and to accept such casualties as could be transferred from assault convoys and naval covering forces. According to the local situation she would then either return to the United Kingdom or be sent forward to whichever port might need her most, if necessary disembarking her sick and wounded at Gibraltar beforehand.

(b) H.M.H.S. *Amarapoora* was to pass Gibraltar 48 hours after the assaults and was to accept her orders from there, and was to have in mind Oran as her probable destination.

(c) H.M.H.S. *Newfoundland* was to pass Gibraltar 24 hours after the assaults with Algiers as her probable destination.

The duties of hospital ships would be to be placed alongside in occupied ports as early as possible, to evacuate casualties, and to return to the United Kingdom.

In addition to the above hospital ship arrangements, the personnel ship *Argentina* was to be specially staffed and stored as a casualty evacuation ship for Oran, and was to proceed from there directly to the United States about one week after the assaults.

It is of historical interest that medical planning did not include the use of American hospital ships, as it was understood that these would not be available before the spring of 1943. It was, however, placed on record that it would be desirable for American hospital ships to be available by that date in order that British hospital ships could then be released for return to their normal fleet duties elsewhere.*

Fifty-one medical officers were attached to the assault and personnel ships, and to them were issued advance instructions on the following lines:

(a) It was considered probable that some officers and ratings would not have completed inoculation and vaccination. Medical officers were to make sure that there were no defaulters in this respect and that such inoculations and vaccinations as might be necessary should be completed early on the outward voyage.

(b) The immediate necessities in the ships themselves were to be:
  (i) The formation of medical action stations.
  (ii) The organisation for abandoning ship, and the safety of casualties or sick during such a procedure.

(c) As regards the embarkation of casualties, the primary duty of the medical staffs in the care of casualties which might occur during

---

* Hospital ships for Operation 'Torch' were on loan to the Army. They were not naval commitments from the point of view of their requirement, but only as regards their movements.

the assault phases was to organise arrangements to receive them on board their parent ships with the minimum of delay. The variety of ships involved did not permit of any hard and fast rules being laid down, but medical officers were advised to review the following methods of receiving such casualties:

(i) By hoisting landing craft to the deck level of the parent ship, and then evacuating casualties into the latter directly.
(ii) By direct entry through sally-ports.
(iii) By the use of Neil-Robertson stretchers.
(iv) By the use of ships' lifeboats lowered into the water in readiness.

It was emphasised that the responsibility for the whole treatment of these casualties would devolve, normally, on the medical officers of the ships receiving them. It was considered most unlikely that any local transfer of casualties to hospital ships would be possible. However, should the severity and number of casualties demand it, the following alternatives were made available:

(a) A report should be made to the Senior Naval Officer of the landing, who would be empowered to direct a local transfer to another ship less heavily burdened.
(b) Should the burden of casualties be overwhelming, it would be possible to obtain permission from the Naval Commander to divert the particular ship to Gibraltar, where a hospital ship would be specially retained for the purpose of transferring the more seriously wounded. But casualties not so transferred were to be held and treated on board until arriving in the United Kingdom.

As regards casualties occurring on the beaches and beyond, organised evacuation through the beaches was not envisaged. The treatment of such casualties would be accepted as an Army commitment and they would be held for evacuation through the ports by hospital ships some three days after the initial landings. On the other hand, should the casualty situation be such that adequate care could not be given ashore, or should the movement into ports be delayed or impossible, local evacuation from the beach areas might be implemented at the discretion of the Senior Army Medical Officer ashore. The latter would operate such a local evacuation in co-operation with the Principal Beach Master who would arrange to make the necessary craft available for the purpose. But it was pointed out that such evacuation would inevitably be attended by some delay.

Additional instructions to these medical officers concerned hygiene and sanitation, and pointed out that the elementary principles of such matters were almost unknown to ratings who had not been accustomed to hot climates with a native environment. Experience had already shown that even in a peaceful atmosphere a period of one month was necessary in order to get accustomed to tropical or sub-tropical conditions ashore. But where active opposition might be encountered from the moment of landing, the necessity for a thorough knowledge of hygiene matters in advance was paramount. Medical officers were therefore to warn personnel in advance of the conditions which they might be likely to encounter, and how dangers might be combated. Warnings were recommended to be on the following broad lines:

(a) *Food*

This was to be protected at all times from flies and dust. Cooks were to be warned to be most careful in their personal cleanliness and health, with special reference to such matters as diarrhoea and skin diseases. Local meat supplies, especially pork, might well be infected, and local milk, especially goats' milk, might be highly dangerous unless boiled.

(b) *Water*

There would be no separate naval organisation for the purification of water. Beach parties would be supplied with Halazone outfits. In the ports naval water supplies would be from Army sources. All water which was not definitely known to have been purified was to be boiled. Local beverages such as mineral waters were not to be imbibed.

(c) *Tropical Diseases*

(i) Intestinal Diseases

Diarrhoea, dysentery, typhoid and cholera were to be borne in mind as of the first importance. Their prevention would depend on rigid discipline in the supplies of water, ice and vegetables, and on the most vigorous methods in preventing the breeding of flies and their access to food.

(ii) Malaria

The malarial season was normally from April to November, so that excessive incidence of this disease was not expected. Nevertheless, constant vigilance was to be observed, and suppressive therapy with mepacrine was to be instituted for one week before arrival, and was to be continued for a period after arrival. Preventive measures would include the supply of mosquito netting, anti-mosquito cream, mechanical sprays and insecticide fluids.

(iii) Typhus Fever

Preventive inoculation would not be possible before embarking. Personal methods of disinfestation were to be taught and practiced by all personnel, and a supply of A.L.63 Powder would be included with medical stores. It would be the aim of the Army to establish disinfesting stations where every man could be disinfested once weekly, and arrangements ashore would be made to allow naval personnel to use these facilities.

(iv) Plague
Rat destruction and the rat proofing of stores was to be borne in mind.

(v) Venereal Diseases
Personnel were to be warned that infection might well be regarded locally as 100 per cent. In so far as the prevention of these diseases might be regarded as partly a medical matter, a supply of prophylactic material would form part of the stores to be carried by medical officers to cover the early days and to supplement the bulk stores which would arrive later. Arrangements would be made for Early Treatment Centres to be established ashore in naval bases.

(iv) Sunstroke and avitaminosis were also mentioned as possible medical factors to be considered.

SPECIAL INSTRUCTIONS FOR MEDICAL OFFICERS IN OCCUPIED PORTS

The original planning included 10 naval medical officers for permanent duty on shore after the occupation. The occupied port under the command of a Flag Officer in Charge (F.O.I.C. Port) would have appointed to it 1 surgeon lieutenant commander, 1 surgeon lieutenant and 6 sick berth ratings. A port under the command of a Naval Officer in Charge (N.O.I.C. Port) would have appointed to it 1 surgeon lieutenant and 4 sick berth ratings.

These medical officers were instructed that their first duties would be to initiate health, hygiene, care of the sick, medical transport and medical liaison in the case of all naval personnel ashore. They were to work in co-operation with the medical officers of ships entering harbour, with the Army medical authorities ashore, and with the local Civil medical authorities, according to the political situation in the case of the latter.

More in the nature of a general directive than as an exact commitment, local conditions and progress being the deciding factor, the following principles of shore naval medical organisation were laid down:

(a) It was proposed that a small sick quarters would be established in each occupied port to serve naval needs; 25 beds should be available in a F.O.I.C. Port and 15 beds in a N.O.I.C. Port. Each sick quarters should be established in the most convenient place for the purpose, and if possible adjacent to local naval headquarters, since supplies, food, etc., would have to come from the latter. In the selection of a building for the purpose heating facilities, fly-proofing, water supply, lighting, and protection against bomb blast were to be considered.

(b) During the phase of consolidation ashore, naval medical officers and sick berth staffs were to be placed at the disposal of the Army medical authorities ashore. Later, when port consolidation was completed, all hospital and specialist treatment for naval personnel would be provided by the Army.

In these instructions, the Fleet Medical Officer required short written reports of local and allied conditions to be rendered to him within 48 hours of landing. He also stressed the importance of accurate record keeping, especially of wounds and injuries which might call for subsequent compensation. He sensibly drew attention to that constant watch which would be required to make sure that records were accurate in an environment in which a large moving Service population was to be expected and no naval hospital would be available.

MEDICAL STORES AND EQUIPMENT

Each port party on landing would carry two Field Service Valises, four Neil-Robertson stretchers and the following additional stores:

Large field service dressings	50
Small field service dressings	25
Elastoplast dressing sets	2
Gentian violet tubes	2
Pulv. bismuth co., tins	4
Pulv. sulphonamide, 1-oz. tins	4
Acid boric, 4-oz. tins	1
Nicamide ampoules	6
Omnopon tubunic ampoules	50
Anusol suppositories	25
Elastoplast, 3 in. Roll	1
Benzedrine tablets	200
Sulphapyridine tablets	200
Sulphaguanidine tablets	200
Phenobarbitone tablets	100
Potassium permanganate pellets	1,000
Calomel cream outfits	1,000
Irrigator E.D.	2
India rubber tubing	12 ft.
Spring clips	2
Urethral tubes	6
Condoms	1,000
Mepacrine tablets	3,000

Bulk medical stores and equipment were planned to follow in the first supply convoy as follows:

For each F.O.I.C. Port

A Double No. 1 Set with special and extra stores up to war scale with folding operating table, 4 Neil-Robertson stretchers, 4 ambulance stretchers and 4 Thomas splints.

In addition:

Mepacrine tablets	25,000
Pamaquin tablets	1,500
Quinine bihydrochloride tablets	15,000
Ascorbic acid tablets	2,500
Ascaridole B.W.	100 c.cm.
Anti-mosquito paste, tins	1,000
A.L.63, tins	1,500
Stebophan B.W., boxes	6
E.B.I. tablets	200
Sulphaguanidine tablets	1,500

In addition to purely medical stores, each F.O.I.C. Port was to be supplied with naval and victualling stores on the following scale:

Blankets	100
Sheets	100
Pillow cases	60
Coverlets	50
Short towels	250
Long towels	30
Wash basins	5
Ewers	5
Dressing buckets	5
Oxtail soup	270 lb.
Chicken broth	360 lb.
Bovril	600 oz.
Pearl barley	100 lb.
Benger's food	50 lb.
Mechanical sprays	10
Flysol	60 gall.
Insecticide powder	600 lb.

Anti-mosquito netting was the subject of a separate special supply to cover all personnel landed. Allowance was also made for supplies of fly-swats and fly-papers from Army sources ashore.

For each N.O.I.C. Port

A Double No. 2 Set of equipment was supplied with extra stores to bring up to war scale with folding operating table, 4 Neil-Robertson stretchers, 2 ambulance stretchers and 4 Thomas splints.

In addition:

Mepacrine tablets	5,000
Pamaquin tablets	500
Quinine bihydrochloride tablets	2,500
Ascorbic acid tablets	1,000
Ascaridole B.W.	100 c.cm.
Anti-mosquito paste, tins	500
A.L.63, tins	750
Stebophan B.W., boxes	3
E.B.I. tablets	100
Sulphaguanidine tablets	750

Naval and victualling stores were supplied as in the case of F.O.I.C. Ports, but on a slightly lesser scale.

THE OPERATIONS

To the historical account of these items of planning must be added, as will be read below, the story of the medical impact of Operation 'Torch' on the large number of British men-of-war, whose duty it was to escort the assault forces and to render sea support and protection during the few weeks which followed the actual occupation.

The approach of the immense initial convoys involved in Operation 'Torch', and guarded by ships of the Royal and United States Navies, was carried through with casualties in only one man-of-war and only one troopship. H.M.S. *Panther* was straddled by bombs from enemy aircraft on November 7, on passage to Oran, with the loss of 2 men killed, 28 missing, and 19 wounded, of whom one died later. The U.S.S. *Thomas Stone* was also torpedoed by a U-boat near Cartagena on the same day, but was later safely towed to Algiers.

But if the approach was quiet, the actual assaults and initial occupation were fiercely opposed by the French for some hours, and naval casualties occurred. On November 8, the cutters *Hartland* and *Walney* were sunk by shellfire from the shore batteries at Oran with the loss of 10 killed, 100 missing and 62 wounded, one proving fatal. The survivors from these ships became temporary prisoners-of-war ashore. H.M.S. *Boadicea* was also damaged by direct shellfire from a French destroyer at Oran with the loss of 1 man killed and 4 wounded.

On the same day H.M.S. *Malcolm* was shelled and hit by French shore batteries while trying to ram the boom at Algiers, and was forced to retire with 4 men wounded in her engine room. Meanwhile, H.M.S. *Broke* succeeded in breaking the boom. She faced strong shellfire and ultimately had to be abandoned. She suffered 9 men killed and 5 wounded, and the latter were transferred to H.M.S. *Zetland* during the course of the action. The *Broke* eventually foundered on November 9.

While these assaults were taking place, H.M. ships were carrying out off-shore anti-aircraft patrols in anticipation of early active enemy intervention from Corsica, Sardinia and Sicily. Such intervention began early on November 9 and off Algiers H.M.Ss. *Sheffield* and *Palomares* both sustained casualties and damage. The *Sheffield* had one man wounded, while the *Palomares* lost 23 killed, 2 missing and 11 wounded.

The shellfire incidents during this assault phase merit some study, since this was one of the few occasions when this weapon was employed in a sea action up to this stage in the war.* Analysis of the wounds caused by shells of the French ships and shore batteries brings to light little of peculiar significance which has not already been recorded. Some 70 per cent. of wounds were due to shell splinters and were evenly distributed over the body, including the feet and ankles. Only three cases of burns were recorded but these were believed to be due to local fires on board damaged ships and not to shell explosions. Traumatic amputations occurred and were severe in some cases. For example, in the *Hartland* one sailor lost both arms, another one arm, another a foot, and a fourth half of one foot.

An interesting effect of shellfire in the case of H.M.S. *Boadicea* was that all wounds were coloured green. This phenomenon was believed to be due to a dye used by the French in their ammunition for the purpose of spotting the fall of shots.†

---

* The other chief occasions were the Battle of the River Plate and the sinking of the *Bismarck*.

† This effect is believed to have been observed previously during the Syrian campaign.

During the weeks immediately following these landings, the Royal Navy's task was concerned with off-shore patrols, the maintenance of sea supply routes, and the escorting of troop and supply convoys in support of our forces established ashore at Bougie and Bone. As the enemy developed his efforts to oppose these measures of supply and support, British men-of-war embarked upon long periods of arduous activity in which losses occurred. On November 10, H.M.S. *Martin* was torpedoed and sunk by a U-boat with the loss of 152 men. On the same day H.M.S. *Ibis* was sunk by an aircraft torpedo while in company with H.M.S. *Scylla*, ten miles north of Algiers. She lost 106 men, with 7 wounded; 107 survivors of the *Ibis* were rescued by the *Scylla*.

On November 11, H.M.S. *Hecla* was torpedoed and sunk by a U-boat near Gibraltar, with the loss of 8 killed, 273 missing, and 3 wounded, of whom one died later. On the same day H.M.S. *Roberts* was bombed near Bougie and lost 17 men and suffered 14 wounded.

On November 12, H.M.S. *Tynwald* was sunk by a mine at Bougie, with 21 men missing and 3 wounded. Also on this day, H.M.S. *Bicester* was bombed near Algiers with the loss of 6 killed and 5 wounded, one of whom died later.

On November 15, the aircraft carrier *Avenger* was torpedoed by a U-boat and sunk 110 miles west of Gibraltar with the loss of 507 of her complement. Further ships damaged by air attacks during the rest of November included H.M.Ss. *Spey*, *Delhi* and *Ithuriel*, with total casualties of 13 killed and 32 wounded.

During December, H.M.S. *Quentin* was sunk by an aircraft torpedo, north of Bone, and H.M.Ss. *Blean* and *Partridge* were torpedoed and sunk by U-boats off Oran. The casualties in these three ships amounted to 126 killed and missing and 43 wounded, of whom 11 died later. In addition, H.M.S. *Marigold* was damaged by enemy aircraft off Algiers on December 9, and lost 46 men and suffered 5 wounded. The cruiser *Argonaut* was also damaged by aircraft torpedoes and lost 4 of her complement.

The official report of the Senior Medical Officer of H.M.S. *Roberts* gives an impression of the circumstances preceding and immediately following the landings at Algiers:

> 'On the night of November 5, at 2330, we left Gibraltar. By the following morning we found ourselves part of the escort of a vast number of ships in convoy, and we steered east and nothing occurred on that or the following day to disturb the serenity of our passage.
>
> 'On November 7, at about 2130, we arrived in the bay of Algiers, our task being to patrol outside and await the capitulation or to carry out bombardment should that prove necessary.
>
> 'On November 9, we continued our patrol duties and early in the day two small scale enemy air attacks were made on our shipping. At 1400 a heavy attack was made by Ju.88s, and smaller sporadic raids occurred until 2030.

'The forenoon of November 10 brought several more small scale air attacks, but the day was a fairly quiet one and we joined up with a troop-ship convoy proceeding further east. At 1700, a heavy attack by Ju.88s was fought off. The convoy arrived at the entrance to the harbour of Bougie at 0600 on November 11, and Allied troops and equipment were landed at various points without opposition.

'We anchored at noon, but at 1430, we were attacked by a very heavy formation of torpedo bombers and Ju.88s. Such enemy air attacks continued until we weighed anchor and recommenced patrol duties at 1535.

'At 1715, a direct attack was made on the *Roberts* and we were soon straddled by a stick of bombs. The ship was first damaged by a near miss, the bomb exploding practically under her bottom. A second bomb entered the ship's port side amidships. A third entered through the main galley and incinerator room on the starboard side of the upper deck, and penetrated to the main deck where it caused extensive damage and several deaths.

'Fires broke out, and very soon communication between the forward and after medical stations was impossible owing to fumes and oil fuel. Secondary lighting had to be used and the water supply failed.

'Casualties began to arrive at the two medical stations immediately after the explosions. I soon received a message from my surgeon lieutenant to the effect that fire and fumes had made it necessary to evacuate the after medical station, and various messdecks had to be taken over to accommodate the injured. Unfortunately this meant replacing a number of patients in Neil-Robertson stretchers in order to transfer them. Many willing helpers from the ship's company soon accomplished this difficult task with a minimum of discomfort to the patients, and when I was eventually able to make my way aft I was very favourably impressed by the way in which everything had been done which possibly could have been done for their comfort.

'We had 16 killed, 1 missing and 14 wounded; 5 of the latter suffered burns from the flash of the explosions, in addition to which 6 suffered fractures. The remainder had splinter lacerations.* There was also a number of men suffering from minor injuries, including contusions due to being thrown about by blast.

'This particular attack began at 1715 and lasted until 1840. Further attacks occurred throughout the night by the light of flares dropped by enemy aircraft, and two other ships in our group were hit.

'At 0545 on November 12, we picked up 30 survivors from H.M.S. *Tynwald* which had sunk close to us. Two of these men had to be treated for exposure and shock. At the same time the sight of two large transports, one on either side of us, each blazing furiously from stem to stern, and with frequent explosions taking place, will remain one of my most vivid memories of the war.

'By this time the *Roberts* had developed a very heavy list to port and it was decided to enter harbour and take the ship alongside. In spite of

---

* A relatively unusual occurrence was that 3 of these 14 wounded suffered serious eye injuries.

continuous air attacks on the harbour area, we landed our casualties safely and discharged them to a shore hospital at 1230.*

'At 1440, the Burial Service was read by our captain over the bodies of our dead comrades, and these were then lowered into an invasion barge and taken out to sea for burial.

'We found that this period of days had a most strained effect on our nerves following the very frequent calls to action, lack of sleep and irregular feeding. We were all very glad when we received orders to depart for Gibraltar.'

H.M.S. *Palomares*, unlike the *Roberts*, was unable to discharge her casualties ashore, and this meant that a number of surgical procedures had to be carried out on board under conditions of considerable difficulty. Her Medical Officer recorded:

'After taking part in the initial landings at Algiers, the *Palomares* was engaged on anti-aircraft patrol duties in Algiers Bay. At 1700 on November 9, enemy aircraft attacked and the ship received a direct hit by a 500-lb. bomb directed from a high level. A fire broke out, there was a great deal of damage and ammunition began to explode. The sick bay was badly damaged, all its lights were extinguished, and it was ankle deep in water. Casualties lay about all over the after part of the ship, both below and above decks. The wardroom was taken over as a temporary sick bay and the wounded were conveyed there, while medical stores and dressings were salvaged from other parts of the ship.

'Some time had to be spent in sorting out our 23 dead from the wounded. The immediate needs of the latter were attended to as quickly as possible and they were then put into sequence for operation. My sick berth petty officer assisted me and an R.N.R. Executive Officer maintained anaesthesia very efficiently after I had induced it in each patient. When I was half way through my "list", the Medical Officer of H.M.S. *Lamerton* arrived on board to help me.

'The operations included a traumatic pneumothorax and one amputation of leg through the thigh.'†

During this same period, H.M.S. *Scylla* was part of a Task Force operating off Algiers and Bougie. This force was subject to heavy enemy air attacks on November 8, 9, 10 and 11. The *Scylla* was herself directly involved on the latter three days.

During a torpedo bombing attack by enemy aircraft at dusk on November 10, H.M.S. *Ibis* was struck by a torpedo which exploded between the boiler rooms. The ship at once took on an alarming list and there was a large fire amidships. A large number of badly scalded and burned ratings made their way to the sick bay in a matter of two minutes. The ship rapidly turned over and her Medical Officer was

---

* This was an Army casualty clearing station. These casualties eventually reached Algiers by ambulance train.

† The Medical Officer and sick berth petty officer of the *Palomares* were mentioned in dispatches.

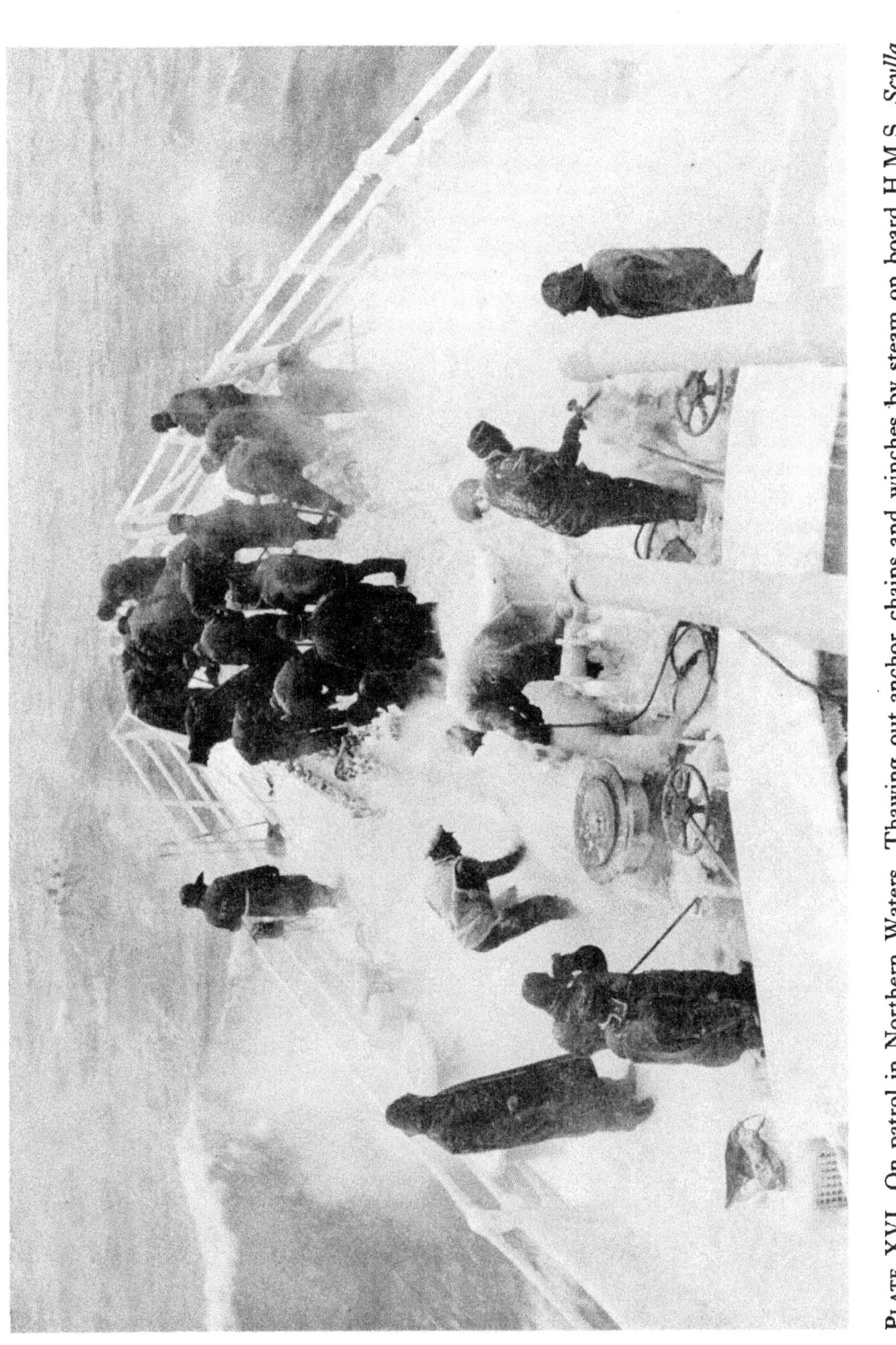

PLATE XVI. On patrol in Northern Waters. Thawing out anchor chains and winches by steam on board H.M.S. *Scylla* during a cold spell on patrol in the Arctic.

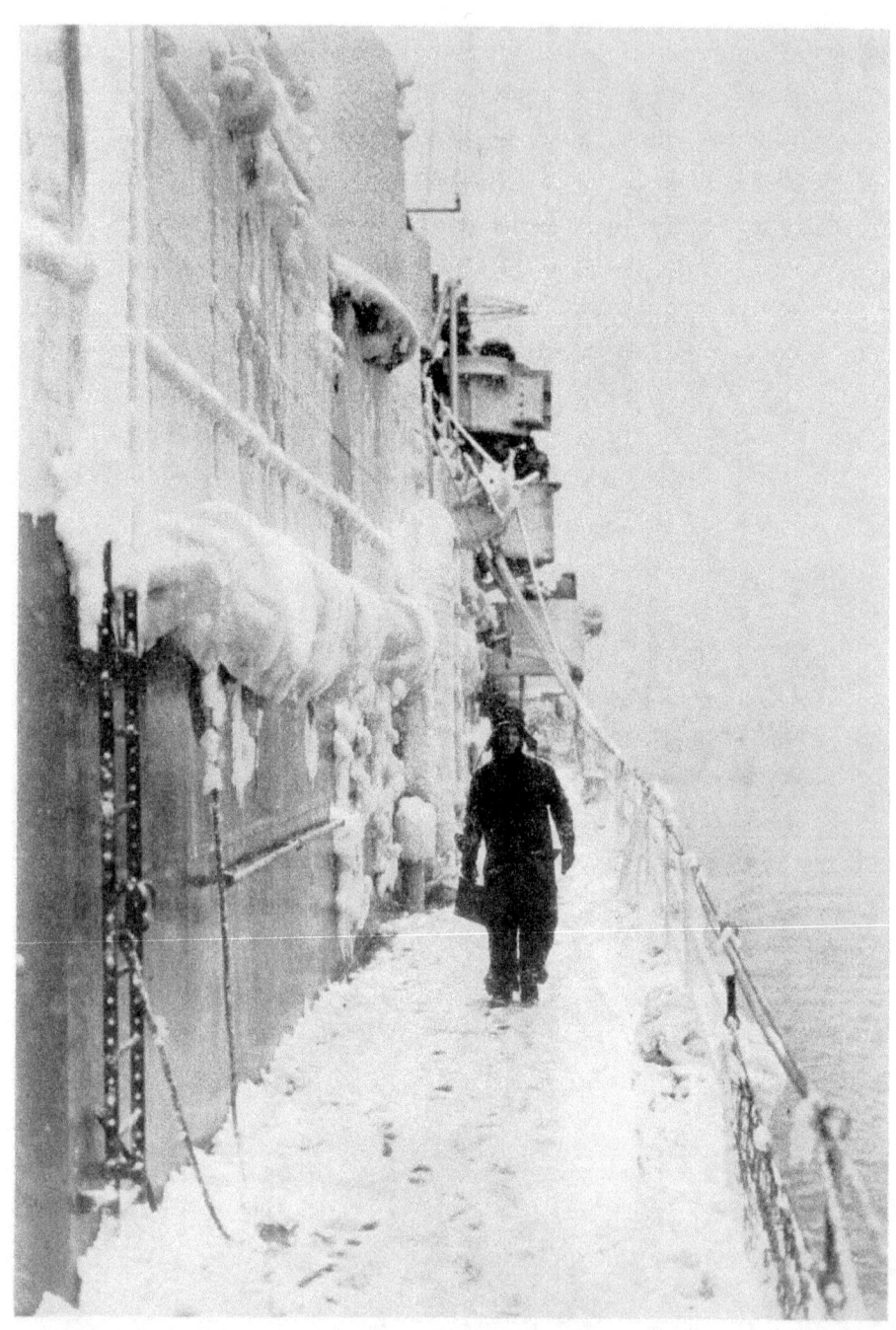

PLATE XVII. Arctic Convoy. Conditions on deck.

forced to abandon, but before he did so he removed his own lifebelt and placed it round one of his casualties and lowered the man into the water.*

Records suggest that a number of ratings of the *Ibis* had no time to blow up their lifebelts. These men found that after jumping into oil fuel on the surface of the sea they were unable to grip the air valve of the lifebelt, and when the valve could be opened, the mouthpiece became so clogged with fuel that air could not be forced through. Few of those whose lifebelts were not inflated could have survived.

The First Lieutenant of the *Ibis* was wearing a patent proprietary life-saving waistcoat which he inflated before abandoning ship. He crawled down the ship's side and lowered himself into a layer of oil fuel. The waistcoat promptly billowed out from below, and the slippery state of the oil fuel was such that, in a matter of seconds, every button on the waistcoat slipped back through its buttonhole. The result was that the officer sank through his waistcoat and was almost drowned by it, and it became more of a hindrance than a help.†

A total of 102 ratings and 5 officers were rescued by the *Scylla*.‡ All were suffering from a mild degree of exposure and oil fuel poisoning. The Commanding Officer of the *Ibis* and one rating were unconscious, and prolonged artificial respiration failed to revive them. They were buried at sea the following day.

MEDICAL ORGANISATION ASHORE

A brief outline of the medical organisation ashore after the landings may be given as follows:

ALGIERS

The port of Algiers became the main British naval base in North Africa, naval headquarters there being known as H.M.S. *Hannibal*.

For the first few days there was some difficulty in making adequate medical provision, particularly as the future attitude of the local French authorities was uncertain. To add to the difficulties of setting up first-aid posts for the treatment of air-raid casualties and of organising sick bays for the routine care of naval personnel ashore, there was the immediate commitment of finding accommodation for casualties who soon began to be brought in from ships' actions afloat.

---

* This Medical Officer is now deceased. A surgeon lieutenant, R.N.V.R., he was awarded the Albert Medal in Gold for this gallant act. The sick berth attendant of the *Ibis* received the same award posthumously.

† These facts were represented later to the manufacturer of this particular type of life-saving waistcoat, with the recommendation that buttons and buttonholes should be replaced by clamps or hooks.

‡ The Senior Medical Officer of H.M.S. *Scylla* was awarded the Distinguished Service Cross for 'outstanding conduct in the face of the enemy'.

The arrival of the Base Medical Officer was delayed, and for the first forty-eight hours his duties were taken over by the Senior Medical Officer of H.M.S. *Bulolo*. The latter reported as follows:

'H.M.S. *Bulolo* entered Algiers Harbour on the morning of November 9. Unfortunately she grounded some 20 yards from the quay and communication with the shore was therefore difficult for the next 48 hours until she had been refloated. This rather complicated the early work ashore which very largely devolved upon this ship.

'During the morning H.M.S. *Othello* arrived with wounded from a destroyer. Fortunately the weather was mild and fine, as there was no available cover of any sort where these men were landed. I at once contacted the Army authorities and found that so far there was no Service medical organisation in the city, neither were any ambulances yet available.

'I therefore acquired a business house close to the quay and equipped it as an emergency sick bay, removing to it the whole of the equipment of one of my ship's main dressing stations including twenty mattresses. I accommodated the destroyer's casualties here and their treatment was begun.

'As this accommodation, while useful, was by no means ideal, I made contact with the local French Military Hospital and Red Cross Organisation. They were extremely helpful, and the hospital agreed to take the casualties, while the Red Cross at once lent me three ambulances.

'While the evacuation of these men was proceeding I was informed that the American transport *Leedstown* had been torpedoed and that a number of wounded survivors was being landed at a point about 6 miles away. As soon as I could I detached my ambulances to deal with this new situation. Some of these latter casualties were dealt with in the French Military Hospital and others were accommodated in the occupied aerodrome at Maison Blanche which was not far from the point where they had been landed.

'By November 10, it was obvious that unless some assistance was given by the Army medical authorities in the near future, a naval organisation on a considerable scale would have to be set up as an emergency measure. During the afternoon I contacted the local British A.D.M.S. and the O.C., 5th Field Hospital. This was a hospital in name only, as it had as yet no building in which to operate. I then procured a car and during the rest of the afternoon found and visited the Headquarters of the 78th Division and the American 168th Combat Team, but I was unable to locate any casualty clearing station. I found out later that this was still about 15 miles from the town in the opposite direction!

'When I returned to the harbour I found that a further batch of wounded had been placed on board H.M.S. *Keren* which had just come alongside. These included men from the destroyer *Broke* and from an Italian submarine. I again procured ambulances from the local French Red Cross and sent 8 of the more seriously wounded men to the French Military Hospital.

'At this point the Base Medical Officer arrived and together we visited the French Military Hospital. We found that conditions were not very good, but they were undoubtedly much better than anything which could have been obtained elsewhere at this time.

'By 2000 on the same day, the British Army had taken over 200 beds in the Mustapha Civil Hospital, which was now ready to receive cases. The first use was made of this organisation two hours later, when the casualties of H.M.S. *Palomares* arrived. The Army now was able to supply ambulances.'

It will be seen, therefore, that for seventy-two hours H.M.S. *Bulolo* maintained a constant medical service both ashore and on board. In addition to the casualties referred to above, a very large number of men received attention for injuries of a minor nature. These ran into some hundreds including, not only men of the British Navy and Army and the American Army, but also French and Italian prisoners.

By November 14 the Base Medical Officer was able to report that the local naval sick bay was working well and this, which was in the dock area, became the future local Naval Medical Headquarters.

Very soon a Royal Naval Barracks was established two miles from the harbour in the Lycée Bugeaud, and here a naval sick quarters was formed with accommodation for twenty cot cases, and with its own medical officer and sick berth staff. Unfortunately, at 0650 hours on November 24, during a heavy air raid, a bomb penetrated five storeys of this barracks and 12 naval ratings were killed and 40 injured. This meant that the sick quarters had to be abandoned for the time being, and it was not working again before the end of the year.

However, by November 20, the local British Army Medical Organisation was a fully established and running concern, and the majority of naval casualties were being received by the 159th Field Hospital and the 8th Casualty Clearing Station. Also the 94th General Hospital was set up in a large orphanage about 7 miles out of Algiers, and it was to this permanent establishment that all naval cases were transferred in due course, as the field hospital and casualty clearing station moved eastward in the wake of the advancing army.

BOUGIE

A naval Base Medical Officer reached this port on the day of its occupation, but repeated severe enemy air attacks made it impracticable to set up a naval sick bay ashore until some months later. Meanwhile an efficient Army C.C.S. was soon established outside the town, and its full facilities were offered to naval casualties who were ultimately evacuated by ambulance train to Algiers.

BONE

Here, too, difficulties were encountered due to constant heavy enemy air attacks. The first available medical stores in this port were those which were salvaged from H.M.S. *Ithuriel*, which had had to be abandoned in the harbour. The stores and equipment of this ship were used to set up a naval sick quarters ashore from where casualties were eventually transferred to the 5th General Hospital which was established by the Army locally under canvas.

ORAN

Medical provision ashore at Oran was intended to be an American commitment. However, even as late as December 1, it was obvious that things were not yet running smoothly. On this date the Senior Medical Officer of H.M.S. *Nelson* called a conference of all medical officers serving in British ships in the harbour at Mers-el-Kebir, the local port of Oran. The situation was discussed and it was decided that medical arrangements locally for the Royal Navy were far from good. There was no doubt that the local United States medical authorities were well prepared to undertake naval medical commitments as soon as possible. But, unfortunately, there had been a lack of liaison owing to the unexpected death of the intended Naval Officer in Charge. In consequence local arrangements had taken a little time to develop; in addition to which, typhus was endemic ashore, and the American authorities were having a difficult task in making the local civil hospitals habitable and sanitary by Service standards. Therefore, special arrangements were made for naval personnel in ships at Mers-el-Kebir. H.M.Ss. *Nelson*, *Renown*, *Formidable* and *Furious* were to keep 'medical guards' and receive emergency cases for operation and after-care. The Surgeon Lieutenant of the *Nelson* (a F.R.C.S., Eng.) was appointed as surgical specialist afloat.*

In due course a Royal Naval Medical Officer was appointed for liaison duties at Oran, but this was not put into effect until the beginning of 1943. Meanwhile American hospitals were assisted and guided in the disposal and administration of British naval personnel by a naval medical officer who visited Oran from Algiers from time to time.

COMMENTARY

Fortunately for the purposes of this History and for the purposes of combined operational planning on an even larger scale during the subsequent two years, the Fleet Medical Officer prepared meticulous reports which were both instructive and constructive in their criticism.

Generally speaking, the medical arrangements which were made for Operation 'Torch' appear to have been satisfactory. From the medical aspect the naval side of a combined operation of such a nature was not an outstandingly large commitment, but during the planning stage many points had to be considered in full appreciation of the problems and uncertainties which were faced by the operational planners themselves.

---

* The local anchorage at Mers-el-Kebir was unsuitable for the permanent basing of a hospital ship.

THE CHIEF NAVAL EVENTS, 1942–1943

CASUALTIES IN H.M. SHIPS, NOVEMBER 8–DECEMBER 31, 1942

H.M. Ship Lost L Damaged D		Weapon	Date	Total casualties			
				Killed	Missing	Died of wounds	Wounded
			1942:				
Panther	D	Bomb	November 7	2	28	1	18
Cowdray	D	Bomb	November 8		5		27
Hartland	L	Shellfire—shore batteries	November 8	1	29	1	40
Walney	L	Shellfire—shore batteries	November 8	9	71		21
Sheffield	D	Shellfire and bombs	November 8				1
Malcolm	D	Shellfire—shore batteries	November 8				4
Boadicea	D	Shellfire	November 8	1			4
Broke	L	Shellfire—ashore and bullets	November 9	9			5
Palomares	D	Bomb	November 9	23	2		11
Martin	L	Torpedo	November 10		152		
Ibis	L	Aircraft torpedo	November 10		106		7
Scylla		? Shell splinter from own forces	November 11				1
Roberts	D	Bomb	November 11	16	1		14
Hecla	L	Torpedoes	November 11/12	8	273	1	2
Marne	L	Torpedo	November 11/12	12	1		4
Tynwald	L	Mine	November 12		21		3
Bicester	D	Bomb	November 12	6		1	4
Avenger	L	Torpedo	November 15		507		
Spey		Bomb	November 16				2
Delhi	D	Bombs	November 20	2		2	7
Ithuriel	D	Bombs	November 27/28				13
Quentin	L	Aircraft torpedo	December 2	2	9	2	8
Marigold	L	Bomb	December 9		46	4	1
Blean	L	U-boat torpedo	December 11	6	80	1	
Argonaut	D	Aircraft torpedoes	December 13		4		
Partridge	L	U-boat torpedo	December 18		29	8	24
				97	1,364	21	221

As regards the medical arrangements for the occupied ports, the uncertainty as to the actual conditions likely to be encountered and the size of the prospective port parties, made it difficult to determine exactly what provision should be made. Experience to date had suggested the need for fairly large naval medical staffs in occupied ports, but some reduction was considered practicable because full Army medical co-operation would be available. There was also an overall need to reduce non-combatant personnel to a minimum. Nevertheless, certainly in the case of Algiers, the big factor was that lack of opposition allowed the port to be occupied immediately, while, in expectation of opposition, the hospital ship and the convoy carrying the main medical supplies had been routed to arrive forty-eight hours later. During this period the casualties were almost entirely those landed from ships, i.e. assault troops and naval personnel. Until late on the second day there was no Army hospital set up to receive these men. But although unexpected, this situation was covered by the presence of two medical officers in all the larger ships present in the harbour, who were able to deal with casualties.

Summarising the situation in retrospect, some years later, the Fleet Medical Officer's view was:

'I think nobody realised how big the naval organisation would rapidly become, and as a consequence the base organisations set up were too small. From the day of occupying a port there was a flood of ships and personnel in numbers which were infinitely larger than anything which had been visualised or seriously considered. Casualties and survivors from naval ships were high. Merchant Navy sick and survivors were a serious commitment. All this means that the immediate establishment of a base sick bay is absolutely vital because Army medical formations were outside the town, and in any case in an operational area their system is to evacuate everybody who can move, which would tend to include key naval personnel with minor complaints. We did, fortunately, lay on some immediate organisation for maintaining sanitary control, but its scope was much smaller than we had anticipated the need to be, and there was no assistance whatever from local authorities.'*

An operation of this nature obviously called for the use of hospital ships, and much thought and discussion revolved around this subject during the planning stages. A minimum number of three hospital ships was called for and since only one was available from Army sources, two were loaned by the Royal Navy. These hospital ships were taken from other needed employment for this purpose, and it was especially noted that the naval hospital ships loaned for this operation should be released as soon as possible and that three hospital ships of the large carrier type would be provided by the United States, one by January 1943, and the other two in the spring of 1943.†

The disposition of the three hospital ships was planned so that one would be retained at Gibraltar in reserve and to cover casualty reception requirements there, while the remaining two ships should pass Gibraltar at a time which would make them available to proceed to any North African port to which they might be directed not later than three days after the actual landings. In point of fact, two of the hospital ships were delayed by fog for forty-eight hours, so that only one ship was

---

* Personal communication to the Editor.
† Records show that the provision of these ships was delayed.

available on the date stated. A signal was made to Oran and Algiers asking each port what its requirements were within twenty-four hours of the landings, but, either through poor communication or misreading of this signal, no reply was received until the message had been repeated two days later. Replies were then received from Algiers and Oran that hospital ships were not needed as the local Army medical organisation had already been built up. However, as has been noted above, the port of Algiers was open on November 9, and had the hospital ship at Gibraltar gone straight there she would have proved most valuable. But, unfortunately, she was not asked for.

With the exception of some minor difficulties in the case of occasional sanitary requirements, the Fleet Medical Officer reported that the supply of medical stores and equipment to the occupied ports was most satisfactory and he paid tribute to the persons responsible for originating these supplies in the Medical Department of the Admiralty. Casualties during the landing operations were fewer than was expected. Nevertheless, the Army Commander of one Task Force commented on the sketchy nature of the medical personnel ashore in the early stages, on the paucity of morphine syrettes and on the need for earlier V.D. prophylaxis. By contrast, the tubunic ampoules used by naval medical officers were both convenient and adequate in supply. Also, anti-V.D. equipment was landed by advance naval medical parties within twenty-four hours.

Referring to the preparation of naval personnel for a landing operation of this nature, the Fleet Medical Officer recorded the vital necessity of up-to-date inoculation and vaccination. Naturally this need was included in the orders to personnel, and, in general, was effectively carried out. However, there seems no doubt that a considerable number of personnel in small ships, independent parties, etc., could not be provided with inoculation and vaccination, and it is probable that a number of Staff Officers was also missed. It would also have been desirable to give anti-typhus inoculation, but this proved to be impracticable.

Two matters of the greatest importance which came to light in assessing the various records of Operation 'Torch' were the inexperience of the Medical Branch of the Navy in Staff Operational Planning, and in addition the consequences of the very high degree of security which was observed. The former omission has been rectified by the inclusion of medical officers in Naval Staff Courses in the post-war years. But for the benefit of future operational planners it is considered of importance that the security question should here be studied in some detail. That the high degree of secrecy which had to be maintained could embarrass, and actually did embarrass the medical planning is very obvious. The Fleet Medical Officer himself has commented on the great difficulty he experienced in actually getting any orders to the medical officers of the various assault ships and he recorded that:

'Although I did meet them all before the Operation, I was not in a position to tell them very much.'

In further relation to this question of security, for a period before and after the Operation the Fleet Medical Officer was at Gibraltar. It was evident to him that should there be a large number of casualties, especially in the Naval Covering Forces,* the medical facilities at Gibraltar would be fully used. Hospital facilities at Gibraltar were entirely in the hands of the Army, and the Fleet Medical Officer recorded that:

'A little awkwardness was occasioned by the fact that the A.D.M.S. was not aware of the plan, and although I had to find out what facilities there were, I could not give him any information until the assaults had commenced. Also there was no Army medical officer on the Allied Force Staff at Gibraltar. Therefore, not understanding that this was a combined operation, the A.D.M.S. was never quite clear as to why I should be so interested in the hospital facilities inside his area. The point was of course entirely clarified once the North African assaults had commenced, and the A.D.M.S. was then able to brief his hospital commanding officers whose only regret was that more actual work did not come their way. Had there been more casualties they could have been accepted without difficulty and with enthusiasm by the Gibraltar Army Hospitals.'

The Operation itself confirmed what had been already noted following some of the Malta Convoys, which was that the actual landing of casualties from ships at Gibraltar was not always easy, and that there was an urgent need for a better and more reliable hospital boat to visit ships anchored in the bay. The Fleet Medical Officer paid high tribute, as did many other medical officers, to the services given by the Naval Medical Liaison Officer, Gibraltar, during this period.† This officer was on duty night and day and his organisation provided for all contingencies to the fullest possible extent.

A number of damaged ships from the Naval Covering Forces arrived in Gibraltar during the course of the Operation, and where casualties occurred the work done by medical staffs afloat was in all cases commented upon most favourably. In his reports the Fleet Medical Officer commended nine medical officers for their services afloat, and these included the Senior Medical Officer of H.M.S. *Scylla*, the Medical Officers of H.M.Ss. *Hecla* and *Ibis* and a Polish Army Medical Officer who was attached to the Naval Covering Forces.

Apart from the reports of the Fleet Medical Officer, attention has been drawn to other aspects of the impact of security on the medical

---

* Casualties in the Naval Covering Forces amounted to 1,703.
† The late Surgeon Captain M. P. Button, O.B.E., R.N.

organisation for Operation 'Torch', particularly in relation to preventive medicine in occupied ports and action organisation in the Naval Covering Force and escorts.

As regards the latter, the high degree of security which was observed caused embarrassment to a number of medical officers in men-of-war. Many of these ships had been diverted for the Operation at short notice, and some had recently been involved in other Operations from which they had barely had time to recover. It is therefore necessary to draw attention to the predicament in which their medical officers were placed when they realised, all too late, that their ships were taking part in an Operation of such magnitude as 'Torch' proved to be, during and following which naval casualties had amounted to 1,703 by the end of the year.

For example, one medical officer, whose stores and equipment were badly depleted during earlier recent operations, considered that the whole of Operation 'Torch' represented a period of anxiety during which he was constantly 'begging, borrowing or stealing' essential medical supplies from other ships in order to meet the new action commitments about which his department had been given no warning at all.

Another doctor, senior medical officer of a cruiser which became heavily engaged during and subsequent to the landings, recorded that he had no knowledge of any impending Operation or of the likelihood of enemy action until precisely half an hour before the landings were carried out. In his own words, in his Action Report, he stated:

> 'A brilliantly lighted port was visible in the distance, which I later discovered to be Algiers. At 0030 I was informed that we were part of a force for the invasion of North Africa. The beaches were actually occupied half an hour later.'

The next day this same medical officer recorded how he sent a hand message to a neighbouring cruiser asking the latter's medical officer if he could spare some extra emergency dressings.

Likewise, the Senior Medical Officer of H.M.S. *Scylla* recorded that in spite of the fact that the Flag Officer directing the Operation was actually on board this ship between the United Kingdom and Gibraltar, 'I have no knowledge of the ship's destination or future commitments, which makes planning ahead very difficult'. He goes on to report:

> 'I sincerely consider that there is a great need to bring the ship's medical department inside the general framework of information when something is being planned. Otherwise, like today, the tendency is that the doctors of ships get left out of things until the last moment, or until they are suddenly expected to advise upon some medical or hygiene problem without reasonable warning.'

As regards preventive medicine in occupied ports, study of post-war literature also suggests that local health conditions ashore were not sufficiently promulgated to Medical Officers of all the Services, whose immediate task was to undertake measures of preventive medicine once the landings were effected. It has also been suggested that more information had been promulgated to American Medical Officers than to those of the British Armed Forces.

Three months after the occupation had been effected the Fleet Medical Officer was able to report upon a number of matters of medical interest under the following headings:

Typhus Fever. 'The greatest present menace is undoubtedly typhus fever. This is a winter disease, January to May, and the incidence is expected to reach a high peak in March. In 1942 38,000 natives and 2,700 Europeans contracted the disease, and the overall mortality was 29 per cent. being higher among older people and among Europeans; 29 doctors were infected of whom 18 were unprotected; 15 of them, all unprotected, died. The mortality rate among protected persons is practically nil.

'While typhus is prevalent in all larger towns, there is a particularly high incidence in Algiers and Oran. Three cases have been seen among native dockyard workers by the Base Medical Officer at Bone.

'A total of 15,000 c.c. of non-living vaccine was available at the Pasteur Institute, and 5,000 naval personnel in the ports and small ships based thereon are now receiving inoculations. But it is not considered feasible to provide inoculations for personnel of all the ships using the ports. Normal attention to hygiene and the better washing facilities on board ship should prevent cases occurring. French Army Authorities who use the vaccine on 100 per cent. of their personnel still consider it to be secondary in importance to ordinary personal prophylactic measures. British and United States Army Authorities are using American vaccine. A signal has been made to Admiralty requesting that, when possible, personnel drafted to this station should receive protective inoculation against typhus before sailing.'

Study of these remarks of the Fleet Medical Officer and other reports from various medical authorities makes it obvious that the position of the invading Allied Force could well have been rendered precarious by the existence of this epidemic of typhus fever at the time of the landings. In point of fact, the epidemic in Algiers at this time was the worst since the year 1868. Fortunately American Forces had been vaccinated before leaving their home country but records suggest that, probably due to the high degree of security measures, the senior British Hygiene Authorities were not fully admitted into the preliminary discussions on the projected Allied landings, which therefore represented an unknown venture both geographically and epidemiologically. The British Forces, including the many shore-based naval personnel, from the beginning had to rely on self-discipline, cleanliness and A.L.63. Propaganda was intensified. As a consequence, though often having to live in close contact with native populations, in 1942 and

1943 there were only 36 cases in the British Forces compared with 9 cases in the American Forces. Admittedly 32 per cent. of the British cases were fatal, whereas all the American cases were mild. Mobilisation of native labour companies in the port areas meant that large numbers of Arabs were under the supervision and control of the Royal Naval Medical Authorities. Frequent and stringent powdering with insecticide was carried out, and as an added precaution dock workers were vaccinated with a single dose of the living murine vaccine of Blanc-Baltazard.*

Smallpox. 'Three cases of smallpox have occurred in Algiers among naval personnel, of which one was fatal. One of these was in the submarine depot ship, one in the naval barracks and one in a small craft afloat. A period of 14 days has now elapsed since these cases were reported and no fresh cases have developed. Unfortunately men are still arriving on the station who report that they have not been vaccinated for a number of years. Vaccine has been obtainable from the Pasteur Institute and a large number of vaccinations has been carried out. But the vaccine does not find universal favour owing to its rather crude appearance. However, it is doubtless effective.'

Cerebro-Spinal Fever. 'One case has been reported.'

The Enteric Fevers. 'The most heavily infected area is Algiers, but no cases have been reported among naval personnel to date. A few Army cases have occurred. The risk of typhoid is less serious than other diseases owing to universal successful inoculation and the comparative simplicity of prophylactic measures. Dysentery of both types has occurred, but is uncommon.'

Rabies. 'Rabies is common, and there were 2,500 cases in Algeria in 1942. Jackals, dogs, cats, monkeys, camels, donkeys and sheep have been considered sources of infection. Efficient treatment is available at the Pasteur Institute in Algiers. There have been no cases to date among naval personnel.'

Malaria. 'An anti-malarial campaign has been planned by the Army Force Surgeon, whose meetings are attended by naval representatives. The Navy accepts local military precautions in each area.'

Venereal Diseases. 'The incidence of venereal diseases among naval personnel has not been unduly high. Unfortunately, the gonococcal infection found in this area does not respond to sulphapyridine medication nearly as well as to sulphathiozal. Supplies of this drug have been called forward from Gibraltar.'

Miscellaneous Ailments. 'Of these jaundice and pharyngitis have been the most troublesome.'

Smoke Complaints. 'Reports have been made that the smoke used for the screening of land areas as anti-aircraft precaution is leading to a number of complaints. The smoke used is hexachlorethane, and while admitted to be

---

* The reader is referred to the account of the Algerian epidemic of typhus, 1941 to 1943, in the *Journal of the Royal Naval Medical Service*, 1953, by Surgeon Commander C. V. Harries, R. N., who was the first Base Medical Officer in Algiers.

temporarily unpleasant, it is stated to be quite harmless unless the concentration is such that suffocation occurs. Naval experience is that certain persons may be idiosyncratic and may therefore develop bronchial irritation which may be distressing for a period up to 48 hours after even mild exposure.'

First-Aid Equipment in Ships. 'Casualty experiences suggest that the present packings of first-aid equipment could be improved upon, and the need has been stated for watertight cupboards on the upper deck, while black japanned boxes have been suggested to replace the ordinary haversacks. In my opinion the difficulties of carrying the latter would outweigh any possible advantages.'

INTER-SERVICE CO-OPERATION

In closing this chapter of this History it is of importance to record that the Fleet Medical Officer stresses, in relation to inter-Service co-operation, how completely the medical facilities of the Army had been placed at the disposal of the Navy. In his own words:

'There has been a constant stream of demands on the Army's time and experience, and in return they have made every effort to help us.'

CHAPTER 5
MEDICAL ASPECT OF THE CHIEF NAVAL EVENTS 1944–1945
Minor Naval Operations, 1944

STUDY of Admiralty records has not been of very great assistance in compiling a medical operational narrative during the year 1943. Likewise, little of outstanding interest has been set on record to cover the period from the beginning of 1944 up to the closing stages of the war. This is not to suggest that the Royal Navy had in any way ceased to shoulder a heavy operational burden, because indeed the reverse would be the case. British men-of-war were offensively engaged in every theatre of the war during the period covered by this chapter and casualties of many kinds still continued to occur afloat. Few of the many incidents, however, afforded material of sufficient medical interest to justify their inclusion in this History, but some of those of special interest have been recorded.

The part that the Naval Medical Service played in the large amphibious operations, which took place largely under Army control, is fully recorded.

INCIDENTS OF MEDICAL INTEREST

Two interesting references have been made to the condition known as 'immersion blast' which was by now established as a special hazard associated with service at sea.

On January 7, 1944, H.M.S. *Tweed* was carrying out an anti-submarine patrol in the Atlantic in fine and calm weather. At 1615 hours the alarm was sounded, and fifteen seconds later the ship was hit by a torpedo and at once started to sink by the stern. The *Tweed* sank in three minutes. No boat could be got away in time, and unfortunately only one Carley float escaped damage. Nevertheless, in spite of the suddenness of the whole incident, the messdecks seem to have been cleared completely and very few men went down with the ship. Two stokers actually swam out of the engine room skylight as it reached sea level.

In the words of the *Tweed's* Medical Officer:

> 'While we were swimming away from the ship, and while the bow was yet sticking out of the water, one depth charge exploded, probably at 250 ft. This was responsible for all the casualties, either directly or indirectly, as everyone was in the water at the time. The furthest man away could not have been more than a hundred yards from the centre of the

explosion. The force of the explosion was considerable, and felt as though something had squeezed the chest and abdomen tightly and suddenly. The majority of men immediately began to cough up bright blood and became incontinent of urine and faeces. Some must have been killed instantly while a number obviously commenced to drown. The survivors soon became spread out over an area of about 300 yards square, which was covered with a considerable amount of oil and wreckage. One group of about 20 men gathered together on and around the Carley float; another dozen or so clung to a large spar; the rest were supported by their lifebelts or odd pieces of wreckage.'

Fifty-three survivors of the *Tweed* were picked up by H.M.S. *Nene* just before sunset. One was dead when rescued and two others died a few hours later.

All these survivors complained of crampy abdominal pains, diarrhoea, melaena and some haemoptysis. It was noted that fat or well covered men were less affected than thinner ones, while those wearing lifebelts and swimming on their backs seem to have suffered less from the effects of underwater blast.

On February 24, 1944, H.M.S. *Wishart* carried out a depth charge attack over a German U-boat. The U-boat surfaced and was abandoned by her crew. At the same moment, while these men were in the sea, an Allied aircraft dropped a pattern of depth charges which exploded among them. The *Wishart* rescued 38 survivors, most of whom complained of little except feeling dazed. However, 5 of these Germans soon showed signs of extreme shock. They complained of severe abdominal pain and began to vomit blood fairly profusely. They were given morphia and were discharged to the Military Hospital at Gibraltar within a few hours. Of these 5 men, one died almost immediately he reached hospital, two survived only a few days, while the others recovered very slowly.

Although those who died showed no outward sign of any injury, post-mortem examination revealed extensive blast injuries to the lungs and multiple perforations of the intestinal tracts.

On January 29, 1944, H.M.S. *Spartan* was struck by a glider bomb, off the west coast of Italy and eventually sank. Her records give an interesting account of the widespread damage and casualties which could be caused by this relatively new form of weapon.

The glider bomb struck the *Spartan* abaft the after funnel, passed through the upper deck, and eventually burst in the region of the after boiler room and the main electrical switchboard room. Just before it passed through the upper deck the bomb struck the port torpedo tubes and burst the air reservoirs of a number of torpedoes. The air pressure in these reservoirs was 2,600 lb. per sq. in., and their bursting caused disintegration of the torpedo warheads with the scattering of their explosive contents all over the upper deck of the ship. When the bomb exploded, besides causing fire below decks, the scattered explosive from the torpedo warheads became ignited and caused further serious fires on the upper deck. These upper deck fires in turn enveloped various ammunition lockers around gun emplacements, with consequent further explosions.

The main electrical switchboard room and the after boiler room were wrecked by the explosion and most of the occupants of these spaces were either killed outright or scalded to death. It would seem that although anti-flash clothing was being worn, most men had not drawn up their socks over the bottoms of their trousers. In consequence, the steam passed up the legs of the trousers, then spread out over abdomens and chests and so in several instances scalded practically the entire body surface.

The wounded and survivors from H.M.S. *Spartan* were rescued by H.M.Ss. *Dido* and *Delhi*, and were eventually discharged to Army hospitals in the Naples area. Twelve of the *Spartan's* complement were killed, 65 were missing and 49 were wounded and injured. Of the latter, burns, scalds and blast constituted the main type of injury, but here again immersion blast was a feature as enemy aircraft also dropped a number of bombs which exploded in the vicinity of survivors swimming in the water.*

A further case of probable immersion blast was reported by the Medical Officer of H.M.S. *Savage*, following the rescue of a survivor from H.M.S. *Lapwing* which was torpedoed and sunk on March 20, 1945. In the words of the Medical Officer:

'The man was unconscious but he moved an arm and there was some movement of his eyes. His face was cyanosed. There were no signs of external injury. He was immediately turned to the prone position and tilted head downwards. A small quantity of water issued from the mouth. Artificial respiration by Schafer's method was carried out from then onwards, but was changed to Eve's method after ten minutes. An airway was placed in the mouth and oxygen and CO_2 were administered. Nicamide was given intravenously and intramuscularly. Meanwhile the clothes were cut off, the man's body was dried, and hot water bottles were packed around him. These measures were continued, but, unfortunately, without success, and after the first hour *rigor mortis* had begun to set in.'

On March 25, 1944, H.M.S. *Emerald* rescued 32 survivors from the S.S. *Nancy Moller* which had been torpedoed and sunk by a Japanese submarine a week before. The account of these survivors gives an extraordinary picture of the conduct of the Japanese Commanding Officer who was responsible for sinking the *Nancy Moller*.

It would seem that though the ship sank within two minutes, about 40 officers and men reached the rafts. Shortly afterwards the Japanese

---

* The Sick Berth Petty Officer of H.M.S. *Spartan* was awarded the British Empire Medal for his devotion to duty on this occasion.

submarine surfaced and took on board one English seaman, two Chinese seamen and some Indians. The English seaman was conducted below and retained on board the submarine as a prisoner-of-war. The Chinese were shot in the back. One was killed instantly, the other was rescued from the sea by his fellow survivors. When taken on board the *Emerald* he had a perforated gunshot wound of the chest which had entered below the left scapula and had emerged in front three inches below the left clavicle in the mid-clavicular line. The only first aid which this man had received was a piece of white lint applied to the wound; nevertheless he made a good recovery!

The Indians taken on board the Japanese submarine were immediately kicked overboard, after which the submarine's crew opened fire on the *Nancy Moller's* rafts for a period of some ten minutes.

In April 1944, the Medical Officer of H.M.S. *Affleck* reported ear damage in the case of a number of men due to the blast of the 3-in. calibre guns of this ship, which would seem to have been due in some part to possible freak circumstances of atmosphere, wind and weather at the time.

This ship was in action with two German submarines during an operational cruise. The action with the second submarine took place on the surface and began very suddenly and unexpectedly. Most upper deck personnel were concussed to some degree by the blast of the *Affleck's* own guns. Four ratings suffered rupture of one tympanic membrane, and 2 suffered rupture of both tympanic membranes.

One officer suffered rupture of both tympanic membranes, after which he was lowered over the side of the ship on a life-line to aid in the rescue of survivors from a German U-boat. In consequence this officer's damaged ears were exposed to salt water and oil fuel soon after injury. He quickly developed an external and middle otitis, and it is of interest to note that he was the only person to develop any complication among those whose ears were so injured.

AN INTERNATIONAL INCIDENT

Early in April 1944, units of the Hellenic Navy in Alexandria were in a state of mutiny, and a number of Greek ships was under the control of personnel holding complex political views of the situation and unrest in their own country. For about three weeks the situation remained substantially unaltered, after which the Greek Government appointed a new Commander-in-Chief of their Fleet who adopted stern measures. On the night of April 23, three ships were captured under his direction by armed boarding parties of loyal Greeks who employed torrential small arms fire and inflicted a number of casualties. The following night the remaining disaffected ships surrendered unconditionally in the face of the threat of similar force.

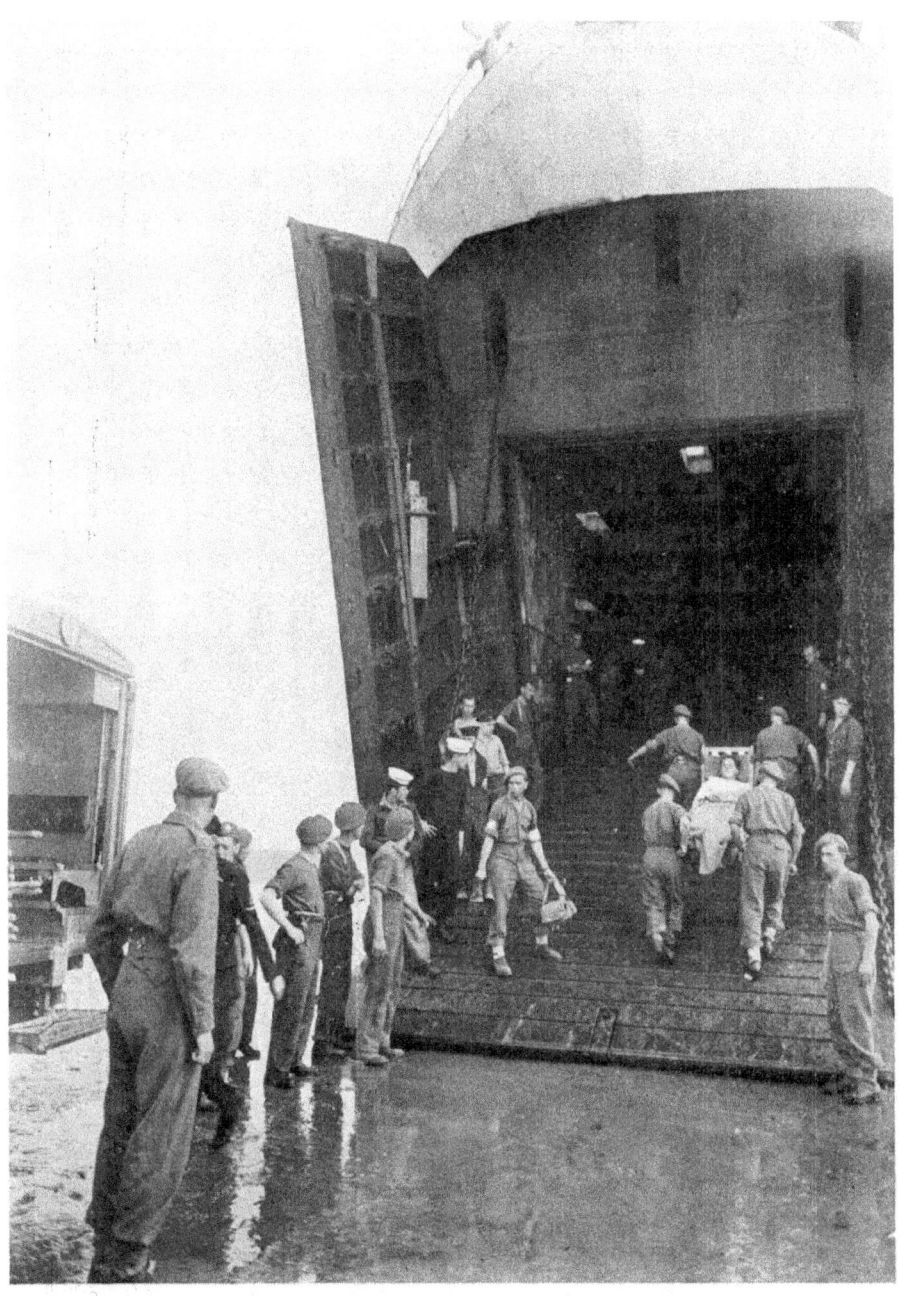

PLATE XVIII. Normandy Landings, with a Hospital L.S.T. Beach scenes as wounded men were being transferred from ambulances to the L.S.T. at low tide.

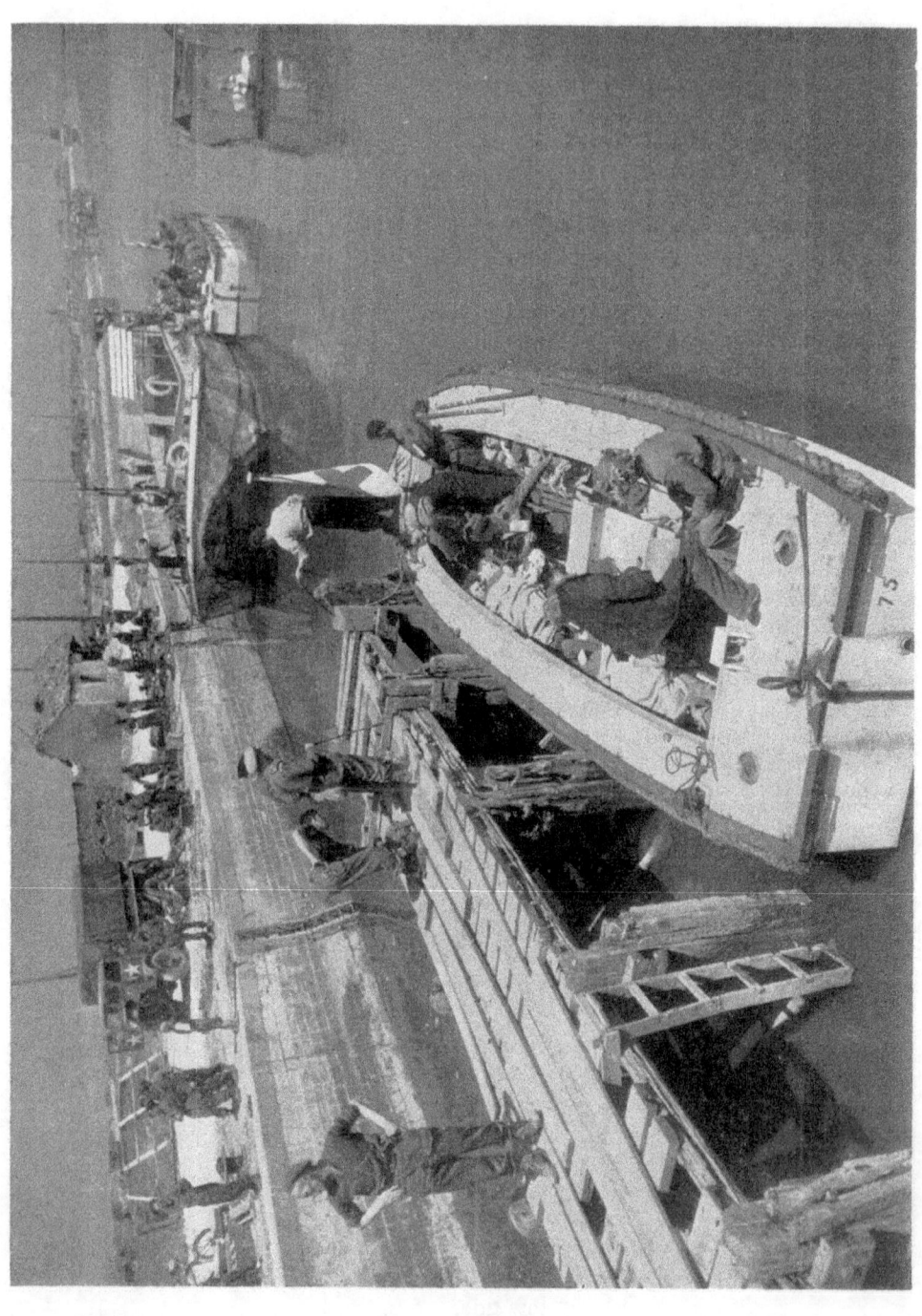

PLATE XIX. Off the Invasion Coast. Courseulles Canal scene as wounded were being embarked in a barge for transport to an awaiting hospital ship.

During this time H.M.S. *Phoebe* was alongside the Mahmoudieh Quay at Alexandria, and two small Greek warships were made fast along the *Phoebe's* outboard side. These two small ships were involved in the mutiny. The result was the somewhat peculiar one that the final armed assault in which 'Greek met Greek' was launched across the decks of the *Phoebe*. Moreover, all the casualties from these ships passed through the sick bay of the *Phoebe* which was employed as a casualty clearing station. It therefore came about that the medical organisation of one of H.M's. cruisers was the only British involvement in this tragic episode.

On April 22, the Senior Medical Officer of the *Phoebe* was informed that an assault upon the two Greek warships had been planned, and that he might expect casualties in his own sick bay in consequence. With true naval thoroughness, and in true medical tradition, this medical officer made ready to receive casualties of another nation whose political differences were no concern of his. He arranged for ambulances to be at hand on the quayside and borrowed a surgical specialist from the local naval hospital to assist him on board his own ship.

The Greeks launched their attack on their own ships in the small hours of April 24, and at about 0245 hours an extremely brisk outburst of small arms fire opened and continued for a period of thirty minutes. Thirty-five Greek casualties were brought to *Phoebe's* sick bay, all of them suffering from bullet wounds. Very few of these men could speak English, but a Greek naval medical officer acted as interpreter and also rendered medical assistance. First aid was quickly applied in each case after which the men were carried to a shed on the quayside where the ambulances were in attendance. Emergency surgery was only employed in two cases, for the extraction of superficial foreign bodies. Plasma transfusion was administered to one officer who was suffering from multiple bullet wounds including one which had entered the abdomen and had passed out of the body under the opposite axilla. Unfortunately this patient died while being transferred to an ambulance.

One other casualty died before admission to hospital, and three Greeks were killed outright. All patients had been cleared by 0430 hours.

The whole incident furnished the medical organisation of the *Phoebe* with valuable experience during an emergency which proved more extensive than had been anticipated. The Greek Commander-in-Chief later expressed his appreciation of the medical work carried out.

In closing this short account it is of importance to observe that the only British personnel to be involved were the naval medical and sick berth staff of the *Phoebe*, acting in a strictly non-combatant capacity.

CASUALTIES CAUSED BY NOXIOUS FUMES

Naval medical records of the Second World War show three detailed accounts of casualties being caused by noxious fumes following explosive damage in men-of-war in the course of enemy action. The first incident occurred in the year 1942 and the others in 1944. But all three have here been included in this chapter of the volume in order that a correct assessment and comparison may be made of the particular hazards involved. Also, of special importance and value is the fact that the first two accounts are based upon reports made by a single naval medical officer who, by coincidence, happened to be senior medical officer of each of the ships which were so affected.*

H.M.S. PHOEBE

H.M.S. *Phoebe* was hit by a U-boat torpedo at 0750 hours on Friday, October 23, 1942, at a point six miles off Pointe Noire, in French Equatorial Africa. The weather was calm, but a heavy rainstorm was in progress at the time.

The torpedo hit on the port side and damaged and flooded compartments across the whole width of the ship. The compartments particularly affected were the port provision room, the CO_2 machine compartment, the switchboard room, the three cold storage meat rooms and the armament store. Above these spaces two messdecks were holed. That is to say, a number of compartments was damaged which could have been the source of noxious fumes which escaped into living spaces overhead. The explosion of the torpedo was followed by an immediate column of smoke which was noticed to be particularly yellow. It was very acrid and choking.

Within a short space of time the ship had taken on a list to port and was considerably down by the bow. However, damage control was successful and the ship was able to enter harbour three hours later.

A first hand account of the presence of fumes following the explosion is given in the words of one seaman:

'I was standing by the meat room hatch. There was a loud bang and I saw a column of bright brown smoke rising. In the split second before the lights went out this column seemed to be about 6 ft. high. I did not realise that we had been hit until I felt water over my ankles. The lights came on again and the messdeck was then full of choking smoke. I ran up the ladder and found that the alleyway above was also full of smoke. At the top of the ladder I saw a scuttle and I ran to it, put my head out and took several gulps of air before climbing through it on to the upper deck.'

Seven bodies were removed from this man's messdeck, and it is interesting to note that he did not remember feeling any blast. Other men climbed out of the scuttles in the Marines' messdeck. It was soon realised that men were being gassed there, but rescue was almost impossible, and it was some time before the smoke had cleared

---

* Passing reference to noxious fumes has been made in the case of a number of other ships, but not in any detail or in connexion with casualties of any great magnitude.

sufficiently for bodies to be recovered. It was observed that a small number of men put on anti-gas respirators and appeared to escape without any ill effects.

Thirteen men died on the Marines' messdeck. It was decided to bury them at sea almost immediately, so that no more than a very perfunctory examination could be carried out. None of these men showed any visible or palpable injury. There was no definite evidence that carbon-monoxide had been a major factor, as their colour was on the whole blue rather than pink, and all were dribbling bloodstained froth from their mouths and noses, which seemed to indicate intense and immediate pulmonary irritation. It was observed that dependent parts became discoloured a remarkably short time after death. Post-mortem staining around their necks was noticeable.

Within about an hour of the explosion, bodies began to be recovered from elsewhere in the ship. But all of these showed signs of gross physical injury, so that it was impossible to attribute their deaths merely to the effects of gas poisoning of some kind. About 90 minutes after the torpedo had struck many men began to report complaining that they found difficulty in breathing. They were all cyanosed in varying degrees. New cases continued to report for a period of 16 hours after the explosion. In these cases the delayed action was most marked, as all these men, after some initial choking at the beginning, had recovered and had performed many hours of hard work before the symptoms proper began to be noticed.

In all 64 cases were treated, and from this series it was possible to divide their progress into the following stages:

(1) Initial choking, retching and vomiting. Recovery from this stage was more or less rapid.
(2) The latent period, lasting up to 16 hours after exposure to the gas. During this period the patient felt quite well apart from slight nausea in some cases. The longer the latent period, the better the prognosis.
(3) A period of apathy, occupying the last hour or so of the latent period.
(4) Cyanosis, with difficulty in breathing and a feeling of pectoral constriction. This started in the upper chest and gradually spread to the lung bases.
(5) Onset of the classical symptoms of pulmonary oedema, with painful spasmodic cough, production of bloodstained frothy sputum and vomiting after each paroxysm of coughing. This stage showed increasing restlessness and apprehension, particularly when it became known to the patient that other men had already died from the condition. Some patients now passed from a state of blue to grey asphyxia.
(6) A quieter period, in which the physical signs became more gross, the sputum increased, the respirations became more gasping and the heart began to fail.

(7) This stage was of two types. More usually, patients who had been remarkably clear minded became comatose, and this coma deepened until death. But in a proportion of cases a stage of cerebral irritation ensued followed by death in about 30 minutes. Only one case recovered after passing into Stage 6.

Eighteen of these patients died. The remainder recovered fairly quickly. It is of interest that during the following weeks other men reported with vague symptoms of difficulty in breathing. Some of these men were obviously merely suffering from anxiety symptoms, but 3 men did develop cough with some evidence of bronchial spasm.

At the time of onset it was only possible to give an opinion that all these men had been affected by some form of choking gas. It was not until much later, after damage had been inspected and combined with clinical data, that any decision could be reached in relation to the type of gas involved and its probable source. The conclusions reached were recorded by the Senior Medical Officer as follows:

(1) Carbon-monoxide, chlorine, phosgene and nitric and nitrous fumes were considered in turn. The compartments damaged and their contents, as well as the nature of the explosion, made it necessary to take each of these gases into account.

(2) Carbon-monoxide, chlorine and phosgene were eliminated on investigation and it was established that the casualties were caused by gassing by nitric and nitrous fumes.

(3) As regards the source of these fumes it was considered unnecessary to look further than the actual explosion of the torpedo itself, combined with a cordite fire which took hold in one of the adjacent magazine compartments.

Further clinical observations of value which were made by the Senior Medical Officer were:

(1) At the time, it was impossible to do more than treat cases symptomatically.

(2) Owing to the high degree of bronchial and alveolar irritation, and probable actual destruction of lung tissue, not all the maxims normally applicable to pulmonary oedema could be operated in these cases.

(3) Oxygen was valuable. Adrenalin and atropine were of doubtful value since the irritation was too intense to allow them to deal effectively with the amount of fluid exuded into the lungs. The most valuable drug was morphine.

(4) It is doubtful if the value of venesection was as high in these cases as it would have been in cases of pulmonary oedema without gross irritation or destruction of lung tissues.

(5) In a proportion of cases there was a terminal stage resembling cerebral irritation. This raises the question as to a possible central nervous effect of nitric and nitrous acids.

(6) As well as a clinical picture resembling that of phosgene poisoning, there was an immediate form simulating chlorine poisoning.

(7) With one exception, once the full syndrome of pulmonary oedema was established, the case went on to a fatal termination.

(8) As regards the aftermath, one of the difficulties was the psychological effect of these cases upon the remainder of the ship's company.

H.M.S. ALBATROSS

H.M.S. *Albatross* was damaged by an underwater explosion at 0650 hours on August 11, 1944, while lying in the anchorage of the British Assault Area, off Courseulles, Normandy. The sea was calm, there was no wind, and later there was hot sunshine which undoubtedly helped in the treatment of shock. The explosion was heavy and the ship was holed forward on the port side. Two messdecks and storerooms below took the main force of the explosion. The time was unfortunate in that the messdecks were crowded with men, many of whom were still in their hammocks.

The area involved was immediately filled with a dense grey white smoke which spread at once to adjacent compartments. This gas smelt of nitrous fumes, and it is considered that the symptoms and signs produced by exposure to it could all be attributed to nitrous fumes and carbon-monoxide.

Sixty-two casualties were treated of whom 4 died before evacuation. Two other bodies were recovered immediately. Sixty-one men were missing of whom only 58 were recovered from the messdecks a week later. Of the casualties treated and the bodies recovered, very few showed any signs of physical injury. All the casualties however were shocked, and showed signs of having been gassed. The course and progress of the affection was not quite so clear cut as in the case of the *Phoebe's* casualties. Nevertheless, the various stages were all recognisable.

Undoubtedly the concentration of fumes was not so high as in the case of the *Phoebe*, and after five or six hours only a small proportion of the cases were showing frank pulmonary oedema. Not one man reported sick after a latent period following his exposure to the gas. Owing to the fact that all the casualties were evacuated from the ship within seven hours, the progress of cases could not be observed in full. Also, the number of casualties made observation and recording difficult. In the case of the *Albatross* there was more flooding than in the *Phoebe* disaster. This meant that partial drowning confused the clinical picture in some cases. But, undoubtedly, in most cases, particularly in those killed, the three factors which were at work in varying degrees were blast, gas and water.

In the cases terminating in death the stages which were passed through were:

(1) Initial choking and vomiting.
(2) A period of comparative well-being.

(3) A short period of depression and apathy.
(4) Onset of pulmonary oedema with blue asphyxia and right sided congestion.
(5) Grey asphyxia with cardiac failure.
(6) A terminal period of cerebral irritation.
(7) Death.

Of the 58 casualties discharged from the ship 57 passed through two or more of these stages. Many other men not discharged as casualties, and including practically every member of the rescue parties, experienced symptoms of stage 1 to some degree. Stage 2 was not clearly defined owing to the effects of carbon-monoxide. There was very little 'well-being', and the vast majority remained shocked and weak after stage 1 had passed off. Most of these men were decidedly pink in colour and no case at this stage could have been said to have been cyanosed. Owing to the modified form of stage 2, the apathy of stage 3 was not always perceptible. Stage 4 was beginning in a few cases before they were evacuated.

In the *Albatross* disaster stage 6 was an early sign in several cases. Four men needed a great deal of physical restraint even after large doses of morphine. This early feature is considered to have been due probably to early anoxaemia consequent upon carbon-monoxide poisoning.

With his experience in the *Phoebe* behind him, the Senior Medical Officer of the *Albatross* regarded rest as the first essential in these gassed cases. Every man who showed any sign of stage 1 was made to lie down and to continue resting despite his protests that he felt better. Every man brought out of damaged compartments was so treated.

Large numbers of casualties from the involved messdecks were wet from the incoming sea, and this increased the shock which was fairly severe in most cases. This shock was combated by five or more blankets per patient and hot drinks. Morphine was given to the majority of patients, but was withheld in cases in which depression of respiration was considered to outweigh the usual advantages. Oxygen could only be given to the most severe cases owing to lack of apparatus. Atropine and adrenalin were not given on this occasion. The majority of these patients had to be left exposed on the upper deck which did at least ensure the maximum amount of fresh air which they so obviously required.

In the case of the *Albatross* the visible gas was a dense, grey white cloud, smelling of nitrous fumes and other products of an explosion. This was in marked contrast to the cloud of gas in *Phoebe* which was of an orange brown colour. In both his reports the Medical Officer concerned has discussed at length the chemistry of nitrous fumes produced by an explosion, and of importance is his quotation from the Torpedo Manual of the Royal Navy, which states that T.N.T. exploding under water produces 32·7 per cent. of nitrous fumes. In the case of the *Albatross* there was no evidence that any further lethal gases, other than carbon-monoxide were produced. But in the case of the *Phoebe* disaster there did seem to be evidence that cordite burning in one of the magazines added quantities of nitrogen peroxide to the gases of the explosion itself. This is of interest in view of the fact that in the case of the *Albatross*, all ammunition and charges in a nearby magazine were found to be intact and so cannot have made any addition to the fumes produced by the explosion.

In the case of the *Albatross*, investigation was made into the possibility of carbon tetra-chloride, which might have generated phosgene, or of any other gas-producing substance being stowed in the involved area, but this line of enquiry was unproductive. It is also of interest to note that cigarettes remained palatable to those who had been subjected to the fumes which, it was considered, would not have been the case had phosgene been present. However, in the *Albatross* a 'Foamite' machine was damaged by the explosion and immediately produced large quantities of foam. Many casualties were covered with this foam, and there seems no doubt that a certain quantity of CO_2 was liberated, but it must be remembered that no case was cyanotic when brought out of the damaged spaces. The Medical Officer took pains to record that as 'Foamite' contains only hexamine and molasses, presumably, even in a combination with products of the explosion, the 'Foamite' could not have played a part in producing a lethal gas. It will be seen therefore, that prolonged investigation once again led to the conclusion that in the *Albatross*, as in the case of the *Phoebe*, nitrous fumes with the possible addition of carbon-monoxide were responsible for the majority of the casualties which occurred.

In concluding this subject, the Medical Officer has furnished a number of miscellaneous details which are of undoubted interest both from the physical and psychological viewpoints:

(1) In the *Phoebe* at least a dozen men in the involved messdecks saved their lives by having their anti-gas respirators at hand and by putting them on immediately. In the *Albatross* no man is known to have used his respirator.

(2) In the *Phoebe* several men escaped through scuttles. In the *Albatross* only one man escaped in this way and was later picked up from the sea. But another man who tried to follow him did so as the ship listed further, and he was pushed back by an inrush of water.

(3) An officer of the *Albatross*, for some days beforehand, had had a premonition that something was about to happen to the ship which would radically alter her programme. At first he placed this future happening as likely to occur 'in a few days'. He then narrowed it down to 'within 48 hours'. During the evening prior to the explosion this officer was so obsessed with the idea that he could

not stop talking about it. At 1800 his presentiment was one of a disaster, and he did not sleep that night, having forecast that 'it would happen' within about 12 hours. In point of fact the damage to the *Albatross* occurred after 12 hours and 50 minutes!

(4) A stoker of the *Albatross*, who always slept on one of the messdecks involved in the explosion, had a dream a week beforehand. In his dream a torpedo hit the ship in that particular position. In consequence the man moved his sleeping billet after which he stoutly maintained, with some justification, that he owed his life to having done so!

(5) The *Albatross* was brought hurriedly out of reserve in May 1944. At that time the ship was badly infested with rats, so much so that it was commonplace for most officers to see them frequently about their cabins at night, and they were also plentiful on the messdecks. The *Albatross* was damaged early on the morning of August 11. During the evening of August 10, as part of the usual sea-going routine, watertight doors were closed throughout the ship, including those leading from the messdecks which were damaged by the explosion a few hours later. It is on record that when these latter doors were closed, large numbers of rats attempted to escape through them from the messdeck. It would seem that these animals scratched and fought at the doors in order to try to get through and that when chased away they returned again and again to their efforts!

In relation to these miscellaneous items, the Medical Officer stated in his report:

'These stories are, I know, similar to many others which are heard after any event, and the last two became current only after the explosion. However, I can myself vouch for the authenticity of the presentiment of the officer which, even if lacking in scientific principles, is at least of interest.'

H.M.S. STEVENSTONE

H.M.S. *Stevenstone* was on patrol off Flushing on the evening of November 30, 1944. At 1822 hours she was struck by an enemy mine. The ship did not sink, and was eventually escorted to Sheerness where she arrived twenty-four hours later.

When the *Stevenstone* was struck, the ship seemed momentarily to lift out of the water, after which she started to settle by the bow. The explosion had occurred in the forward half of the ship and immediate investigation showed that the main effects had been felt under the stokers' messdeck. The whole fore part of the ship was at once filled with fumes of oil and cordite, but, fortunately, the lights continued to function so that it was possible quickly to appreciate the extent of the damage. The after part of the messdeck concerned was found to be full of casualties, numbering about 30. Some of these men were in considerable pain, were foaming at the mouth and finding great difficulty in breathing. Others appeared to be deeply unconscious and seemed partially asphyxiated. As fast as possible the accessible casualties were removed and placed on the upper deck. Owing to the presence of noxious fumes of some kind removal of these men was difficult. It was not possible to stay down in the messdeck for more than a few seconds without being overcome by these fumes. The Medical Officer and several rescuers attempted to remain longer on the messdeck, but they were themselves quickly rendered unconscious in the process. When there was no further sign of life on the messdeck, which was already flooding, and when the water level had risen to near the hatch, the order was given to batten down the hatch, thereby isolating the affected messdeck from the rest of the ship.

A muster of the ship's company now showed that 14 men were missing and 18 incapacitated. As regards the latter, the ship's Medical Officer recorded:

> 'Several stokers coming out of the flooding messdeck fell unconscious at the top of the hatch. I arranged for casualties to be moved into the fresh air, and many of those who had been brought out unconscious soon began to recover. Those who were physically wounded had only suffered superficially. The unconscious state of these men had obviously been caused by fumes of some kind. After an hour all but 18 men had recovered sufficiently to be able to carry on by themselves. Among the 18 remaining, 3 men became very violent while recovering consciousness and had to be given morphine in order to restrain them. In all these men the clinical picture was roughly as follows:
>
> (1) When first seen the patient was deeply unconscious and ashen grey in appearance. All reflexes were absent. The pulse was thin and rapid and the rate 120. Respirations were very shallow and at a rate of 40.
> (2) After 15 minutes the respirations had returned to normal, the pulse was stronger and had fallen to 90. The general condition had improved and colour was returning. The man could be roused, albeit with difficulty.
> (3) After 30 minutes there was some mental confusion, complete disorientation, and active resistance to any physical interference.
> (4) After 1 hour the mental state seemed normal and the man could easily be roused. But headache and vomiting were severe, and were followed by deep, natural sleep.
> (5) After 24 hours there seemed to be no after effects.'

The Medical Officer rightly considered that the general picture presented by these unconscious men was similar to any case of surgical anaesthesia carried to a deep level. His conclusion was that these men had been poisoned by fumes of methyl chloride, the source of which was probably damage to the ship's refrigeration system. When first reported, his conclusions were doubted by some authorities, mainly, it would seem, on two grounds:

(1) The fact that no post-mortem examination was ever conducted on seven bodies later recovered from the affected messdeck, and
(2) Absence of that lachrymation which, it was considered, would certainly have been present had the poisoning been due to fumes of methyl chloride.

However, quite apart from the view of the Medical Officer, the opinion of the *Stevenstone's* Commanding Officer was quite definite in his official report of the incident in which he stated:

'Undoubtedly some of the deaths occurred through men becoming unconscious on the messdeck through the escape of methyl chloride gas from the ship's damaged refrigerator plant. One or two breaths were probably sufficient to render these men unconscious, after which they were drowned by the inrush of sea water. All who managed to get to the top of the hatch did so as they were about to be overcome by the gas. A few others were rescued, while unconscious, just before they would have been drowned by the rising water.'

In a later paragraph of his report the Commanding Officer gives the following most interesting account of the fortunate survival and escape of a stoker who was left behind on the messdeck while unconscious:

'About two hours after the distorted hatch to the messdeck had been closed, shouting was heard. It seemed that one of those overcome by gas had survived. The clips of the hatch were eased back to test for water pressure and then the hatch was lifted. A stoker was found standing at the top of the ladder under the hatch with his head and shoulders just above the level of the water. He could give little explanation about what had happened, except that at the time of the explosion he was sitting on a table at the forward end of the messdeck. He would seem at once to have been gassed, after which he must have fallen back unconscious on the messdeck table. The table itself was wrenched from its fittings by the explosion. With the unconscious stoker upon it it must have floated to the small space between the water and the deckhead above, where it remained. As the fumes cleared the unconscious stoker recovered and he was eventually awakened by the noise of hammering by damage control parties overhead. He then found himself under the hatch and started to shout.'

This account of the mining of H.M.S. *Stevenstone* may best be concluded by an official report made to the Admiralty on January 18, 1945, which reads:

'H.M.S. *Stevenstone* has now entered dry dock. On examination of the ship's refrigeration compartment it was found that the bulkhead was split, and that the pipes containing methyl chloride were fractured. This would have resulted in the damaged messdeck becoming filled with this gas.'

THE LOSS OF THE RESCUE SHIP PINTO

During 1944 the work of escorting convoys of merchant ships across the Atlantic continued to be a heavy burden for the Royal Navy. Outstanding work also continued to be performed by the rescue ships attached to these convoys.

On August 27, 1944, a convoy of 97 vessels left Halifax. The rescue ship attached to this convoy was the M.V. *Pinto*. Nothing unusual occurred until 0510 hours on September 8, when the S.S. *Empire Heritage* was sunk by a U-boat torpedo. The *Pinto* at once altered course to rescue survivors of the *Empire Heritage*. The ship itself had sunk, but many life-jacket lights could be seen flashing in the sea, so the *Pinto* stopped, lowered a boat, dropped her scrambling nets and prepared to receive survivors on board. Two survivors had actually been received when the rescue operations were interrupted by an alarm that a submarine's periscope had been sighted a short distance away. The periscope was obviously that of a U-boat which passed close ahead of the *Pinto* and through the wreckage and rafts from the *Empire Heritage*. The *Pinto* was quite prepared to engage this U-boat with her 12-pounder gun, but it was impossible to do this because of the danger of shells falling among the many survivors in the water. Almost immediately the U-boat fired a torpedo which struck the *Pinto* on the starboard side directly under the bridge. The engine room was flooded immediately, the mainmast collapsed, the ship took a heavy list to starboard and sank, stern first, within a few minutes. At the time of the explosion the *Pinto* was lowering a rescue basket over the starboard side with a seaman in it to assist the survivors on board. This seaman was not seen again.

Of her crew of 62 the *Pinto* lost 21 who went down with the ship. Those lost included her Master and Chief Engineer. Also lost were the two survivors of the *Empire Heritage* who had just been taken from the sea. The survivors of the *Pinto* were picked up by H.M.S. *Northern Wave* about two hours later. In his official report the senior surviving officer of the *Pinto* recorded that:

> 'Our doctor did magnificent work for the survivors. Although he was trapped under the shrouds of the foremast as the ship sank and was consequently badly shaken, he continued to attend to the wounded on board the *Northern Wave* for some hours, without even stopping to change into dry clothing. His unselfish action set a very fine example.'*

The *Pinto's* medical staff consisted of a naval medical officer and 2 sick berth attendants. The following report of the Medical Officer is

---

* The *Pinto's* Medical Officer, a surgeon lieutenant, R.N.V.R., was mentioned in dispatches for his outstanding conduct on this occasion.

considered worthy of a place in this History as a tribute to the gallant work of convoy rescue ships as a whole:

'I was awakened by the sound of an explosion and the ringing of the ship's alarms. I mustered my S.B.As. and learned that the *Empire Heritage* had been torpedoed. In accordance with our routine I sent the senior S.B.A. away in the rescue boat when it was lowered so that he could render immediate first aid to survivors picked up by the boat. The other S.B.A. helped me to prepare the ship's hospital for the reception of casualties.

'Many lights could be seen blinking in the water, and the rescue boat had started to pick up men. Others were beginning to attempt to come aboard by the scrambling nets. But it was very dark and the hauling up of survivors was difficult, and only two men were completely aboard before we ourselves were sunk. These men were uninjured.

'I was making my way to the ship's hospital and had got to a point near the coal locker when there was a rushing noise which blended into a tremendous explosive crash. The ship shuddered and the whole deck seemed to jump up. Smoke and water were all around and much of the ship's superstructure seemed to be disintegrated. I was flung against the rails and was temporarily dazed by large quantities of debris, including a considerable amount of coal, which landed on my head and back. I tried to locate the S.B.A. and could hear his voice from somewhere outside. The ship was already heeling over and water was rushing along the alleyway. I went in to make sure that the hospital was clear and then went to report to the Master. I found him standing outside the entrance to his cabin shouting to men to get over the side. Some were getting into the dinghy which was slung overboard. I next went down the ladder to have another look round and the ship then seemed to make a sudden drop. I was now standing on the deck up to my waist in water and I was then carried down a long way and became jammed against the rigging. When I got free I began to rise and on reaching the surface I found that the ship had gone.

'When I surfaced I saw three rafts full of men, and when I had recovered my breath I managed to swim to one of them. The rafts kept fairly close together but the sea was getting rough and kept drenching us.

'I cannot say how long it was before we were picked up, but I should think about two hours. My watch had stopped. It began to get light quite quickly and we heard an aircraft overhead. Later on H.M.S. *Northern Wave* appeared and picked up survivors with great difficulty as the seas were very heavy. Our raft was the fourth to be cleared and it was amazing that there were not further casualties during the manoeuvre of getting aboard.

'Once aboard I was told that there were some casualties needing attention in the *Northern Wave's* sick bay. I was pleased to see my senior S.B.A. already aboard and found him assisting the S.B.A. of the *Northern Wave* to look after the wounded. My junior S.B.A. had been in the alleyway almost directly above the torpedo when it struck the *Pinto*. But somehow he managed to escape, and he too turned up on board the *Northern Wave* about half an hour later. I was thus fortunate to have three sick berth ratings to assist me.

'There were 10 hospital cases in all, largely Merchant Navy personnel. I landed them at Londonderry where we were met by the Port Medical Officer.'

The Normandy Landings

Reference has already been made in this History to naval medical co-operation with the other Services in the various operations which aimed at the liberation of Northern Europe, in June 1944.*

In attempting to give any historical account of the part played by the Royal Naval Medical Service in the Normandy landings and the events which followed these landings, it is first necessary to emphasise that naval medical commitments should be kept in their proper perspective. That is to say that the work done by naval doctors and nurses, though valuable, should not be exaggerated. In fact, it must be remembered that the part played by the Navy was a relatively minor rôle in a vast medical operational organisation which was essentially a far greater Army commitment once the initial stages had been passed.

THE SEABORNE EVACUATION OF CASUALTIES

The Senior Naval Medical Officer who served on the Staff of the Allied Naval Forces Commander on this occasion has himself given a broad account of what was involved, as follows:

'†For such a vast operation, the naval medical commitments fell roughly into two categories, one relatively static and the other mobile. In the first category, which involved naval forces lying off the enemy beaches, were included all the bombarding ships, the protecting destroyers, the depot ships, and the minesweeping flotillas which moved in the area. In the second category were the personnel ships and the Landing Ship (Tanks), which were constantly in transit across the Channel.

'As regards the first category, it was an extraordinary sight to see a hundred and more ships of all sizes anchored off the coast, and spread out as if for some mammoth review. On the British front the assault had been made on three beaches, designated from East to West as "Sword", "Juno" and "Gold". The ships and landing craft had been subjected to shelling, there were constant incidents through ships striking mines, and in addition, the ordinary risks had to be considered of weather which had not been uniformly favourable. Casualties which occurred among these off-shore ships were either ferried inshore to join the main casualty evacuation stream, or else were sent direct to a hospital fitted L.S.T. which was

---

* *See* Volume I, Chapters 9 and 14.
† Extracted from a Paper read by Surgeon Captain W. B. D. Miller, D.S.C., R.N.V.R., at an Inter-Allied Conference on War Medicine, organised by the Royal Society of Medicine on October 2, 1944.

shortly due to leave the area. The depot ships had accommodation for upwards of fifty cot cases apiece. But early evacuation from these depot ships was always desirable as unfortunately the shipping casualties were rather heavy in the early stages. This off-shore medical commitment operated by itself and, though several times extended, was never oppressed.

'The greater interest was focused on the second category, because this represented the medium through which the bulk of the seaborne evacuation of casualties had to be effected. Up to this stage in the war such evacuation of casualties had always been one of the biggest problems when considering future amphibious warfare. To surmount the problem much careful planning had been carried out by all three branches of the British Services with the assistance of the United States. Staff Officers had held many meetings, numerous experiments had been conducted, and we had pooled our knowledge to one common end.

'For the British sector 70 L.S.Ts. had been fitted for casualty evacuation; 40 of these were medically manned by the Royal Navy and 30 by the Royal Army Medical Corps. (*See* Plate XVIII).

'Briefly, the modifications made to a L.S.T. to render it suitable for medical requirements consisted of adjustable racks to carry three tiers of stretchers on either side of the tank deck. The tank deck accommodation itself allowed 144 stretchers to be placed there. Previous experience of these craft at Anzio had demonstrated that stretchers laid on the tank deck were quite acceptable for a relatively short journey, and when suitably arranged they gave ready access for nursing attention. On the other hand the troop spaces in these ships were difficult of access, but they were quite suitable for walking wounded and could accommodate upwards of 150 patients.

'At the after end of the tank deck a small dressing station was constructed out of canvas over a light tubular steel framework of dimensions 18 ft. × 8 ft. × 8 ft. The dressing station was fitted with heating, additional lighting, drainage, and a hot and cold water supply.

'These medically fitted landing craft had been supplied with drugs and equipment on a basis devised by the consulting surgeons to the three Services. In addition, adequate replenishments were prepared and waiting at the various disembarkation points in the United Kingdom.

'It was not considered feasible for these particular craft to be beached, far less to dry out, so preliminary training aimed at casualties being transferred to them from smaller craft and D.U.K.W. However, in practice, it was found that these craft dried out very quickly, which made the direct loading of casualties relatively simple.

'At the shore end of the operation a naval medical liaison officer was appointed to each beach whose task was to effect the smooth working of the evacuation of casualties. But at the end of the first week, the D.D.M.S., Second Army, decided to canalise all the evacuation of casualties through the centre beachhead. This greatly simplified matters because, by then, it was realised that it was impossible to guarantee that medically manned landing craft would be available at each tide at all three beachheads. The establishing of the Army's Central Casualty Evacuation Point, with a holding capacity of upwards of 1,000 beds, solved this difficulty.

'A further important line of evacuation of casualties was the hospital carrier. Naturally in many ways these ships were infinitely better than the rapidly converted L.S.T. Nevertheless their accommodation for patients was frequently limited, and they suffered from the added disadvantage that, at all events to begin with, there were no quays or wharves alongside which they could lie and load. However, once the Casualty Evacuation Point had been established, ambulance convoys were organised from it to the small harbour of Courseulles. When the tide was favourable these casualties were then carried to the hospital carriers by L.C.P.(S). The latter were Landing Craft Personnel (Small), designed to be hoisted at ordinary ship's davits. The dimensions of these craft were 28 ft. long × 8 ft. 6 in. beam, of shallow draught, 6 in. forward and 1 ft. 9 in. aft. Each was powered by a Chrysler Crown 30-h.p. engine. These L.C.P.(S) were modified to carry six stretcher cases and ten walking wounded. The crew consisted of 3 Merchant Navy seamen and 1 R.A.M.C. orderly. When fully loaded with casualties and crew the craft could be hoisted to the deck level of the hospital carrier. These L.C.P.(S) were admirable in fair weather but they were apt to bump alarmingly in a moderate swell which also made them difficult to hoist into the parent ship. (*See* Plate XIX).

'The D.U.K.W. was also used to load hospital carriers but this meant stretcher cases being hauled through the sally-port of the carrier, which was always a hazardous procedure if any kind of sea was running.

'Landing Craft Tanks (L.C.T.) were also used to load casualties into hospital carriers. These craft varied from 108 ft. to 191 ft. in length, with an open deck. The difficulty with them was that individual slinging of cot cases into the carrier was necessary, and this tended to be a lengthy process even when carried out by well-trained personnel.

'But in spite of the difficulties involved, the hospital carrier mode of evacuating casualties did have the tremendous advantage that the carrier could disembark alongside in Southampton directly into a hospital train.

'Fortunately, many of the problems of casualty evacuation, particularly that of speed, were soon solved by the use of Dakota aircraft which, operating from the airstrip at Banville, were capable of carrying eighteen stretcher and six walking cases apiece.

'Perhaps the greatest difficulties encountered by the Navy in evacuating casualties from the beaches were the natural elements of tides, weather and darkness. Though predictable, tides did create difficulty in that time schedules of evacuation had to be varied in advance each 24 hours, and once fixed, had to be rigidly adhered to. In this respect the slightest delay might ultimately lead to the loss of a tide and the complete dissolution of the plans for that particular evacuation.

'The weather was something which could never be predicted with accuracy. This is not meant to refer to bad weather of severe magnitude, but merely to the existence of mild breezes, a shallow swell or a choppy sea surface, all of which factors could cause acute discomfort to wounded personnel, and could make their transfer by sea in small craft extremely difficult if not actually hazardous.

'Darkness was an element which could not be solved because each beach had soft patches and holes in unexpected places. Illumination of the beaches was impracticable and also unsafe in view of enemy aircraft, and L.S.T. could only be illuminated by faint blue lights. The result was that any attempts to carry out casualty evacuation by sea at night had to be abandoned.'

It is of interest that, some months after the landings, the Staff Medical Officer gave it as his opinion that:

'The task was greatly facilitated by the intimate integration of all the Services from the early planning stages onwards and, on the transport side, by those three modern developments, the D.U.K.W., the Dakota and the Landing Ship Tank.'

It would be impossible, in the space available, to record in this History every medical incident which arose during the Normandy landings. Instead, an attempt to give the reader some idea of the various events has been made by recording sample reports extracted from those of the great number of ships which took part in the diverse phases of the operation.

THE NAVAL OFF-SHORE FORCE

Some idea of the events which concerned the off-shore naval units is given in the official report of the Senior Medical Officer[*] of H.M.S. *Scylla*, flagship of the Naval Commander of the Eastern Task Force.[†]

'The *Scylla* supported the Normandy landings between June 5 and June 23, 1944.

'During this period the health of the ship's company was extremely good. Only one illness of major importance occurred, which was a severe haematemesis in a seaman under treatment for symptoms suggesting peptic ulcer. The chief complaint among personnel was lack of sleep, due to the constant high degree of readiness for action and damage control which had to be maintained.

'Accommodation on board was extremely overcrowded, particularly after a large number of additional personnel, including those of the Army and R.A.F., had joined the ship. Over the period, an average number of 94 officers and 750 ratings was victualled on board each day, this figure representing an increase of 25 per cent. over the normal ship's company.

'It is noteworthy that prior to D-day, a large number of trivial, and sometimes imaginary complaints were reported, prompted perhaps by a general anxiety for the future and the stress of an impending operation of great magnitude. But the number of men attending for advice fell considerably once the operation had started, and minor complaints seemed to be forgotten in the general excitement of events. Three known cases of well-developed anxiety state gave no trouble during the operation and, in fact, emerged with a newly acquired confidence in their ability to work and live under such conditions in the same way as their more robust shipmates.

---

[*] The late Surgeon Lieutenant Commander G. D. Channell, R.N.V.R., who was mentioned in dispatches for his outstanding conduct during the course of these operations.

[†] Rear Admiral, now Admiral of the Fleet, Sir Philip Vian, G.C.B., K.B.E.

'In the early phases the *Scylla* herself suffered no damage or casualties, so that for all practical purposes our medical organisation functioned as that of a reception centre to deal with casualties and sick brought to us from elsewhere.

'After the loss of H.M.S. *Lawford*, 106 survivors were accommodated, 7 of whom were wounded; 3 M.T.B. ratings, killed in action, were received on board and buried from the ship, as was the body of an officer of the Royal Canadian Air Force which was recovered from the sea; 15 other serious casualties were dealt with on board and were received from all three Services.

'On June 23, the *Scylla* herself struck a mine, the explosion taking place just aft of midships. There were 11 casualties, 3 moderately serious and 8 of a minor nature. In the sick bay a number of bottles were broken and their contents scattered in all directions. In the main medical distributing station a methyl chloride container in a domestic refrigerator was damaged. This damage released a large quantity of methyl chloride gas which rendered the station temporarily untenable. But once the gas was cleared from the area, the station was able to function again with all its facilities unimpaired.*

'The casualties were easily treated in the ship's sick bay, without using either of the auxiliary dressing stations or any of the first-aid posts. It is of interest that the portable X-ray machine, though severely shaken and well within the area affected by the explosion, suffered no damage.

'During the period under review, one soldier was received on board from the M.T. *Samnesse*, with a 24 hour history of abdominal pain and nausea. His condition was diagnosed as acute appendicitis. Operation was undertaken on board and a gangrenous appendix was removed. This patient made a good recovery and remained on board until the *Scylla* managed to make her way back to England in her damaged state, after which he was discharged to the Royal Naval Hospital, Chatham.'

The cruiser *Belfast* was also involved in numerous medical incidents between June 5 and July 8, 1944.

When it became known that this ship was to take part in the assaults on the French coast, her medical organisation was reviewed in relation to the probability of prolonged periods having to be spent at action stations. All her medical stores and equipment were brought up to full strength and were dispersed between the two medical distributing stations and five first-aid posts throughout the ship. Steps were taken to make sure that every man in the ship was aware of the position of the first-aid post nearest to his action station. Nine officers in different parts of the ship were given supplies of tubunic ampoules of omnopon, and were instructed in their use.

On June 6 the ship took part in the initial bombardment of the Normandy coast. She was engaged by shore batteries in reply, but suffered no casualties. During the day calls for medical assistance were

---

* *See* the account of the mining of H.M.S. *Stevenstone*, in this Chapter.

received from a number of landing craft which had sustained casualties in the landings. Seven Army casualties were received on board from landing craft and were treated and transferred to H.M.S. *Orion* for passage to the United Kingdom. Two of these men died within a few hours and were buried at sea from the *Orion*.

On June 8, a landing craft was engaged on the dangerous task of transporting a cargo of German landmines from the beach in order to jettison them in the sea. In the course of this operation the mines detonated and the craft sank a short distance away from the *Belfast*. Three of her crew were lost and the remainder were brought on board the *Belfast* where they were treated.

On June 9, the anchorage was attacked by German aircraft. A number of bombs fell near the *Belfast* but she sustained no damage or casualties. However, her Senior Medical Officer recorded that:

'Several ratings sustained minor injuries in their hurry to take cover!'

On June 22, casualties were received in the *Belfast* from a damaged minesweeper, and on June 24, 14 casualties were brought on board from H.M.S. *Swift* which was mined and sunk nearby. On the same day a casualty was received on board from a neighbouring merchant ship which had been hit by a shell from a shore battery. All these casualties were transferred to medically equipped landing craft for passage to the United Kingdom.

On June 30, the *Belfast* herself was hit on the port side by fragments of shrapnel and sustained 3 casualties.

This period spent off the Normandy coast proved most strenuous for the ship's company of the *Belfast*. For some twenty days they were in a sustained degree of readiness for action, sleeping in their clothes, and at their action stations. In any case very little sleep could ever be obtained as the ship was exposed to enemy air attack, to desultory shelling from the shore, to the danger of mines, and to the prospect of attacks by U-boat and E-boat. However, the fact that the ship herself carried out periodic bombardments of the enemy coast did much to maintain the morale of the ship's company at a high level despite the discomforts.

As regards specific discomforts, one of the most trying features of this period was the restricted ventilation below decks which was necessitated by rigid damage control measures with a view to the safety of the ship herself.

Apart from the many medical incidents which arose from circumstances of action, the records of the *Belfast* show that on June 19, 1944, a stoker came under treatment suffering from diphtheria. Under the very adverse conditions existing on board this patient was isolated and treated with anti-diphtheritic serum. He developed a mild palatal palsy. Unfortunately, owing to heavy seas, it was five days before he could be transferred to another ship for passage to the United Kingdom. He eventually made a complete recovery.

At 2315 hours on June 24, 1944, H.M.S. *Nith* was bombed while serving with the off-shore force. Extra interest was added by the fact that not only was the ship herself struck by a bomb of the anti-personnel type, but at the same moment the German aircraft which had released the bomb crashed and exploded alongside. Nine seamen were killed outright and 17 were wounded, 7 seriously. The explosion caused temporary failure of both main and secondary lighting, so that measures of first aid and resuscitation had to be effected by torchlight.

The ship herself remained afloat and all her wounded had been dealt with by 0300 hours on June 25. A medically equipped landing craft was then asked for and at 0730 hours the U.S.S. *L.S.T.* 336 was made available, and the casualties were transferred to her in an American coastguard cutter.

THE NAVAL ESCORTING FORCE

The type of incident in which units of the naval escorts for the landings were likely to find themselves involved is illustrated by the following extract from a report of the Medical Officer of H.M.S. *Wrestler*:

'The *Wrestler* left Portsmouth at 2100 on June 5 in company with the naval escort to a force of landing craft.

'I slept until 0500 on June 6. I was busy deciphering in the sick bay when, at 0637, there was the heavy concussion of an underwater explosion.

'The sick bay was completely wrecked, all cupboards and drawers were overthrown and all bottles were smashed. The lights went out, and the door was blown in, and I could see nothing through dense smoke. I had one seaman sick in a cot with German measles. He was stunned by a blow on the head by a deck-head beam. He quickly recovered, so I put his lifebelt on him and pushed him out on to the forecastle.

'I left the sick bay and tried to get along the starboard alley, but fire was so fierce in the area that any hope of rescuing possible casualties had to be abandoned.'

Thirty casualties in this ship suffered severe burns. Such burns were known to be uncommon from the flash of exploding mines detonating under water. However, subsequent investigation showed that the mine explosion had detonated cordite and a certain amount of ammunition in the ship's forward magazine. The bulkheads and deck-head of the magazine were shattered, and it was considered that the cases of burns were actually caused by the exploding cordite.

In view of these cases of burns, particularly at this relatively late stage of the war afloat, it is of tragic interest to record a further extract from the Medical Officer's report in which he states:

'In spite of ceaseless propaganda from myself and the ship's executive officers, none of the severely burned men was, at the time of the explosion, wearing anti-flash gear. The majority of these men had worn this gear during the night but had removed it when their breakfast was served at 0630. One casualty himself volunteered the statement:

"I took it off, Sir, in spite of what you always said, because it was difficult to eat and drink with it on. But this has taught me a lesson which I shall never forget." '

EVACUATION OF CASUALTIES BY LANDING CRAFT

The following report of the Senior Medical Officer of H.M. *L.S.T.* 363 illustrates the work performed by medically equipped and manned landing craft during the period of the Normandy landings:

'The period covered by this report is from D-day to June 30th, 1944.

'The complete staff had joined only five days before D-day, and a great deal had to be done to evolve an efficient medical organisation. We had to use our own initiative as, unfortunately, the official Army publication for our guidance was not received on board until the day after the operation had commenced.*

'Fortunately one surgeon lieutenant had been on board for three weeks and had done much useful work in obtaining stocks of sterile dressings and towels. In spite of repeated demands, the D.U.K.W. ramp was not forthcoming from the local dockyard. However, in due course the ship's Christchurch ramps proved excellent for unloading the D.U.K.Ws.

'We found it necessary to make further small structural additions and modifications to the medical arrangements already provided. For example, our shipwright made two small tables for the operating theatre. These tables were fitted with "fiddles",† and were secured to the pipes in the operating theatre and they proved most useful and safe as instrument tables. They were indeed appreciated on our fourth voyage when the weather was very rough and 279 casualties had been embarked.

'Our ship's engineers provided securing bolts for trestles in the operating theatre. We also found it necessary to arrange for additional lighting in the operating theatre because a L.S.T. has no secondary lighting circuit. However, an adequate supply of battery lamps was made available, and these were put to good use particularly on our fourth voyage, when the main light failed while an amputation was in progress.

'We found it helpful to sew large canvas pockets on the insides of the operating theatre's screens. These proved most useful for holding bandages, wool and non-sterile dressings, which could not spill in rough weather.

'On the whole our basic medical equipment and stores proved excellent. On our first journey we found it necessary to apply a large number of plasters. It was also necessary to replace some plasters which had been hastily applied elsewhere. This meant that our supplies of plaster-of-paris were soon depleted, and for a time had to be replenished from private

---

* The reference here appears to be to ' Instructions to Medical Officers Manning L.S.T.'

† A device whereby a raised edge can be fitted to a table in a ship, so that in rough weather articles placed on the table are prevented from sliding off it.

sources. We also found a need for a larger number of self-retaining catheters and 8 in. haemostats.

'As regards cold storage space, our engineer officer kindly placed a complete refrigerator room at our disposal. Here we were able to store our blood, plasma, sera and penicillin. This was a most essential requirement because in a L.S.T. the temperature cannot be automatically regulated, so that if other ships' stores are in the same refrigerator room as medical stores, the coming and going of supply personnel cause undesirable changes in temperature from time to time. To begin with we had assumed that our refrigerator room would remain at an even temperature of around 40° F. But what we did not realise was that it was necessary constantly to watch the temperature dial on the outside of the refrigerator, and to regulate the valve which controlled the inside temperature. Our ignorance of this led to the deterioration of one complete batch of blood. From then onwards a S.B.A. was kept constantly on watch at the indicator and valve.

'As regards the conversion of the tank deck for medical use, we always found that we had ample time to do this while the vehicles themselves were being disembarked. On all our journeys we were ready to receive casualties long before they arrived.

'On our first visit to Normandy our casualties arrived by D.U.K.W., three at a time. Each D.U.K.W. drained for thirty seconds on the ramp before entering the tank deck, and we found that very little water was taken on board. On subsequent journeys the method of loading casualties varied, and sometimes D.U.K.Ws. were used and sometimes ambulances which unloaded at our bow doors. There seemed no doubt that when the ship was beached, loading by D.U.K.W. was considerably quicker than by ambulance. We found, too, that casualties seemed to stand the rough journey by D.U.K.W. remarkably well.

'Naturally, with experience our loading time improved, and on our last trip we embarked 279 casualties in exactly two hours. Only on one journey did we have to carry stretchers on deck. On this occasion our 150 stretcher racks were filled, which meant that 38 deck stretchers had to be accommodated. However, these patients fared extremely well and, although the weather was rough, we did not find it necessary to secure these deck stretchers in any way.

'The time during which our casualties were retained on board for the cross Channel journey varied from trip to trip. Our first batch of casualties were on board for thirty hours, the second twenty-six hours, but the fourth only fourteen hours. This latter great reduction in time was the result of improved unloading facilities at our point of disembarkation in the United Kingdom. On this occasion an Army surgical specialist was present to assist in assessing the transportability of the casualties and in directing their transfer to special centres.* On most occasions the turn round period in the United Kingdom was brief and our needs were rapidly met by the local naval medical officer-in-charge of replenishment units.

---

* The many reports of naval medical officers serving in L.S.T. are unanimous in describing the disembarkation arrangements of the Royal Army Medical Corps as 'excellent'.—Editor.

'As regards resuscitation of casualties on board, our efforts proved lifesaving on several occasions. We used whole blood and plasma in about equal amounts. One case of serious haemorrhage from a compound fracture of femur was moribund on arrival, but he was completely revived after four pints of whole blood, followed by ligation of the bleeding vessels and application of plaster. We found the small rubber bulbs included in the ship's American-stocked sick bay most valuable in accelerating blood transfusion. In one case of very serious haemorrhage transfusions thus accelerated were given into both arms simultaneously.

'Surgery on board was performed under pentothal anaesthesia and was reserved for urgent cases only. The need for operation fell steadily with succeeding voyages, largely due to the fact that the Royal Army Medical Corps' facilities for dealing with casualties on the far shore became more established. Twenty operations were performed on our first journey. Most of these were compound fractures of the lower extremities, though one case was a compound fracture of skull. Eighteen operations were performed on the second journey and included compound fractures and one penetrating wound of abdomen. On the fourth journey only seven operations were performed, two of which were amputations. The total number of operations performed on board was 45.

'During the period under review we were exposed to sporadic bombing and shelling on the beaches, and to some E-boat activity while at sea. Fortunately our few psychiatric cases carried seemed oblivious of such encounters with the enemy, having been liberally dosed with phenobarbitone before embarkation.

'Our experience of transporting casualties across the Channel by L.S.T. showed that the welfare of wounded does not depend merely upon doctors and clinical procedures. We found that the goodwill of the ship's officers and crew went far towards assisting us in our task. In this respect, good nursing and adequate victualling were of importance. For instance the casualties of our first journey had not had solid food for more than 24 hours when we received them, and the cases embarked on our second journey had starved for three days. In dealing with these men we received the utmost co-operation from our ship's galley staff, and all our casualties who were permitted to eat had soon received a satisfying hot meal.

'H.M. *L.S.T.* 363 made five round voyages in all and carried altogether 560 casualties. All these casualties were transported in the course of three voyages, the ship returning empty on two occasions. The numbers transported were as follows:

First Voyage
- Cot cases . . . 112
- Walking cases . . 73

Total 185

Second Voyage
- Cot cases . . . 84
- Walking cases . . 12

Total 96

Fourth Voyage
    Cot cases .   . 188
    Walking cases   . 91

                             Total   279

'There were three deaths on board. All three cases were moribund on arrival and failed to respond to measures of resuscitation.'

Study of further reports of medical officers attached to medically equipped landing craft reveals other matters of interest worthy of inclusion in this History. For example, it was the unanimous opinion that the morale among Army wounded was of the highest order. However, one medical officer recorded that he found a number of paratroops most despondent. This was due to the fact that after a long and arduous training, they had been eliminated, without ever firing a shot, because of injuries due to accidents on landing. Also unanimous was the view that the initial treatment of casualties on shore, under conditions of exceptional difficulty, reflected the greatest credit on Army doctors and nursing staff. As regards anaesthetics for operations carried out on cross Channel journeys, pentothal would seem to have been the anaesthetic of choice. Although large quantities of ether and chloroform had been provided, no medical officer found their use a practical proposition.*

Some medical officers remarked on difficulties associated with the provision of urine bottles and bedpans. For example:

'As soon as the casualties came on board there was a general request for a bottle or receptacle into which they could micturate. This had been foreseen to some extent, and a fair number of utensils was available. But what had not been foreseen was the difficulty which was experienced in very many cases in getting severely wounded stretcher patients into a position in which this could be done. It was practically a whole time job for several men, during the whole night, to attend to this need. In some cases there was difficulty in providing a bedpan at short notice. Some of the men with severe back and buttock wounds had a terrific desire to defecate, and it was surprisingly troublesome to arrange for them to do this.'

Adverse criticism by naval medical officers is scanty save in one respect, reference to which has already been made in this Volume.† Complaints revolved chiefly around the fact that medical officers were appointed for duty in landing craft only a few days before the operation

---

* *See* Chapter 1 of this Volume. The inclusion of ether in the stores of these craft is puzzling at this stage in the war. Anaesthetic ether had already been largely eliminated from most men-of-war, some of whose Commanding Officers adhered rigidly to the principle that unless of vital necessity, all material likely to provide a source of fire should be dumped overboard before going into action. In many ships this rule was even made to apply to 'pocket cigarette lighters', the use of which was prohibited by implication.—Editor.

† *See* Chapter 4 of this Volume.

was due to commence. The same short period applied in the case of sick berth staff, which meant that there was little if any opportunity for preparation or training of any kind. For example, one senior medical officer reported:

> 'Some recently qualified medical officers obviously lacked experience in dealing with casualties. This is difficult to remedy, but a few lectures in naval barracks, while newly joined and awaiting first appointments, from persons with actual experience of action stations would have been far more valuable than the handbooks which were provided. It is important for the authorities to realise that active service medicine and surgery is not part of the teaching curriculum in civilian hospitals.'

In addition many medical officers complained bitterly that they had been inadequately 'briefed' and had no definite knowledge of the overall medical arrangements in force for the operation. Some went so far as to suggest that it was most fortunate that the casualty rate was generally low, the implication being that, had it been of great magnitude, the ignorance of medical officers concerning the general organisation for the reception and evacuation of casualties might have led to grave difficulties.

MEDICAL ORGANISATION OF THE PORT PARTIES*

Details of the naval medical organisation in occupied ports are conspicuous only by their absence in Admiralty records. This lack of documentation may well be due to the rather unsettled atmosphere surrounding an invading force, as well as to the administrative inexperience of many of the medical officers serving in the Royal Navy at this period of the war.

Fortunately however, the Senior Medical Officer of Port Party No. 1500 was an officer possessing great capabilities, not the least of which was his realisation of the importance of maintaining documentation on an efficient working basis, even in circumstances of action. The result was that meticulous records were forwarded to the Admiralty, which permit the story to be followed of the building up of the medical organisation in what was, at least for a time, the most important supply port connected with the Normandy landings.

Port Party No. 1500 was assembled in the United Kingdom, at Barnet, in April 1944. The party there carried out the preliminary training required for its future function which, at that time, was not definitely known to the bulk of its members. The medical staff consisted of 2 medical officers and 5 sick berth ratings. A month before the Senior Medical Officer had undergone a course in Military Sanitation and Field Hygiene at Mychett.

---

* Largely compiled from the records of Surgeon Commander J. Carlton, R.N., who later became Staff Medical Officer to Flag Officer, Schleswig-Holstein.

During the training period at Barnet, all members of the party were inoculated against typhoid and typhus, and vaccinated against smallpox. Frequent lectures and first-aid demonstrations were given, and particular stress was laid on teaching cooks and stewards the elementary principles of field hygiene. Exercises included Field Days, both by day and by night, the local Home Guard co-operating in the latter. During these exercises personnel were given the opportunity of dealing with casualties under conditions of land warfare which were strange to the Navy.

A special group of men was trained in advanced principles of first aid and field sanitation. The members of this group were attached to the Hygiene Medical Officer, and a time came when many of them acted independently and achieved a very high standard of efficiency. In point of fact, this particular phase of training obviously proved to be of paramount importance, as during the course of the operations ahead men were embarked upon detached duties where they had to apply the principles of sanitation and hygiene without the supervision of a doctor.

In one of his early reports, the Senior Medical Officer emphasises the fact that, as regards this training period, he obtained the wholehearted co-operation of the Commanding Officer of the Party and also from the Commanding Officer of the Royal Marine Detachment. In his own words:

> 'Their personal interest and co-operation with me were always unfailing in securing the maximum medical welfare for their Commands.'

As soon as the liberation of Europe was imminent, the prime function of Party No. 1500 was revealed, which was to assist in the building of the prefabricated port of Arromanches, and to operate it on its completion.

The main party, with the Senior Medical Officer and 4 sick berth ratings, was carried from the United Kingdom in H.M.S. *Despatch*. The remaining medical members were embarked in H.M.S. *Aristocrat*. The function of the latter was to remain in Arromanches waters where the planting of blockships and caissons was directed. The medical stores allocated to the party were divided between the two medical officers, care being taken that each had sufficient equipment to act independently in the event of one or the other becoming a casualty, or allowing for the loss of equipment. Kit bags, plainly marked with a red cross, were filled with emergency first-aid supplies, sterilisers, instruments, drugs and sera. These bags were distributed among the various landing parties, each of which had a sick berth attendant attached to it. Selected officers were given tubunic ampoules of morphine, together with detailed instruction for their use.

The main party, with the Senior Medical Officer, disembarked and waded through the water on to the beaches of Arromanches on the evening of D-day+2. Fighting was going on just outside the village, where the Army was pushing back and destroying pockets of enemy resistance. Medical stores were got ashore as rapidly as possible by man-handling, and a sick bay was established in the cellar of a house. Within the shortest possible time a first-aid post had been established and the Army Medical Officer of the Arromanches sector gave assistance in dealing with the casualties of the party which, miraculously, were negligible. With nightfall enemy aircraft attacked Arromanches but fortunately most of the bombs fell clear of the personnel of the party. On the following day naval reinforcements were landed and the task of establishing a prefabricated naval base was begun.

While the work of building the prefabricated harbour was in progress, increasing numbers of naval personnel were landed, and the next problem became the establishing of a central Naval Headquarters, with its attendant auxiliaries of billets, signal station, fire station and sick bay. As many of the local habitations had been destroyed by bombing, a great deal of improvisation became necessary. The future expansion and development of the Naval Party had been foreseen, and it soon became obvious that this measure would have to be undertaken. A house, in fairly good condition, was selected as a sick bay and these premises were rapidly equipped, opportunities being taken during lulls in the enemy attacks to land the more bulky equipment such as bedding, medical chests and reserve stores. Emergency lighting was provided by means of accumulators, and a small operating theatre was equipped.

In a distant part of Arromanches an emergency first-aid post and dressing station was established in an underground cellar under the control of the junior medical officer. Here reserve medical stores were stowed. Part of yet another house was used for the accommodation of yet a third reserve of medical stores which now were considered to have been distributed adequately as a precaution against damage. Routes to the sick bay were clearly signposted at various points on the beaches and in the village.

Meanwhile, while these preparations were being made, sanitation had been catered for by constructing deep trench latrines, and measures had been taken to control the water supply by constant supervision and super-chlorination. When it became possible to foresee that a naval base would have to be developed at Arromanches on a permanent basis, plans were put into operation for the construction and consolidation of a permanent camp site. The Senior Medical Officer was at once co-opted in order to advise on the hygiene and sanitation aspects of such planning and building. Several Nissen huts were erected, and a large recreation hall was built with an annexe for rest rooms, canteens, etc. During this planning phase great attention was paid to cooking, drainage, and bathing facilities, and hot and cold running water was installed whenever possible. Roads were constructed inside the camp area, and the main drainage of the area was connected up with the town drainage system after the latter had been repaired and made to function efficiently by the discharge of effluent into the sea. Heating was arranged by installing coal burning stoves. When the camp was eventually completed it proved a most efficient and comfortable accommodation for the large numbers borne which, as time passed, came to include W.R.N.S. personnel for whom separate medical arrangements were made.

One of the major medical commitments of the port of Arromanches was that of dealing with the large numbers of survivors who were constantly landed after the loss of their ships by enemy action, particularly after mining disasters. As a result of close and harmonious liaison with the Army, adequate ambulance transport and hospital accommodation were always available for the survivors. Wounded personnel were sent directly to hospital to be cared for by the Army. Uninjured personnel were looked after by the Navy locally in a separate Naval Reception Camp, where they could be accommodated until arrangements had been made for their return to the United Kingdom. In due course a prominent feature of the Arromanches area was the Normandy Fleet Club, which was established a few miles away at Ryes. This Fleet Club became a rest and recreation centre in which officers and men could be accommodated away from the immediate surroundings of the port and from their numerous small ships and craft in Arromanches harbour.

After six months, the Senior Medical Officer of Port Party No. 1500 was in a position to submit a number of remarks for Admiralty consideration. These remarks, which were most valuable and constructive in their nature, were listed as follows:

(1) *Training*

Where possible, a far longer time should be given to the formation of Port Parties so as to ensure constant practice and exercising in field hygiene and the medical requirements of land warfare. In particular, all medical personnel, including doctors and sick berth staff, should receive a full course of military hygiene at an Army Hygiene School.

(2) *Medical Stores and Equipment*

Where these are to be landed on open beaches by carriers and handlers who have to wade through water, they should not be packaged in large packing cases. Instead, medical stores and equipment should be packed in boxes and panniers of a standard suitable size which can easily be carried. The scale of contents of such standard containers should be carefully worked out, and there should be drastic abolition of many of those unnecessary articles which have come to be included by custom but which, in fact, are hardly ever used and are largely outmoded. Those containers intended for immediate use on landing should contain sterile dressings, bandages, sera, minor instruments, pentothal, and an abundance of morphia, these being the articles most constantly used at the beginning. The containers themselves should be provided with a type of handle which causes the minimum of discomfort to the carrier, and they should not have rope handles, which abrade the hands and cause unnecessary fatigue. It is also of importance that the lid of the container should not be screwed down, but should be readily detachable so that the contents may be accessible within the shortest possible time.

The landing of more bulky medical equipment should be delayed until such time as the particular beachhead has been finally and permanently established.

The planned equipment should include a portable generator which would make a medical centre on shore completely independent of other forms of auxiliary lighting. An X-ray apparatus should also be included.

(3) *Transport of Casualties*

The War Office type of stretcher was found to be cumbersome, heavy and exhausting to carry over rough beaches. Its replacement by the American light, steel frame pattern stretcher is strongly recommended.

Despite the high degree of liaison and co-operation with the Army Medical Authorities, it would nevertheless be of value that the Navy should be provided with its own ambulances, thus eliminating constant reliance on the Army for medical road transport.

(4) *Hospitals*

In any major operation, where large numbers of naval personnel become involved, both afloat and ashore, serious consideration should be given to the establishment of either a separate naval hospital or at least to the establishment of naval casualty clearing stations. The temporary attachment of a naval hospital ship was never found to be a satisfactory alternative owing to the risk of damage by enemy action in congested waters. Also such a hospital ship means the added complication of boat work which may be embarrassed by bad weather and the state of tides.*

(5) *Secrecy of planning*†

As has been frequently recorded in the Administration and

---

* This Senior Medical Officer took pains to emphasise that these recommendations in his reports were not meant to reflect adversely on Army hospitals, 'whose courtesy, consideration and unfailing help were always placed at the disposal of the Royal Navy'.

† *See ante.*

Operational Volumes of the Royal Naval Medical History of the War, the constant complaint of naval medical officers was that they were excluded from the main picture of events. No less than his colleagues in the Royal Naval Medical Service, the Senior Medical Officer of Port Party No. 1500 has recorded similar views in his recommendation which reads:

'It is fully realised that in all intended naval and military operations, secrecy is absolutely essential and vital but this principle of secrecy can be carried too far. This is particularly so when officers, whose special departments are expected to play a major part in the success of an enterprise, are not fully informed of the object for which they have to plan. My own experience of the Normandy landings was that I had to make repeated requests before I could be fully informed of my responsibilities and future commitments. By contrast, my Army opposite numbers, with whom I was in daily consultation in combining our mutual medical welfare, were always possessed of full information about what lay ahead'.

NAVAL MEDICAL ORGANISATION FOR THE RECEPTION OF CASUALTIES IN THE UNITED KINGDOM*

Although the treatment of casualties from the Normandy landings was largely a Civilian and Army commitment, in many cases their actual reception in the United Kingdom, before onward transit elsewhere, was a task performed by the Royal Navy. To organise the reception of an unknown, but possibly large influx of such casualties, meant that the particular naval port involved had to develop not only an efficient organisation for receiving them, but also a complete reorganisation of the internal domestic naval medical arrangements of the area.

In the Portsmouth area, early in 1944, a programme was secretly promulgated with a view to revising the local domestic medical arrangements of the port on a future date, as yet unknown. The basic elements of these revised arrangements were that in order to provide accommodation for urgent casualties arriving from the Continent, local Service hospital routine would fall into abeyance, which meant that local Service establishments must make provision for holding and treating their own sick as far as possible.

The organisation laid down that the usual routine of reception in the Royal Naval Hospital, Haslar, of hospital cases from naval establishments for treatment, consultations, medical boards, etc., would be suspended. At the same time routine pulmographic examinations were to fall into abeyance in the port.

---

* Compiled in part from the records of the late Surgeon Captain E. St. G. S. Goodwin, R.N.

Naval establishments in the Portsmouth area were to make arrangements to accommodate and treat all cases not requiring urgent hospital or specialist treatment. It was realised that this might mean additional, improvised accommodation for local naval sick, on the assumption that it might be necessary to hold such cases for an indefinite period pending the cessation of the expected flow of Normandy casualties through the port.

With a view to mutual medical aid and assistance, naval establishments in the Portsmouth and Gosport areas were grouped into three Sectors as follows:

Sector A

This extended from Portsmouth to Bedhampton, and included the Royal Naval Barracks, H.M. Dockyard, miscellaneous naval units inside Portsmouth itself, the Royal Marine Barracks, Eastney, and establishments at Stamshaw, Belmont, Stockheath and Hayling Island.

As regards Service personnel in these places, during the expected period of emergency, only serious casualties and urgent hospital cases would be admitted to local hospitals.

Within Sector A the Principal Medical Officer of the Royal Naval Barracks, Portsmouth, would act as Co-ordinating Officer, and would be responsible for issuing local instructions and orders as necessary to cover medical aid and assistance within the area.

Sector B

This extended over Gosport, Lee-on-Solent and Fareham, and included the Submarine Depot in H.M.S. *Dolphin*, the Coastal Forces Depot in H.M.S. *Hornet*, a number of ancillary dockyard establishments, the Royal Naval Air Station, Lee-on-Solent, the Training Centre H.M.S. *Collingwood*, and a large number of miscellaneous naval units.

As in the case of Sector A, only serious and urgent cases were to be accepted by local hospitals. The Co-ordinating Officer for this Sector was to be the Medical Officer-in-Charge of the Royal Naval Hospital, Haslar.

Sector C

This covered naval establishments not already included in the arrangements for Sectors A and B. Such establishments were situated in outlying districts, and they were to make arrangements with their nearest local hospitals for the reception of serious and urgent cases, it being emphasised that such cases from these districts were on no account to be sent into either the Portsmouth or Gosport areas during the period of the pending operation.

These arrangements were intended to apply to all naval personnel including those of the W.R.N.S.

Special arrangements for the disposal of cases of infectious disease were evolved for all three Sectors. As regards diphtheria, scarlet fever and C.S.M., cases from Sector A were to be sent to Milton Infectious Diseases Hospital, those from Sector B to Haslar, and those from Sector C to local isolation hospitals. As regards cases of chicken pox, measles, mumps and rubella, these were to be isolated and treated by their own establishments. In addition, the usual rigid Service precautions for the control of contacts of infectious diseases were greatly modified, and although such men were to be examined daily by a medical officer, quarantine was not to be observed in the absence of a definite epidemic of some kind.

As regards the actual reception of casualties from Normandy at the port of Portsmouth, the arrangements were planned by the Principal Medical Officer of the Royal Naval Barracks, in accordance with his function as Co-ordinating Officer of Sector A.*

This officer found the planning of what was likely to be involved far from easy. Although he had been warned, as far back as January 1944, that he should make preparations for certain eventualities, he received no further definite information of what was likely to be required from him until April 3. He was then informed that he would be responsible for the reception of casualties arriving in Portsmouth Dockyard, and that he must achieve mutual medical co-operation for the ultimate disposal of these casualties with the Army and Civilian Medical Services.

Although the official view was that it was unlikely that any large number of casualties would be landed in Portsmouth Dockyard, the Co-ordinating Officer allowed for a large influx, and acted promptly. Three senior naval medical officers were detailed to take charge of the disembarkation of casualties and six junior naval medical officers, each with two sick berth ratings, were held in readiness. Contact was made with the Army Medical Services, and especially with the Assistant Director of Medical Services, Fareham, and the Officer Commanding 'B' Company, 207 Field Ambulance, Clarence Barracks, Portsmouth.

On June 3, 1944, a conference was held at the Royal Naval Barracks, Portsmouth, and was attended by the Assistant Director of Medical Services (Evacuation). At this conference a plan of disembarkation of casualties was discussed, and a general scheme was agreed for the classification of organised and unorganised casualties into Port Cases and Transit Cases. Details of documentation and checking at the gangways were formulated.

It was decided that Port Cases, i.e., casualties so urgently in need of treatment as to require immediate hospital attention, would be diverted

---

* *See* footnote on page 318 of Volume I.

either to the Royal Naval Hospital, Haslar, or to local E.M.S. Hospitals. Transit Cases, i.e. those of less urgency, would be transferred at once to ambulance trains. But should train accommodation not be immediately available, these Transit Cases would be sent to a holding depot at the Advance Dressing Station, Clarence Barracks, or alternatively to the Queen Alexandra Hospital, Cosham, or possibly to the naval sick bay established at Portsmouth Grammar School.

Also at this conference, the discussion allowed for the possibility that during the period for which the arrangements were being made, enemy air activity might be heavy over the port of Portsmouth itself. This might mean that the holding of casualties owing to delay in evacuation might present a formidable problem. With such a prospect in view, another local Portsmouth school was sited, and also the gymnasium of the local naval Physical Training Establishment. The Army undertook to provide the necessary nursing staffs should such a contingency arise.

Meanwhile, in connexion with the actual landing of casualties in H.M. Dockyard, the Co-ordinating Officer established a Central Control Office. The planning conceived that messages regarding the arrival of ships and craft carrying casualties would be received through the Captain of the Dockyard or the King's Harbour Master. It was anticipated that thirty minutes' warning would then be given to the Central Control Office, the function of which was to transmit the information to the various port departments likely to be concerned. For example, the Co-ordinating Officer, Senior Medical Officers of Medical Parties, and the A.D.M.S. (Evacuation) were to be informed immediately, as was the local Senior Naval Stores Officer, whose task it was to control the provision of stretchers and bedding, and also to supervise the allocation of vehicles from the local Ambulance Pool.

The system put into practice was that once the ship or craft came alongside, a Boarding Medical Officer checked the number of her casualties. Should the cases be unorganised they were then classified by the Boarding Medical Officer as Port Cases or Transit Cases.

Walking cases for transit were sent ashore first and accommodated for transport in buses. These buses, which were under the direction of a R.A.M.C. officer on the jetty, conveyed these walking casualties to either Clarence Barracks or the Queen Alexandra Hospital, Cosham.

The next to be landed were seriously wounded Port Cases, who were sent at once to port hospitals.

Following on this the remainder of the stretcher cases were landed and sent to the Transit Hospital at Cosham. However, where warning was received that the number of stretcher cases for transit was large, they were sent direct to Fratton Station (Southsea), where a hospital train was provided by the Army.

In actual practice it was found desirable for an Army Surgical Specialist to be present on the arrival of casualties in any great number. Apart from his assistance in classifying casualties in order of priority, experience proved that occasional cases showed signs of gas gangrene, which necessitated them being diverted into a local port hospital. In addition, experience prompted the immediate admission of cases of head injury into the Portsmouth Royal Hospital.

The actual handling of casualties from landing craft arriving in Portsmouth Dockyard was based upon mutual co-operation between the Naval and Army Medical Services which worked most smoothly in practice. For example, in L.S.T., casualties were carried by the ships' army stretcher-bearers to the lifts, where they were then taken over by naval parties and brought to the upper deck, 17 cases at a time. From the upper deck the naval parties would transfer the stretchers to the jetty where they would be taken over by army stretcher-bearers for shipment into ambulances. Meanwhile the ships' stretcher-bearers would be gathering further cases into the lifts, thus avoiding delay.

In addition to his organisation for the actual reception of casualties, the Co-ordinating Officer was responsible for the replenishment of depleted medical stores and equipment in all ships entering Portsmouth harbour, which he did from local naval sources.

THE CASUALTIES—PORTSMOUTH AREA

Following the Normandy landings, casualties were received in H.M. Dockyard, Portsmouth, in the following numbers, between 0800 hours on one day and 0800 hours on the day following:

	Wounded	*Dead*
June 6–7	6	
June 7–8	35	
June 8–9	1	6
June 9–10	27	
June 10–11	615	
June 11–12	297	2
June 12–13	444	7
June 13–14	297	2
June 14–15	613	1
June 15–16	162	6
June 16–17	14	1
June 17–18	Nil	
June 18–19	138	
June 19–20	311	
June 20–21	Nil	
June 21–22	Nil	
June 22–23	Nil	
June 23–24	Nil	
June 24–25	48	
June 25–26	232	
June 26–27	523	
June 27–28	523	

		Wounded	Dead
June 28–29		177	
June 29–30		18	
Total for the month of June 1944	Wounded	4,471	
	Dead	25	
	Total	4,496	

From the end of June 1944, casualties were recorded, according to time, ship and place of landing as follows:

Date	Time	Ship	Place	Casualties
June 30–July 1	0805	L.S.T.80	South Railway Jetty	279
June 30–July 1	0805	L.S.T.423	,, ,, ,,	117
July 1–2	2250	L.S.T.236	,, ,, ,,	380
July 2–3	2315	L.S.T.367	Pitch House Jetty	282
July 3–4				Nil
July 4–5	2020	L.S.T.324	South Railway Jetty	209
	0150	L.S.T.212	,, ,, ,,	129
July 5–6	1830	L.S.T.367	,, ,, ,,	125
July 6–7	0940	L.S.T.(?)	,, ,, ,,	131
	0645	H.M.S. *Stevenstone*,,	,, ,,	12
Total casualties up to week ending July 7				6,160
July 7–8	1005	H.M.S. *Burdock*	South Railway Jetty	14
	2050	L.S.T.324	,, ,, ,,	199
July 8–9	2015	L.S.T.365	,, ,, ,,	131
July 9–10	2000	L.S.T.62	,, ,, ,,	226
July 10–11	0940	L.S.T.363	,, ,, ,,	230
	2130	L.S.T.9	,, ,, ,,	226
	0530	L.S.T.239	,, ,, ,,	129
July 11–12	2225	L.S.T.415	,, ,, ,,	2
	2225	L.S.T.430	,, ,, ,,	122
July 12–13	1950	L.S.T.361	,, ,, ,,	402
	0250	L.S.T.324	,, ,, ,,	150
July 13–14	1955	L.S.T.9	,, ,, ,,	248
Total casualties up to week ending July 14				8,239*
July 14–15	2215	L.S.T.425	South Railway Jetty	146
July 15–16				Nil
July 16–17				Nil
July 17–18				Nil
July 18–19	1830	L.S.T.180	South Railway Jetty	244
	2245	Frigate	Buoy at Spithead	9
July 19–20	2045	L.S.T.322	South Railway Jetty	291
	2045	L.S.T.163	,, ,, ,,	273
July 20–21				Nil
Total casualties up to week ending July 21				9,202†

* Including 29 German prisoners-of-war.   † Including 42 German prisoners-of-war.

July 21–22	0845	L.S.T.430	South Railway Jetty		334
	2000	L.S.T.427	,,	,, ,,	429
July 22–23	0905	L.S.T.365	,,	,, ,,	181
	1945	L.S.T.367	,,	,, ,,	297
	0400	L.S.T.364	,,	,, ,,	272
July 23–24	0755	H.M.S. *Minico*	At Spithead		1
	0855	H.M.S. *Forester*	Asia Pontoon		9
	2000	L.S.T.164	South Railway Jetty		224
July 24–25					Nil
July 25–26					Nil
July 26–27	0800	L.S.T.164	South Railway Jetty		225
July 27–28	0850	H.M.S. *Talybent*	Asia Pontoon		18
Total casualties up to week ending July 28 .					11,192*†
July 28–29	1955	L.S.T.419	South Railway Jetty		109
	1955	L.S.T.423	,,	,, ,,	129
July 29–30	0840	L.S.T.65	,,	,, ,,	43
	1400	H.M.S. *Talybent*	At Spithead		3
	1830	H.M.S. *Chalmer*	Asia Pontoon		23
	2105	L.S.T.425	South Railway Jetty		68
July 30–31					Nil
July 31–August 1	2215	L.S.T.302	,,	,, ,,	126
August 1–2					Nil
August 2–3					Nil
August 3–4	2020	L.S.T.239	,,	,, ,,	248
	2020	L.S.T.302	,,	,, ,,	120
Total casualties up to week ending August 4 .					12,061§‡

At this point a Progress Report was made by the Co-ordinating Officer, and it is of some interest to record that this report would seem to have been prompted owing to the mistaken impression in the Department of the Medical Director-General of the Navy that the flow of casualties into Portsmouth harbour had ceased, or in any event was no longer a local naval medical reception commitment. Thus, at the commencement of his report, the Co-ordinating Officer drew attention to the fact that the flow and disembarkation of casualties had by no means ceased to be a naval medical commitment, neither did there seem to be any prospect of cessation for an indefinite period.

This report also makes it obvious that the unexplained lack of appreciation of the local situation by the Admiralty had led to a number of medical officers being appointed away from the Portsmouth area at a time when their presence was necessary, a procedure which must undoubtedly have affected the reception organisation of the Co-ordinating Officer.

---

* Including 136 German prisoners-of-war. † Including 5 dead.
‡ Including 13 German prisoners-of-war. § Including 3 dead.

The report makes mention of the smooth working and close co-operation established with the Army Medical Services and expresses appreciation of the valuable assistance of all ranks of the Royal Army Medical Corps with the reception and rapid disposal of casualties.

Mention is also made of the valuable support rendered by naval dental officers of the Royal Naval Barracks, Portsmouth, and tribute is paid to the sick berth and W.R.N.S. clerical staff of the barracks whose task was to maintain accurate records.

It is considered of interest to record extracts from this report which indicate that even some five weeks after the Normandy landings, the normal internal domestic medical arrangements of the port of Portsmouth were still in abeyance. In this respect the Co-ordinating Officer stated:

> 'Co-ordination of the internal domestic arrangements inside the port still proves to be a pressing problem, and pulmographic examinations, specialists' consultations and medical boards are greatly in arrears. A constant and close liaison has had to be maintained with the medical officers of local naval establishments and with the Superintendents of the various E.M.S. Hospitals. It is most essential that the extra accommodation for the sick locally should be retained time being, particularly as considerable provision has had to be made for isolation of cases of chicken-pox and mumps. Accommodation of such cases has also been complicated by the fact that a number of W.R.N.S. has been affected.'

That the burden of responsibility carried by the Co-ordinating Officer and his staff in Portsmouth was by no means quickly eased, is shown from the following statistics for August 1944:

				Casualties
August 4–5	1950	L.S.T.402	South Railway Jetty	218
August 5–6				Nil
August 6–7	1955	L.S.T.239	Pitch House Jetty	272
August 7–8				Nil
August 8–9	2110	L.S.T.324	,, ,, ,,	112
August 9–10	0604	L.S.T.302	,, ,, ,,	225
	0604	L.S.T.268	,, ,, ,,	268
August 10–11	2215	L.S.T.364	,, ,, ,,	281
	2215	L.S.T.415	,, ,, ,,	287
Total casualties up to week ending August 11 . .				13,724*
August 11–12				Nil
August 12–13	1420	L.S.T.428	South Railway Jetty	152
August 13–14				Nil
August 14–15	1830	H.M.S. *Saumarez* Asia Pontoon		4
August 15–16				Nil
August 16–17	1710	L.S.T.320	South Railway Jetty	154
	1710	L.S.T.160	,, ,, ,,	153

---

* Including 92 German prisoners-of-war.

August 17–18	1835	L.S.T.329	South Railway Jetty		287
	1835	L.S.T.80	,, ,, ,,		245
Total casualties up to week ending August 18 .				.	14,719*
August 18–19	1820	L.S.T.405	South Railway Jetty		241
	1820	L.S.T.420	,, ,, ,,		217
August 19–20	1945	L.S.T.304	,, ,, ,,		228
	1945	L.S.T.363	,, ,, ,,		218
August 20–21					Nil
August 21–22					Nil
August 22–23	0850	L.S.T.361	,, ,, ,,		91
	2045	L.S.T.180	,, ,, ,,		252
	2045	L.S.T.367	,, ,, ,,		162
August 23–24	2105	L.S.T.324	,, ,, ,,		206
	2105	L.S.T.304	,, ,, ,,		159
	2105	L.S.T.363	,, ,, ,,		74
August 24–25	1720	L.S.T.239	,, ,, ,,		208
	1720	L.S.T.408	,, ,, ,,		220
Total casualties up to week ending August 25 .				.	16,995†
August 25–26	1815	L.S.T.367	South Railway Jetty		209
August 26–27					Nil
August 27–28					Nil
August 28–29	0850	L.S.T.363	,, ,, ,,		334
August 29–30					Nil
August 30–31					Nil
August 31–September 1					Nil
Total casualties up to week ending September 1				.	17,538‡

However, the flow of casualties into Portsmouth declined very rapidly at the beginning of September 1944, as is shown in the following figures:

			Casualties
September 1–2			Nil
September 2–3			Nil
September 3–4			Nil
September 4–5			Nil
September 5–6			Nil
September 6–7	1250	H.M.S. *Middleton* Asia Pontoon	7
September 7–8			Nil
Total casualties up to week ending September 8		.	17,545§

---

* Including 82 German prisoners-of-war.
† Including 598 German prisoners-of-war.
‡ Including 482 German prisoners-of-war.
§ Including 1 dead.

From then onwards the port of Portsmouth ceased to be a major reception centre for casualties from the Continent, and the local domestic medical organisation gradually reverted to normal.

In his final Progress Report the Co-ordinating Officer again pays tribute to the valuable work of his local naval medical and dental officers and sick berth staff, and again emphasises the close degree of co-operation and mutual support which was achieved with the Royal Army Medical Corps.

In his comments he mentions one unforeseen factor which arose during the reception of casualties, which was that on occasions medical officers and parties had to be sent out to Spithead and the Solent in order to deal with casualties which they frequently found had been removed elsewhere on the instructions of another medical authority by the time they arrived! However, study of records shows that here there was no true duplication of effort, and such a situation need not have arisen had the Co-ordinating Officer adhered rigidly to his original plan which was that the scope of the casualty clearing organisation at Portsmouth was not intended to include casualties other than those actually landed in Portsmouth Dockyard. Any departure from this plan, e.g., by sending medical staff to Spithead or the Solent could only result, as it did result, in encroachment upon a commitment of another medical organisation with consequent waste of time and duplication of medical assistance.

The Co-ordinating Officer ends his final Progress Report with comments on the co-ordination of the domestic medical activities of the area which are of importance in this History and which read as follows:

'It was not known until approximately April 3, 1944 that R.N. Hospital, Haslar, would become a Port Hospital and would therefore not be in a position to accept cases, however urgent, from the eastern side of Portsmouth harbour. Neither would specialist consultations, medical boards and other routine work be carried out by the hospital. Accordingly, contact was made with all the Senior Medical Officers of naval establishments in the Portsmouth area and also with the civilian Medical Officer of Health and the Superintendents of local civil hospitals.

'From May 25 onwards no cases of any nature were accepted by R.N. Hospital, Haslar. In consequence arrangements were made to send all urgent naval cases to local hospitals, and cases of the more severe infectious diseases to the Isolation Hospital at Milton. Accommodation in this latter hospital presented a problem as, although cabin and ward space were available for naval patients, the hospital was short of nursing and domestic staff. This problem was solved by supplying the hospital with 10 naval V.A.Ds. and 2 W.R.N.S. domestic staff.

'Regarding the Hayling Island area, the Senior Medical Officer of H.M.S. *Northney* arranged for urgent naval cases to be admitted either to Emsworth Hospital or to Havant War Memorial Hospital.

'As far as possible information was sent to outlying establishments and to the Medical Superintendents of the E.M.S. Hospitals at Mount Vernon, Stoke Mandeville and Park Prewett not to send discharged naval cases into the Portsmouth area for the time being. Arrangements were made for naval cases awaiting discharge from these hospitals to be sent to R.N. Auxiliary Hospital, Sherborne.

'With regard to the treatment of members of the W.R.N.S., local Service accommodation proved sufficient with, perhaps, the exception of a small number of infectious cases.

'On the whole the local arrangements worked very well as regards personnel urgently or mildly ill. But the problem which really became formidable was that of the large number awaiting specialist consultations, pulmographic examination, medical boards and the like for which facilities normally offered by the Royal Naval Hospital, Haslar, were suspended for a time.

'It is worthy of comment that in putting into effect the arrangements for receiving casualties from the Continent at the naval port of Portsmouth, it has been found that by far the most formidable task has been the reorganisation of the local domestic medical arrangements. This reorganisation was necessary in order that the flow of battle casualties through the port should not be impeded in any way. What has been most evident is that this side of the work, though less spectacular, occupied a considerable amount of time, energy and patience in dealing with the numerous problems which arose in association with it.'

Events of Special Interest, 1945

Copious naval medical records are available for the year 1945. Nevertheless, in bringing this Operational Volume to a close, it is only intended to include a very small number of events which have a special bearing or interest.

That naval medical organisation was generally embarrassed during the whole of 1945 has already been illustrated earlier in this History, the personnel problem having always been paramount.*

LANDING CRAFT INFANTRY (CASUALTY CLEARING SHIPS)

Mention has already been made, in connexion with the Normandy landings, of the use of landing craft for the ferrying of casualties from the beaches to hospital ships anchored off shore. In the light of this experience, by 1945, plans had been advanced for equipping and staffing particular landing craft for this special purpose.

Although it was intended that such craft should be available for use during the proposed assaults against the Japanese in the Far Eastern theatre of the war, the need for such a vessel and its value were

---

* *See* Chapters 2 and 15 of Volume I.

demonstrated following representations made by the Army for naval medical assistance during the disturbances in Greece early in 1945.

From the Army viewpoint, medical arrangements in the Athens-Piraeus region had to allow for the rapid evacuation of casualties. In this respect air evacuation was uncertain at the time because of weather conditions in Italy. The Hospital Ship *Maine* was available, but was anchored so far away as to make her inaccessible by the smaller type of craft in bad weather. The Army facilities ashore were of no higher level than field ambulances. The result was that by late December 1944 and early January 1945 the unevacuated Army casualties on shore were higher than had been expected, and many of these required urgent operation and resuscitation. To these men the arrival of H.M. *L.C.C.S.* 253 proved to be life saving.

This ship, which was specially equipped and staffed with a surgical team, performed most valuable work in the following ways:

(1) As a small, advance operational hospital. By being placed alongside small jetties, she was able to accept and treat serious surgical cases, thus allowing full facilities in inaccessible areas which otherwise would not have been available.

(2) As a clearing ship from the beaches, ferrying casualties out to a hospital ship anchored some distance away.

(3) As a surgical holding and treatment centre at times when the weather was too rough to permit the sea journey to the hospital ship to be made in safety.

Altogether H.M. *L.C.C.S.*253 dealt with some 300 casualties and an appreciation of her value was given by an Army spokesman in the following words:

'I am of the opinion that in the newly instituted casualty clearing ship the Navy has developed an organisation which has been proved in action to be first class. It can provide very early surgery, it can save many lives, and it undoubtedly has a very good effect on morale. The conception of this type of craft has been most opportune and its further developments will be watched with interest.'

'KAMIKAZE' ATTACKS

In the Far Eastern Theatre, in 1945, attacks on British men-of-war by Japanese 'suicide' aircraft constituted virtually a new type of weapon which called for special medical measures afloat, particularly with regard to resuscitation and the emergency treatment of burns.*

Among the ships affected by this form of enemy attack were H.M.Ss. *Sussex* and *Vestal*, and the aircraft carriers *Formidable* and *Victorious*.

On July 26, 1945, a British naval force was operating off Puket Island, Malaya, when a 'suicide' aircraft was sighted making for the cruiser *Sussex*. Fortunately it was shot down into the sea by the ship's

---

* *See* Chapter 15 of Volume I.

own armament. However, on striking the surface of the water the aircraft ricocheted and hit the *Sussex* on her starboard quarter. Some minor damage was caused above the water-line, but there were no casualties.

Within half an hour a second 'suicide' aircraft was observed heading towards the *Sussex*. This aircraft manoeuvred around the ship in the face of intense gunfire. It then suddenly changed course and delivered its final attack on H.M.S. *Vestal*, hitting the ship abaft the bridge. There was a violent explosion and an uncontrollable fire broke out in the *Vestal* which had to be abandoned. Casualties from burns were numerous and serious. Many men jumped into the sea while others were deliberately thrown into the sea to avoid being burned to death.

On May 9, 1945, H.M.S. *Victorious*, while operating in the Ryuku Pacific Combat area, was attacked by two 'suicide' aircraft. The first aircraft carried with it a 500-lb. bomb and struck the fore port area of the flight deck, causing blast from the explosion and fire from the machine's cargo of petrol. The second aircraft carried no bomb and struck the after port area of the flight deck, with moderate blast and fire in consequence.

In the case of the first aircraft the explosion caused metal from the aircraft and her bomb to pierce the armour of the ship's deck and to pass vertically through five other decks beneath. A fragment of the armoured flight deck, one foot square, was also projected a similar distance inside the ship.

A neighbouring gun turret was directly involved in the explosion and two men were killed by shrapnel and blast, three were seriously wounded by shrapnel and flash burns, while fourteen others suffered from moderate burns and miscellaneous shrapnel wounds.

In the case of the other aircraft an area of burning petrol spread over the after end of the flight deck and reached three of the ship's company one of whom died of his burns later in the day.

As regards the treatment and disposal of these casualties there is little upon which to comment. But again it is of importance to note that the Senior Medical Officer of the *Victorious* drew the attention of his Commanding Officer to the fact that anti-flash gear was not being properly worn, and that 25 per cent. of the cases of burns had received their injuries for this reason.

At 1130 hours on May 4 H.M.S. *Formidable* was attacked by a 'suicide' aircraft. At the time of the attack aircraft were being taxied forward on her flight deck which was fairly crowded with aircraft handling parties, pilots and observers.

The 'suicide' aircraft dropped a 1,000-lb. bomb just before itself hitting the *Formidable's* flight deck. Large fires were immediately started on the flight deck and in the hangar and torpedo shop between decks. One effect was to put out of action the ventilation fan in the engine room, and this constituted an extra hazard under tropical conditions. The fires between decks were soon extinguished, and the fire on the flight deck was under control in about half an hour. At this point it is interesting to note that there were no cases of burns among the fire parties.

It is also of interest to record that the Senior Medical Officer of the *Formidable* had made an important alteration in the action distribution of his medical personnel only a few days beforehand. He had in fact noted that the practice of maintaining a medical officer and party on constant duty immediately adjacent to the flight deck itself was attended by grave risk. Incidents had already occurred in aircraft carriers almost alongside the flight deck first-aid post with the result that the first casualties to be suffered were among the medical personnel. Therefore, the flight deck first-aid post in the *Formidable* had been moved to a more inboard position, and what had been the old first-aid post was occupied, on May 4, 1945, by the ship's Air Intelligence Department. At the time of the incident, the old first-aid post was crowded with personnel of this latter department with tragic consequences. The bomb exploded almost abreast the outer door of the old first-aid post and completely wrecked it. It also started a fire which prevented exit on to the flight deck. One officer was killed outright and another died a few minutes later. All the other occupants of the old first-aid post were injured, some seriously, by blast and fire. Some managed to escape by climbing through a scuttle on the side away from the fire. A midshipman suffered blast injury and penetrating wounds of the chest, and another naval officer sustained a perforating wound of the left eye which necessitated its enucleation.

At the time of the incident an officer of the Fleet Air Arm was about to take off from the flight deck in an aircraft. His aircraft took fire and he was enveloped in flame. But he managed to extricate himself from the cockpit, albeit terribly burned.*

Among the aircraft handlers wounded was a petty officer who suffered multiple injuries and died 72 hours after the incident.

Apart from the fatal cases, there were 33 other casualties in the *Formidable* of whom 13 were badly burned.

The second 'Kamikaze' incident in which H.M.S. *Formidable* was involved took place at 1700 hours on May 9, 1945. This time the 'suicide' aircraft again hit the flight deck in the mid line at a point within a few feet of the former attack. Although the material damage caused was very similar, on this occasion the flight deck was relatively clear of personnel, with the result that casualties were far fewer.

One rating was killed instantaneously by being decapitated by the wheel of an aircraft which was hurled through the air by the force of

---

* This officer died on board H.M.H.S. *Oxfordshire* on May 16, 1945.

the explosion. There were four cases of burns, all of whom recovered. It is of some interest to note that the men who suffered burns were wearing overalls and anti-flash gear at the time. The burns which they suffered were on their shoulders and backs, due to the fact that the necks of their overalls were gaping behind and that the wearers were bending forward, with their heads down, at the moment when the explosion occurred.

SURVIVAL AT SEA

It is considered fitting that this volume of the Navy's Medical Operational History should be concluded with yet a final reference to survival of the shipwrecked, particularly in view of modern views and current thoughts which have come to hand during the course of the preparation of this narrative.*

On February 28, 1945 H.M.S. *Activity* rescued 20 survivors from a lifeboat. These survivors were passengers and members of the crew of the American S.S. *Peter Silvester*.

The ages of the survivors varied from 19 to 25 years. They had been adrift for twenty-two days. During this time they had existed on the following diet:

> *Water*. Fortunately, owing to supplies in the lifeboat itself, supplemented by occasional rain, a ration of one pint of water per man per day was possible.
> *Food*. For the first fourteen days three meals per day were taken comprising:
> > One three inch square biscuit, one-third chocolate bar or one-fourth tin of pemmican.
>
> After the first fourteen days this daily ration was cut by half.

During the whole period fish were plentiful around the boat, especially when the sea was calm. But only one small fish was ever caught with a line. Also, although a harpoon was available, it was never used with success.

These survivors were rescued in a position approximately 101° E., and 26° S., and their weather conditions had been favourable most of the time.

There were no deaths in their boat, and when rescued their general condition was remarkably good. All had lost weight and were unsteady on their feet.

Total constipation was the rule, and without exception these men complained of painful feet with constant aching which was aggravated by exercise.

---

* See *The Bombard Story*, 1953.

One man was suffering from mumps which had been prevalent in the *Peter Silvester* at the time of her sinking.

All the survivors recovered quickly, the main feature during their recovery period being insomnia for which sedation was required for some days.

This story of the work of the Naval Medical Services in the Second World War aims at fulfilling a dual purpose. Firstly, to set on proud record for posterity the work of naval doctors and nurses. Secondly, to provide a work of reference should the successors of these doctors and nurses ever be called upon to play a similar rôle on behalf of their country and their professions.

Future generations of naval medical administrators may have different problems to solve in time of war. But even so, they may be glad to borrow a measure of guidance from this history of the past, wisely applying that professional axiom which says:

> 'Be not the first by whom the new is tried,
> Nor yet the last to cast the old aside.'

J. L. S. C.

INDEX

Achilles, H.M.S., 288
Active service afloat, strain of, 114
Air attack, effects of, 341, 395
    medical aspects of enemy, 88
Air raids affecting Naval shore establishments, 342, 387
Ajax, H.M.S., 288
Albatross, H.M.S., casualties from noxious fumes on, 501
Algiers, medical organisation at, 481
Arctic Convoy battles, 441
Arctic Convoys (*Plates XVI, XVII*), 417
    repatriation of survivors, 463
    rescue organisation, 449
Armed merchant cruisers, actions involving, 333
Asiatic Hospital at Royal Naval Base, 159
Athelstone, R.F.A., loss of, 408

Barrow-in-Furness area, air raids on, 389
Bilge keel casualties, 397
Bismarck, sinking of, 359
Bombing attacks, effect of, in Norwegian campaign, 303
British Expeditionary Force, casualties among (*see* Casualties)
    evacuation of, from continent, 308
Burial of dead, 85
Burma, operations in, 142

Calabria, action off, 331
Cannon-fire at sea, effects of, 342
Cape Spada, Crete, action off, 331
Casualties among B.E.F., clinical assessment of, 322
    reception and disposal of, in England, 319
    treatment on board destroyers, 325
    types of wounds, 323
Casualties, assessment of, Norwegian operations, 302, 307
    caused by noxious fumes, 497
    effects of oil fuel on (*Plate VIII*), 81
    evacuation of, by landing craft, Normandy, 516
    in destroyers during evacuation, 1940, 329
    in Greek and Cretan operations, 370, 374
    in H.M. ships during evacuation, 1940, 330
    in H.M. ships, occupation of North Africa, 485
    in Operation 'Excess', clinical assessment of, 355
    in sinking of *Bismarck*, clinical assessment of, 361

Casualties (*cont.*)
    reception of, from Normandy, in Portsmouth area, 529
    in U.K., 525
    sea-borne evacuation of, Normandy (*Plates XVIII, XIX*), 509
    transfer of, at sea (*Plates IV–VII*), 46
Casualty-clearing ships, 535
Casualty, danger of transport of, during action, 16
Ceylon, Naval operations off, 400
Clinical practice in convoy, 344
Convoy, clinical practice in, 344
Convoys to North Russia, 1942–1943, (*Plates XVI, XVII*), 417
Cornwall and *Dorsetshire*, H.M.Ss., loss of, 401
Cretan and Greek operations, 364
    assessment of casualties, 370, 374
Crete, action off Cape Spada, 331
    active operations on, 126
    Naval operations at, 367
Cyphering duties, employment of medical officers on, 3

Daily journal of Naval M.O., 31–76
    lessons to be learned from, 77–119
Dakar, operations off, 332
Damage control organisation (*Plates II, III*), 18
Dead, burial of, 85
Dental service, 114
Depth charges, effects of, 341, 397
Destroyers, casualties in, during evacuation, 1940, 329
Destroyer flotillas, medical officers of, 9
Destroyers, treatment of B.E.F. casualties on board, 325
Diego Suarez, Naval operations at the capture of, 410
Dieppe, raid on (*Plates XIV, XV*), 415
Diet, 104
Distributing Stations in H.M. Ships, 14, 28, 30
Dorsetshire and *Cornwall*, H.M.Ss., loss of, 401
Dry dock, refitting in, 115
'Dynamo' operation, 309

East Africa, Red Sea and Persian Gulf, operations in, 375
Egypt, disposal of wounded in, 373
Evacuation of British Expeditionary Forces from Continent, 308

INDEX

Evacuation of casualties, Normandy, by landing craft, 516
    sea-borne (*Plates XVIII, XIX*), 509
'Excess', Operation (*Plate XII*), 347
    casualties in, clinical assessment of, 355
Executive, relations between Medical Department and, 113
Exeter, H.M.S., 286
    loss of, and subsequent events, 202

Fatigue, mental, 99
First aid in action, 79
First-aid posts, in H.M. Ships, 14, 28
First-aid training of officers and men, 7, 16
Flying personnel, care of (*Plate IX*), 117
Fumes, noxious, casualties caused by, 497

Gloucester, H.M.S., loss of, and subsequent events, 176
Greece, Naval operations at, 365
Greek and Cretan operations, 364
    assessment of casualties, 370, 374

Hermes, Vampire and *Hollyhock*, H.M.Ss., loss of, 408
Hollyhock, Hermes and *Vampire*, H.M.Ss., loss of, 408
Hong Kong, fall of, 256
    report of Principal Medical Officer of R.N. Hospital at, 258
Hospital ships, occupation of North Africa, 471

'Kamikaze' attacks, 536
King's Regulations on duties of medical officers in action, 6

Landing craft, evacuation of casualties by, Normandy, 516
    infantry, 535
Landlock, H.M.S., 164
Landswell, H.M.S., 151
Lighting systems, emergency, 22

Machine-gun attacks and sniping, Norwegian campaign, 304
Machine-gun fire at sea, effects of, 342
Malaya, service in, 173
Maldive Islands, operations in, 139
Malta, air raids on, 390
Marooned on Tjebia Island, 232
Medical aspect of chief Naval events, 1939–1941 (*Plates XII, XIII*), 283–399
    1942–1943, 400–492
    1944–1945 (*Plates XVIII, XIX*), 493–540
Medical aspects of enemy air attacks, 88
Medical Department, relations between Executive and, 113

Medical events of special interest, ashore, 176–282
Medical operations ashore (*Plates X, XI*), 120–176
Medical organisation, action, in sinking of *Bismarck*, 361
    afloat, North Russian convoys (*Plates XVI, XVII*), 418
    ashore, North Africa, 481
        North Russia, 429
        Norwegian operations, 299
    for evacuation of B.E.F., 319
    for reception of casualties from Normandy in U.K., 525
    occupation of North Africa, 469
    of H.M. Ships in war (*Plates II, III*), 1–31 of Port Parties, Normandy, 520
Medical posts in H.M. Ships, 14
Medical stores and equipment, 110
    North Africa, 475
    Norwegian operations, 300
Medical transport, Norwegian operations, 301
Mental fatigue, 99
Merchant cruisers, armed, actions involving, 333
Mines, effects of, 339, 392

Mobile Landing Craft Advanced Bases (MOLCAB), 150
Mobile Naval Base Defence Organisation (M.N.B.D.O) (*Plates X, XI*), 120
M.N.B.D.O. (2), 144
MOLCAB, 150
MOLCAB 1, 151
MOLCAB 2, 164
Molde, 298
Morale, 94
    in Norwegian campaign, 304
    in North Russian convoys, 464

Namsos, operations around, 296
Narvik, battle of, first, 291
    casualties at, 302
    second, 293
    casualties at, 303
Naval Air Arm, Norwegian Campaign, 305
Naval escorting force, Normandy, 515
Naval establishments ashore, air raids affecting, 342, 387
Naval Medical Officer afloat, daily journal of, 31–76
    in war-time (*Plates II–IX*), 1–119
Naval Medical Officer on active service ashore (*Plates X, XI*), 120–282
Naval Medical Officers, training of newly joined, 5, 8
Naval medical personnel captured by enemy, narratives of, 176–282
Naval off-shore force, Normandy, 512
Naval operations at capture of Diego Suarez, 410
Naval operations, Crete, 367
    Greece, 365
    minor, 1942, 400
    minor, 1944, 493

INDEX

Naval operations off Ceylon, 400
Normandy landings (*Plates XVIII, XIX*), 509
North Africa, occupation of, 468
North African coastal operations, 1940–1941, 376
Norwegian operations, 290–308
    assessment of casualties, 302, 307
    medical lessons of, 306
    medical organisation ashore, 299
    medical stores and equipment, 300
    medical transport, 301
    morale in, 304

Oil fuel, effects of, on casualties (*Plate VIII*), 81

Persian Gulf, East Africa and Red Sea, operations in, 375
Phoebe, H.M.S., casualties from noxious fumes on, 498
Pinto, Rescue Ship, loss of, 507
Plymouth area, air raids on, 388
Portsmouth area, air raids on, 387
    reception of casualties from Normandy into, 529
Port Parties, Normandy, medical organisation of, 520
'Primrose', Operation, 297
Prince of Wales and *Repulse*, H.M.Ss., loss of, 383
Prisoners-of-war, naval medical personnel as, 176
Psychological effects on casualties among B.E.F., 327

Reception and disposal of B.E.F. casualties in England, 319
Red Sea, East Africa and Persian Gulf, operations in, 375
Refitting in dry dock, 115
Repulse and *Prince of Wales*, H.M.Ss., loss of, 383
Rescue organisation, Arctic Convoys, 449
Rescue Ship *Pinto*, loss of, 507
Rescues at sea (1940), 343
River Plate, battle of, 285
Royal Naval Base, Singapore, Asiatic Hospital at, 159
Royal Naval Hospital, Hong Kong, report of Matron of, 269
    report of P.M.O. of, 258
Royal Naval Tented Hospital, First, 124, 136
    Second, 135
'Rupert', Operation, 294

Russia, North, convoys to, 1942–1943 (*Plates XVI, XVII*), 417

St. Nazaire, attack on, 413
    evacuation from, 318
Sea, survival at, 539
Sea-borne evacuation of casualties, Normandy (*Plates XVIII, XIX*), 509
Security, 112
Shellfire, effects of, 335
Ships in harbour, air raids affecting, 387
Shore establishments, Naval, bombing of, 342, 387
'Sickle', Operations, 297
Singapore, escape from, 223
Singapore Naval Base, Asiatic Hospital at, 159
Special Operations Executive, activities with, 168
Stavangar, 299
Stevenstone, H.M.S., casualties from noxious fumes on, 504
Strain of active service afloat, 114
Stretchers, use and types of, 20
Survival at sea, 539
Survivors, reception of, 77
    repatriation of, from Arctic Convoys, 463

Tjebia Island, discussion of high mortality on, 246
    marooned on, 232
'Torch', Operation, 468
Torpedoes, effects of, 337, (*Plate XIII*), 395
Tropical diseases, occupation of North Africa, 473, 490

United Kingdom, air raids affecting Naval establishments ashore and ships in harbour, 387

Vampire, *Hermes* and *Hollyhock*, H.M.Ss., loss of, 408

Warships, casualties in, during evacuation, 1940, 330
Weapons, effects of particular, 335, (*Plate XIII*), 392
Wounded, disposal of, in Egypt, 373

Yugoslavia, service in, 169

www.ingramcontent.com/pod-product-compliance
Lightning Source LLC
Chambersburg PA
CBHW060452300426
44113CB00016B/2560